Ticks and Tick-Borne Pathogens

Ticks and Tick-Borne Pathogens

Editor: Remo Hemsworth

AMERICAN
MEDICAL PUBLISHERS
www.americanmedicalpublishers.com

AMERICAN
MEDICAL PUBLISHERS
www.americanmedicalpublishers.com

Cataloging-in-Publication Data

Ticks and tick-borne pathogens / edited by Remo Hemsworth.
p. cm.
Includes bibliographical references and index.
ISBN 979-8-88740-512-4
1. Tick-borne diseases. 2. Tick-borne diseases--Pathogenesis.
3. Tick-borne diseases--Diagnosis. 4. Tick-borne diseases--Treatment.
5. Communicable diseases. I. Hemsworth, Remo.
RA641.T5 T533 2023
614.433--dc23

American Medical Publishers,
41 Flatbush Avenue,
1st Floor, New York,
NY 11217, USA

ISBN 979-8-88740-512-4 (Hardback)

Contents

Preface

Ticks are obligate ectoparasites which feed on the blood of their hosts. They cause physical damage to their hosts by injuring skin and sucking blood. Furthermore, majority of the species of tick have the capability to transmit pathogens to their hosts. They are often more active in warmer months and a change in the populations of their hosts affects tick populations. Tick-borne diseases are those diseases that afflict humans and animals, and are caused by infectious agents transmitted by tick bites. Various pathogens comprising rickettsia and other types of bacteria, viruses, and protozoa are the primary causes of the infection resulting in diseases. There are various symptoms a person may feel after being bitten by a tick such as body aches, fever, fatigue, joint pain or rashes. This book provides comprehensive insights on ticks and tick-borne pathogens. It presents researches and studies performed by experts across the globe. Those with an interest in these pathogens would find this book helpful.

This book has been the outcome of endless efforts put in by authors and researchers on various issues and topics within the field. The book is a comprehensive collection of significant researches that are addressed in a variety of chapters. It will surely enhance the knowledge of the field among readers across the globe.

It gives us an immense pleasure to thank our researchers and authors for their efforts to submit their piece of writing before the deadlines. Finally in the end, I would like to thank my family and colleagues who have been a great source of inspiration and support.

Editor

1

Tick Salivary Compounds for Targeted Immunomodulatory Therapy

Hajer Aounallah[1,2†], Chaima Bensaoud[3†], Youmna M'ghirbi[1], Fernanda Faria[2], Jindřich Chmelař[4] and Michail Kotsyfakis[3,4]*

[1] Institut Pasteur de Tunis, LR19IPTX, Service d'Entomologie Médicale, Université de Tunis El Manar, Tunis, Tunisia,
[2] Innovation and Development Laboratory, Innovation and Development Center, Instituto Butantan, São Paulo, Brazil,
[3] Institute of Parasitology, Biology Centre, Czech Academy of Sciences, České Budějovice, Czechia, [4] Department of Medical Biology, Faculty of Science, University of South Bohemia in České Budějovice, České Budějovice, Czechia

***Correspondence:**
Michail Kotsyfakis
mich_kotsyfakis@yahoo.com

† These authors have contributed equally to this work

Immunodeficiency disorders and autoimmune diseases are common, but a lack of effective targeted drugs and the side-effects of existing drugs have stimulated interest in finding therapeutic alternatives. Naturally derived substances are a recognized source of novel drugs, and tick saliva is increasingly recognized as a rich source of bioactive molecules with specific functions. Ticks use their saliva to overcome the innate and adaptive host immune systems. Their saliva is a rich cocktail of molecules including proteins, peptides, lipid derivatives, and recently discovered non-coding RNAs that inhibit or modulate vertebrate immune reactions. A number of tick saliva and/or salivary gland molecules have been characterized and shown to be promising candidates for drug development for vertebrate immune diseases. However, further validation of these molecules at the molecular, cellular, and organism levels is now required to progress lead candidates to clinical testing. In this paper, we review the data on the immuno-pharmacological aspects of tick salivary compounds characterized *in vitro* and/or *in vivo* and present recent findings on non-coding RNAs that might be exploitable as immunomodulatory therapies.

Keywords: tick saliva, salivary glands, host immunity, immunomodulation, drug discovery

INTRODUCTION

The vertebrate immune system is a sophisticated and highly developed network of cells, tissues, and organs that together identify and neutralize foreign and endogenous threats. Immunodeficiencies represent a breakdown in these highly organized processes caused by a lack or dysfunction of specific immune cell subpopulations or soluble effectors (1). Immune disorders also arise due to

Abbreviations: AAS, *Amblyomma americanum* serpin; BIF, B cell inhibitory factor; BIP, B cell inhibitory protein; BMDCs, mouse bone marrow-derived dendritic cells; BMDMs, mouse bone marrow-derived macrophages; CD, cluster of differentiation; CFA, complete freund's adjuvant; DC, dendritic cells; EAE, experimental autoimmune encephalomyelitis; HIV, human immunodeficiency viruses; HL-p36, *Haemaphysalis longicornis* p-36; IFN-γ, interferon gamma; IL, interleukin; Irac, *Ixodes ricinus* anticomplement; IRS-2, *Ixodes ricinus* Serpin- 2; Isac, *Ixodes scapularis* salivary anticomplement; LPS, lipopolysaccharide; MBL, mannose-binding lectin; MC, Mast cells; MCP-1 monocyte chemoattractant protein 1; MHC-I, -II, major histocompatibility complex-I, -II; MIF, macrophage migration inhibitory factor; MS, mass spectrometry; NGS, next-generation sequencing; OmCI, *Ornithodoros moubata* complement inhibitor; PDAC, pancreatic ductal adenocarcinoma; PGE_2, prostaglandin E2; Ra-HBPs, *Rhipicephalus appendiculatus* histamine-binding proteins; RmS-3, *Rhipicephalus microplus* serpin 3; Salp, salivary protein; SHBP, serotonin and histamine-binding protein; TCR, T cell receptor; TdPI, Tick-derived protease inhibitor; TGF-β, transforming growth factor-beta; Th, T helper; TLR, toll-like receptors; TNF, tumor necrosis factor; TSLPI, tick salivary lectin pathway inhibitor.

excessive immune responses, such as in allergic reactions or autoimmunity (2), usually as a result of dysregulation or overexpression of specific cytokines and their related immune signaling pathways (3). The human immune system is also affected, and often weakened, by stress, malnutrition, and age-related changes, which increase susceptibility to infectious diseases and other pathologies such as cancer (4–6). Current therapies for immune-related illnesses usually have side-effects or suboptimal efficacy (7, 8), leading to efforts to identify alternative therapies that might naturally inhibit and/or modulate specific immune system targets without significant off-target effects (9), including bioactive molecules derived from natural sources (10). Compounds with therapeutic potential have traditionally been extracted from plants (phytotherapy) (11), but other sources have included scorpion and snake venom (12, 13) and arthropods (14). However, substances extracted from natural sources and applied in practice remain limited, and their clinical utility is hampered by the risk of contamination with impurities (15). More positively, drug discovery has been assisted by the development of new protein production methods using various expression systems (16–18), and advances in new technologies such as next-generation sequencing (NGS) and mass spectrometry (MS) have revolutionized screening for novel natural substances (19, 20).

Tick salivary glands are now recognized as a rich source of pharmaco-active molecules (21). Tick saliva contains a rich cocktail of bioactive molecules including protein and lipid derivatives with a remarkable binding affinity, avidity, and selectivity for their targets in various host defense systems (22). Ticks are obligatory hematophagous that, in order to feed, must overcome the evolutionarily sophisticated immune defense systems of their vertebrate hosts. To achieve this, they secrete a wide variety of molecules in their saliva with immunomodulatory, anti-inflammatory, anti-clotting, and anti-platelet effects (23, 24).

Despite the identification of a large number of bioactive tick salivary molecules, their investigation for therapeutic purposes remains in its outset. Only a limited number of tick salivary compounds, mostly proteins, have been tested pre-clinically (25, 26). Here we discuss the literature on therapeutically valuable tick salivary molecules with function(s) known to be directly related to host immune responses. In doing so, we identify the most promising salivary candidates with drug development potential, including newly discovered non-coding (nc) RNAs.

TICK SALIVA TARGETS AT THE TICK-HOST INTERFACE

Ticks are obligate hematophagous ectoparasites of amphibians, reptiles, birds, and mammals that cause host blood loss and skin damage (27). Compared to other blood feeders, tick feeding behavior is unique. Hard ticks discretely and solidly attach to their hosts for several days to weeks to complete their blood uptake (28), with the skin representing the main interface where tick salivary compounds meet host defense systems (29, 30) (**Figure 1**). Furthermore, the skin is the site of multiplication and persistence of several tick-borne pathogens (31, 32). In the local environment of the skin, the tick-host molecular interaction can be viewed as a competition between host defense mechanisms against the ectoparasite and tick evasion strategies (30). To ensure an uninterrupted blood meal, ticks have developed myriad strategies to overcome the complex homeostatic and immune responses that are raised against them (22). As long-term pool feeders, they create an immunologically privileged micro-environment in the host's skin, in which they secrete an impressive mixture of proteins, peptides, and non-peptide molecules (**Figure 1**), thereby modulating wound healing, hemostasis, inflammation, and both the innate and adaptive immune responses (33). These molecules interfere with various host molecules including enzymes, cytokines, complement components, antibodies, cell signaling molecules, and immune cell receptors (33).

Hemostasis is triggered within seconds of tissue damage and is the product of the triad of blood coagulation, platelet aggregation, and vasoconstriction, a process mainly controlled by serine proteases (34). The anti-hemostatic properties of tick salivary secretions are reviewed elsewhere (23, 35). In addition to hemostasis, complement components and inflammatory mediators are also initial tick saliva targets (36, 37). When tick mouthparts are inserted into the skin, pre-positioned sentinel leukocytes of the epidermis and dermis, including mast cells (MCs), eosinophils, dendritic cells (DCs), and macrophages, as well as keratinocytes and endothelial cells, are activated by mediators released from damaged skin cells or expressed by pathogens transmitted by ticks (38). The resident macrophages release pro-inflammatory chemokines and cytokines including interleukin-8 (IL-8), tumor necrosis factor (TNF), and IL-1β (38). These chemoattractants recruit blood-borne innate immune cells such as neutrophils and monocytes to the bite site, which intensify the stimulation of local and infiltrating innate immune cells (30, 39). Monocytes secrete growth hormones that induce fibroblast proliferation and extracellular matrix deposition, thus contributing to wound healing (39). Given their parasitic lifestyle, ticks must overcome innate immunity during their primary infestation and both innate and adaptive immunity during secondary or subsequent infestations (22). Following tick feeding, tick-derived antigens may be presented to naïve B and T cells by activated DCs that have acquired foreign antigens and have migrated to skin-draining lymph nodes (40). Both the humoral and cellular branches of host adaptive immunity are activated, thereby resulting in the generation of antigen-specific antibodies and T lymphocytes (40). In subsequent infestations, activated memory T and B lymphocytes secrete cytokines and produce specific antibodies that target tick salivary or mouthpart-derived antigens in an effort to reject the tick (41).

IMPACT OF TICK SALIVARY COMPOUNDS ON HOST IMMUNE RESPONSES

The complex mixture of tick salivary compounds specifically and selectively targets host immune reactions, subverting the rejection and death of the tick (24). This specificity and selectivity

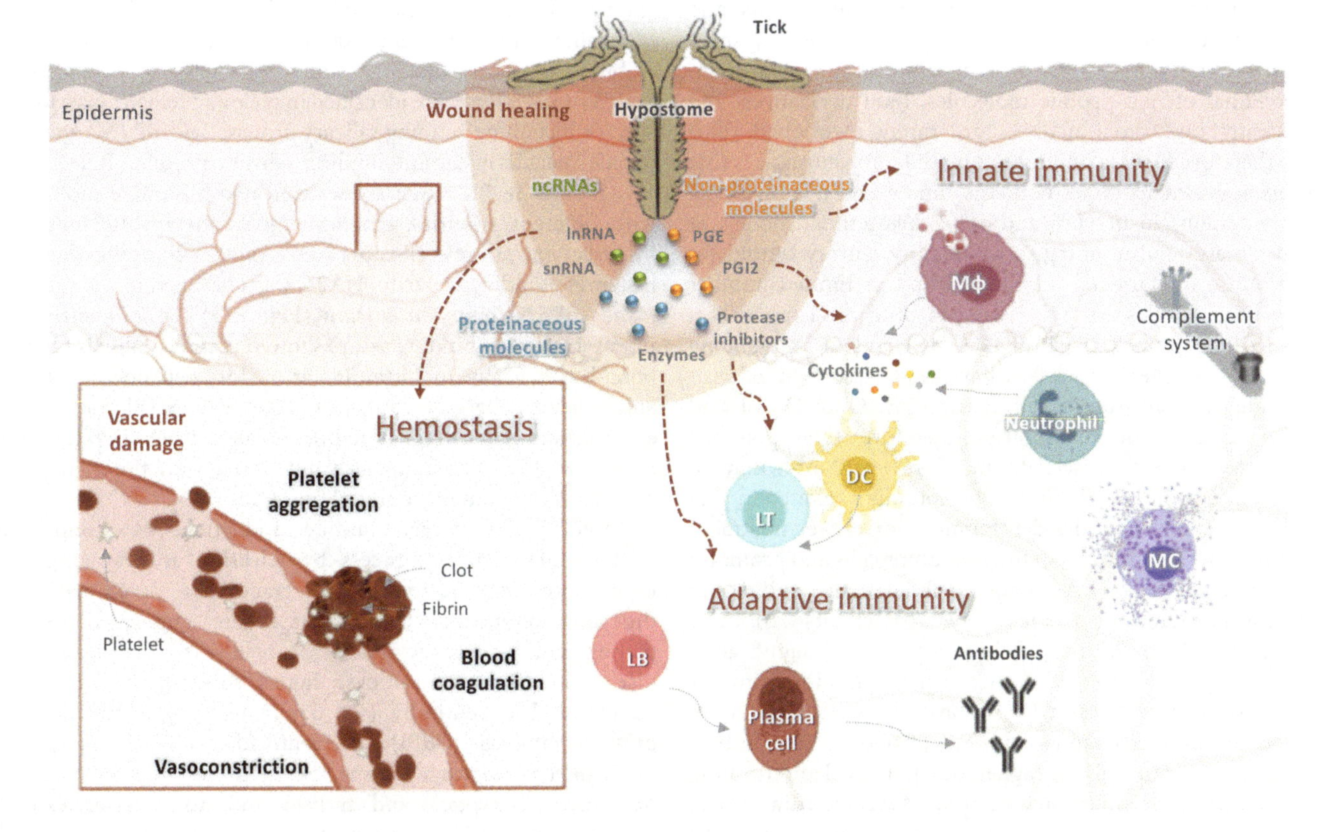

FIGURE 1 | Obstacles faced by ticks at the host-tick interface when taking a blood meal. Ticks initiate feeding by inserting their hypostomes into host skin, resulting in tissue and vascular damage. The host has developed several mechanisms to prevent blood loss including activating hemostasis, innate and adaptive immunity, the complement pathway, and inflammatory responses leading to wound healing and tissue remodeling, all of which disrupt tick feeding. Ticks, in turn, secrete saliva at the bite site that contains proteinaceous molecules (enzymes, lipocalins, protease inhibitors, etc.), non-proteinaceous molecules (prostaglandins, prostacyclins), and ncRNAs (miRNAs and lncRNAs). These molecules display anticoagulatory, antiplatelet, vasodilatory, anti-inflammatory, and immunomodulatory activities to counter host reactions and to guarantee a successful blood meal. DC, dendritic cells; LT, lymphocyte T; LB, lymphocyte T; Mφ, macrophage.

may therefore be exploited for diseases in which dysfunction of the same host immune reactions is implicated in their pathogenesis, for instance the innate immune system in Sjögren's syndrome (42), adaptive immunity in Tregopathies (43) and autoimmune encephalomyelitis (44), and complement activation in local and/or systemic inflammation, tissue damage, and disease (45).

Some tick salivary components have immune system specificity at different steps of immune recognition (21). Despite this specificity, tick salivary component targets often show redundancy at the molecular, cellular, and functional level (i.e., may be targeted by more than one tick salivary molecule) (29). Furthermore, several tick salivary compounds are pleiotropic, targeting both hemostatic and immune system components (29). For instance, Salp15, a multifunctional protein, was shown to bind specifically to dendritic cell, inhibit CD4 + T cell activation and proliferation, and block the liberation of interleukin 2 (IL-2) (46). Apart from its immunomodulatory activities, it has also been described to modulate host coagulation (47). This pleiotropicity could be problematic in targeted immunotherapy, which relies mainly on single target drugs and is often considered as a serious limitation in drug conception. Nevertheless, this issue does not exclude the possibility of using these salivary components in other therapeutic applications. Multi-target drugs, also known as multifunctional drugs or network therapeutics are more suitable as potential therapeutic solutions in diseases of complex etiology, such as Alzheimer's disease, Parkinson's disease, and neglected tropical diseases (48). Single-target drugs, although highly selective and specific, may not necessarily have better efficacy in these cases (49). Indeed, multi- target drugs tend to be beneficial to face complex disorders, multifactorial health conditions and drug resistance issues (50, 51). Some studies trend to changing paradigm from "one target one ligand" toward "multi-target" as they does not provide a complete solution for multifactorial diseases (49). Therefore, tick salivary compounds with broad-spectrum targets might be useful in these diseases mediated by multiple processes.

The immunomodulatory properties of whole tick saliva and/or salivary gland extracts were previously reviewed by Kotál and colleagues (52), and some comprehensive and recent reviews have focused on the composition and role of saliva in tick feeding and tick-host-pathogen interactions (21, 53, 54). These articles have tended to focus on proteinaceous salivary component families including lipocalins, protease inhibitors such as Kunitz-type domains containing proteins, serpins, and cystatins, metalloproteases, basic tail secreted proteins, small peptide inhibitors, and some protein families unique to ticks. The potential of non-peptide molecules, lipid derivatives, and the recently discovered ncRNAs are rarely mentioned. This review therefore focuses on immunomodulatory substances that have been shown to target both the innate and adaptive host immune systems in *in vitro* and/or *in vivo* animal models of human diseases and in doing so we identify salivary candidates with promise for targeted immunotherapy. A limited number of salivary molecules are progressing in preclinical trials. This includes Amblyomin-X, Ir-CPI, TAP, OmCI, and Ra-HBP, among others. Most of these molecules have been described as anti-hemostatic and anti-tumor candidates (55). Only OmCI and Ra-HBP target immune responses, therefore, their potential applications will be discussed later in this review. Amblyomin-X, a Kunitz-type protease inhibitor, is profoundly exploited in pre-clinical testing and is under development for cancer treatment (26). It selectively induces apoptosis in tumor cells and promotes tumor reduction *in vivo* in melanoma animal models and reduce metastasis and tumor growth in *in vivo* experiments (56). In its pre-clinical evaluation, this protein was proven to significantly decrease lung metastasis in a mice orthotopic kidney tumor model (25). More interestingly, Amblyomin-X does not seem to cause any mortality; and symptoms of toxicity were subtle, reversible, and seen only at higher doses, thus demonstrating a safety profile for injection in mice. More recently, it was investigated on Amblyomin-X-treated horse melanomas showing significant reduction in the tumor size (57). Ir-CPI (*Ixodes ricinus* contact phase inhibitor), an antithrombotic protein, has proven its effectiveness in inhibiting the contact phase of the coagulation cascade in preclinical trials, preventing clotting in catheter and arteriovenous shunt rabbit models during Cardiopulmonary Bypass (58). TAP, a Kunitz domain protease inhibitor from *Ornithodoros moubata*, has been described as an anticoagulant candidate, showing promising results in *in vivo* models of venous and arterial thrombosis (59). Its efficacy on blood coagulation has been approved in preliminary preclinical experiments; however, it has never been inquired in humans mainly due to its antigenicity (59).

Innate Immune Responses

The host innate immune response forms the first and immediate line of defense to tick attachment (52). Activated resident cells in the cutaneous barrier including MCs, macrophages, and DCs stimulate host awareness to the injury followed by removal of feeding ticks (**Figure 2**).

Itch and Pain

Mast cells and basophils degranulate to release soluble mediators such as histamine and serotonin, which cause local itch and pain at the infestation site (60). However, ticks alleviate itch and pain through salivary components that sequester histamine and/or serotonin or modulate MC function. RmS-3, a novel serpin extracted from the salivary glands of *Rhipicephalus microplus* (61), has been shown to modulate MC function by inhibiting chymase and vascular permeability in acute inflammation (**Figure 2**). The hard tick *Rhipicephalus appendiculatus* uses the histamine-binding proteins Ra-HBPs (in the lipocalin family) to bind histamine with high affinity during early feeding (62). Different Ra-HBPs were identified in male and female ticks: male-specific histamine-binding salivary protein Ra-HBP (M) and two female-specific histamine-binding salivary proteins RaHBP(F)-1,2 (**Figure 2**). Ra-HBP2 sequestered two histamine molecules with different affinities, emphasizing its therapeutic potential by targeting multiple effectors (63). Another lipocalin showing histamine binding capacity, HA24, was identified in the salivary glands of *Hyalomma asiaticum* (**Figure 2**) (64). *In vitro* and *in vivo* histamine binding assays showed that recombinant HA24 bound specifically to histamine in a dose-dependent manner and relieved allergic asthma in mice (64). SHBP (serotonin and histamine-binding protein), isolated from *Dermacentor reticulatus* (65), simultaneously interfered with the activity of both serotonin and histamine (**Figure 2**).

In addition to biogenic amine production, MCs contribute to the inflammatory process by releasing a wide range of highly bioactive effectors after degranulation, tryptases being the most abundant (66). Tryptases are implicated in the pathogenesis of allergic inflammatory diseases, cardiovascular disease, lung fibrosis, and even cancer, so their inhibition may be useful therapeutically (66, 67). Interestingly, tick-derived protease inhibitor (TdPI) was identified in the salivary glands of *R. appendiculatus* and was shown to suppress the activity of human β-tryptase and trypsin and, to a lesser extent, plasmin (68). TdPI accumulates in the cytosolic granules of mouse MCs, presumably blocking the autocatalytic activation of tryptase, thereby suppressing inflammation in the host animal's skin (**Figure 2**) (69). Tryptogalinin, an *Ixodes scapularis* salivary Kunitz-type protein, was also found to inhibit β-tryptase (**Figure 2**) and other MC serine proteases such as α-chymotrypsin, plasmin, matriptase, and elastase and participated in inflammation and tissue remodeling (70). β-tryptases are MC-specific serine proteases with roles in inflammation that are used clinically as biomarker of MCs and their activation (67). Both tryptogalinin and TdPI could be engineered as highly specific pharmacological inhibitors of MC tryptases for the treatment of allergic inflammatory disorders like asthma (67–70).

Recruitment of Blood-Borne Innate Immune Cells

Within the first few hours after attachment, blood-borne leukocytes are recruited to the site of injury, triggered by a set of mediators including complement components, eicosanoids, chemokines, and cytokines (71). Neutrophil and monocyte recruitment has been shown to be strongly suppressed by tick salivary compounds. A homolog of the vertebrate macrophage migration inhibitory factor (MIF) was identified in *Amblyomma americanum* (72, 73) and *Haemaphysalis longicornis* (74). In both ticks, functional *in vitro* assays revealed that MIF inhibited the migration of human monocytes, suggesting that it might decrease monocyte recruitment *in vivo*. Ir-LBP from *I. ricinus* inhibited neutrophil chemotaxis and activation *in vitro* by binding specifically and with high affinity to leukotriene B4, an important inflammatory mediator (75). Ir-LBP was also shown to inhibit inflammatory responses in rabbits by decreasing

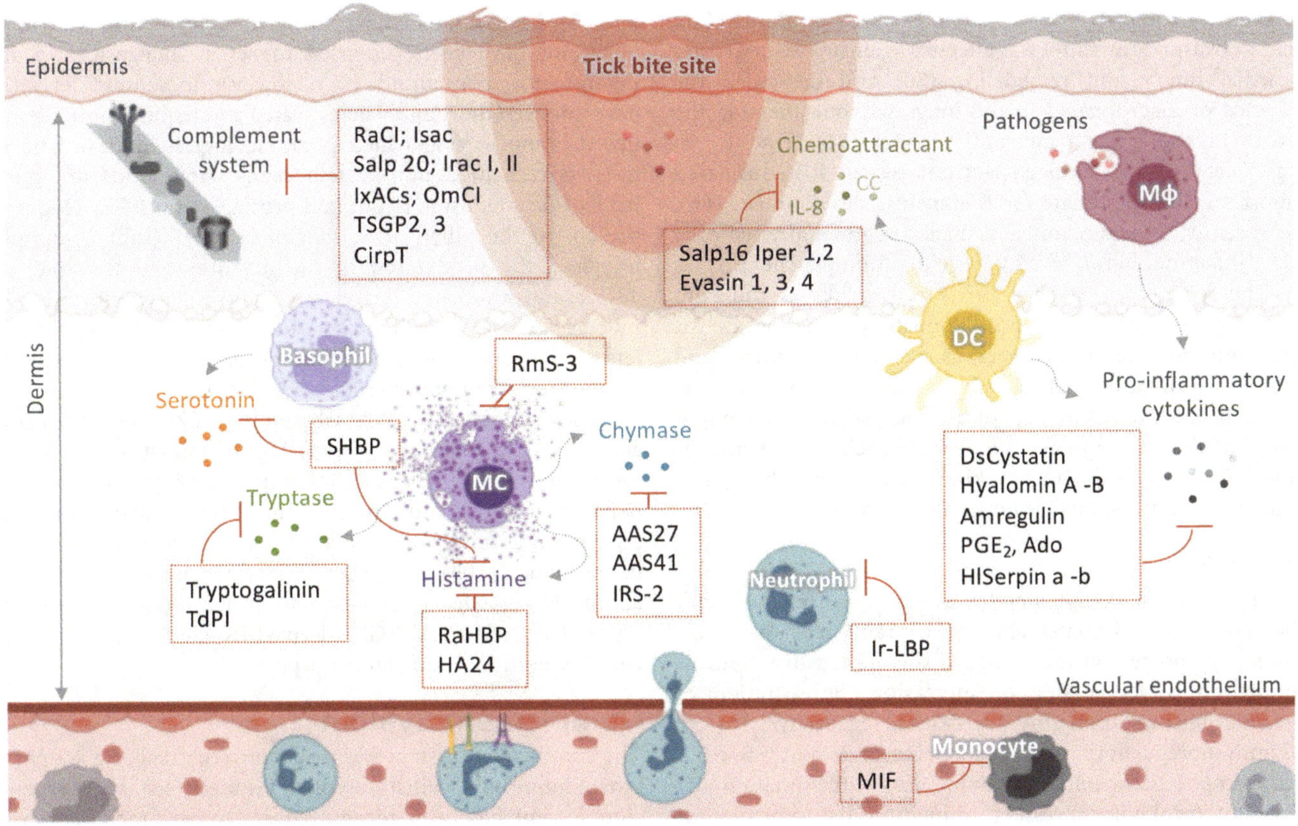

FIGURE 2 | Schematic representation of tick salivary molecules implicated in the modulation of the complement system and innate immunity. Activated resident cells in the dermis stimulate host awareness of injury and removal of the feeding ticks. Tick saliva neutralizes itch and pain through salivary components that sequester histamine and/or serotonin (such as SHBP, Ra-HBPs, and HA24) or modulate MC function (such as RmS-3). TdPI and Tryptogalinin inhibit tryptase released by MCs. AAS27, AAS41, and IRS-2 inhibit chymase liberated by MCs. Neutrophil and monocyte recruitment is suppressed by MIF and Ir-LBP. Moreover, ticks manipulate the host cytokine network by inhibiting cytokines and chemokines using Salp16 Iper 1,2; Evasin 1, 3, 4; DsCystatin; Hyalomin-A, –B; Amregulin; PGE_2; Ado; and HlSerpin-a, –b. Several anti-complement molecules have been identified in tick salivary glands including RaCl; Isac; Salp 20; Irac I, II; IxACs; OmCI; TSGP2, 3; and CirpT. AAS: *Amblyomma americanum* serpin; DC: dendritic cells; IL: interleukin; Irac: *I. ricinus* anticomplement; IRS-2: *I. ricinus* Serpin-2; Isac: *I. scapularis* salivary anticomplement; IxACs: *Ixodes* anticomplement proteins; MIF: macrophage migration inhibitory factor; Mφ: macrophage; OmCI: *O. moubata* complement inhibitor; PGE_2: prostaglandin E2; Ra-HBPs: *R. appendiculatus* histamine-binding proteins; RmS: *Rhipicephalus microplus* serpin; Salp: salivary protein; SHBP: serotonin- and histamine-binding protein; TdPI: tick-derived protease inhibitor.

the number of neutrophils located at the tick bite site (75). Therefore, Ir-LBP may have therapeutic use in inflammatory diseases or illnesses associated with increased leukotriene B4 production. Moreover, ticks employ salivary inhibitors of CXCL8 (IL-8) and CC chemokines to manipulate the host cytokine network. Salp16 Iper1 and Salp16 Iper2 (**Figure 2**), salivary proteins from *Ixodes persulcatus*, have been shown to have anti-IL-8 activity, thereby impairing neutrophil chemotaxis (76). A very recent review summarized the data on Evasins, which are secreted by hard ticks and bind to host chemokines to inhibit their activation of chemokine receptors (77). Of the Evasins, three from *Rhipicephalus sanguineus* (Evasin-1, -3, and -4) were selective for different chemokines (78). Evasin-1 bound to the CC chemokine members CCL3, CCL4, and CCL18 (78) and inhibited neutrophil, T cell, and macrophage migration and the production of inflammatory cytokines *in vitro* (78). Russo and colleagues demonstrated the high efficiency of Evasin-1 in reducing CCL3-induced influx of neutrophils in murine bleomycin-induced lung fibrosis (79). Evasin-1 has also been shown to reduce graft-versus-host disease in mice, which may be particularly useful in patients undergoing bone marrow transplantation (80). Moreover, the administration of recombinant Evasin-1 reduced skin inflammation and decreased mortality in mice deficient in the chemokine receptor D6, which renders then highly susceptible to inflammation (81). Evasin-3 is specific for the CXC chemokines CXCL8 and CXCL1 and was recently found to disrupt the interaction between CXCL8 and glycosaminoglycans and CXCR2 (**Figure 2**), which modulate neutrophil migration (82). Several studies have demonstrated the effectiveness of Evasin-3 in different neutrophil-dependent disease models. A single administration of Evasin-3 during mouse myocardial ischemia/reperfusion injury effectively reduced infarct size and decreased CXC chemokine-induced neutrophil recruitment (83). Evasin-3 also reduced atherosclerotic vulnerability to ischemic stroke in an *in vivo* murine model (84) and inhibited neutrophil-mediated pancreatic and lung inflammation in a mouse model of acute pancreatitis (85). Evasin-4 interacts with at least 18 CC chemokines (78). Similar to Evasin-3, Evasin-4 was effective against post-infarction myocardial injury and remodeling (86) and decreased the abundance of macrophages in the lungs without affecting the pancreas in the acute pancreatitis model (85). Due to its broad CC chemokine-binding spectrum, Evasin-4 is considered the most suitable candidate for therapeutic development (86). More recently, Evasin-inspired artificial peptides dramatically reduced inflammation *in vivo* by targeting multiple chemokines (87). These peptides might therefore provide a route to the development of new anti-inflammatory therapeutics for chronic autoimmune diseases such as rheumatoid arthritis and inflammatory diseases such as atherosclerosis. Moreover, the mechanism of action of these peptides suggests that they might also be useful in acute infectious diseases such as influenza or COVID-19, where exuberant cytokine responses are thought to be at least partially responsible for tissue injury (87).

Inflammation

Activated resident cells secrete several pro-inflammatory mediators, which initiate and then reinforce the local inflammatory process at the damaged site. Tick saliva controls inflammation by decreasing or increasing the secretion of pro- and anti-inflammatory cytokines, respectively (29). Two immunoregulatory peptides, Hyalomin-A and –B from *H. asiaticum asiaticum*, overcome host inflammation by modulating cytokine expression, inhibiting the secretion of pro-inflammatory TNF-α, MCP-1, and IFN-γ and stimulating the secretion of the immunosuppressant cytokine IL-10 (88). Amregulin from *Amblyomma variegatum* saliva was found to suppress the *in vitro* production of TNF-α, IL-1, IL-8, and IFN-γ in a dose-dependent manner (89). Hyalomin-A and –B and Amregulin significantly inhibited adjuvant-induced paw inflammation in mouse models *in vivo* (88, 89). HlSerpin-a and –b, novel serpins from the hard tick *H. Longicornis*, suppressed the expression of TNF-α, IL-6, and IL-1β from LPS-stimulated mouse bone marrow-derived macrophages (BMDMs) or mouse bone marrow-derived dendritic cells (BMDCs) (90). Three salivary gland serpins, AAS27 and AAS41 from *A. americanum* (91, 92) and IRS-2 from *I. ricinus* (93), inhibited inflammation by targeting chymase (**Figure 2**), an enzyme produced by activated MCs. IRS-2 also inhibited Cathepsin G, which is involved in tissue remodeling during inflammation and modulates the production of IL-6 by DCs, which subsequently impairs Th17 differentiation and maturation. DsCystatin from *Dermacentor silvarum* salivary glands was shown to impair the expression of the inflammatory cytokines IL-1β, IFN-γ, TNF-α, and IL-6 from mouse BMDMs (94), and the authors proposed that DsCystatin might be useful for the treatment of inflammatory diseases since it suppressed joint inflammation induced by complete Freund's adjuvant (CFA) and *Borrelia burgdorferi* in a mouse arthritis model (95).

Another category of anti-inflammatory compounds are non-proteinaceous substances. It is important to point out that bioactive lipidic salivary component despite being abundant in the saliva of hard ticks; mainly prostaglandins PGE_2 and $PGF_{2\alpha}$, only a few studies describe their pharmaceutical use (96, 97). Cannabinoids have also been detected in *Amblyomma* ticks and have been proposed to act as analgesic and anti-inflammatory compounds (98). However, these lipid derivatives have not been thoroughly investigated and require more rigorous investigation to assess their pharmacological interest. The two most documented non-proteinaceous compounds are purine nucleoside adenosine (Ado) and prostaglandin PGE_2 (**Figure 2**) present in the saliva of *R. sanguineus* (99). Both compounds impaired the production of pro-inflammatory IL-12p40 and TNF-α and stimulated the release of anti-inflammatory IL-10 by murine DCs (99). In humans, Ado is a homeostatic regulator and a "danger signal" for cells and organs, since it is expressed during trauma or stress (100, 101). The therapeutic potential of Ado is well documented elsewhere (100–102). Ado is protective against several pathologies including inflammation and various forms of neuronal hyperexcitability and/or toxicity including hypoxia, seizures, and chronic pain (101). Similarly, PGE_2 has pharmacological proprieties *in vitro* and *in vivo* associated with inflammation (103) and cancer (97) influencing cell proliferation, apoptosis, angiogenesis, inflammation, and immune surveillance (104). Thus, Ado and PGE_2 derived from *R. sanguineus* saliva could be used for therapeutic purposes.

Complement System

The complement system was originally regarded as a support to innate immunity against microbial invaders (45). More recently, complement has been recognized as having functions beyond microbial elimination such as clearance of immune complexes (105), complementing T and B cell immune functions (36), and tissue regeneration (106). Complement links the host innate and adaptive immune responses and is activated via three pathways (alternative, classical, and lectin) (31, 85). The excessive activation of complement components is responsible for a wide range of immune-mediated diseases (107) including autoimmune diseases, Alzheimer's disease, schizophrenia, atypical hemolytic-uremic syndrome, angioedema, macular degeneration, and Crohn's disease (108). Since the introduction of the first complement-specific drug, eculizumab, into the clinic, over 20 candidate drugs are now being evaluated in clinical trials and additional agents are in preclinical development (109). Several molecules with promising anti-complement activities were identified in tick salivary glands. For instance, Isac from *I. scapularis* (110) and its paralogs IRAC I and II from *I. ricinus* (111) specifically blocked binding of complement factor B to complement C3b *in vitro*, inhibiting the formation of the C3 convertase of the alternative pathway. Since convertases mediate nearly all complement effector functions, they are ideal targets for therapeutic inhibition (112). Selective inhibition of complement precursors and regulators is also of great therapeutic interest (109). Salp20 from *I. scapularis* (113) and IxACs from *I. ricinus* (114) inhibit the alternative pathway by binding properdin, a positive regulator of the pathway. Soft ticks have been reported to inhibit the classical complement pathway, with the lipocalins OmCI from *O. moubata* (115, 116) and TSGP2 and TSGP3 from *Ornithodoros savignyi* (117) specifically targeting C5 activation. The recombinant version of OmCI (also known as

Coversin or rEV576) has been tested in several animal models of complement-mediated diseases and has shown efficacy in a clinical trial (115, 118, 119). By inhibiting C5 activation, OmCI significantly reduced excessive inflammatory reactions associated with severe forms of influenza virus A (IAV) in mice (116). In addition to its effect on C5, OmCI significantly decreased leukotriene B4 levels in septic pigs (120). In the same study, combined inhibition of complement C5 by OmCI and CD14 with anti-CD14 antibodies significantly attenuated inflammation, thrombogenicity, and hemodynamic abnormalities (115, 120), suggesting OmCI might be useful for the treatment of sepsis. OmCI was also effective in preventing experimental autoimmune myasthenia gravis induced by passive transfer in normal Lewis rats (118). RaCI, from *R. appendiculatus* salivary glands, bound human C5 and blocked C5a generation and membrane attack complex formation (121). RaCI exhibits cross-species reactivity, allowing it to be used in disease models to test therapeutic effectiveness. An OmCI and RaCI homolog, CirpT, is a new class of complement inhibitor identified in *Rhipicephalus pulchellus* saliva that binds C5 *in vitro* via a unique binding site that does not overlap with other known inhibitors (122). Eculizumab, an antibody against C5, is currently prescribed for diseases characterized by excessive activation of the alternative pathway, including paroxysmal nocturnal hemoglobinuria and atypical hemolytic uremic syndrome (123, 124). Despite its effectiveness, eculizumab is one of the most expensive drugs in the world (121). Nevertheless, these other proteins derived from tick saliva offer exciting prospects for C5-targeted therapeutics of complement-mediated diseases and could be alternatives to eculizumab. In addition to the alternative pathway, the lectin pathway is also targeted by the tick salivary lectin pathway inhibitor (TSLPI), identified from the salivary glands of *I. scapularis* (125). The lectin pathway is activated in an antibody and C1-independent manner, upon the interaction of Mannose-binding lectin (MBL) with hyper glycosylated pathogen-associated molecular patterns (PAMPs) on microbial surfaces (126). TSLPI was described to directly inhibit MBL complement pathway activation (125). Additionally, both TSLPI and its ortholog from *I. ricinus* were shown to protect *Borrelia burgdorferi* sensu lato from complement-mediated killing, by inhibiting MBL function (127, 128). MBL appears to influence the severity of several diseases including pancreatic ductal adenocarcinoma (PDAC) (129). During a Pancreatic Cancer, MBL is required for oncogenic progression, whereas inhibition of MBL by TSLPI could be protective against tumor growth.

Acquired Immune Responses

During the first encounter with ticks, antigen-presenting cells, mainly DCs, present salivary immunogens to lymphocytes, which trigger cell-mediated and antibody responses (22). Sets of immunoglobulins and long-lived memory T and B cells are induced in the host (**Figure 3**). In subsequent contacts with the same tick, acquired immunity is quickly activated to yield a more specific protective response. It has been reported that tick saliva suppresses adaptive immunity in various ways (33). Some tick salivary compounds interfere with DCs and alter their capacity to present antigens. Other compounds prevent lymphocyte proliferation or T cell cytokine production.

Antigen Processing and Presentation

Several tick salivary molecules target DCs, thereby preventing the initiation of adaptive immunity. PGE_2 has been described as the major DC inhibitor (**Figure 3**) in both *I. scapularis* (130) and *Amblyomma sculptum* saliva (131). RHS2 from *Rhipicephalus haemaphysaloides* can inhibit the differentiation of BMDCs into DCs *in vitro* and promote their differentiation into macrophages (132). RHS2 also inhibits the expression of CD80, CD86, and the major histocompatibility complex class II (MHCII), thereby preventing DC maturation. DC differentiation from monocytes is blocked by Japanin (**Figure 3**), a salivary gland lipocalin from *R. appendiculatus* (133). Moreover, Japanin was found to reprogram DC responses to a broad variety of stimuli *in vitro*, radically altering the expression of co-stimulatory and co-inhibitory molecules and modifying the production of diverse cytokines (134).

Humoral Immunity

Tick salivary components also disarm host humoral immunity by inhibiting B cells responses, including their production of specific anti-tick antibodies (134). BIP (B cell inhibitory protein) (**Figure 3**) derived from *I. ricinus* inhibited B lymphocyte proliferation induced by *B. burgdorferi* lipoproteins (135). Similarly, BIF (B cell inhibitory factor) from *H. asiaticum asiaticum* salivary glands (**Figure 3**) was found to suppress B cell responses (136).

Cell-Mediated Immunity

Numerous inhibitors of T cell functions have been identified in tick saliva and salivary glands. Three immunosuppressant salivary proteins, p36 from *Dermacentor andersoni* (137, 138), HL-p36 from *H. longicornis* (139), and RH36 from *R. haemaphysaloides* (140) suppressed T lymphocyte proliferation *in vitro*. Recombinant HL-p36 and RH36 also directly inhibited the proliferation of several mitogen-stimulated cells *in vivo* and the expression of several cytokines such as IL-2, IL-12, and TNF-α (141, 142). In addition to its effect on DCs, RHS2 can prevent the activation of $CD4^+$ and $CD8^+$ T cells, leading to inhibition of the Th1 immune response (132). Two salivary cystatins from *I. scapularis*, Sialostatin L and Sialostatin L2, have shown promising anti-inflammatory and immunosuppressive activity *in vitro* and *in vivo* (141, 142). Sialostatin L was immunosuppressive in mammalian models of immune-related diseases, suppressing the proliferation of both CD4 and CD8 T cells, neutrophil migration in severe inflammation, and the secretion of cytokines by MCs, DCs, and lymphocytes (130, 141). Sialostatin L reduced the release of IL-9 by Th9 cells, which might explain its suppression of airway hyperresponsiveness and eosinophilia in an experimental asthma model (143). In the experimental autoimmune encephalomyelitis (EAE) mouse model of multiple sclerosis, *in vivo* administration of Sialostatin L significantly prevented disease symptoms (144). Furthermore, Sialostatin L effectively altered lysosomal cysteine cathepsins L, C, V, S, X and papain activity, critical elements

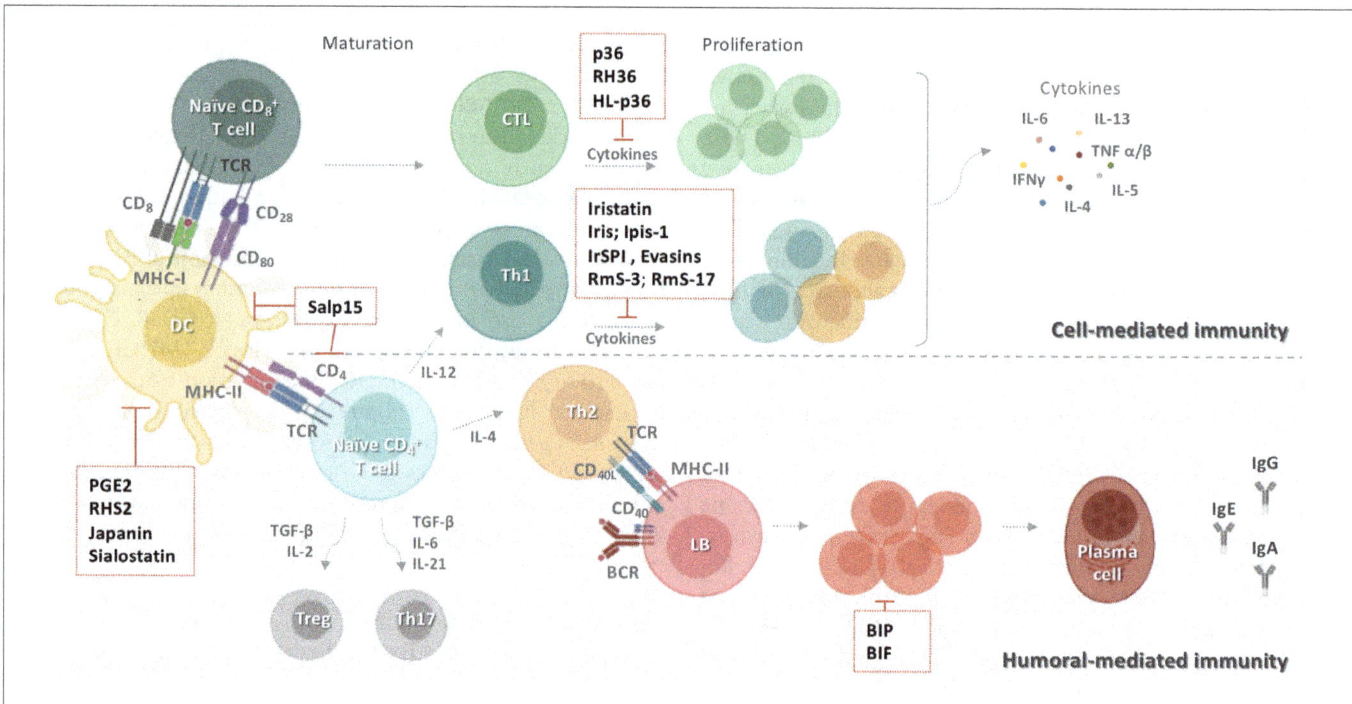

FIGURE 3 | Schematic representation of tick salivary molecules targeting adaptive immunity. During the primary contact with ticks, dendritic cells present salivary antigens to lymphocytes, which trigger cell- and humoral-mediated responses. Some tick salivary molecules prevent the initiation of adaptive immunity by targeting DCs, including Salp15, PGE_2, RHS2, Japanin, and sialostatin. Other compounds block the proliferation of lymphocytes and/or inhibit the production of T cell cytokines such as p36, RH36, HL-p36, Iristatin, Iris, Ipis-1, IrSPI, Evasins, RmS-3, and RmS-17. However, BIP and BIF disarm humoral host immunity by inhibiting B cell responses, including the production of specific anti-tick antibodies. BCR: B cell receptor; BIF: B cell inhibitory factor; BIP: B cell inhibitory protein; CD: cluster of differentiation; CTL: cytotoxic T lymphocyte; DC: dendritic cells; HL-p36: *Haemaphysalis longicornis* p-36; IFN-γ: interferon gamma; Ig: immunoglobulin; IL: interleukin; LB: lymphocyte B; MHC: major histocompatibility complex; PGE_2: prostaglandin E2; RmS: *Rhipicephalus microplus* serpin; Salp: salivary protein; TCR: T cell receptor; TGF-β: transforming growth factor-beta; Th: T helper; TNF: tumor necrosis factor; Treg: regulatory T cell.

in antigen presentation (141). Sialostatin L2 suppressed IFN-β-mediated immune reactions in murine DCs (145), and was also found to inhibit cathepsins C, L, S, and V and decrease IL-1β and IL-18 secretion by macrophages (146). Similar to sialostatins, Iristatin, a novel type 2 cystatin from *I. ricinus*, inhibited the proteolytic activity of cathepsins L and C (147) and diminished IL-2, IL-4, IL-9, and IFN-γ production by different T cell populations, IL-6 and IL-9 production by MCs, and nitric oxide production by macrophages. Iristatin inhibited OVA antigen-induced $CD4^+$ T cell proliferation and leukocyte recruitment *in vivo* and *in vitro* (**Figure 3**). With such a wide spectrum of immunosuppressive activities, Iristatin may be exploitable as an immunotherapeutic.

T cell inhibitory salivary molecules also include Iris and IrSPI from *I. ricinus* (148), Ipis-1 from *I. persulcatus* (149), RmS-3 and RmS-17 from *R. microplus* (61), and Salp15 from *I. scapularis* (47). Iris was found to suppress T cell proliferation, promote a Th2-type response, and bind to monocytes/macrophages, inhibiting their ability to secrete pro-inflammatory cytokines IL-6 and TNF-α (150). Similarly, IrSPI suppressed proliferation of $CD4^+$ T lymphocytes and pro-inflammatory cytokine secretion (**Figure 3**) from splenocytes and macrophages (151). The Iris homolog Ipis-1 inhibited cellular proliferation and the production of IFN-γ in bovine peripheral blood mononuclear cells, suggesting that Ipis could directly interact with T cells and inhibit their functions (149). RmS-3 and RmS-17 inhibited the metabolic activity of lymphocytes, decreasing lymphocyte proliferation (61). One of the most extensively studied components of tick saliva is Salp15, an immunosuppressive cysteine-rich glycoprotein (47). Salp15 binds specifically to CD4 co-receptors on the surface of T lymphocytes, interfering with TCR-mediated signaling transduction and impeding IL-2 secretion in a dose-dependent manner (47, 148, 149). A subsequent study reported that Salp15 interacts with DC-SIGN on DCs, triggering a novel Raf-1/MEK-dependent signaling pathway, thereby impairing cytokine production and T cell proliferation (152). Apart from its effect on adaptive immunity, Salp15 inhibited TLR2-dependent keratinocyte inflammation *in vitro* (153). Together, these findings make this salivary protein a potential candidate for the treatment of T cell-mediated autoimmune diseases. Indeed, the immunomodulatory effect of Salp15 has been investigated in various models *in vivo*. Paveglio and colleagues (154) were the first to show that Salp15 has a therapeutic effect in a mouse model of allergic asthma. The specific binding of Salp15 to CD4 inhibited the proliferation and differentiation of $CD4^+$ T cells toward Th2 cells and suppressed the production of inflammatory cytokines, significantly reducing symptoms of allergic asthma in treated mice. Moreover, Salp15 prevented the association of HIV-1 gp120 and CD4 in an experimental HIV infection (155).

gp120 is an HIV-1 envelope glycoprotein which, by binding to CD4, promotes penetration of HIV-1 into the host cell (156). The authors suggested that Salp15 competes with gp120 for an association with CD4 due to its ability to interact with CD4 on T cells. Another investigation showed the opposite effect in murine EAE/multiple sclerosis (157). The occurrence and progression of EAE is associated with myelin-specific $CD4^+$ T cell activation and secretion of IL-17 and INF-γ by Th17 and Th1 cells, respectively (158). Unexpectedly, Salp15 worsened the pathology in mice upon induction of EAE. A possible reason for this might be that Salp15 promoted Th17 activation, increasing IL-17 levels *in vivo*, and it also enhanced Th17 differentiation in the presence of IL-6 and absence of TGF-β *in vitro* (157). More recently, it was shown that Salp15 binding to CD4 is persistent and induces a long-lasting immunomodulatory effect in a murine model of hematopoietic transplantation (159). Based on these results, Salp15 could provide important opportunities for the development of novel and sophisticated therapies for human disease mainly those mediated by multiple processes.

TICK NON-CODING RNAs: NEW ALTERNATIVES IN TARGETED IMMUNOMODULATORY THERAPY?

Tick salivary molecules are pluripotent (i.e., one molecule may affect more than one host cell population) and show considerable functional redundancy (i.e., the same host cell population may be targeted by more than one tick salivary molecule) (160). Tick saliva not only contains proteins and metabolites but also non-proteinaceous species including nucleic acids (22, 161) and RNA silencing signals, which are now recognized as crucial for cross-species communication across diverse biological niches (162, 163). With respect to the tripartite tick-pathogen-host interaction, recent transcriptomic and proteomic projects, facilitated by rapid developments in high-throughput sequencing, have revealed several tick genes/transcripts of unknown function or transcripts without an open reading frame (ORF) (160). These projects have also revealed a significant number of ncRNAs in tick saliva that are predicted to be functionally involved in the vector-host interaction (164). ncRNAs are important in vector-host interactions at the tick-host interface: ticks use ncRNAs, broadly divided by length into long non-coding RNAs (lncRNAs) (>200 nucleotides (nt) long) and small non-coding RNAs (sncRNAs) (<200 nt long), to hijack host defense mechanisms (165). They are suggested to be secreted via exosomes (166, 167) and released in the host cells, to manipulate gene expression and deregulate host defense pathways (165). LncRNAs are not translated into proteins and include mRNA-like intergenic transcripts (lincRNAs), antisense transcripts of protein-coding genes, and primary RNA polymerase II (Pol II) transcript-derived unconventional lncRNAs (168). LncRNAs are involved in numerous important biological phenomena such as imprinting genomic loci, shaping chromosome conformation and allosterically regulating enzymatic activity (169). On the other hand, sncRNAs represent a diverse set of molecules that control the expression of most vertebrate genes and include small-interfering RNAs (siRNAs), microRNAs (miRNAs), and piwi-interacting RNAs (piRNAs) (170). miRNAs have been extensively studied in several organisms and their function in gene regulation is well understood. The first attempt to identify host targets of tick ncRNAs was performed by Hackenberg and colleagues (171). Their *in silico* study showed that saliva-specific miRNAs from *I. ricinus* might have combinatorial effects on the host targetome: different tick miRNAs may target vertebrate host genes in the same host homeostatic pathway, and the expression of a given host gene may also be regulated by more than one saliva-specific tick miRNA (171). The authors suggested combinatorial effects of vector miRNAs on host target genes, which may be of importance in evolutionary terms to maintain robust regulation of host genes and pathways important in the tick-host interaction. miR-8-3p, bantam-3p, mir-317-3p, and miR-279a-3p from *I. ricinus* were predicted to target host KEGG pathways such as "gap junction" and "inflammatory mediator regulation of TRP channels," which play a role in the host homeostatic response (**Figure 4A**).

The huge number of ncRNA sequences revealed by high-throughput projects suggests that tick ncRNAs might also modulate host gene expression by binding to regulatory host miRNAs involved in host immune cell responses. Tick ncRNAs could regulate protein-coding genes through mRNA cleavage and/or direct translational repression and/or mRNA destabilization. We hypothesize that lncRNAs compete with host mRNAs for host miRNA binding by acting as "sponge" molecules that inhibit host miRNA interactions with host mRNAs, thus affecting host homeostatic responses to tick feeding (**Figure 4B**). *In silico* predictions now need to be validated using systems-based approaches in order to characterize tick ncRNAs and to understand their involvement in tick-host interactions. Various academic and commercial research groups are now exploring ncRNA-based therapies and exploring the potential of miRNA therapeutics, as miRNAs are the most studied ncRNAs to date (172). A few miRNAs have entered preclinical and clinical testing, so might soon be available on the market for use in humans. As tick ncRNAs are likely to be less immunogenic by their intrinsic ability to hijack and bypass host immunity, we strongly believe that this flourishing field might lead to ncRNA therapeutics useful for the treatment of various diseases. Emerging data on the possible regulatory function of ncRNAs, the vector, the pathogen, and the host, the role of ncRNA in the vector or host-pathogen remain quite challenging, due to several biological and technical aspects. For example, the used techniques for ncRNAs study can generate several biases in the results. New scRNA-seq technology that is showing its efficiency to counter this issue, but sufficient read depths of rarely expressed RNAs can also be misleading, and vector, host or pathogen-derived RNAs information could be easily lost. LncRNAs data analyses also remain controversial due to the lack of accurate transcript models in current annotations. LncRNAs could also be pluripotent, and just as the salivary proteins, this would also be a serious limitation in any potential therapeutic applications. Overall, given the arising data on the ability of ncRNAs produced in tick salivary glands and also the

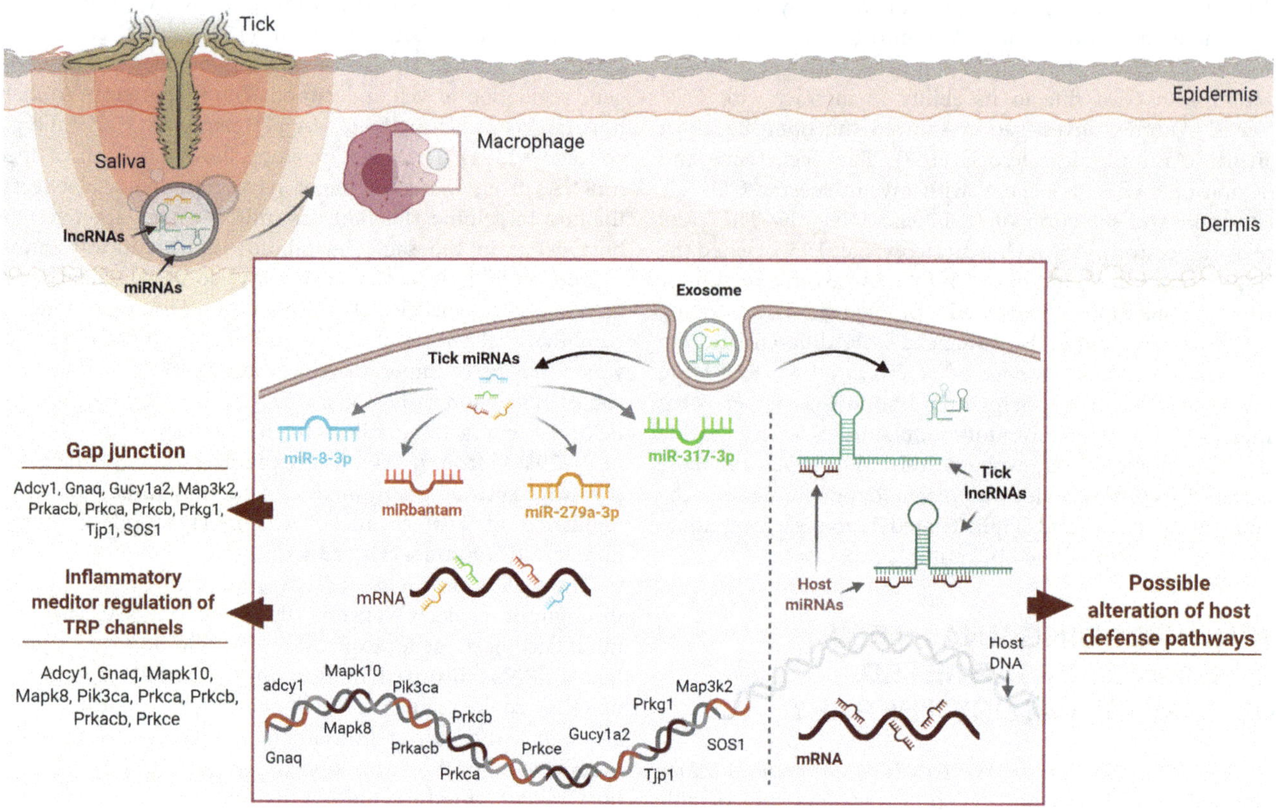

FIGURE 4 | Possible strategies used by tick ncRNAs in host cells. (A) miR-8-3p, bantam-3p, mir-317-3p, and miR-279a-3p from *Ixodes ricinus* have been predicted to target gap junctions and inflammatory mediator regulation of TRP channels, which play a role in host homeostatic responses. (B) Host miRNAs regulate protein coding genes through mRNA cleavage and/or direct translational repression and/or mRNA destabilization. Ticks secrete exosomes in their saliva containing lncRNAs, which may compete with host mRNAs for host miRNA binding by acting as "sponge" molecules that inhibit host miRNA interactions with host mRNAs, thus affecting host homeostatic responses to tick feeding.

possible regulatory function of cellular RNAs on the vector, pathogen or host, the role of ncRNA in the vector or host-pathogen crosstalk might be even more sophisticated than what is expected. Development of research projects that employ single-cell/single molecule sequencing methodologies and do not require nucleic acid amplification will definitely enable less biased and reliable data output.

CONCLUDING REMARKS

Inflammatory, autoimmune, metabolic, and neurodegenerative diseases remain critical health problems worldwide, creating an enormous need for new, effective, and specific medicines. Over the last few decades, ticks have shown their "good side" as promising sources of new drugs targeting distinct pathophysiological pathways in mammals. In this review, we summarized potential drug candidates from tick salivary glands that might have therapeutic use in immune disorders and other related diseases. We have also highlighted that tick ncRNAs are possible new alternatives for targeted immunomodulatory therapy. The molecules described in this review have been tested *in vitro* and/or in various animal models of human disease and have shown encouraging results. However, only a few of them have advanced to (pre-)clinical investigations, and further in-depth molecular and cellular studies are required to further develop candidates for clinical trials. The major challenges to drug development are (i) specificity and efficacy, since broad-spectrum targets can generate unwanted side-effects; and (ii) safety, with drug-induced toxicity and immunogenicity critical limitations of many drug candidates. Addressing these challenges, tick salivary molecules, at least in theory, might have a somewhat higher clinical success rate than molecules from other origins, since many tick-derived products have an intrinsically low risk of toxicity and immunogenicity and high target specificity to execute their intended functions. From the pharmaceutical perspective, some molecules might be unstable or have a short half-lives, so pharmacokinetic, dose optimization, and modification studies are critical research priorities. While experimental validation and ultimately clinical trialing remain the cornerstone of successful therapeutic development, computational methods might play a role as time-saving, cost-effective, and productive approaches to design and discover novel lead compounds for associated disease targets.

Modeling and simulation of preclinical and clinical trials could also be used to bridge the gap between the early stages of drug development and their potential effects on humans.

AUTHOR CONTRIBUTIONS

All authors searched and read the literature and edited the manuscript. HA, CB, and MK wrote the manuscript.

FUNDING

This study was financed by the Coordenação de Aperfeiçoamento de Pessoal de Nível Superior - Brazil (CAPES) - Finance Code 001; by FAPESP (CETICS: 2013/07467-1) and Fundação Butantan. It was also financed by the Grant Agency of the Czech Republic (Grant19-382 07247S to MK and 19-14704Y to JC) and by ERD Funds, project CePaVip OPVVV (No. 384 CZ.02.1.01/0.0/0.0/16_019/0000759 to MK).

REFERENCES

Raje N, Dinakar C. Overview of immunodeficiency disorders. *Immunol Allergy Clin North Am.* (2015) 35:599–623. doi: 10.1016/j.iac.2015.07.001

Wang L, Wang FS, Gershwin ME. Human autoimmune diseases: a comprehensive update. *J Int Med.* (2015) 278:369–95. doi: 10.1111/joim.12395

Bogdanos DP, Smyk DS, Rigopoulou EI, Mytilinaiou MG, Heneghan MA, Selmi C, et al. Twin studies in autoimmune disease: genetics, gender and environment. *J Autoimmun.* (2012) 38:J156–69. doi: 10.1016/j.jaut.2011.11.003

Mahoney EJ, Veling MC, Mims JW. Food allergy in adults and children. *Otolaryngol Clin North Am.* (2011) 44:815–33. doi: 10.1016/j.otc.2011.03.014

Peden DB. Effect of pollution on allergy/immunology. *J Allergy Clin Immunol.* (2018) 141:878–9. doi: 10.1016/j.jaci.2018.01.017

Nikolich-Žugich J. The twilight of immunity: emerging concepts in aging of the immune system. *Nat Immunol.* (2018) 19:10–9. doi: 10.1038/s41590-017-0006-x

Krones E, Högenauer C. Diarrhea in the immunocompromised patient. *Gastroenterol Clin North Am.* (2012) 41:677–701. doi: 10.1016/j.gtc.2012.06.009

Girish MB. Emerging drugs for the treatment of human immunodeficiency virus. *Recent Pat AntiInfect Drug Discov.* (2012) 7:45–52. doi: 10.2174/157489112799829729

Bucktrout SL, Bluestone JA, Ramsdell F. Recent advances in immunotherapies: from infection and autoimmunity, to cancer, and back again. *Genome Med.* (2018) 10:79. doi: 10.1186/s13073-018-0588-4

Li G, Lou H-X. Strategies to diversify natural products for drug discovery. *Med Res Rev.* (2018) 38:1255–94. doi: 10.1002/med.21474

Lautié E, Russo O, Ducrot P, Boutin JA. Unraveling plant natural chemical diversity for drug discovery purposes. *Front Pharmacol.* (2020) 11:397. doi: 10.3389/fphar.2020.00397

Uzair B, Bint-e-Irshad S, Khan BA, Azad B, Mahmood T, Rehman MU, et al. Scorpion venom peptides as a potential source for human drug candidates. *Protein Pept Lett.* (2018) 25:702–8. doi: 10.2174/0929866525666180614114307

Perumal Samy R, Stiles BG, Franco OL, Sethi G, Lim LHK. Animal venoms as antimicrobial agents. *Biochem Pharmacol.* (2017) 134:127–38. doi: 10.1016/j. bcp.2017.03.005

Franchin M, Freires IA, Lazarini JG, Nani BD, da Cunha MG, Colón DF, et al. The use of Brazilian propolis for discovery and development of novel anti-inflammatory drugs. *Eur J Med Chem.* (2018) 153:49–55. doi: 10.1016/j.ejmech.2017.06.050

Katz L, Baltz RH. Natural product discovery: past, present, and future. *J Ind Microbiol Biotechnol.* (2016) 43:155–76. doi: 10.1007/s10295-015-1723-5

Gileadi O. Recombinant protein expression in *E. coli*: a historical perspective. *Methods Mol Biol.* (2017) 1586:3–10. doi: 10.1007/978-1-4939-6887-9_1

Baghban R, Farajnia S, Ghasemi Y, Mortazavi M, Zarghami N, Samadi N. New developments in *Pichia pastoris* expression system, review and update. *Curr Pharm Biotechnol.* (2018) 19:451–67. doi: 10.2174/1389201019666180718093037

Rozov SM, Permyakova NV, Deineko EV. Main strategies of plant expression system glycoengineering for producing humanized recombinant pharmaceutical proteins. *Biochemistry.* (2018) 83:215–32. doi: 10.1134/S0006297918030033

Metzker ML. Sequencing technologies the next generation. *Nat Rev Genet.* (2010) 11:31–46. doi: 10.1038/nrg2626

Wingfield J, Wilson ID. Advances in mass spectrometry within drug discovery. *J Biomol Screen.* (2016) 21:109–10. doi: 10.1177/1087057115623454

Chmelar J, Kotál J, Kovaríková A, Kotsyfakis M. The use of tick salivary proteins as novel therapeutics. *Front Physiol.* (2019) 10:812. doi: 10.3389/fphys.2019.00812

Francischetti IMB, Sa-Nunes A, Mans BJ, Santos IM, Ribeiro JMC. The role of saliva in tick feeding. *Front Biosci.* (2009) 14:2051–88. doi: 10.2741/3363

Chmelar J, Calvo E, Pedra JHF, Francischetti IMB, Kotsyfakis M. Tick salivary secretion as a source of antihemostatics. *J Proteomics.* (2012) 75:3842–54. doi: 10.1016/j.jprot.2012.04.026

Boulanger N. [Immunomodulatory effect of tick saliva in pathogen transmission]. *Biolo Aujourd'hui.* (2018) 212:107–17. doi: 10.1051/jbio/2019001

Maria DA, Will SEAL, Bosch RV, Souza JG, Sciani JM, Goldfeder MB, et al. Preclinical evaluation of Amblyomin-X, a Kunitz-type protease inhibitor with antitumor activity. *Toxicol Rep.* (2019) 6:51–63. doi: 10.1016/j.toxrep.2018.11.014

Boufleur P, Sciani JM, Goldfeder M, Faria F, Branco V, Chudzinski- Tavassi AM. Biodistribution and pharmacokinetics of Amblyomin-X, a novel antitumour protein drug in healthy mice. *Eur J Drug Metab Pharmacokinet.* (2019) 44:111–20. doi: 10.1007/s13318-018-0500-z

Jongejan F, Uilenberg G. The global importance of ticks. *Parasitology.* (2004) 129:S3–14. doi: 10.1017/S0031182004005967

Sonenshine DE. Biology of ticks. *Vet Clin North Am Small Anim Pract.* (1991) 21:1–26. doi: 10.1016/S0195-5616(91)50001-2

Nuttall PA. Wonders of tick saliva. *Ticks Tick Borne Dis.* (2019) 10:470–81. doi: 10.1016/j.ttbdis.2018.11.005

Castelli E, Caputo V, Morello V, Tomasino RM. Local reactions to tick bites. *Am J Dermatopathol.* (2008) 30:241–8. doi: 10.1097/DAD. 0b013e3181676b60

Bernard Q, Grillon A, Lenormand C, Ehret-Sabatier L, Boulanger N. Skin interface, a key player for *Borrelia* multiplication and persistence in lyme borreliosis. *Trends Parasitol.* (2020) 36:304–14. doi: 10.1016/j.pt.2019.12.017

Hermance ME, Thangamani S. Tick–virus–host interactions at the cutaneous interface: the nidus of flavivirus transmission. *Viruses.* (2018) 10:362. doi: 10.3390/v10070362

Kazimírová M, Štibrániová I. Tick salivary compounds: their role in modulation of host defences and pathogen transmission. *Front Cell Infect Microbiol.* (2013) 3:43. doi: 10.3389/fcimb.2013.00043

Versteeg HH, Heemskerk JWM, Levi M, Reitsma PH. New fundamentals in hemostasis. *Physiol Rev.* (2013) 93:327–58. doi: 10.1152/physrev.00016.2011

Chudzinski-Tavassi AM, Faria F, Flores MPA. Anticoagulants from hematophagous. In: Mijovski MB editor. *Anticoagulant Drugs.* London: InTech. (2018). doi: 10.5772/intechopen.78025 .

Carroll MC, Isenman DE. Regulation of humoral immunity by complement. *Immunity.* (2012) 37:199–207. doi: 10.1016/j.immuni.2012.08.002

Dunkelberger JR, Song WC. Complement and its role in innate and adaptive immune responses. *Cell Res.* (2010) 20:34–50. doi: 10.1038/cr.2009.139

Wikel S. Ticks and tick-borne pathogens at the cutaneous interface: host defenses, tick countermeasures, and a suitable environment for pathogen establishment. *Front Microbiol.* (2013) 4:337. doi: 10.3389/fmicb.2013.00337

Glatz M, Means T, Haas J, Steere AC, Müllegger RR. Characterization of the early local immune response to *Ixodes ricinus* tick bites in human skin. *Exp Dermatol.* (2017) 26:263–9. doi: 10.1111/exd.13207

Buczek A, Bartosik K. [Tick-host interactions]. *Przegl Epidemiol.* (2006) 60(Suppl. 1):28–33.

Krause PJ, Grant-Kels JM, Tahan SR, Dardick KR, Alarcon-Chaidez F, Bouchard K, et al. Dermatologic changes induced by repeated *Ixodes scapularis* bites and implications for prevention of tick-borne infection. *Vector Borne Zoonotic Dis.* (2009) 9:603–10. doi: 10.1089/vbz.2008.0091

Kiripolsky J, McCabe LG, Kramer JM. Innate immunity in Sjögren's syndrome. *Clin Immunol.* (2017) 182:4–13. doi: 10.1016/j.clim.2017.04.003

Cepika AM, Sato Y, Liu JMH, Uyeda MJ, Bacchetta R, Roncarolo MG. Tregopathies: monogenic diseases resulting in regulatory T-cell deficiency. *J Allergy Clin Immunol.* (2018) 142:1679–95. doi: 10.1016/j.jaci.2018.10.026

Anderton SM. Peptide immunotherapy in experimental autoimmune encephalomyelitis. *Biomed J.* (2015) 38:206–14. doi: 10.4103/2319-4170.158510

Morgan BP, Harris CL. Complement, a target for therapy in inflammatory and degenerative diseases. *Nat Rev Drug Discov.* (2015) 14:857–77. doi: 10.1038/nrd4657

Anguita J, Ramamoorthi N, Hovius JWR, Das S, Thomas V, Persinski R, et al. Salp15, an *Ixodes scapularis* salivary protein, inhibits CD4(+) T cell activation. *Immunity.* (2002) 16:849–59. doi: 10.1016/s1074-7613(02)00325-4

Wen S, Wang F, Ji Z, Pan Y, Jian M, Bi Y, et al. Salp15, a multifunctional protein from tick saliva with potential pharmaceutical effects. *Front Immunol.* (2019) 10:3067. doi: 10.3389/fimmu.2019.03067

Yang T, Sui X, Yu B, Shen Y, Cong H. Recent advances in the rational drug design based on multi-target ligands. *Curr Med Chem.* (2020) 27:4720–40. doi: 10.2174/0929867327666200102120652

Kumar A, Tiwari A, Sharma A. Changing paradigm from one target one ligand towards multi-target directed ligand design for key drug targets of alzheimer disease: an important role of *in silico* methods in multi-target directed ligands design. *Curr Neuropharmacol.* (2018) 16:726–39. doi: 10.2174/1570159X16666180315141643

Talevi A. Multi-target pharmacology: possibilities and limitations of the "skeleton key approach" from a medicinal chemist perspective. *Front Pharmacol.* (2015) 6:205. doi: 10.3389/fphar.2015.00205

Talevi A. Tailored multi-target agents. applications and design considerations. *Curr Pharm Des.* (2016) 22:3164–70. doi: 10.2174/1381612822666160308141203

Kotál J, Langhansová H, Lieskovská J, Andersen JF, Francischetti IMB, Chavakis T, et al. Modulation of host immunity by tick saliva. *J Proteomics.* (2015) 128:58–68. doi: 10.1016/j.jprot.2015.07.005

Almazan C, Tipacamu GA, Rodriguez S, Mosqueda J, Perez de Leon A. Immunological control of ticks and tick-borne diseases that impact cattle health and production. *Front Biosci.* (2018) 23:1535–51. doi: 10.2741/4659

Šimo L, Kazimirova M, Richardson J, Bonnet SI. The essential role of tick salivary glands and saliva in tick feeding and pathogen transmission. *Front Cell Infect Microbiol.* (2017) 7:281. doi: 10.3389/fcimb.2017.00281

Štibrániová I, Bartíková P, Holíková V, Kazimírová M. Deciphering biological processes at the tick-host interface opens new strategies for treatment of human diseases. *Front Physiol.* (2019) 10:830. doi: 10.3389/fphys.2019.00830

Schmidt MCB, Morais KLP, Almeida MES, Iqbal A, Goldfeder MB, Chudzinski-Tavassi AM. Amblyomin-X, a recombinant Kunitz-type inhibitor, regulates cell adhesion and migration of human tumor cells. *Cell Adh Migr.* (2020) 14:129–38. doi: 10.1080/19336918.2018.1516982

Lichtenstein F, Iqbal A, de Lima Will SEA, Bosch RV, DeOcesano-Pereira C, Goldfeder MB, et al. Modulation of stress and immune response by Amblyomin-X results in tumor cell death in a horse melanoma model. *Sci Rep.* (2020) 10:6388. doi: 10.1038/s41598-020-63275-2

Pireaux V, Tassignon J, Demoulin S, Derochette S, Borenstein N, Ente A, et al. Anticoagulation with an inhibitor of factors XIa and XIIa during cardiopulmonary bypass. *J Am Coll Cardiol.* (2019) 74:2178–89. doi: 10.1016/ j.jacc.2019.08.1028

Yeh CH, Fredenburgh JC, Weitz JI. Oral direct factor Xa inhibitors. *Circ Res.* (2012) 111:1069–78. doi: 10.1161/CIRCRESAHA.112.276741

Borriello F, Iannone R, Marone G. Histamine release from mast cells and basophils. In: Hattori Y, Seifert R editors. *Handbook of Experimental Pharmacology*. New York: Springer. (2017). p. 1–19. doi: 10.1007/164_2017_18

Coutinho ML, Bizzarro B, Tirloni L, Berger M, Freire Oliveira CJ, Sá- Nunes A, et al. *Rhipicephalus microplus* serpins interfere with host immune responses by specifically modulating mast cells and lymphocytes. *Ticks Tick Borne Dis.* (2020) 11:101425. doi: 10.1016/j.ttbdis.2020.101425

Paesen GC, Adams PL, Harlos K, Nuttall PA, Stuart DI. Tick histamine- binding proteins: isolation, cloning, and three-dimensional structure. *Mol Cell.* (1999) 3:661–71. doi: 10.1016/S1097-2765(00)80359-7

Paesen GC, Adams PL, Nuttall PA, Stuart DL. Tick histamine-binding proteins: lipocalins with a second binding cavity. *Biochim Biophys Acta.* (2000) 1482:92–101. doi: 10.1016/S0167-4838(00)00168-0

Wang Y, Li Z, Zhou Y, Cao J, Zhang H, Gong H, et al. Specific histamine binding activity of a new lipocalin from *Hyalomma asiaticum* (Ixodidae) and therapeutic effects on allergic asthma in mice. *Parasit Vectors.* (2016) 9:506. doi: 10.1186/s13071-016-1790-0

Sangamnatdej S, Paesen GC, Slovak M, Nuttall PA. A high affinity serotonin- and histamine-binding lipocalin from tick saliva. *Insect Mol Biol.* (2002) 11:79–86. doi: 10.1046/j.0962-1075.2001.00311.x

Mohajeri M, Kovanen PT, Bianconi V, Pirro M, Cicero AFG, Sahebkar A. Mast cell tryptase – marker and maker of cardiovascular diseases. *Pharmacol Ther.* (2019) 199:91–110. doi: 10.1016/j.pharmthera.2019.03.008

Ni WW, Da Cao M, Huang W, Meng L, Wei JF. Tryptase inhibitors: a patent review. *Expert Opin Ther Pat.* (2017) 27:919–28. doi: 10.1080/13543776.2017.1322064

Paesen GC, Siebold C, Harlos K, Peacey MF, Nuttall PA, Stuart DIA. Tick protein with a modified kunitz fold inhibits human tryptase. *J Mol Biol.* (2007) 368:1172–86. doi: 10.1016/j.jmb.2007.03.011

Valdés JJ, Schwarz A, Cabeza de Vaca I, Calvo E, Pedra JHF, Guallar V, et al. Tryptogalinin is a tick kunitz serine protease inhibitor with a unique intrinsic disorder. *PLoS One.* (2013) 8:e62562. doi: 10.1371/journal.pone.0062562

Sommerhoff C, Schaschke N. Mast cell tryptase β as a target in allergic inflammation: an evolving story. *Curr Pharm Des.* (2006) 13:313–32. doi: 10.2174/138161207779313579

Andrade BB, Teixeira CR, Barral A, Barral-Netto M. Haematophagous arthropod saliva and host defense system: a tale of tear and blood. *An Acad Bras Cienc.* (2005) 77:665–93. doi: 10.1590/S0001-37652005000400008

Jaworski DC, Jasinskas A, Metz CN, Bucala R, Barbour AG. Identification and characterization of a homologue of the pro- inflammatory cytokine macrophage migration inhibitory factor in the tick, *Amblyomma americanum. Insect Mol Biol.* (2001) 10:323–31. doi: 10.1046/j.0962-1075.2001.00271.x

Bowen CJ, Jaworski DC, Wasala NB, Coons LB. Macrophage migration inhibitory factor expression and protein localization in *Amblyomma americanum* (Ixodidae). *Exp Appl Acarol.* (2010) 50:343–52. doi: 10.1007/s10493-009-9324-5

Umemiya R, Hatta T, Liao M, Tanaka M, Zhou J, Inoue N, et al. *Haemaphysalis longicornis*: molecular characterization of a homologue of the macrophage migration inhibitory factor from the partially fed ticks. *Exp Parasitol.* (2007) 115:135–42. doi: 10.1016/j.exppara.2006.07.006

Beaufays J, Adam B, Menten-Dedoyart C, Fievez L, Grosjean A, Decrem Y, et al. Ir-LBP, an *Ixodes ricinus* tick salivary ltb4-binding lipocalin, interferes with host neutrophil function. *PLoS One.* (2008) 3:e3987. doi: 10.1371/ journal.pone.0003987

Hidano A, Konnai S, Yamada S, Githaka N, Isezaki M, Higuchi H, et al. Suppressive effects of neutrophil by Salp16-like salivary gland proteins from *Ixodes persulcatus* Schulze tick. *Insect Mol Biol.* (2014) 23:466–74. doi: 10.1111/imb.12101

Bhusal RP, Eaton JRO, Chowdhury ST, Power CA, Proudfoot AEI, Stone MJ, et al. Evasins: tick salivary proteins that inhibit mammalian chemokines. *Trends Biochem Sci.* (2020) 45:108–22. doi: 10.1016/j.tibs.2019.10.003

Frauenschuh A, Power CA, Déruaz M, Ferreira BR, Silva JS, Teixeira MM, et al. Molecular cloning and characterization of a highly selective chemokine-binding protein from the tick Rhipicephalus sanguineus. *J Biol Chem.* (2007) 282:27250–8. doi: 10.1074/jbc.M704706200

Russo RC, Alessandri AL, Garcia CC, Cordeiro BF, Pinho V, Cassali GD, et al. Therapeutic effects of evasin-1, a chemokine binding protein, in bleomycin-induced pulmonary fibrosis. *Am J Respir Cell Mol Biol.* (2011) 45:72–80. doi: 10.1165/rcmb.2009-0406OC

Castor MGM, Rezende B, Resende CB, Alessandri AL, Fagundes CT, Sousa LP, et al. The CCL3/Macrophage inflammatory protein-1a-binding protein evasin-1 protects from graft-versus-host disease but does not modify graft-versus-leukemia in mice. *J Immunol.* (2010) 184:2646–54. doi: 10.4049/jimmunol.0902614

Déruaz M, Frauenschuh A, Alessandri AL, Dias JM, Coelho FM, Russo RC, et al. Ticks produce highly selective chemokine binding proteins with antiinflammatory activity. *J Exp Med.* (2008) 205:2019–31. doi: 10.1084/jem. 20072689

Denisov SS, Ippel JH, Heinzmann ACA, Koenen RR, Ortega-Gomez A, Soehnlein O, et al. Tick saliva protein Evasin-3 modulates chemotaxis by disrupting CXCL8 interactions with glycosaminoglycans and CXCR2. *J Biol Chem.* (2019) 294:12370–9. doi: 10.1074/jbc.RA119.008902

Montecucco F, Lenglet S, Braunersreuther V, Pelli G, Pellieux C, Montessuit C, et al. Single administration of the CXC chemokine-binding protein evasin-3 during ischemia prevents myocardial reperfusion injury in mice. *Arterioscler Thromb Vasc Biol.* (2010) 30:1371–7. doi: 10.1161/ATVBAHA.110.206011

Copin JC, Da Silva RF, Fraga-Silva RA, Capettini L, Quintao S, Lenglet S, et al. Treatment with Evasin-3 reduces atherosclerotic vulnerability for ischemic stroke, but not brain injury in mice. *J Cereb Blood Flow Metab.* (2013) 33:490–8. doi: 10.1038/jcbfm.2012.198

Montecucco F, Mach F, Lenglet S, Vonlaufen A, Gomes Quinderé AL, Pelli G, et al. Treatment with Evasin-3 abrogates neutrophil-mediated inflammation in mouse acute pancreatitis. *Eur J Clin Investig.* (2014) 44:940–50. doi: 10.1111/eci.12327

Braunersreuther V, Montecucco F, Pelli G, Galan K, Proudfoot AE, Belin A, et al. Treatment with the CC chemokine-binding protein Evasin-4 improves post-infarction myocardial injury and survival in mice. *Thromb Haemost.* (2013) 110:807–25. doi: 10.1160/TH13-04-0297

Darlot B, Eaton JRO, Geis-Asteggiante L, Yakala GK, Karuppanan K, Davies G, et al. Engineered anti-inflammatory peptides inspired by mapping an evasin-chemokine interaction. *J Biol Chem.* (2020) 295:10926–39. doi: 10.1074/jbc.ra120.014103

Wu J, Wang Y, Liu H, Yang H, Ma D, Li J, et al. Two immunoregulatory peptides with antioxidant activity from tick salivary glands. *J Biol Chem.* (2010) 285:16606–13. doi: 10.1074/jbc.M109.094615

Tian Y, Chen W, Mo G, Chen R, Fang M, Yedid G, et al. An immunosuppressant peptide from the hard tick *Amblyomma variegatum. Toxins.* (2016) 8:133. doi: 10.3390/toxins8050133

Wang F, Gong H, Zhang H, Zhou Y, Cao J, Zhou J. Lipopolysaccharide-induced differential expression of mirnas in male and female *Rhipicephalus haemaphysaloides* ticks. *PLoS One.* (2015) 10:e0139241. doi: 10.1371/journal. pone.0139241

Kim TK, Tirloni L, Berger M, Diedrich JK, Yates JR, Termignoni C, et al. *Amblyomma americanum* serpin 41 (AAS41) inhibits inflammation by targeting chymase and chymotrypsin. *Int J Biol Macromol.* (2020) 156:1007–21. doi: 10.1016/j.ijbiomac.2020.04.088

Tirloni L, Kim TK, Berger M, Termignoni C, Da Silva Vaz I, Mulenga *Amblyomma americanum* serpin 27 (AAS27) is a tick salivary anti-inflammatory protein secreted into the host during feeding. *PLoS Negl Trop Dis.* (2019) 13:e0007660. doi: 10.1371/journal.pntd.0007660

Chmelar J, Oliveira CJ, Rezacova P, Francischetti IMB, Kovarova Z, Pejler G, et al. A tick salivary protein targets cathepsin G and chymase and inhibits host inflammation and platelet aggregation. *Blood.* (2011) 117:736–44. doi: 10.1182/blood-2010-06-293241

Páleníková J, Lieskovská J, Langhansová H, Kotsyfakis M, Chmelaø J, Kopeck? J. *Ixodes ricinus* salivary serpin IRS-2 affects Th17 differentiation via inhibition of the interleukin-6/STAT-3 signaling pathway. *Infect Immun.* (2015) 83:1949–56. doi: 10.1128/IAI.03065-14

Sun T, Wang F, Pan W, Wu Q, Wang J, Dai J. An immunosuppressive tick salivary gland protein DsCystatin interferes with toll-like receptor signaling by downregulating TRAF6. *Front Immunol.* (2018) 9:1245. doi: 10.3389/fimmu.2018.01245

Dickinson RG, O'Hagan JE, Schotz M, Binnington KC, Hegarty MP. Prostaglandin in the saliva of the cattle tick *Boophilus microplus. Aust J Exp Biol Med Sci.* (1976) 54:475–86. doi: 10.1038/icb.1976.48

Ruan D, So S-P. Prostaglandin E2 produced by inducible COX-2 and mPGES-1 promoting cancer cell proliferation *in vitro* and *in vivo. Life Sci.* (2014) 116:43–50. doi: 10.1016/j.lfs.2014.07.042

Fezza F, Dillwith JW, Bisogno T, Tucker JS, Di Marzo V, Sauer JR. Endocannabinoids and related fatty acid amides, and their regulation, in the salivary glands of the lone star tick. *Biochim Biophys Acta.* (2003) 1633:61–7. doi: 10.1016/s1388-1981(03)00087-8

Oliveira CJF, Sá-Nunes A, Francischetti IMB, Carregaro V, Anatriello E, Silva JS, et al. Deconstructing tick saliva: non-protein molecules with potent immunomodulatory properties. *J Biol Chem.* (2011) 286:10960–9. doi: 10.1074/jbc.M110.205047

Della Latta V, Cabiati M, Rocchiccioli S, Del Ry S, Morales MA. The role of the adenosinergic system in lung fibrosis. *Pharmacol Res.* (2013) 76:182–9. doi: 10.1016/j.phrs.2013.08.004

Jarvis MF. Therapeutic potential of adenosine kinase inhibition–revisited. *Pharmacol Res Perspect.* (2019) 7:506. doi: 10.1002/prp2.506

Cai Y, Feng L, Wang X. Targeting the tumor promoting effects of adenosine in chronic lymphocytic leukemia. *Crit Rev Oncol Hematol.* (2018) 126:24–31. doi: 10.1016/j.critrevonc.2018.03.022

Honda T, Matsuoka T, Ueta M, Kabashima K, Miyachi Y, Narumiya S. Prostaglandin E2-EP3 signaling suppresses skin inflammation in murine contact hypersensitivity. *J Allergy Clin Immunol.* (2009) 124:809–27. doi: 10.1016/j.jaci.2009.04.029

Nakanishi M, Rosenberg DW. Multifaceted roles of PGE2 in inflammation and cancer. *Semin Immunopathol.* (2013) 35:123–37. doi: 10.1007/s00281- 012-0342-8

Łukawska E, Polcyn-Adamczak M, Niemir ZI. The role of the alternative pathway of complement activation in glomerular diseases. *Clin Exp Med.* (2018) 18:297–318. doi: 10.1007/s10238-018-0491-8

Thorgersen EB, Barratt-Due A, Haugaa H, Harboe M, Pischke SE, Nilsson PH, et al. The role of complement in liver injury, regeneration, and transplantation. *Hepatology.* (2019) 70:725–36. doi: 10.1002/hep.30508

Tichaczek-Goska D. Deficiencies and excessive human complement system activation in disorders of multifarious etiology. *Adv Clin Exp Med.* (2012) 21:105–14.

Ricklin D, Reis ES, Lambris JD. Complement in disease: a defence system turning offensive. *Nat Rev Nephrol.* (2016) 12:383–401. doi: 10.1038/nrneph. 2016.70

Ricklin D, Mastellos DC, Reis ES, Lambris JD. The renaissance of complement therapeutics. *Nat Rev Nephrol.* (2017) 14:26–47. doi: 10.1038/nrneph.2017.156

Valenzuela JG, Charlab R, Mather TN, Ribeiro JMC. Purification, cloning, and expression of a novel salivary anticomplement protein from the tick *Ixodes scapularis. J Biol Chem.* (2000) 275:18717–23. doi: 10.1074/jbc. M001486200

Schroeder H, Daix V, Gillet L, Renauld JC, Vanderplasschen A. The paralogous salivary anti-complement proteins IRAC I and IRAC II encoded by *Ixodes ricinus* ticks have broad and complementary inhibitory activities against the complement of different host species. *Microb Infect.* (2007) 9:247–50. doi: 10.1016/j.micinf.2006.10.020

Zwarthoff SA, Berends ETM, Mol S, Ruyken M, Aerts PC, Józsi M, et al. Functional characterization of alternative and classical pathway C3/C5 convertase activity and inhibition using purified models. *Front Immunol.* (2018) 9:1691. doi: 10.3389/fimmu.2018.01691

Hourcade DE, Akk AM, Mitchell LM, Zhou HF, Hauhart R, Pham CTN. Anti-complement activity of the *Ixodes scapularis* salivary protein Salp20. *Mol Immunol.* (2016) 69:62–9. doi: 10.1016/j.molimm.2015.11.008

Couvreur B, Beaufays J, Charon C, Lahaye K, Gensale F, Denis V, et al. Variability and action mechanism of a family of anticomplement proteins in *Ixodes ricinus. PLoS One.* (2008) 3:e1400. doi: 10.1371/journal.pone.0001400

Barratt-Due A, Thorgersen EB, Lindstad JK, Pharo A, Lissina O, Lambris JD, et al. *Ornithodoros moubata* complement inhibitor is an equally effective C5 Inhibitor in pigs and humans. *J Immunol.* (2011) 187:4913–9. doi: 10.4049/jimmunol.1101000

Nunn MA, Sharma A, Paesen GC, Adamson S, Lissina O, Willis AC, et al. Complement inhibitor of C5 activation from the soft tick *Ornithodoros moubata*. *J Immunol.* (2005) 174:2084–91. doi: 10.4049/jimmunol.174.4.2084

Mans BJ, Ribeiro JMC. Function, mechanism and evolution of the moubatin-clade of soft tick lipocalins. *Insect Biochem Mol Biol.* (2008) 38:841–52. doi: 10.1016/j.ibmb.2008.06.007

Hepburn NJ, Williams AS, Nunn MA, Chamberlain-Banoub JC, Hamer J, Morgan BP, et al. *In vivo* characterization and therapeutic efficacy of a C5-specific inhibitor from the soft tick *Ornithodoros moubata*. J Biol Chem. (2007) 282:8292–9. doi: 10.1074/jbc.M609858200

Kuhn N, Schmidt CQ, Schlapschy M, Skerra A. PASylated coversin, a C5-specific complement inhibitor with extended pharmacokinetics, shows enhanced anti-hemolytic activity *in vitro*. *Bioconjug Chem.* (2016) 27:2359–71. doi: 10.1021/acs.bioconjchem.6b00369

Barratt-Due A, Thorgersen EB, Egge K, Pischke S, Sokolov A, Hellerud BC, et al. Combined inhibition of complement (C5) and CD14 markedly attenuates inflammation, thrombogenicity, and hemodynamic changes in porcine sepsis. *J Immunol.* (2013) 191:819–27. doi: 10.4049/jimmunol.1201909

Jore MM, Johnson S, Sheppard D, Barber NM, Li YI, Nunn MA, et al. Structural basis for therapeutic inhibition of complement C5. *Nat Struct Mol Biol.* (2016) 23:378–86. doi: 10.1038/nsmb.3196

Reichhardt MP, Johnson S, Tang T, Morgan T, Tebeka N, Popitsch N, et al. An inhibitor of complement C5 provides structural insights into activation. *Proc Natl Acad Sci USA.* (2020) 117:362–70. doi: 10.1073/pnas.1909973116

Yuan X, Gavriilaki E, Thanassi JA, Yang G, Baines AC, Podos SD, et al. Small-molecule factor D inhibitors selectively block the alternative pathway of complement in paroxysmal nocturnal hemoglobinuria and atypical hemolytic uremic syndrome. *Haematologica.* (2017) 102:466–75. doi: 10.3324/haematol.2016.153312

Rother RP, Rollins SA, Mojcik CF, Brodsky RA, Bell L. Discovery and development of the complement inhibitor eculizumab for the treatment of paroxysmal nocturnal hemoglobinuria. *Nat Biotechnol.* (2007) 25:1256–64. doi: 10.1038/nbt1344

Schuijt TJ, Coumou J, Narasimhan S, Dai J, Deponte K, Wouters D, et al. A tick mannose-binding lectin inhibitor interferes with the vertebrate complement cascade to enhance transmission of the lyme disease agent. *Cell Host Microbe.* (2011) 10:136–46. doi: 10.1016/j.chom.2011.06.010

Dommett RM, Klein N, Turner MW. Mannose-binding lectin in innate immunity: past, present and future. *Tissue Antigens.* (2006) 68:193–209. doi: 10.1111/j.1399-0039.2006.00649.x

Wagemakers A, Coumou J, Schuijt TJ, Oei A, Nijhof AM, van 't Veer C, et al. An *Ixodes ricinus* tick salivary lectin pathway inhibitor protects borrelia burgdorferi sensu lato from human complement. *Vector Borne Zoonotic Dis.* (2016) 16:223–8. doi: 10.1089/vbz.2015.1901

Coumou J, Wagemakers A, Narasimhan S, Schuijt TJ, Ersoz JI, Oei A, et al. The role of mannose binding lectin in the immune response against *Borrelia burgdorferi sensu lato*. *Sci Rep.* (2019) 9:1431. doi: 10.1038/s41598-018-37922-8

Kaz′mierczak-Siedlecka K, Dvoˇrák A, Folwarski M, Daca A, Przewłócka K, Makarewicz W. Fungal gut microbiota dysbiosis and its role in colorectal, oral, and pancreatic carcinogenesis. *Cancers.* (2020) 12:1326. doi: 10.3390/cancers12051326

Sá-Nunes A, Bafica A, Lucas DA, Conrads TP, Veenstra TD, Andersen JF, et al. Prostaglandin E 2 is a major inhibitor of dendritic cell maturation and function in *Ixodes scapularis* Saliva. *J Immunol.* (2007) 179:1497–505. doi: 10.4049/jimmunol.179.3.1497

Esteves E, Bizzarro B, Costa FB, Ramírez-Hernández A, Peti APF, Cataneo AHD, et al. Amblyomma sculptum salivary PGE 2 modulates the dendritic cell *Rickettsia rickettsii* interactions *in vitro* and *in vivo*. *Front Immunol.* (2019) 10:118. doi: 10.3389/fimmu.2019.00118

Xu Z, Lin Z, Wei N, Di Q, Cao J, Zhou Y, et al. Immunomodulatory effects of *Rhipicephalus haemaphysaloides* serpin RHS2 on host immune responses. *Parasit Vectors.* (2019) 12:341. doi: 10.1186/s13071-019-3607-4

Preston SG, Majtán J, Kouremenou C, Rysnik O, Burger LF, Cabezas Cruz A, et al. Novel immunomodulators from hard ticks selectively reprogramme human dendritic cell responses. *PLoS Pathog.* (2013) 9:e1003450. doi: 10.1371/journal.ppat.1003450

Hannier S, Liversidge J, Sternberg JM, Bowman AS. *Ixodes ricinus* tick salivary gland extract inhibits IL-10 secretion and CD69 expression by mitogen-stimulated murine splenocytes and induces hyporesponsiveness in B lymphocytes. *Parasit Immunol.* (2003) 25:27–37. doi: 10.1046/j.1365-3024.2003.00605.x

Hannier S, Liversidge J, Sternberg JM, Bowman AS. Characterization of the B-cell inhibitory protein factor in *Ixodes ricinus* tick saliva: a potential role in enhanced *Borrelia burgdoferi* transmission. *Immunology.* (2004) 113:401–8. doi: 10.1111/j.1365-2567.2004.01975.x

Yu D, Liang J, Yu H, Wu H, Xu C, Liu J, et al. A tick B-cell inhibitory protein from salivary glands of the hard tick, *Hyalomma asiaticum asiaticum*. *Biochem Biophys Res Commun.* (2006) 343:585–90. doi: 10.1016/j.bbrc.2006. 02.188

Dk B, Mj P, Mj C, Jd R, Sk W. Isolation and molecular cloning of a secreted immunosuppressant protein from *Dermacentor andersoni* salivary gland. *J Parasitol.* (2000) 86:516–25.

Alarcon-Chaidez FJ, Müller-Doblies UU, Wikel S. Characterization of a recombinant immunomodulatory protein from the salivary glands of *Dermacentor andersoni*. *Parasit Immunol.* (2003) 25:69–77. doi: 10.1046/j.1365-3024.2003.00609.x

Konnai S, Nakajima C, Imamura S, Yamada S, Nishikado H, Kodama M, et al. Suppression of cell proliferation and cytokine expression by HL-p36, a tick salivary gland-derived protein of *Haemaphysalis longicornis*. *Immunology.* (2009) 126:209–19. doi: 10.1111/j.1365-2567.2008. 02890.x

Wang F, Lu X, Guo F, Gong H, Zhang H, Zhou Y, et al. The immunomodulatory protein RH36 is relating to blood-feeding success and oviposition in hard ticks. *Vet Parasitol.* (2017) 240:49–59. doi: 10.1016/j. vetpar.2017.03.017

Kotsyfakis M, Horka H, Salat J, Andersen JF. The crystal structures of two salivary cystatins from the tick *Ixodes scapularis* and the effect of these inhibitors on the establishment of *Borrelia burgdorferi* infection in a murine model. *Mol Microbiol.* (2010) 77:456–70. doi: 10.1111/j.1365-2958.2010.07220.x

Kotsyfakis M, Sá-Nunes A, Francischetti IMB, Mather TN, Andersen JF, Ribeiro JMC. Antiinflammatory and immunosuppressive activity of sialostatin L, a salivary cystatin from the tick *Ixodes scapularis*. *J Biol Chem.* (2006) 281:26298–307. doi: 10.1074/jbc.M513010200

Horka H, Staudt V, Klein M, Taube C, Reuter S, Dehzad N, et al. The tick salivary protein Sialostatin L Inhibits the Th9-derived production of the asthma-promoting cytokine il-9 and is effective in the prevention of experimental asthma. *J Immunol.* (2012) 188:2669–76. doi: 10.4049/jimmunol.1100529

Sá-Nunes A, Bafica A, Antonelli LR, Choi EY, Francischetti IMB, Andersen JF, et al. The immunomodulatory action of Sialostatin L on dendritic cells reveals its potential to interfere with autoimmunity. *J Immunol.* (2009) 182:7422–9. doi: 10.4049/jimmunol.0900075

Lieskovská J, Páleníková J, Širmarová J, Elsterová J, Kotsyfakis M, Campos Chagas A, et al. Tick salivary cystatin sialostatin L2 suppresses IFN responses in mouse dendritic cells. *Parasit Immunol.* (2015) 37:70–8. doi: 10.1111/pim. 12162

Chen G, Wang X, Severo MS, Sakhon OS, Sohail M, Brown LJ, et al. The tick salivary protein sialostatin L2 inhibits caspase-1-mediated inflammation during *Anaplasma phagocytophilum* infection. *Infect Immun.* (2014) 82:2553–64. doi: 10.1128/IAI.01679-14

Kotál J, Stergiou N, Buša M, Chlastáková A, Beránková Z, Rˇ ezácˇová P, et al. The structure and function of Iristatin, a novel immunosuppressive tick salivary cystatin. *Cell Mol Life Sci.* (2019) 76:2003–13. doi: 10.1007/s00018-019-03034-3

Leboulle G, Crippa M, Decrem Y, Mejri N, Brossard M, Bollen A, et al. Characterization of a novel salivary immunosuppressive protein from *Ixodes ricinus* ticks. *J Biol Chem.* (2002) 277:10083–9. doi: 10.1074/jbc.M11139 1200

Toyomane K, Konnai S, Niwa A, Githaka N, Isezaki M, Yamada S, et al. Identification and the preliminary *in vitro* characterization of IRIS homologue from salivary glands of *Ixodes persulcatus* schulze. *Ticks Tick Borne Dis.* (2016) 7:119–25. doi: 10.1016/j.ttbdis.2015. 09.006

Prevot PP, Beschin A, Lins L, Beaufays J, Grosjean A, Bruys L, et al. Exosites mediate the anti-inflammatory effects of a multifunctional serpin from the saliva of the tick *Ixodes ricinus*. *FEBS J*. (2009) 276:3235–46. doi: 10.1111/j. 1742-4658.2009.07038.x

Blisnick AA, Šimo L, Grillon C, Fasani F, Brûlé S, Le Bonniec B, et al. The immunomodulatory effect of IrSPI, a tick salivary gland serine protease inhibitor involved in *Ixodes ricinus* tick feeding. *Vaccines*. (2019) 7:148. doi: 10.3390/vaccines7040148

Garg R, Juncadella IJ, Ramamoorthi N, Ashish, Ananthanarayanan SK, Thomas V, et al. Cutting edge: CD4 is the receptor for the tick saliva immunosuppressor, Salp15. *J Immunol*. (2006) 177:6579–83. doi: 10.4049/ jimmunol.177.10.6579

Marchal C, Schramm F, Kern A, Luft BJ, Yang X, Schuijt TJ, et al. Antialarmin effect of tick saliva during the transmission of Lyme disease. *Infect Immun*. (2011) 79:774–85. doi: 10.1128/IAI.00482-10

Paveglio SA, Allard J, Mayette J, Whittaker LA, Juncadella I, Anguita J, et al. The tick salivary protein, Salp15, inhibits the development of experimental asthma. *J Immunol*. (2007) 178:7064–71. doi: 10.4049/jimmunol.178.11. 7064

Juncadella IJ, Garg R, Bates TC, Olivera ER, Anguita J. The *Ixodes scapularis* salivary protein, salp15, prevents the association of HIV-1 gp120 and CD4. *Biochem Biophys Res Commun*. (2008) 367:41–6. doi: 10.1016/j. bbrc.2007.12. 104

Liu Q, Acharya P, Dolan MA, Zhang P, Guzzo C, Lu J, et al. Quaternary contact in the initial interaction of CD4 with the HIV-1 envelope trimer. *Nat Struct Mol Biol*. (2017) 24:370–8. doi: 10.1038/nsmb.3382

Juncadella IJ, Bates TC, Suleiman R, Monteagudo-Mera A, Olson CM, Navasa N, et al. The tick saliva immunosuppressor, Salp15, contributes to Th17-induced pathology during experimental autoimmune encephalomyelitis. *Biochem Biophys Res Commun*. (2010) 402:105–9. doi: 10.1016/j.bbrc.2010. 09.125

Robinson AP, Harp CT, Noronha A, Miller SD. The experimental autoimmune encephalomyelitis (EAE) model of MS. utility for understanding disease pathophysiology and treatment. *Handb Clin Neurol*. (2014) 122:173–89. doi: 10.1016/B978-0-444-52001-2.00008-X

Tomás-Cortázar J, Martín-Ruiz I, Barriales D, Pascual-Itoiz MÁ, de Juan VG, Caro-Maldonado A, et al. The immunosuppressive effect of the tick protein, Salp15, is long-lasting and persists in a murine model of hematopoietic transplant. *Sci Rep*. (2017) 7:10740. doi: 10.1038/s41598-017-11354-2

Chmelaˇr J, Kotál J, Karim S, Kopacek P, Francischetti IMB, Pedra JHF, et al. Sialomes and mialomes: a systems-biology view of tick tissues and tick-host interactions. *Trends Parasitol*. (2016) 32:242–54. doi: 10.1016/j.pt.2015.10. 002

Lefebvre FA, Lécuyer E. Small luggage for a long journey: transfer of vesicle-enclosed small RNA in interspecies communication. *Front Microbiol*. (2017) 8:377. doi: 10.3389/fmicb.2017.00377

Knip M, Constantin ME, Thordal-Christensen H. Trans-kingdom cross-talk: small RNAs on the move. *PLoS Genet*. (2014) 10:e1004602. doi: 10.1371/ journal.pgen.1004602

Weiberg A, Bellinger M, Jin H. Conversations between kingdoms: small RNAs. *Curr Opin Biotechnol*. (2015) 32:207–15. doi: 10.1016/j.copbio.2014. 12.025

Barrero RA, Keeble-Gagnère G, Zhang B, Moolhuijzen P, Ikeo K, Tateno Y, et al. Evolutionary conserved microRNAs are ubiquitously expressed compared to tick-specific miRNAs in the cattle tick *Rhipicephalus* (Boophilus) microplus. *BMC Genomics*. (2011) 12:328. doi: 10.1186/1471-2164-12-328

Bensaoud C, Hackenberg M, Kotsyfakis M. Noncoding RNAs in parasite–vector–host interactions. *Trends Parasitol*. (2019) 35:715–24. doi: 10.1016/j. pt.2019.06.012

Chávez ASO, O'Neal AJ, Santambrogio L, Kotsyfakis M, Pedra JHF. Message in a vesicle – trans-kingdom intercommunication at the vector-host interface. *J Cell Sci*. (2019) 132:jcs224212. doi: 10.1242/jcs.224212

Hackenberg M, Kotsyfakis M. Exosome-mediated pathogen transmission by arthropod vectors. *Trends Parasitol*. (2018) 34:549–52. doi: 10.1016/j. pt.2018. 04.001

Yao R-W, Wang Y, Chen L-L. Cellular functions of long noncoding RNAs. *Nat Cell Biol*. (2019) 21:542–51. doi: 10.1038/s41556-019-0311-8

Quinn JJ, Chang HY. Unique features of long non-coding RNA biogenesis and function. *Nat Rev Genet*. (2016) 17:47–62. doi: 10.1038/nrg.2015.10

Gomes AQ, Nolasco S, Soares H. Non-coding RNAs: multi-tasking molecules in the cell. *Int J Mol Sci*. (2013) 14:16010–39. doi: 10.3390/ijms140816010

Hackenberg M, Langenberger D, Schwarz A, Erhart J, Kotsyfakis M. *In silico* target network analysis of de novo-discovered, tick saliva-specific microRNAs reveals important combinatorial effects in their interference with vertebrate host physiology. *RNA*. (2017) 23:1259–69. doi: 10.1261/rna. 061168.117

Christopher AF, Kaur RP, Kaur G, Kaur A, Gupta V, Bansal P. MicroRNA therapeutics: discovering novel targets and developing specific therapy. *Perspect Clin Res*. (2016) 7:68–74. doi: 10.4103/2229-3485.179431

2

Deciphering Biological Processes at the Tick-Host Interface Opens New Strategies for Treatment of Human Diseases

Iveta Štibrániová[1], Pavlína Bartíková[1], Viera Holíková[1] and Mária Kazimírová[2]*

[1] *Biomedical Research Center, Institute of Virology, Slovak Academy of Sciences, Bratislava, Slovakia,* [2] *Institute of Zoology, Slovak Academy of Sciences, Bratislava, Slovakia*

Correspondence:
Pavlína Bartíková
virupaca@savba.sk

Ticks are obligatory blood-feeding ectoparasites, causing blood loss and skin damage in their hosts. In addition, ticks also transmit a number of various pathogenic microorganisms that cause serious diseases in humans and animals. Ticks evolved a wide array of salivary bioactive compounds that, upon injection into the host skin, inhibit or modulate host reactions such as hemostasis, inflammation and wound healing. Modulation of the tick attachment site in the host skin involves mainly molecules which affect physiological processes orchestrated by cytokines, chemokines and growth factors. Suppressing host defense reactions is crucial for tick survival and reproduction. Furthermore, pharmacologically active compounds in tick saliva have a promising therapeutic potential for treatment of some human diseases connected with disorders in hemostasis and immune system. These disorders are often associated to alterations in signaling pathways and dysregulation or overexpression of specific cytokines which, in turn, affect mechanisms of angiogenesis, cell motility and cytoskeletal regulation. Moreover, tick salivary molecules were found to exert cytotoxic and cytolytic effects on various tumor cells and have anti-angiogenic properties. Elucidation of the mode of action of tick bioactive molecules on the regulation of cell processes in their mammalian hosts could provide new tools for understanding the complex changes leading to immune disorders and cancer. Tick bioactive molecules may also be exploited as new pharmacological inhibitors of the signaling pathways of cytokines and thus help alleviate patient discomfort and increase patient survival. We review the current knowledge about tick salivary peptides and proteins that have been identified and functionally characterized in *in vitro* and/or *in vivo* models and their therapeutic perspective.

Keywords: tick saliva, immunomodulation, host defense, pharmacological molecules, immunological disorders

INTRODUCTION

For centuries, humans have exploited arthropods (insects, scorpions, spiders, centipedes, ticks) and other invertebrates (leeches, hookworms, snails, etc.) and their products (honey, royal jelly, venom, propolis, etc.) or biologically active substances derived from them as valuable resources to treat various diseases (Cherniack, 2010, 2011; Chen et al., 2018; Koh et al., 2018). Their properties range from immunomodulatory, analgesic, anti-bacterial, anti-coagulant, anticancer, diuretic and anesthetic to anti-rheumatic. Many human cultures, especially in Asia, Africa and South America, have used arthropods in traditional medicine and highly appreciated their therapeutic potential. In some cases, whole organisms, in others individual ingredients have been used. The capabilities of maggots (larvae of blowflies) feeding on necrotic tissues to heal wounds are among well-studied medical application of insects (maggot therapy) (Wolf and Hansson, 2003). Of other invertebrates, medicinal leeches have been applied, e.g., in reconstructive microsurgery, and in treatment of phlebitis (Eldor et al., 1996) or osteoarthritis (Michalsen et al., 2002). Anticoagulants designed based on their product, hirudin and its derivatives, have been used as antithrombotics (Markwardt, 2002; Chudzinski-Tavassi et al., 2018; Koh et al., 2018). Endoparasitic helminths have been used to cure inflammatory bowel diseases (Buning et al., 2008), and cantharidin, a derivate from blister beetles, has been applied for warts, molluscum contagiosum (Moed et al., 2001) and in anticancer therapy (Efferth et al., 2005; Liu and Chen, 2009). The enormous richness and diversity of arthropods, the wide range of biological activities exerted by their products, the use of some species and their products or derivatives as drugs against common and important diseases suggest that arthropods are a rich, and yet unexplored and unexploited source of potentially useful compounds for development of new therapeutic agents for modern medicine (Pemberton, 1999).

Among blood-feeding arthropods, ticks occupy a unique position. Their parasitic lifestyle resulted in development of a wide spectrum of evasive and disarming mechanisms of host defense reactions. Tick salivary glands produce and secrete into the feeding site in the host skin an impressive amount and variety of bioactive molecules modulating hemostatic, inflammatory and immune responses as well as wound healing. The composition of tick saliva is highly complex and changes through the feeding process. There are a few comprehensive and recent reviews on the composition and role of saliva in tick feeding and tick-host-pathogen interactions (Francischetti et al., 2009; Kotal et al., 2015; Blisnick et al., 2017; Šimo et al., 2017; Nuttall, 2018; Wikel, 2018). They all highlight the fact that only an integrated understanding of the physiological roles of tick bioactive molecules and their mode of action can elucidate complex changes in the mammalian hosts, leading to immune disorders and cancer, and disclose therapeutically valuable molecules. This review is focused on identified tick salivary peptides and proteins with known structure and function(s) which are promising candidates for development of drugs and their recombinant forms have been tested in disease models *in vitro* and/or *in vivo*. Non-peptide molecules (e.g., nucleosides, lipids) contained in tick saliva are beyond the scope of this paper.

TICKS AND PHARMACOLOGICAL PROPERTIES OF THEIR SALIVA

Ticks are blood feeders and bioactive compounds in their saliva have a promising therapeutic potential for treatment of some human diseases associated with hemostatic and immunological disorders (Mans, 2005; Hovius et al., 2008; Francischetti, 2010; Štibrániová et al., 2013; Sousa et al., 2015; Bonvin et al., 2016; Chudzinski-Tavassi et al., 2016, 2018; Chmelar et al., 2017; Murfin and Fikrig, 2017; Parizi et al., 2018). Tick salivary glands, a paired organ consisting of acini in grape-like clusters, produce saliva secreted by the feeding tick into the host primarily to enable blood feeding by suppressing local hemostatic and host immune responses (Francischetti et al., 2009; Kazimírová and Štibrániová, 2013; Wikel, 2013; Kotal et al., 2015; Šimo et al., 2017; Nuttall, 2018). Tick feeding, in addition, enables host infection with pathogenic microorganisms carried by ticks. Cutting-edge high-throughput technologies used during the last decade for studying composition and function of tick saliva have revealed its complexity (Ribeiro et al., 2006; Francischetti et al., 2011; Radulovič et al., 2014; Kotsyfakis et al., 2015; Tan et al., 2015; Xu et al., 2015; de Castro et al., 2016; Mans, 2016; Bonnet et al., 2018); not surprisingly, considering the tick's biology and their parasitic lifestyle, i.e., strict hematophagy, short-term (soft ticks) to long-lasting feeding (hard ticks) on the vertebrate host, and broad spectrum of hosts. The composition of tick saliva is complex and changes with biological factors such as gender, developmental stage, feeding stage and/or the presence/absence of microorganisms, pathogenic as well non-pathogenic (Liu et al., 2014; Ayllón et al., 2015; Kotsyfakis et al., 2015; Yu et al., 2015; Bonnet et al., 2017, 2018).

Tick saliva is a mixture of proteins, peptides and non-peptide molecules that interfere with various components of hemostasis, wound healing, and both arms of the immune system of the vertebrate hosts, including enzymes, cytokines, complement, antibodies, cell signaling components, immune cells (Francischetti et al., 2009; Mans, 2016; Nuttall, 2018; Wikel, 2018). In addition, cytotoxic and cytolitic activities acting against different cell types, impairment of cancer cells migration and signaling pathways, as well as anti-angiogenic properties have been demonstrated for saliva of different hard tick species (Kazimirova et al., 2006; Poole et al., 2013; Holíková et al., 2018; Sousa et al., 2018; de Sá Jr. et al., 2019; Gradowski do Nascimento et al., 2019), showing that tick saliva is an important source for designing new anticancer drugs (Kazimírová, 2011; Sousa et al., 2015; Chudzinski-Tavassi et al., 2016). Proteinaceous components of the tick saliva are grouped into families like lipocalins, proteins with Kunitz type domain, metalloproteases, serpins, cystatins, basic-tail secreted proteins, small peptide inhibitors, some protein families unique to ticks, and proteins and peptides of unknown structure and function (Ribeiro et al., 2006; Francischetti et al., 2009; Chmelar et al., 2012). Interestingly, a high redundancy and multifunctionality of the tick salivary compounds has been revealed, whereby many of them can target multiple components of hemostasis and, in addition, also components of the immune system (Francischetti et al., 2009; Chmelar et al., 2016; Šimo et al., 2017).

PROTEASE INHIBITORS

Transcriptome and proteome studies of tick salivary glands (SGs) discovered an enormous protein diversity and unique proteins belonging to novel protein families with unknown functions (Francischetti et al., 2011; Radulovič et al., 2014;

Kotsyfakis et al., 2015; Mans, 2016; Esteves et al., 2017). Many of these proteins are differentially expressed during the feeding process (Mans et al., 2008; Kotsyfakis et al., 2015).

Enzyme activity inhibitors represent a very abundant group and include, among others, protease inhibitors containing the Kunitz domain, serine protease inhibitors (serpins), cysteine proteinase inhibitors (cystatins), peptides of the hirudin-like/madanin/variegin superfamily, and basic tail proteins (de Miranda Santos et al., 2004; Francischetti et al., 2005, 2009; Ribeiro et al., 2006; Garcia et al., 2014; Liu and Bonnet, 2014; Parizi et al., 2018).

Kunitz Domain Containing Proteins

Members of the Kunitz domain family, the one of the larger protein families expressed in tick salivary glands, have been functionally characterized primarily as anti-hemostatic agents that block or inhibit host blood coagulation and/or platelet aggregation (Corral-Rodriguez et al., 2009; Chmelar et al., 2012; Parizi et al., 2018), but some of them have been found to display multiple functions, e.g., ixolaris (de Oliveira et al., 2012) or Amblyomin X (Chudzinski-Tavassi et al., 2010).

Hemostasis is the first line of defense against the tick bite and the first stage of wound healing. It comprises a series of physiological processes that stop bleeding at the site of vascular injury by formation of a hemostatic plug. Three major mechanisms are involved in hemostasis: (i) vasoconstriction – termination of bleeding from damaged blood vessels, (ii) coagulation – production of a fibrin clot, (iii) formation of a platelet plug. The enzymes in the coagulation cascade are activated through different pathways, depending on various endogenous and exogenous factors (Hoffman et al., 2009). Ticks have evolved various and effective countermeasures against the different mechanisms of the vertebrate hemostatic system and can target single or multiple host coagulation factors (Maritz-Olivier et al., 2007; Francischetti et al., 2009; Kazimírová et al., 2010; Chmelar et al., 2012; Šimo et al., 2017). Thrombin is the main target for majority of the identified tick anticoagulants (**Table 1**) and inhibition of thrombin generation is one of the main strategies to prevent thrombosis (Kazimírová et al., 2010; Chmelar et al., 2012). However, drugs that target other coagulation factors, e.g., factor Xa (FXa) would be an alternative treatment when thrombin generation has already occurred (Yeh et al., 2012). In spite of the wide range of different identified inhibitors derived from tick salivary glands, due to strict criteria for clinical use, only a limited number passed pre-clinical and clinical tests. For example, only preliminary validations of the tick anticoagulant peptide (TAP) has been performed *in vivo* using animal models, but TAP has never been tested in humans due to a slow onset of action and because its antigenicity, and a single study performed for ixolaris in a rat model awaits future validation (Maritz-Olivier et al., 2007). However, as tick anticoagulants bind specifically to their target molecules, they are important molecular tools to study and increase our understanding of the mechanisms of host blood coagulation. Examples include the mapping of thrombin exosites by ornithodorin derived from *Ornithodoros moubata* (van der Locht et al., 1996), understanding the prothrombinase complex formation by using ixolaris from *I. scapularis* (Monteiro et al., 2005), or characterization of the molecular mechanisms that maintain the procofactor state of circulating FV and the conversion of FV to active cofactor FVa by means of recombinant TIXC-5 from *I. scapularis* (Aleman and Wolberg, 2013; Schuijt et al., 2013). In addition, information on the structure and function of tick-derived anticoagulants can be used in designing synthetic peptides as a basis for development of novel drugs (Maritz-Olivier et al., 2007; Koh et al., 2018).

The **tick anticoagulant peptide TAP** is the first Kunitz-domain protease inhibitor identified in tick saliva that was functionally characterized and prepared in recombinant form. It was originally isolated from the soft tick *O. moubata* (Waxman et al., 1990). TAP is a single Kunitz domain direct slow, tight-binding competitive inhibitor of FXa, with a unique binding mode and high affinity to FXa (Wei et al., 1998). Recombinant forms of TAP (rTAP) have been tested in a variety of animal models of venous and arterial thrombosis showing that the molecule was more effective than heparin and was at least as effective as hirudin, but produced less bleeding (Yeh et al., 2012). For example, in an *in vivo* study, following an infusion into rhesus monkeys rTAP inhibited generation of fibrinopeptide A induced by thromboplastin (Neeper et al., 1990). In another study, the antithrombotic effect of rTAP was tested and compared with heparin in a baboon model of arterial thrombosis. The results also demonstrated the antithrombotic effect of rTAP without alterations of primary hemostasis (Schaffer et al., 1991). In a mouse carotid artery thrombosis model, TAP-antibody targeting activated platelets fusion protein was more effective than enoxaparin without prolonged bleeding time in comparison to conventional anticoagulants (Stoll et al., 2007). These results initiated speculations that drugs targeting FXa could be safer than thrombin inhibitors, although TAP has not been tested in humans (Yeh et al., 2012). In addition, direct FXa inhibitors, including TAP, could potentially be used in prevention of other diseases, such as atherosclerosis or atrial fibrillation, because FXa as well as thrombin are involved in mediation of protease-activated receptor signaling and modulation of cellular mechanisms in the abovementioned pathophysiological processes (Spronk et al., 2014).

Ornithodorin from *O. moubata* was the first thrombin inhibitor identified in a soft tick. It has two domains of the Kunitz basic pancreatic trypsin inhibitor (BPTI) family. The N-terminal domain binds to the active site of thrombin, the C-terminal domain binds at the fibrinogen recognition exosite. Ornithodorin is a slow, tight-binding, competitive inhibitor of thrombin (van der Locht et al., 1996).

Another tick Kunitz domain protease inhibitor with promising antithrombotic and anti-tumor therapeutic usage, **Ixolaris,** a two-Kunitz domain inhibitor that displays homology to the tissue factor (TF) pathway inhibitor (TFPI), was obtained by screening the cDNA library derived from salivary glands of *Ixodes scapularis* (Francischetti et al., 2002, 2004). Ixolaris inhibits factor VIIa (FVIIa)/TF–induced factor (FX) activation by binding to the FXa exosite (Francischetti et al., 2002) and also binds plasmatic FX, decreases heparin-catalyzed inhibition by antithrombin III, and impairs binding of FXa to plasmatic

TABLE 1 | Examples of tick salivary molecules of therapeutic interest in human diseases.

Molecule	Main function: Target(s) Proposed drug	Tick species	References
Protease inhibitors			
Serine protease inhibitors - Kunitz domain containing proteins			
TAP	Anticoagulant: FXa Antithrombotic	*Ornithodoros moubata*	Waxman et al., 1990; Corral-Rodriguez et al., 2009
Ornithodorin	Anticoagulant: thrombin Antithrombotic	*O. moubata*	van der Locht et al., 1996
Ixolaris	Anticoagulant: inhibitor of contact system proteins (VIIa/tissue factor-induced FX, FXa) Antithrombotic, antitumor (glioblastoma, melanoma)	*Ixodes scapularis*	Francischetti et al., 2002; Nazareth et al., 2006; Carneiro-Lobo et al., 2009; de Oliveira et al., 2012
Amblyomin-X	Anticoagulant: FXa, FVIIa/TF complex activity, prothombin conversion Antitumor, anti-angiogenetic	Amblyomma sculptum (formerly *A. cajennense*)	Batista et al., 2010; Drewes et al., 2012, 2015; Maria et al., 2013; Pacheco et al., 2014; Branco et al., 2016; Chudzinski-Tavassi et al., 2016
BmTI-A	Anticoagulant: inhibitor of contact system proteins, inhibits plasmin, elastase, and plasma kallikrein Inhibitor of wound healing and vessel formation Anti-angiogenetic	*Rhipicephalus. (Boophilus) microplus*	Tanaka et al., 1999; Soares et al., 2016
Ir-CPI	Anticoagulant: inhibitor of contact system proteins, blocks FXII, FXI, and kallikrein activation Antithrombotic	*Ixodes ricinus*	Decrem et al., 2009
TdPI	Immunomodulation: innate immune responses, inflammation, inhibitor of human skin β-tryptase Anti-inflammatory	*Rhipicephalus appendiculatus*	Paesen et al., 2007
Tryptogalinin	Immunomodulation: innate immune responses, inhibitor of human skin β-tryptase Anti-inflammatory	*I. scapularis*	Valdés et al., 2013
Haemangin	Wound healing, angiogenesis: inhibits angiogenesis and neovascularization Anti-angiogenetic	*Haemaphysalis longicornis*	Islam et al., 2009
Disagregin	Antiplatelet agent: inhibitor of glycoprotein IIb/IIIa (integrin αIIbβ3) Antithrombotic	*O. moubata*	Karczewski et al., 1994
Serine protease inhibitors – Serpin domain family			
Iris	Anticoagulant: thrombin, FXa Immunosuppression: pro-inflammatory cytokines Drug acting in regulation of TNF-alpha overexpression	*I. ricinus*	Leboulle et al., 2002; Prevot et al., 2009
IRS-2	Immunomodulation: innate immune responses – T cells, T17 cells, cathepsin G, chymase Treatment of autoimmune diseases	*I. ricinus*	Chmelar et al., 2011; Palenikova et al., 2015
Cystatins (cysteine protease inhibitors)			
Sialostatin L	Immunomodulation: acquired immune responses – cathepsin L and V, papain, dendritic cells maturation Immunosuppressive drug for asthma attack	*I. scapularis*	Kotsyfakis et al., 2006; Sa-Nunes et al., 2009; Horka et al., 2012; Klein et al., 2015; Lieskovská et al., 2015b
Sialostatin L2	Immunomodulation: acquired immune responses - cathepsin L, V and S, papain, interferon Anti-inflammatory	*I. scapularis*	Kotsyfakis et al., 2007; Chen et al., 2014; Lieskovská et al., 2015a,b
Iristatin	Immunomodulation: innate immune responses Immunotherapeutic	*I. ricinus*	Kotál et al., 2019
DsCystatin	Immunomodulation: cathepsin L and B, pro-inflammatory cytokines, TLR signaling pathway Anti-inflammatory	*Dermacentor silvarum*	Sun et al., 2018

(Continued)

TABLE 1 | Continued

Molecule	Main function: Target(s) Proposed drug	Tick species	References
Hirudin-like/Madanin/Variegin superfamily			
Variegin	Anticoagulant: thrombin Antithrombotic	*Amblyomma variegatum*	Koh et al., 2007, 2011; Kazimírová et al., 2015
Avathrin	Anticoagulant: thrombin Antithrombotic, coating of medical devices	*A. variegatum*	Iyer et al., 2017, 2019|
Sculptin	Anticoagulant: thrombin Antithrombotic	*A. sculptum*	Iqbal et al., 2017
Madanin-1, 2, chimadanin	Anticoagulant: thrombin Antithrombotic	*H. longicornis*	Iwanaga et al., 2003; Thompson et al., 2017
Hyalomin 1	Anticoagulant: thrombin Antithrombotic	*Hyalomma marginatum*	Jablonka et al., 2015
Basic tail-secreted proteins			
Salp14	Anticoagulant: FXa Antithrombotic	*I. scapularis*	Narasimhan et al., 2002
Ixonnexin	Modulator of haemostasis: promotes fibrinolysis Antithrombotic	*I. scapularis*	Assumpção et al., 2018
Lipocalins			
OmCI	Complement: inhibitor of C5 activation Coversin: second-generation complement inhibitor; acute and chronic inflammation	*O. moubata*	Nunn et al., 2005; Roversi et al., 2007; Barratt-Due et al., 2011
Moubatin and other lipocalins of the moubatin clade from soft ticks	Antiplatelet agent: inhibition of platelet aggregation, binds to thromboxane A2 Antithrombotic	*O. moubata*	Waxman and Connolly, 1993; Mans and Ribeiro, 2008; Francischetti, 2010
Ra-HBPs	Innate immune responses: histamine-binding Anti-inflammatory	*R. appendiculatus*	Paesen et al., 1999; Mans, 2005
SHBP	Innate immune responses: histamine and serotonine-binding Anti-inflammatory	*D. reticulatus*	Sangamnatdej et al., 2002
Japanin	Immunomodulation: monocyte-derived dendritic cells, reprogrammes dendritic cell responses Immunotherapeutic (autoimmune disorders, allergies, transplant rejection, acute and chronic inflammatory diseases)	*R. appendiculatus*	Preston et al., 2013; Roversi et al., 2017
HA24	Innate immune responses: histamine-binding Anti-inflammatory	*Hyalomma asiaticum*	Wang et al., 2016
Ixodegrin superfamily			
Variabilin	Antiplatelet agent: inhibitor of glycoprotein IIb/IIIa (integrin αIIbβ3) Antithrombotic	*Dermacentor variabilis*	Wang et al., 1996
YY-39	Antiplatelet agent: blocks platelet adhesion to soluble collagen and bind to glycoprotein IIb/IIIa Antithrombotic	*Ixodes pacificus*	Tang et al., 2015
Metastriate-specific families			
Evasins	Innate immune responses: chemokine binding Anti-inflammatory (myocarditis, arthritis), anti-fibrotic	*Rhipicephalus sanguineus* and other hard ticks	Hajnicka et al., 2005; Frauenschuh et al., 2007; Deruaz et al., 2008; Hayward et al., 2017; Singh et al., 2017; Eaton et al., 2018
Small immunoregulatory peptides			
Hyalomin-A and -B	Innate immune responses: pro-inflammatory cytokine inhibitor Anti-inflammatory	*H. asiaticum asiaticum*	Wu et al., 2010
Amregulin	Innate immune responses: pro-inflammatory cytokine inhibitor Anti-inflammatory	*A. variegatum*	Tian et al., 2016
~8 kDa tick-derived C5 inhibitors			
RaCI	Complement: inhibitor of C5 activation Anti-inflammatory	*R. appendiculatus*	Matthijs et al., 2016

(Continued)

TABLE 1 | Continued

Molecule	Main function: Target(s) Proposed drug	Tick species	References
Prostriate-specific families			
Isac protein family			
Isac	Complement: inhibition of the alternative complement pathway (AP) by destabilizing the C3 convertase Anti-inflammatory	*I. scapularis*	Valenzuela et al., 2000
Salp 20	Complement: inhibits the AP by binding properdin and dissociating active C3 convertase Anti-inflammatory	*I. scapularis*	Tyson et al., 2007; Hourcade et al., 2016
Irac I, II	Complement: inhibition of AP by destabilizing the C3 convertase Anti-inflammatory	*I. ricinus*	Daix et al., 2007
IxACs	Complement: inhibits the AP by binding properdin Anti-inflammatory	*I. ricinus*	Couvreur et al., 2008
Family of 15 kDa salivary proteins			
Salp15	Immunosuppression: multifunctional, $CD4^+$ T cells, dendritic cells Immunosuppressive therapy in transplantation	*I. scapularis*	Anguita et al., 2002; Hovius et al., 2008; Tomás-Cortázar et al., 2017
Putative secreted salivary gland proteins			
TIX-5 (formerly P23)	Anticoagulatio: inhibitor of FXa-mediated FV activation	*I. scapularis*	Schuijt et al., 2011, 2013
EF-hand calcium-binding proteins			
Longistatin	Anticoagulant: plasminogen activator, degrades fibrin clots, antagonist to RAGE and suppresses inflammation during severe tissue injury Antithrombotic RAGE-regulated diseases, e.g.; Alzheimer's disease, psoriasis, diabetic complications and tumorigenesis	*H. longicornis*	Anisuzzaman et al. (2010, 2011, 2014, 2015)
Glycine-rich, or proline-rich, collagen-like superfamily	Glycine-rich cement proteins – cement cone, prevent loss of fluids and secures tick mouthparts in the skin New medical adhesives	Various species of hard ticks	Suppan et al., 2018

TAP, tick anticoagulant peptide; BmTI-A, Boophilus microplus trypsin inhibitor A; Ir-CPI, coagulation contact phase inhibitor from Ixodes ricinus; TdPI, tick-derived peptidase inhibitor; Iris, I. ricinus immunosuppressor; IRS-2, I. ricinus serpin 2; DsCystatin, Dermacentor silvarum cystatin; Ra-HBPs, Rhipicephalus appendiculatus histamine-binding proteins; SHBP, Dermacentor reticulatus serotonin-histamine binding protein; OmCI, Ornithodoros moubata complement inhibitor; HA, Hyalomma asiaticum; RaCI, R. appendiculatus complement inhibitor; Isac, Ixodes scapularis anticomplement; Irac, I. ricinus anticomplement; Salp, salivary protein; IxACs, Ixodes anticomplement proteins; YY-39, ixodegrin from I. pacificus; TIX-5, tick inhibitor of factor Xa toward factor V.

or immobilized heparin (Monteiro et al., 2005). By using a rat model, application of ixolaris resulted in effective antithrombotic activity, without hemorrhage and bleeding (Nazareth et al., 2006). Several evidences showed close correlation between thrombosis and cancer (Timp et al., 2013). Ixolaris was shown to block TF-dependent procoagulant activity in human melanoma cell lines and inhibit their metastatic potential as well as tumor angiogenesis in mice, without evidence of bleeding (de Oliveira et al., 2012). Ixolaris was also associated with reduced tumor vascularization and expression of vascular endothelial growth factor (VEGF) in a human glioblastoma model (Carneiro-Lobo et al., 2009, 2012). All this makes ixolaris a promising agent for anticancer therapy. In a recent study, the therapeutic potential of Ixolaris in chronic infections with immunodeficiency virus (HIV) has been demonstrated (Schechter et al., 2017). Despite effective anti-HIV infection therapy, persistent inflammation involving activated monocytes and their product (e.g., soluble TF) can result in cardiovascular and thromboembolic diseases (Funderburg and Lederman, 2014). In a non-human primate model, pigtail macaques chronically infected with Simian immunodeficiency virus (SIV) exhibited high numbers of monocytes expressing TF and producing proinflammatory cytokines such as tumor necrosis factor (TNF)-α, interleukin (IL)-1β and IL-6, simultaneously leading to coagulopathy and inflammation. *In vitro,* low doses of Ixolaris inhibited TF activity (formation of FXa) in peripheral blood mononuclear cells (PBMCs) derived from chronically SIV-infected macaques and in unstimulated and LPS-stimulated PBMCs originating from anti-HIV therapy naïve and treated HIV^+ suppressed humans, but without effect on TF expression or cytokine production (Schechter et al., 2017). *In vivo,* administration of Ixolaris to pigtails macaques showed reduced levels of IL-17 and decreased expression of Glut-1, CD80 and CD86 (i.e., markers associated with activation of lymphocytes), and resulted in lower concentration of $CD4^+$ and $CD8^+$ T cells (HLA-DR^+, $CD38^+$) and reduced expression of TF by $CD14^+$ monocytes. In addition, Ixolaris-treated animals showed reduced plasma D-dimer levels, indicating cardiovascular comorbidities, lower

SIV viremia and no developing disease up to 100 days after infection. This study has suggested a great potential of Ixolaris in anticoagulant therapy of HIV+ humans and in treatment of other inflammatory diseases (Schechter et al., 2017).

Amblyomin-X is a non-competitive inhibitor of FXa identified in salivary glands of *Amblyomma cajennense* (currently *A. sculptum*) ticks (Batista et al., 2010). It contains a single Kunitz domain and is able to inhibit FXa, prothrombinase and tenase activities (Morais et al., 2014; Branco et al., 2016). In an *in vitro* murine melanoma model, Amblyomin-X decreased tumor mass and reduced metastasis as well as induced apoptosis (Chudzinski-Tavassi et al., 2010; Ventura et al., 2013). It also displays cytotoxic activity on several human tumor cells, among them SK-Mel-28 (human melanoma) or Mia-PaCa-2 (human pancreatic adeno-carcinoma) cell lines, but not on non-tumor cells (Simons et al., 2011), and promotes apoptosis probably by targeting the ubiquitin-proteasome system (Chudzinski-Tavassi et al., 2010). In addition, Amblyomin-X induces apoptosis in murine renal adenocarcinoma (RENCA) cells, mitochondrial damage and the production of reactive oxygen species (ROS) (Akagi et al., 2012; Maria et al., 2013). Amblyomin-X impairs cell migration and causes actin cytoskeleton disruption in human tumor cells (Schmidt et al., 2018). In addition, tumor regression and the reduction of lung metastasis after administration of recombinant Amblyomin-X have been observed in animal models (de Souza et al., 2016). Apart its effects on tumor growth, Amblyomin-X displays antiangiogenic properties and inhibits vascular endothelial growth factor A (VEGF-A)-induced angiogenesis in both the dorsal subcutaneous tissue of mice and the chicken chorioallantoic membrane by modulation of endothelial cell proliferation and adhesion, especially of membrane expression of platelet-endothelial cell adhesion molecule-1 (PECAM-1) (Drewes et al., 2012, 2015), suggesting the possible application of Amblyomin-X as a local inhibitor to undesired neovascularization. Recently, the protein is being developed as anti-tumor drug and is under preclinical evaluations, undergoing pharmacokinetic and toxicity investigations in animals (Boufleur et al., 2019; Maria et al., 2019). These studies revealed that Amblyomin-X did not cause any mortality in mice, toxicity signs were observed only at higher doses, and there was no accumulation of Amblyomin-X in any organ.

Rhipicephalus (Boophilus) microplus possess a trypsin inhibitor A, **BmTI-A**, a two Kunitz domain inhibitor involved in counteracting host hemostasis. BmTI-A blocks neutrophil elastase, plasma kallikrein (Tanaka et al., 1999), trypsin and plasmin and, according to the latest information, it inhibits angiogenesis in a vessel formation assay *in vitro* (Soares et al., 2016). Neutrophil elastase is a serine proteinase secreted by neutrophils and macrophages during inflammation and destroys bacteria. It belongs to the same family as chymotrypsin and is closely related to other cytotoxic immune serine proteases, such as granzymes and cathepsin G. Abnormal expression of neutrophil elastase can cause emphysema, a chronic obstructive pulmonary disease. In elastase-induced experimental emphysema, BmTI-A minimizes parenchymal lesions in mice, suggesting the potential application of this inhibitor in emphysema treatment (Lourenço et al., 2014).

Ixodes ricinus- derived inhibitor of contact phase, **Ir-CPI,** with one Kunitz domain inhibits the intrinsic coagulation pathway by interference with FXIIa, FXIa and kallikrein. In addition, it protects Ir-CPI treated mice against collagen- and epinephrine-induced thromboembolism without increasing bleeding (Decrem et al., 2009).

Tick-derived protease inhibitor, **TdPI,** was identified in salivary glands of *Rhipicephalus appendiculatus* females (Paesen et al., 2007). TdPI is only expressed during the first 4 h after tick attachment and manipulates host immune defenses during the tick feeding process. It is a glycosylated Kunitz-related potent inhibitor of human β-tryptase and trypsin and moderately affects human plasmin (Paesen et al., 2007; Bronsoms et al., 2011). Human β-tryptases, specific serine proteases of mast cells, together with leukocyte elastase and chymase, are involved in inflammation and different aspects of tissue remodeling (Caughey, 2007). Beta-tryptase is a clinically useful marker of mast cells and their activation and in addition, it contributes to the pathogenesis of allergic inflammatory disorders, e.g., asthma. Thus, β-tryptase is a potential therapeutic target of tryptase inhibitors which have therapeutic potential in asthma (Sommerhoff and Schaschke, 2007). TdPI is able to penetrate mouse mast cells and may block the autocatalytic activation of tryptase required for its biological action (Paesen et al., 2007). Thus, TdPI-derived drugs could be used as inhibitors of mast cell tryptase in the control of injury caused by parasites, and in the treatment of allergies.

Tryptogalinin, an *I. scapularis* salivary Kunitz-type protein, was found to inhibit a number of serine proteases involved in inflammation and vertebrate immunity: β-tryptase, β-trypsin, α-chymotrypsin, plasmin, matriptase and elastase, showing a potential broad effect against mast cell proteins and other host enzymes (Valdés et al., 2013). Tryptogalinin is phylogenetically related to TdPI and provides another example when understanding of the structure and function of a tick protein could help in engineering highly specific pharmacological agents.

Haemangin was identified as a salivary Kunitz inhibitor in *Haemaphysalis lonigicornis* which is up-regulated during blood feeding (Islam et al., 2009). It strongly inhibits trypsin, chymotrypsin and plasmin and thereby supporting plasmin-dependent fibrinolysis inhibition and indicating its antiproteolytic potential on angiogenic cascades (Islam et al., 2009). Haemangin also blocks chick aortic explant angiogenesis and neovascularization of chick chorioalantoic membrane, demonstrating that it can inhibit both pre-existing vessel angiogenesis and neovascularization. Haemangin also impedes differentiation, proliferation, and tube formation and significantly induces expression of a variety of genes involved in apoptosis, angiogenesis and wound healing in human umbilical vein endothelial (HUVEC) cells (Islam et al., 2009).

Disagregin is a Kunitz-type protein derived from *O. moubata* that inhibits activation of platelet aggregation through integrin aIIbb3 (Karczewski et al., 1994). It does not contain the RGD motif that binds to the fibrinogen-binding site and thus, it is unique in its sequence as well as function and could serve to design therapeutically useful antithrombotics.

Serine Protease Inhibitors – Serpin Domain Family

Serpins form one of the largest families of serine protease inhibitors ubiquitously distributed in nature, yet abundant in ticks (Francischetti et al., 2009). Several next-generation sequencing transcriptome studies revealed a high number of transcripts, e.g., over 150 in genus *Amblyomma*, around 20 in *Rhipicephalus* and at least 36 in *I. ricinus*, but only 20 tick serpins from different tick species have been functionally characterized. One of their functions is manipulation of host innate immune responses by impacting enzymes released from neutrophils, mast and dendritic cells (DCs).

The first tick serpin affecting host immune defenses was identified in salivary glands of *I. ricinus* and was named **Iris** (Leboulle et al., 2002). It inhibits T cells and splenocytes proliferation and alters cytokines levels of PBMC (Leboulle et al., 2002). It also suppresses coagulation and fibrinolysis by inhibition of thrombin, FXa and tissue plasminogen activator (Prevot et al., 2006). In addition, Iris inhibits secretion of TNF-α after binding on monocyte/macrophage cells (Prevot et al., 2009). Thus, Iris modulates multiple host processes simultaneously via independent mechanisms and potentially can serve for design of therapeutic for TNF-α overexpression induced pathological situations.

Ixodes ricinus serpin 2 **(IRS-2)** is a serine protease inhibitor that specifically inhibits two proteases, cathepsin G and chymase (**Figure 1**) that are secreted in mammals by stimulated neutrophils and mast cells, respectively. Cathepsin G is involved in tissue remodeling during inflammation, thus IRS-2 postpones this process, as well as platelet aggregation resulting in facilitating feeding (Chmelar et al., 2011). IRS-2 also modulates production of IL-6 by DCs, and subsequently differentiation and maturation of T helper 17 cells (Th17) via the IL-6/STAT-3 (Signal Transducer and Activator of Transcription 3) signaling pathway (Palenikova et al., 2015). In addition, IRS-2 impedes the paw edema development and the influx of neutrophils in an animal model of acute inflammation (Chmelar et al., 2011).

Cystatins (Cysteine Protease Inhibitors)

Cystatins represent a large superfamily of reversible and tight-binding inhibitors of papain-like cysteine proteases and legumains (Abrahamson et al., 2003). They regulate diverse vertebrate biological processes such as development of immune system, epidermal homeostasis, antigen presentation, neutrophil chemotaxis during inflammation, or apoptosis. Tick cystatins can interfere with both, innate and adaptive immune responses of the vertebrate host (Lieskovská et al., 2015a,b). Over the last decade, around 20 cystatins from various hard and soft ticks have been identified and biochemically analyzed for their role in the tick's physiology and blood feeding (Schwarz et al., 2012). All these cystatins are effective inhibitors of papain-like cysteine proteases, but not of legumain and belong to two of four existing cystatin subgroups, namely type 1 cystatins/stefins) and type 2 cystatins. While stefins are known to be primarily intracellular cytoplasmic proteins, type 2 are expressed and secreted in salivary glands and midgut and therefore have been more intensively studied in ticks. **Sialostatin L** was found first in the salivary glands of *I. scapularis* ticks by a sialotranscriptome study (Valenzuela, 2002) and later **Sialostatin L2** was described (Kotsyfakis et al., 2007).

Sialostatin L exerts miscellaneous immunosuppressive effects on mammalians. It is a potent inhibitor of lysosomal cysteine cathepsins L, C, V, S, X (**Figure 1**) and papain, proliferation of CD4+ cells and cytotoxic T cells (Kotsyfakis et al., 2006, 2007, 2010; Sa-Nunes et al., 2009), migration of neutrophils during acute inflammation, secretion of cytokines by mast cells, DCs and lymphocytes, and shows preventive potential against autoimmune diseases (Kotsyfakis et al., 2006; Sa-Nunes et al., 2009). On one side, mammalian cathepsins S, L, and V represent key players in the vertebrate immunity through their participation in the antigen presentation processes of DCs and macrophages, on the other hand, they are involved in many pathological processes, such as psoriasis, muscular dystrophy, neurodegenerative disorders, cancer, etc. Sialostatin L strongly decreases the production of IL-9 by Th9 cells, essentially involved in the induction of asthma symptoms. Application of sialostatin L almost completely abrogates airway hyperresponsiveness and eosinophilia in a model of experimental asthma and experimental data suggest its preventing effect in this disease model (Horka et al., 2012), probably by suppressing mast cell-derived IL-9 production by inhibiting IRF4 (Klein et al., 2015). In a mouse model of multiple sclerosis, *in vivo* administration of Sialostatin L during the immunization phase of experimental autoimmune encephalomyelitis pointedly prevents disease symptoms associated with decreased production of IFN-γ and IL-17 and proliferation of specific T cell (Sa-Nunes et al., 2009).

Sialostatin L2 impairs cathepsins C, L, S and V, diminishes secretion of IL-1b and IL-18 by macrophages and inhibits maturation of caspase-1. Upon infection with bacterial agents (e.g., *Anaplasma phagocytophilum*), Sialostatin L2 can significantly attenuate the severity of the disease due to its anti-inflammatory effects (Chen et al., 2014). Sialostatin L2 was found to suppress the interferon mediated immune response and enhance TBEV replication in murine DCs (Lieskovská et al., 2015a) and impair the production of proinflammatory chemokines in murine DCs upon infection with *Borrelia burgdorferi* (Lieskovská et al., 2015a).

Iristatin, a novel type 2 cystatin was identified in *I. ricinus* (Kotál et al., 2019). It suppresses vertebrate cathepsins C and L with similar affinity as sialostatins, production of T-cell derived cytokines, such as pro-inflammatory IFN-γ and IL-2 by stimulated Th1 cells, anti-inflammatory cytokine IL-4 by Th2 cells and IL-2 and IL-9 by Th9 cells, without effect on IL-17 production by Th17 cells. In mast cells, it blocks IL-9 and IL-6 production, but not IL-4. Furthermore, Iristatin inhibits OVA antigen-induced murine CD4+ T-cell proliferation *in vitro* and *in vivo* leukocyte (neutrophils and myeloid cells) recruitment in a mouse model of thioglycollate induced peritonitis. Iristatin with such a broad-spectrum of immunosuppressive activities may be useful in the therapy of immune-mediated diseases.

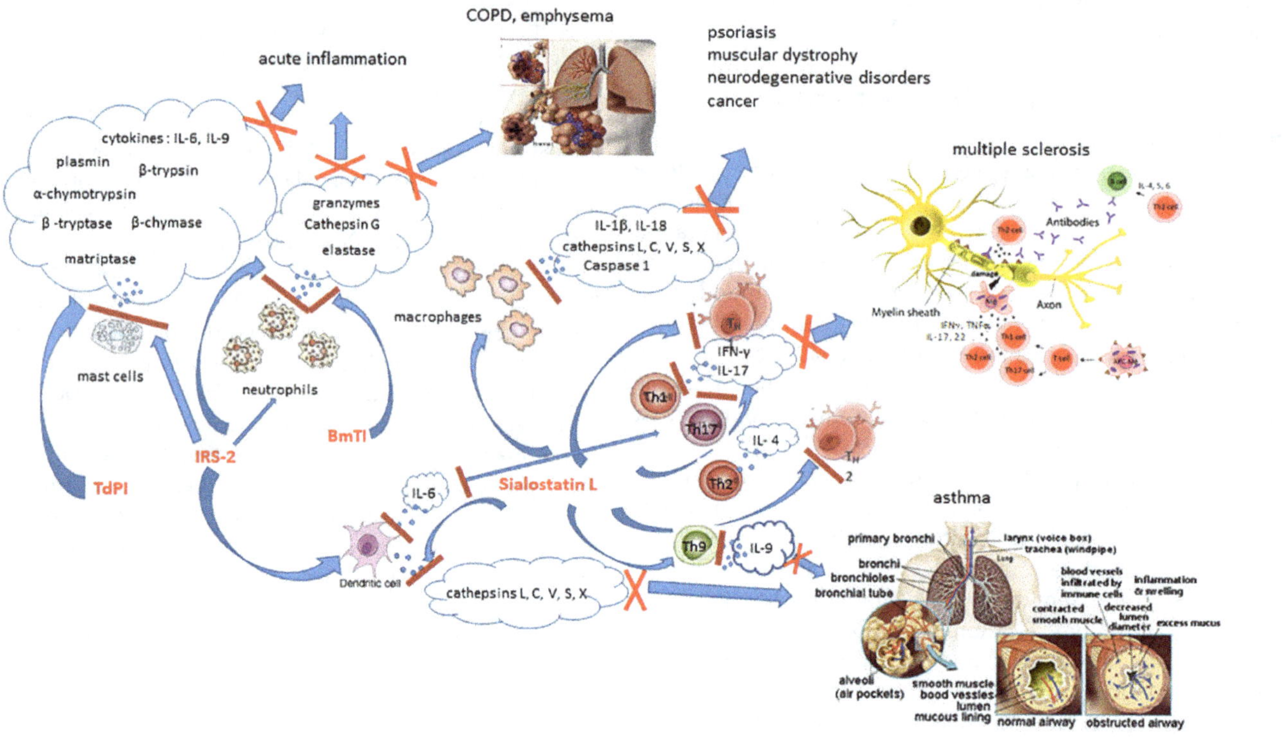

FIGURE 1 | Effects of selected tick salivary proteins on host immune cells and their potential therapeutic usage to treat immunological disorders. IRS-2, BmTI, and Sialostatin L modulate functions of enzymes released by immune cells, resulting in inhibition of their biological and pathological functions.

DsCystatin was identified by screening of the cDNA of *Dermacentor silvarum* salivary glands (Sun et al., 2018). DsCystatin impairs the activities of human cathepsins L and B and the expression of pro-inflammatory cytokines IFNγ, TNFα, and IL6 in mouse bone marrow-derived macrophages. It inhibits activation of mouse bone marrow-derived DCs and activation of NFκB in TLR2 and TLR4 signaling pathways. In a mouse arthritis model, DsCystatin suppresses joint inflammation induced by CFA and *B. burgdorferi*. DsCystatin could potentially be used in the cure of inflammatory diseases.

Small Peptide Inhibitors of the Hirudin-Like/Madanin/Variegin Superfamily

This superfamily comprises mainly small antithrombins and is probably specific to metastriate ticks (Francischetti et al., 2009).

Variegin is a 32-residue peptide derived from the salivary glands of partially fed female *Amblyomma variegatum* ticks. Its C-terminal tail displays homology to hirudin and is one of the smallest thrombin inhibitors in nature (Koh et al., 2007). It is a direct thrombin inhibitor and binds to thrombin from the active site to exosite-I (Koh et al., 2011). Upon binding, variegin is cleaved by thrombin, and its cleavage product continues to inhibit the thrombin active site in a non-competitive manner (Koh et al., 2009). Variegin is structurally and functionally similar to, but is more potent than bivalirudin (hirulog), a drug used for the treatment of patients with acute coronary syndromes (Lincoff et al., 2004; Stone et al., 2006). Pharmacokinetic studies involving rats confirmed that variegin, similar to other small peptide antithrombins, e.g., bivalirudin, was rapidly excreted by the renal route, which makes it suitable for short-lasting intravenous anticoagulation during surgical procedures[1].

Variegin-like thrombin inhibitors are probably synthesized in ticks as larger precursors that can be processed into multiple variants. Iyer et al. (2017) described **avathrin,** a new variegin-like thrombin inhibitor in *A. variegatum*. Similar to variegin, avathrin is a fast, tight-binding competitive inhibitor interacting with the thrombin active site and exosite-I after binding to thrombin. Avathrin is cleaved by thrombin, but the C-terminal cleavage product continues to exert prolonged inhibition. Avathrin prevented thrombosis better than hirulog-1 in a $FeCl_3$-induced murine carotid artery thrombosis model (Iyer et al., 2017, 2019). Variegin-like peptides represent perspective candidates for designing anticoagulants to prevent arterial and venous thrombosis during invasive procedures and for coating of medical devices.

Sculptin, a new thrombin inhibitor was identified in the transcriptome of salivary glands of *Amblyomma sculptum* (formerly *A. cajennense*) (Iqbal et al., 2017). Scupltin consists of 168 amino acid residues, has four similar repeats, shares few similarities with hirudin, but is more similar with serine protease inhibitors of the antistasin family. Sculptin is a novel class of competitive, specific and reversible thrombin

[1]https://patents.google.com/patent/US9217027

inhibitors and its mechanism of inhibition slightly differs from hirudin. Sculptin is cleaved by thrombin, but its fragments have no thrombin inhibitory activity. In contrast, fragments produced after hydrolysis by FXa are able to inhibit thrombin independently. Sculptin and its independent domain(s) have a potential to become novel antithrombotic drugs.

Madanin-1, 2 and **chimadanin** are small, cystein-free (~6 kDa) specific antithrombins isolated from the salivary glands of *H. longicornis* (Iwanaga et al., 2003). These peptides behave as cleavable competitive inhibitors of thrombin, bind to the active site and exosite II of the enzyme, and lose their affinity to thrombin upon proteolysis (Figueiredo et al., 2013; Thompson et al., 2017). Tyrosine sulfation of madanin-1 and chimadanin are crucial for their thrombin inhibitory activity. A dramatic increase in their potency was observed following tyrosine sulfation, with the sulfated tyrosine residues binding to exosite II of thrombin. The importance of tyrosine sulfation and the unique binding mode of these peptides make them promising candidates for the development of next generation thrombin inhibitors (Thompson et al., 2017).

Hyalomin 1, a 59-residue cystein-free peptide was identified in the salivary gland transcriptome of *Hyalomma marginatum rufipes*. The peptide is a selective and competitive inhibitor of thrombin, interacting with both the active site and exosite I of the enzyme (Jablonka et al., 2015). Hyalomin-1 also inhibits the thrombin-mediated activation of FXI, thrombin-mediated platelet aggregation, and the activation of FV by thrombin. It is cleaved by thrombin and cleavage region and the C-terminal fragment inhibited the enzyme similar to the full-length peptide. Testing of hyalomin-1 in a mouse model of thrombosis increased arterial occlusion time, making the peptide as another candidate for development of antithrombotic drugs.

Basic Tail-Secreted Proteins (BTSP)

This family comprises over hundred proteins that were found primarily in *Ixodes* species (Francischetti et al., 2009; Chmelar et al., 2012). In spite some homologs from metastriate ticks were identified, BTSP seem to be typical for prostriate ticks. Most members of this protein family contain a basic carboxy terminus (tail) (Francischetti et al., 2009). Only two BTSP have been functionally characterized. They include anticoagulants with novel mode of action, derived from salivary glands of *I. scapularis*: salivary protein 14 (Salp14), and Ixonnexin.

Salp14, a 9.8 kDa protein, was found to impair the intrinsic pathway of coagulation and specifically inhibit FXa, but it does not inhibit other proteases (Narasimhan et al., 2002).

Ixonnexin is a 11.8 kDa salivary protein, displaying homology to Salp14 (Assumpção et al., 2018). It also interacts with FXa, but in addition, promotes fibrinolysis *in vitro* by enzymatically productive ternary complex through binding to tissue type plasminogen activator (t-PA) and plasminogen. In *in vivo* experiments, ixonnexin was found to inhibit $FeCl_3$-induced thrombosis in mice and appears as a novel modulator of fibrinolysis that can be involved in studies on participation of plasmin in ischemic events, tumor growth and metastasis.

LIPOCALINS

Lipocalins, a family of ubiquitous barrel-shaped proteins with low molecular weight, perform multiple biological functions, including the regulation of cell homeostasis and immune responses via sequestering small hydrophobic molecules such as vitamins, steroids, histamine, serotonin, prostaglandin, involved in modulation of platelet aggregation, vasoconstriction and inflammation (Schlehuber and Skerra, 2005). Lipocalins are a protein family with a large expansion in ticks; in soft ticks they act as anti-complement factors (Nunn et al., 2005; Tambourgi and van den Berg, 2014), inhibitors of platelet aggregation (Keller et al., 1993; Waxman and Connolly, 1993) and toxins (Mans et al., 2003), while in hard ticks they scavenge biogenic amines such as histamine and serotonin (Paesen et al., 1999; Sangamnatdej et al., 2002) or leukotriene B4 (LTB4) (Beaufays et al., 2008). Tick lipocalins are considered outliers since they lack the three structural conserved motifs typical of the general lipocalin family, which are apparently designed to accommodate charged, hydrophilic ligands. Unlike other lipocalins, tick lipocalins harbor two internal binding sites, the H for histamine with high affinity and the L also for histamine but weakly (Paesen et al., 2000).

OmCI (*O. moubata* Complement Inhibitor), a 16.8-kDa protein from *O. moubata,* is the first described natural complement inhibitor from ticks, targeting specifically the C5 activation step in the complement cascade (Nunn et al., 2005; Roversi et al., 2007; Mans and Ribeiro, 2008; Barratt-Due et al., 2011).

The vertebrate complement system is a key member of innate defenses against infection, maintaining tissue homeostasis and orchestrating the crosstalk between adaptive and innate immunity (Harris, 2018). However, it is also involved in common and serious diseases, among them in many autoimmune diseases such as rheumatoid arthritis, diabetes mellitus type 1, systemic lupus erythematosus, multiple sclerosis, and myasthenia gravis (Mollnes et al., 2002). Complement can be activated by four pathways (classical, alternative, lectin, and thrombin) (Duncan et al., 2007; Thiel, 2007; Zipfel et al., 2007a,b). Although, complement association with disease has driven a boom in complement drug discovery based on natural sources, very few drugs have progressed to late-stage clinical studies due to high target concentration and turnover, unwanted side effects and lack of clarity around disease mechanism (Tambourgi and van den Berg, 2014).

OmCI binds directly to C5 and thus inhibits cleavage into anaphylatoxin C5a and C5b, a subunit of the membrane attack complex (MAC; C5b-9) and prevents MAC-mediated lysis and destruction of red blood cells in paroxysmal nocturnal hemoglobinuria (PNH) and tissue destruction in various other complement-mediated inflammatory and autoimmune diseases (Hepburn et al., 2007; Fredslund et al., 2008). In addition, OmCI captures the inflammatory mediator leukotriene B4, a potent chemotactic agent and activator of neutrophils (Yoshikai, 2001). A recombinant form of OmCI (known as Coversin and rEV576) has shown efficacy in numerous animal models of complement-mediated diseases and successfully accomplished a phase Ia clinical trial. The protein is protective in rat experimental models of passive and active autoimmune myasthenia gravis. OmCI-treated animals exhibited fewer symptoms and a markedly attenuated inflammatory response (Hepburn et al., 2007; Soltys et al., 2009). Coversin, if not bound to C5, has a very short plasma half-life and requires frequent dosing. N-terminal conjugation with a 600 amino acid polypeptide composed of Pro, Ala, and Ser has improved the pharmacokinetics of Coversin by extending the half-time, slowing kidney clearance, and considerably reducing background hemolysis of erythrocytes. Moreover, Coversin reduced lysis of erythrocyte as effectively as its non-conjugated form in a clinically relevant *in vitro* model of the complement-mediated disease, PNH (Kuhn et al., 2016).

Moubatin is a lipocalin derived from salivary glands of *O. moubata*. It inhibits platelet aggregation induced by collagen (Keller et al., 1993; Waxman and Connolly, 1993) and binds to thromboxane A_2, a potent platelet aggregation agonist and vasoconstrictor (Mans and Ribeiro, 2008). Moubatin was found to relax rat aorta pre-constricted by U46619 (a thromboxane A_2 mimetic) and inhibit its contraction induced by U46619 (Mans and Ribeiro, 2008).

The hard tick *R. appendiculatus* has two types of salivary lipocalins that are structurally resolved, bind different ligands and have separate functions, namely, *R. appendiculatus*-histamine binding proteins, **Ra-HBPs** (Paesen et al., 1999) and **Japanin** (Preston et al., 2013). The high-affinity Ra-HBPs were identified in both genders of the tick: RaHBP1 and 2 are specific for females, Ra-HBP3 is associated with males. Ra-HBP1 and 2 are around 20 kDa unglycosylated monomeric proteins secreted by the tick females during the early feeding stage, while Ra-HBP3 is a glycosylated dimeric protein produced throughout feeding. Ra-HBP2 and 3 show strong affinity to histamine whereas affinity of Ra-HBP1 is weak. Ra-HBP2 has been proposed for therapeutic use since it sequesters two histamine molecules, with different affinities, thereby reducing inflammatory responses (Paesen et al., 1999, 2000).

Serotonin-histamine binding protein, **SHBP**, identified in *Dermacentor reticulatus* ticks (Sangamnatdej et al., 2002) is a lipocalin simultaneously binding serotonin and histamine. Serotonin represents a key neurotransmitter of the central nervous system and is also involved in a number of neurological disorders (Dinan, 1996). Similarly to histamine, serotonin is a key mediator of inflammation (Askenase et al., 1980) produced by mast cells and platelets.

The described histamine binding proteins and related protein family members were under investigation as potential therapeutic agents for the treatment of various diseases: Ra-HBP2 (as rEV-131) for conjunctivitis (Nuttall and Paesen, 2001b), allergic rhinitis and asthma (Nuttall and Paesen, 2001a), carcinoid syndrome and rheumatoid arthritis (Weston-Davies, 2004), Dr-SHBP for treatment of carcinoid syndrome with high production of serotonin (Schnirer et al., 2003) and post-chemotherapy emesis with nausea and vomiting due to various neurotransmitters involving serotonin. The latter treatment focused on serotonin receptor antagonists (Hesketh, 2004). In both cases, SHBP primarily targets serotonin, with secondary anti-inflammatory effects due to its histamine-binding capabilities.

In a murine allergic asthma model, the intranasal administration of Ra-HBP2 to immunized mice before antigen challenge prevented airway hyper-reactivity by 70%, and also abrogated peribronchial inflammation, pulmonary eosinophilia, mucus hypersecretion, and IL-4 and IL-5 secretion and effectively reduced airway resistance, comparable with budesonide, the conventionally prescribed corticosteroid (Couillin et al., 2004). In a corticosteroid-resistant LPS-induced murine model of acute respiratory distress syndrome, rEV-131 decreased bronchoconstriction, activation and influx of neutrophils. In phase I and II clinical trial this lipocalin showed safety and pharmacological activity in treatment of allergy in humans (Schlehuber and Skerra, 2005).

Japanin is a 17.7 kDa *N*-glycosylated lipocalin which exists in complex with cholesterol (Preston et al., 2013; Roversi et al., 2017). It reprograms DCs, antigen-presenting cells, so they no longer respond to a wide spectrum of stimuli *in vitro* specific for immune recognition. DCs, resident cells within most peripheral tissues (including skin), represent a bridge between innate and adaptive immunity as the important initiators and modulators of T cell responses. Japanin blocks differentiation of DCs from monocytes and on one side impedes upregulation of co-stimulatory molecules and pro-inflammatory cytokines in response to stimuli and on other side it promotes upregulation of co-inhibitory molecules and the anti-inflammatory cytokine IL-10 (Preston et al., 2013). Although the exact mechanism by which Japanin modulates DCs has not been fully described, the molecule may represent a novel tool to modulate DCs with possible therapeutic applications, such as prevention or treatment of transplant rejection or autoimmune diseases.

HA24, identified in the salivary glands of the tick *Hyalomma asiaticum,* represents a new lipocalin protein with particular histamine binding capacity (Wang et al., 2016). Its recombinant form binds specifically to histamine in a dose-dependent manner, and can provide palliation from allergic asthma in mice (Yanan et al., 2016).

IXODEGRIN SUPERFAMILY

Ixodegrins include cysteine-rich proteins containing the RGD (Arg-Gly-Asp) or KGD (Lys-Gly-Asp) motif that interfere with fibrinogen binding to platelets and exert antiplatelet activities (Francischetti et al., 2009). As GPIIb/IIIa inhibitors are widely used clinically during coronary interventions (Hashemzadeh et al., 2008), tick-derived disintegrins could also serve as candidates for drug design.

Variabilin, derived from salivary glands of *Dermacentor variabilis,* is 5-kDa RGD-containing disintegrin and was the first RGD-containing antagonist isolated from ticks (Wang et al., 1996). It blocks ADP-induced platelet aggregation and prevents integrin aIIbb3 binding to immobilized fibrinogen. It also an antagonist of the vitronectin receptor $\alpha v\beta 3$ and attenuates osteosarcoma cell adhesion to vitronectin. Its sequence differs from other known naturally occurring antagonists of GPIIb-IIIa.

Ixodegrins identified in *Ixodes pacificus* and *I. scapularis* salivary gland transcriptomes display sequence homology to variabilin, including the RGD domain (Francischetti et al., 2005, 2009). Using the sequence of ixodegrin in the *I. pacificus* transcriptome (Francischetti et al., 2005), the molecule **YY-39** was synthesized and refolded for studies on its effects on platelets and thrombosis *in vivo* (Tang et al., 2015). YY-39 decreased adenosine diphosphate (ADP)-, thrombin- and thromboxane A_2-induced platelet aggregation. In addition, it inhibited platelet adhesion to soluble collagen and bound to purified GPIIb/IIIa. YY-39 also reduced thrombus weight in an *in vivo* experimental rat arteriovenous shunt model and as well as blocked thrombosis in a carrageenan-induced mouse tail thrombosis model. However, in the tested animal models, YY-39 showed little bleeding complication, which makes the molecule a promising antithrombotic agent.

METASTRIATE-SPECIFIC FAMILIES

Over thirty families of proteins have been found exclusively in metastriate ticks (Francischetti et al., 2009), but only a few have been functionally characterized. These include small immunoregulatory proteins that modulate vertebrate immune responses, mainly acting on cytokines and chemokines.

Cytokines, a diverse group of small secreted proteins (interleukins, growth factors, chemokines), represent key humoral controllers of cells in their interactions and communications and regulators of processes under normal, developmental and pathological conditions (inflammation, wound healing). Cytokine through binding to their specific receptors orchestrate immune responses, including the recruitment of immune cells into the site of inflammation. Uncontrolled expressions of cytokines are associated with inflammatory, autoimmunity even with cancer, thus members of cytokine networks are targets for development of new effective therapeutics. Ticks either suppress production of cytokines by various immune cells or directly inhibit cytokines by binding ligands. However, from all anticytokine activities described in different tick species (Hajnická et al., 2001; Hajnicka et al., 2005, 2011; Vančová et al., 2007, 2010; Peterková et al., 2008; Slovák et al., 2014), only hyalomins (Wu et al., 2010), Amregulin (Tian et al., 2016) and chemokine binding factors named Evasins derived from *Rhipicephalus sanguineus* (Frauenschuh et al., 2007; Deruaz et al., 2008) have been functionally and structurally characterized.

Small Immunoregulatory Peptides

Hyalomin-A and -B were identified in salivary glands of the hard tick *Hyalomma asiaticum asiaticum* (Wu et al., 2010). Both immunosuppressant peptides exert significant anti-inflammatory activities, either directly by inhibiting LPS-induced production of inflammatory cytokines – TNF-α, monocyte chemotactic protein-1and IFN-γ in mouse splenocytes or indirectly by stimulating secretion of immunosuppressant cytokine IL-10. Moreover, both hyalomins scavenge free radical 2,2′-azinobis 3-ethylbenzothiazoline-6-sulfonic acid ($ABTS^{+}$) radicals *in vitro* and inhibit adjuvant-induced arthritis in mice *in vivo*.

Tian et al. (2016) structurally and functionally characterized a small immunosuppressant peptide **Amregulin** from *A. variegatum*. Amregulin inhibits *in vitro* secretion of inflammatory cytokines – TNF-α, IL-8, IL-1 and IFN-γ by LPS stimulated rat splenocytes in a dose-dependent manner. Like hyalomins, this peptide shows concentration dependent antioxidant activity by scavenging free radical $ABTS^{+}$, but not 2,2-diphenyl-1-picrylhydrazyl (DPPH) and by reducing ferric ions (Fe^{3+}) to Fe^{2+}. Amregulin also significantly inhibits Freuds adjuvant-induced paw inflammation in mouse models *in vivo*.

Evasins

Three salivary glycoproteins, found in the brown dog tick *R. sanguineus*, are secreted during a feeding and bind to host chemokines, thus inhibiting the host inflammatory response (Frauenschuh et al., 2007; Deruaz et al., 2008). **Evasin-1** and **-3** are high specific binders of only three CC chemokines (CCL3, CCL4, and CCL18) and a subset of CXC chemokines (CXCL1, -2, -3, -5, -8), respectively, whereas **Evasin-4** demonstrated more promiscuity effect by interaction with at least 18 chemokines of the CC subfamily. Evasin-1 in a dose-dependent manner reduced CCL3-induced influx of neutrophils in a peritoneal cell recruitment assay and showed high efficiency in reducing fibrosis resulted from neutrophil infiltration into the lung after bleomycin treatment, and also decreased the mortality observed in this model (Russo et al., 2011). Evasin-3 is effective in several neutrophil-dependent disease models with regards to its *in vitro* effect mentioned above. Montecucco et al. (2014) demonstrated beneficial effects of Evasin-3 and partially of Evasin-4 on inflammatory processes in pancreas and lungs in a mouse model of acute pancreatitis (AP). Evasin-3 treatment of mice with cerulein-induced AP decreased recruitment of neutrophils, production of ROS and apoptosis in the lungs and inhibited necrosis and apoptosis of neutrophils and macrophages in the pancreas. Evasin-4 only decreased the abundance of macrophages in lungs, without any effects in the pancreas. A dose-dependent Evasin-3 inhibition of CXCL8 induced leukocyte infiltration into the peritoneal cavity is determined. In an antigen-induced arthritis by BSA, intradermal injection of Evasin-3 significantly suppresses disease symptoms. In case of ischemic reperfusion injury, Evasin-3 showed higher efficiency than Evasin-1, even though only Evasin-1 effectively inhibited first DCs recruitment to the site of infection with *Leishmania major*, mediated by CCL3 released from neutrophils (Charmoy et al., 2010). Moreover, Evasin-1 is able to reduce skin inflammation observed in D6−/− mice in response to 12-*O*-tetradecanoylphorbol-13-acetate (Deruaz et al., 2008). Castor et al. (2010) studied effects of Evasin-1 on pathogenesis of acute graft-versus-host disease (GVHD) in mice, induced by transplantation of C57BL/6J murine splenocytes to B6D2F1 mice. GVHD is a complication occurring in allogeneic bone marrow transplantation with significant morbidity and mortality in humans (Ferrara and Deeg, 1991), and is characteristic by CCL3 expression and CCL3-induced recruitment and proliferation of T cells. Although application of Evasin-1 did not interfere with GVH-leukemia in mice, Evasin-1 treatment reduced levels of IFN-γ and

CCL5, but not TNF-α, reduced the number of $CD4^+$ and $CD8^+$ T cells infiltrating the small intestine and the damage of intestine and liver. In addition, Evasin-1 also ameliorated GVHD and provided partial relief from symptoms, whereby the effect was comparable to glucocorticosteroid dexamethasone and was similar to protection observed in $CCL3^{-/-}$ mice. Furthermore, both Evasin-3 and -4 effectively reduce post-infarction myocardial injury and remodeling (Braunersreuther et al., 2013) and Evasin-4 is effective in DSS-induced colitis (Vieira et al., 2009). Because of its broad CC chemokine-binding spectrum, Evasin-4 is considered the most suitable candidate for design of a therapeutic agent. By sequence similarity searches in transcriptomes of hard ticks, mainly of the *Rhipicephalus*, *Amblyomma*, and *Ixodes* genera, over 250 putative evasin sequences were detected (Hayward et al., 2017). Eight of them were expressed in *Escherichia coli* and exhibited high-affinity binding to human chemokines. They were classified into C8 and C6 evasins. By using the yeast surface display method, Singh et al. (2017) detected ten novel polyvalent CC-chemokine binding evasin-like molecules from eight hard tick species of the *Rhipicephalus* and *Amblyomma* genera. One of them, P672 from *Rhipicephalus pulchellus*, was found to bind to CCL8 and its properties could be altered by homology modeling, demonstrating that the function of tick evasins can be manipulated to design novel drugs (Eaton et al., 2018).

~8 kDa Tick-Derived C5 Inhibitors

RaCI (Rhipicephalus appendiculatus C5 Inhibitor) belongs to a novel protein family of ~8 kDa tick-derived C5 inhibitors. It was identified in the transcriptome of *R. appendiculatus* salivary glands (Matthijs et al., 2016) and its sequence shares no similarity to previously characterized tick complement inhibitors. RaCI binds human C5 and blocks the generation of C5a and membrane attack complex formation. RaCI exhibits cross-species reactivity which can be used in disease models on animal to test therapeutic efficacy of drug candidates. The small size of RaCI in comparison with the previously described OmCI and retaining its potency after its further reducing may potentially aid drug administration. As OmCI and RaCI target different sites on C5 (C5d-CUB and C5d-MG1-MG2, respectively), RaCI may be used to tune therapeutic effects of complement 5 inhibitors.

PROSTRIATE-SPECIFIC FAMILIES

Out of the six protein families included in this group, only members of one group, i.e., the Isac protein family, have been characterized functionally. This group comprises salivary anti-complement proteins derived from *I. scapularis* and *I. ricinus* (Francischetti et al., 2009).

Isac Protein Family

Several tick saliva molecules with promising anti-complement activities have been identified and characterized in ticks of the *Ixodes* genus: **Isac** and **Salp20** in *I. scapularis* (Valenzuela et al., 2000; Tyson et al., 2007), **Irac I, Irac II** (Daix et al., 2007), and **IxACs** (Couvreur et al., 2008) in *I. ricinus*. Isac and Irac proteins specifically inhibit the alternative pathway (AP) of complement via blocking C3 convertase, whereby this inhibition can lead to immunosuppression or diminishing of opsonization. On the other hand, depletion of serum C3 detected in neuromuscular junction, an important factor determining severity of myasthenia gravis, is appreciated in some patients with this autoimmune neuromuscular transmission diseases. Salp20, displaying homology to Isac, inhibits the AP by binding properdin, which is a positive regulator of this pathway (Tyson et al., 2008; Hourcade et al., 2016). Couvreur et al. (2008) cloned and expressed proteins from *I. ricinus*, named IxACs, showing 40% identity to Isac and Irac. IxACs also inhibit the AP by binding to properdin.

Family of 15 kDa Salivary Proteins

Salp15, a 15 kDa immunosuppressive cystein-rich glycoprotein, was identified in salivary glands of *I. scapularis* (Anguita et al., 2002). It inhibits directly the activation of CD4+ T cells through binding on the coreceptor CD4, which results in signaling pathway inhibition, reduced IL-2 production and CD25 (IL-2Rα) expression (Juncadella et al., 2007; Garg et al., 2014), and also indirectly via inhibition of DCs functions by binding on lectin type. Salp15 binding to CD4 is persistent and induces a long-lasting immunomodulatory effect, probably due to induction of an increased expression of the ectoenzyme, CD73, in regulatory T cells and increased production of adenosine (Tomás-Cortázar et al., 2017). This immunomodulatory protein is a promising candidate for treatment of T-cell-mediated autoimmune diseases involving asthma or allogeneic transplant tolerance. Paveglio et al. (2007) tested Salp15 in a mouse model of human allergic asthma with typical imbalance of CD4+ T cells toward Th2 cells and overproduction of cytokines IL-4, IL-5, and IL-13, leading to production of IgE, eosinophilpoiesis, production and secretion of mucus. Mice were intra-peritoneally sensitized with OVA in aluminum hydroxide in combination with or without Salp15, followed by OVA-aerosol treatment. Salp15 significantly reduced all features of allergic asthma mentioned above thus effectively prevented the development of experimental asthma. An opposite effect of Salp15 was detected in a mouse model of multiple sclerosis, experimental autoimmune encephalomyelitis (EAE), the progression of which is directly associated with Th17 and Th1 cells secreting IL-17 and IFN-γ, respectively (El-behi et al., 2010). Surprisingly, application of Salp15 led to enhanced activation of Th17 cells and consequently to increased production of IL-17 and development of severe EAE in mice *in vivo* and to induced differentiation of Th17 cells with IL-6 and without TGF-β *in vitro*. Salp15 did neither affect infiltration of T cells to the central nervous system, nor the development of antibody responses against the eliciting peptide $PLP_{139-151}$ or the presence of IFN-γ in the sera. The reported effect can be associated with repression of IL-2 during T cell differentiation, which could be achieved also by TGF-β and/or other immunosuppressants (Juncadella et al., 2010).

Putative Secreted Salivary Gland Proteins

TIX-5 ('Tick Inhibitor of factor Xa toward factor V,' formerly P23) was originally identified as a salivary antigen by screening *I. scapularis* nymphal salivary gland yeast surface display library with nymph-immune rabbit sera (Schuijt et al., 2011). Recombinant P23 demonstrated anti-coagulant activity. The anticoalgulant properties of P23 renamed to TIX-5 were further characterized (Schuijt et al., 2013). The studies show that TIX-5 specifically inhibits FXa-mediated factor V (FV) activation involving the B-domain of FV and reveal that activation of FV by FXa is a crucial event in the initiation of thrombin generation. The data not only elucidate a unique molecular mechanism by which ticks inhibit host blood coagulation, but propose a revised blood coagulation scheme in which direct FXa-mediated FV activation occurs in the initiation phase of coagulation. These findings could potentially results in novel therapeutic approaches for anticoagulation (Aleman and Wolberg, 2013).

EF-Hand Calcium-Binding Proteins

Longistatin was the first EF-hand calcium-binding protein identified and characterized from salivary glands of an ixodid tick, *H. longicornis* (Anisuzzaman et al., 2010). The protein was found to function as an anticoagulant and plasminogen activator, hydrolyze fibrinogen and delay fibrin clot formation (Anisuzzaman et al., 2011). Moreover, longistatin modulates host immune responses and inflammation associated with tick bites by binding to the receptor for advanced glycation end products (RAGE) that mediates immune cell activation and is highly expressed in the host skin at inflammatory sites (Anisuzzaman et al., 2014). Due to its ability to block RAGE, longistatin may be a therapeutic tool against RAGE-regulated diseases such as Alzheimer's disease, psoriasis, diabetic complications and tumorigenesis (Anisuzzaman et al., 2015).

GLYCINE-RICH, OR PROLINE-RICH, COLLAGEN-LIKE SUPERFAMILY

This superfamily of proteins produced in tick salivary glands is subdivided to a number of subgroups and includes, e.g., cuticle proteins, collagens, small and large GGY peptides, metastriate spider-like cement protein, Ixodes-specific collagen-like small peptides, metastriate and argasidae proteins distantly related to Ixodes collagen-like proteins, etc. (for details see Francischetti et al., 2009). Of interest to medical applications are proteins associated with tick cement. The main function of the cement is to anchor mouthparts of the feeding tick to the host skin and seal the feeding lesion during attachment. There are important differences in the strategy of attachment of metastriate and prostriate ticks as well as in the ultrastructure, mechanical properties and chemical composition of their cement (for review see Suppan et al., 2018). Metastriate ticks having shorter mouthparts produce an abundant cement protein cone, whereas prostriate ticks have longer mouthparts that allow mechanical attach into the host dermis, and thus produce less cement.

Considering the adhesive and sealing properties of tick cement, its potential applications as a template for biomimetic tissue adhesives is proposed (Suppan et al., 2018). Currently available tissue glues contain toxic substances, have weak bonding forces, and/or do not cover all possible fields of application in surgery and microsurgery (for review see Suppan et al., 2018). However, to be able replace currently used tissue glues by adhesives developed based on the structure and function of tick cement, the adhesive molecules produced in tick salivary glands need to be further explored.

CONCLUSION

The mammalian hemostatic and immune systems represent robust complex networks, comprising diverse humoral and cellular biological structures and processes that are essential for protection against disease, injuries or any other potentially damaging disturbers. Hemostasis belongs to the first line of defense and prevents from blood loss after damage of blood vessels. Functioning properly, both the hemostatic and the immune system identify a variety of threats and the immune system distinguishes them from the own healthy tissue. Hemostatic and immune pathways are closely interconnected. Any disorders of the immune system can result in immunodeficiency, autoimmune diseases, inflammatory diseases, even cancer, in which events of innate and adaptive immune responses, but also coagulation factors participate. Current treatment options of such diseases have often limited effectiveness, are accompanied by many side effects or are insufficient. Therefore researchers are looking for alternative medicaments derived from nature, for example, from plants, animals, or microorganisms. Ticks are astounding "pharmacologists." Their saliva contains hundreds of proteins and low molecular weight effectors with immunomodulatory, anti-inflammatory, anti-clotting and anti-platelet as well as antitumor and antiangiogenic properties with high affinity, avidity and selectivity for their targets in the host defense mechanisms. Moreover, many of the tick-derived molecules show specific, yet unknown functions and modes of action. Thus, ticks are promising sources for discovering and designing new medical treats targeting various pathways of the mammalian physiology. In addition to their high target specificity, tick-derived products have a low risk of microbial resistance, toxicity and immunogenicity (Simons et al., 2011). However, the exploration and exploitation of the pharmacological potential of ticks is still in its infancy. The candidates for designing novel drugs mentioned in this study have been tested in various animal models of human diseases and have shown promising continues. Unfortunately, only a few of them advanced to pre-clinical investigations, e.g., TAP, Ra-HBP, Dr-SBP, OmCI, or Amblyomin-X. The tick lipocalin RaHBP exhibited high ligand specificity and affinity and data from clinical trial exhibited beneficial effects in human allergy. Lipocalins are promising new therapy candidates based on their natural ligand-binding functions to store and transport small compounds, which together with their structure (small polypeptide chain) led to design of artificial binding proteins "anticalins" with novel specificities, for example as transporters for pharmaceuticals. In general, it is a very long way from basic research to translation to the clinical praxis and, according to Murfin and Fikrig (2017), with many gaps and lacks. It is known that arthropod molecules are unstable, have a short half-life (for example OmCI mentioned in this review) or are cytotoxic, thus they require improved pharmacokinetics, optimization of dosage, delivery way, etc. (Ratcliffe et al., 2014). Another complication in drug development based on tick molecules is the identification of the mode of action of individual molecules within the complex mixture of saliva, where synergistic effect of molecules is presumed in the context of tick feeding. Thus, for therapeutic benefit identification of the interacting partners would be necessary. Last but not least, the high costs of development of new drugs designed on the basis of tick molecules is very relevant, thus the approval processes are not very attractive. However, only profound basic studies of the biological functions of tick molecules can lead to discovery and approval of new therapeutic agents.

AUTHOR CONTRIBUTIONS

PB, IŠ, VH, and MK conducted the literature search and wrote the manuscript. MK prepared the table. IŠ prepared the figure. All authors critically read and revised the manuscript.

FUNDING

This work was supported by the Grant agency of Slovak Republic (VEGA 2/0047/18 and VEGA 2/0172/19) and Slovak Research and Development Agency (APVV-0737-12).

REFERENCES

Abrahamson, M., Alvarez-Fernandez, M., and Nathanson, C. M. (2003). Cystatins. *Biochem. Soc. Symp.* 70, 179–199.

Akagi, E. M., de Sá Júnior, P. L., Simons, S. M., Bellini, M. H., Barreto, S. A., and Chudzinski-Tavassi, A. M. (2012). Pro-apoptotic effects of amblyomin-X in murine renal cell carcinoma "in vitro". *Biomed. Pharmacother.* 66, 64–69. doi: 10.1016/j.biopha.2011.11.015

Aleman, M. M., and Wolberg, A. S. (2013). Tick spit shines a light on the initiation of coagulation. *Circulation* 128, 203–205. doi: 10.1161/circulationaha.113.003800

Anguita, J., Ramamoorthi, N., Hovius, J. W. R., Das, S., Thomas, V., Persinski, R., et al. (2002). Salp15, an *Ixodes scapularis* salivary protein, inhibits CD4+ T cell activation. *Immunity* 16, 849–859. doi: 10.1016/S1074-7613(02)00325-324

Anisuzzaman, Alim, M. A., and Tsuji, N. (2015). Longistatin in tick-saliva targets RAGE. *Oncotarget* 6, 35133–35134. doi: 10.18632/oncotarget.6032

Anisuzzaman, Hatta, T., Miyoshi, T., Matsubayashi, M., Islam, M. K., Alim, M. A., et al. (2014). Longistatin in tick saliva blocks advanced glycation end-product receptor activation. *J. Clin. Invest.* 124, 4429–4444. doi: 10.1172/jci74917

Anisuzzaman, Islam, M. K., Alim, M. A., Miyoshi, T., Hata, T., Yamaji, K., et al. (2011). Longistatin, a plasminogen activator, is key to the availability of blood-meals for ixodid ticks. *PLoS Pathog.* 7:e1001312. doi: 10.1371/journal.ppat.1001312

Anisuzzaman, Islam, M. K., Miyoshim, T., Alim, M. A., Hatta, T., Yamaji, K., et al. (2010). Longistatin, a novel EF-hand protein from the ixodid tick *Haemaphysalis longicornis*, is required for acquisition of host blood-meals. *Int. J. Parasitol.* 40, 721–729. doi: 10.1016/j.ijpara.2009.11.004

Askenase, P. W., Bursztajn, S., Gershon, M. D., and Gershon, R. K. (1980). T cell-dependent mast cell degranulation and release of serotonin in murine delayed-type hypersensitivity. *J. Exp. Med.* 152, 1358–1374. doi: 10.1084/jem.152.5.1358

Assumpção, T. C., Mizurini, D. M., Ma, D., Monteiro, R. Q., Ahlstedt, S., Reyes, M., et al. (2018). Ixonnexin from tick saliva promotes fibrinolysis by interacting with plasminogen and tissue-type plasminogen activator, and prevents arterial thrombosis. *Sci. Rep.* 8:4806. doi: 10.1038/s41598-018-22780-22781

Ayllón, N., Villar, M., Galindo, R. C., Kocan, K. M., Šíma, R., López, J. A., et al. (2015). Systems biology of tissue-specific response to *Anaplasma phagocytophilum* reveals differentiated apoptosis in the tick vector ixodes scapularis. *PLoS Genet.* 11:e1005120. doi: 10.1371/journal.pgen.1005120

Barratt-Due, A., Thorgersen, E. B., Lindstad, J. K., Pharo, A., Lisina, O., Lambris, J. D., et al. (2011). *Ornithodoros moubata* complement inhibitor is an equally effective C5 inhibitor in pigs and humans. *J. Immunol.* 187, 4913–4919. doi: 10.4049/jimmunol.1101000

Batista, I. F. C., Ramos, O. H. P., Ventura, J. S., Junqueira-de-Azevedo, I. L. M., Ho, P. L., and Chudzinski-Tavassi, A. M. (2010). A new factor xa inhibitor from *Amblyomma cajennense* with a unique domain composition. *Arch. Biochem. Biophys.* 493, 151–156. doi: 10.1016/j.abb.2009.10.009

Beaufays, J., Adam, B., Decrem, Y., Prévôt, P. P., Santini, S., Brasseur, R., et al. (2008). Ixodes ricinus tick lipocalins: identifications, cloning, phylogenetic analysis and biochemical characterization. *PLoS One* 3:e3941. doi: 10.1371/journal.pone.0003941

Blisnick, A. A., Foulon, T., and Bonnet, S. I. (2017). Serine protease inhibitors in ticks: an overview of their role in tick biology and tick-borne pathogen transmission. *Front. Cell Infect. Microbiol.* 7:199. doi: 10.3389/fcimb.2017.00199

Bonnet, S., Kazimírová, M., Richardson, J., and Šimo, L. (2018). "„Tick saliva and its role in pathogen transmission"," in *Skin and Arthropod Vectors*, ed. N. Boulanger (Amsterdam: Elsevier), 121–192.

Bonnet, S. I., Binetruy, F., Hernández-Jarguín, A. M., and Duron, O. (2017). The tick microbiome: why non-pathogenic microorganisms matter in tick biology and pathogen transmission. *Front. Cell Infect. Microbiol.* 7:236. doi: 10.3389/fcimb.2017.00236

Bonvin, P., Power, C. A., and Proudfoot, A. E. (2016). Evasins: therapeutic potential of new family of chemokine-binding proteins from ticks. *Front. Immunol.* 7:208. doi: 10.3389/fimmu.2016.00208

Boufleur, P., Sciani, J. M., Goldfeder, M., Faria, F., Branco, V., and Chudzinski-Tavassi, A. M. (2019). Biodistribution and pharmacokinetics of amblyomin-X, a novel antitumour protein drug in healthy mice. *Eur. J. Drug. Metab. Pharmacokinet.* 44, 111–120. doi: 10.1007/s13318-018-0500-z

Branco, V. G., Iqbal, A., Alvarez-Flores, M. P., Sciani, J. M., de Andrade, S. A., Iwai, L. K., et al. (2016). Amblyomin-X having a Kunitz-type homologous domain is a noncompetitive inhibitor of FXa and induces anticoagulation *in vitro* and *in vivo*. *Biochim. Biophys. Acta* 1864, 1428–1435. doi: 10.1016/j.bbapap.2016.07.011

Braunersreuther, V., Montecucco, F., Pelli, G., Galan, K., Proudfoot, A. E., Belin, A., et al. (2013). Treatment with the CC chemokine-binding protein Evasin-4 improves post-infarction myocardial injury and survival in mice. *Thromb. Haemost.* 110, 807–825. doi: 10.1160/TH13-04-0297

Bronsoms, S., Pantoja-Uceda, D., Gabrijelcic-Geiger, D., Sanglas, L., Aviles, F. X., Santoro, J., et al. (2011). Oxidative folding and structural analyses of a Kunitz-Related Inhibitor and its disulfide intermediates: functional implications. *J. Mol. Biol.* 414, 427–441. doi: 10.1016/j.jmb.2011.10.018

Buning, J., Homann, N., von Smolinski, D., Borcherding, F., Noack, F., Stolte, M., et al. (2008). Helminths as governors of inflammatory bowel disease. *Gut* 57, 1182–1183. doi: 10.1136/gut.2008.152355

Carneiro-Lobo, T. C., Konig, S., Machado, D. E., Nasciutti, L. E., Forni, M. F., Francischetti, I. M. B., et al. (2009). Ixolaris, a tissue factor inhibitor, blocks primary tumor growth and angiogenesis in a glioblastoma model. *J. Thromb. Haemost.* 7, 1855–1864. doi: 10.1111/j.1538-7836.2009.03553.x

Carneiro-Lobo, T. C., Schaffner, F., Disse, J., Ostergaard, H., Francischetti, I. M. B., Monteiro, R. Q., et al. (2012). The tick-derived inhibitor ixolaris prevents tissue factor signaling on tumor cells. *J. Thromb. Haemost.* 10, 1849–1858. doi: 10.1111/j.1538-7836.2012.04864.x

Castor, M. G. M., Rezende, B., Resende, C. B., Alessandri, A. L., Fagundes, C. T., Sousa, L. P., et al. (2010). The CCL3/macrophage inflammatory protein-1α–binding protein evasin-1 protects from graft-versus-host disease but does not modify graft-versus-leukemia in mice. *J. Immunol.* 184, 2646–2654. doi: 10. 4049/jimmunol.0902614

Caughey, G. H. (2007). Mast cell tryptases and chymases in inflammation and host defense. *Immunol. Rev.* 217, 141–154. doi: 10.1111/j.1600-065X.2007.00509.x

Charmoy, M., Brunner-Agten, S., Aebischer, D., Auderset, F., Launois, P., Milon, G., et al. (2010). Neutrophil-derived CCL3 is essential for the rapid recruitment of dendritic cells to the site of Leishmania major inoculation in resistant mice. *PLoS Pathog.* 6:e1000755. doi: 10.1371/journal.ppat.1000755

Chen, G., Wang, X., Severo, M. S., Sakhon, O. S., Sohail, M., Brown, L. J., et al. (2014). The tick salivary protein sialostatin L2 inhibits caspase-1-mediated inflammation during *Anaplasma phagocytophilum* infection. *Infect. Immun.* 82, 2553–2564. doi: 10.1128/IAI.01679-14

Chen, N., Xu, S., Zhang, Y., and Wang, F. (2018). Animal protein toxins: origins and therapeutic applications. *Biophys. Rep.* 4, 233–242. doi: 10.1007/s41048-018-0067-x

Cherniack, P. E. (2010). Bugs as drugs, Part 1: insects. the "New" alternative medicine for the 21st century? *Altern. Med. Rev.* 15, 124–135. doi: 10.1128/ 9781555819705

Cherniack, P. E. (2011). Bugs as drugs, part two_ worms, leeches, scorpions, snails, ticks, centipedes, and spiders. *Altern. Med. Rev.* 16, 50–58.

Chmelar, J., Calvo, E., Pedra, J. H. F., Francischetti, I. M. B., and Kotsyfakis, M. (2012). Tick salivary secretion as a source of antihemostatics. *J. Proteomics* 75, 3842–3854. doi: 10.1016/j.jprot.2012.04.026

Chmelar, J., Kotál, J., Kopecký, J., Pedra, J. H. F., and Kotsyfakis, M. (2016). All for one and one for all on the tick-host battlefield. *Trends Parasitol.* 32, 368–377. doi: 10.1016/j.pt.2016.01.004

Chmelar, J., Kotál, J., Langhansová, H., and Kotsyfakis, M. (2017). Protease inhibitors in tick saliva: the role of serpins and cystatins in tick-host-pathogen interaction. *Front. Cell Infect. Microbiol.* 7:216. doi: 10.3389/fcimb.2017.00216

Chmelar, J., Oliveira, C. J., Rezacova, P., Francischetti, I. M. B., Kovarova, Z., Pejler, G., et al. (2011). A tick salivary protein targets cathepsin G and chymase and inhibits host inflammation and platelet aggregation. *Blood* 117, 736–744. doi: 10.1182/blood-2010-06-293241

Chudzinski-Tavassi, A. M., de-Sá-Júnior, P. L., Simons, S. M., Maria, D. A., de Souza Ventura, J., de Fatima Correia Batista, I., et al. (2010). A new tick Kunitz type inhibitor, Amblyomin-X, induces tumor cell death by modulating genes related to the cell cycle and targeting the ubiquitin-proteasome system. *Toxicon* 56, 1145–1154. doi: 10.1016/j.toxicon.2010.04.019

Chudzinski-Tavassi, A. M., Faria, F., and Alvarez Flores, M. P. (2018). "Anticoagulants from hematophagous," in *Anticoagulant Drugs*, ed. M. Božič-Mijovski (Rijeka: IntechOpen), doi: 10.5772/intechopen.78025

Chudzinski-Tavassi, A. M., Morais, K. L. P., Pacheco, M. T. F., Pasqualoto, K. F. M., and de Souza, J. G. (2016). Tick salivary gland as potential natural source for the discovery of promising antitumor drug candidates. *Biomed. Pharmacother.* 77, 14–19. doi: 10.1016/j.biopha.2015.11.003

Corral-Rodriguez, M. A., Macedo-Ribeiro, S., Pereira, P. J. B., and Fuentes-Prior, P. (2009). Tick-derived Kunitz-type inhibitors as antihemostatic factors. *Insect Biochem. Mol. Biol.* 39, 579–595. doi: 10.1016/j.ibmb.2009.07.003

Couillin, I., Maillet, I., Vargaftig, B. B., Jacobs, M., Paesen, G. C., Nuttall, P. A., et al. (2004). Arthropod-derived histamine-binding protein prevents murine allergic asthma. *J. Immunol.* 173, 3281–3286. doi: 10.4049/jimmunol.173.5.3281

Couvreur, B., Beaufays, J., Charon, C., Lahaye, K., Gensale, F., Denis, V., et al. (2008). Variability and action mechanism of a family of anticomplement proteins in *Ixodes ricinus*. *PLoS One* 3:e1400. doi: 10.1371/journal.pone. 0001400

Daix, V., Schroeder, H., Praet, N., Georgin, J. P., Chiappino, I., Gillet, L., et al. (2007). Ixodes ticks belonging to the *Ixodes ricinus* complex encode a family of anticomplement proteins. *Insect Mol. Biol.* 16, 155–166. doi: 10.1111/j.1365-2583.2006.00710.x

de Castro, M. H., de Klerk, D., Pienaar, R., Latif, A. A., Rees, D. J. G., and Mans, B. J. (2016). De novo assembly and annotation of the salivary gland transcriptome of *Rhipicephalus appendiculatus* male and female ticks during blood feeding. *Ticks Tick Borne Dis.* 7, 536–548. doi: 10.1016/j.ttbdis.2016.01.014

de Miranda Santos, I. K. F., Valenzuela, J. G., Ribeiro, J. M. C., de Castro, M. H., Costa, J. N., Costa, A. M., et al. (2004). Gene discovery in *Boophilus microplus*, the cattle tick: the transcriptomes of ovaries, salivary glands, and hemocytes. *Ann. N. Y. Acad. Sci.* 1026, 242–246. doi: 10.1196/annals.1307.037

de Oliveira, A. S., Lima, L. G., Mariano-Oliveira, A., Machado, D. E., Nasciutti, L. E., Andersen, J. F., et al. (2012). Inhibition of tissue factor by ixolaris reduces primary tumor growth and experimental metastasis in a murine model of melanoma. *Thromb. Res.* 130, 163–170. doi: 10.1016/j.thromres.2012.05.021

de Souza, J. G., Morais, K. L. P., Anglés-Cano, E., Boufleur, P., de Mello, E. S., Maria, D. A., et al. (2016). Promising pharmacological profile of a Kunitz-type inhibitor in murine renal cell carcinoma model. *Oncotarget* 7, 62255–62266. doi: 10.18632/oncotarget.11555

de Sá Jr, P. L., Camara, D. A. D., Sciani, J. M., Porcacchia, A. S., Fonseca, P. M. M., Mendonca, R. Z., et al. (2019). Antiproliferative and antiangiogenic effect of *Amblyomma sculptum* (Acari: Ixodidae) crude saliva in endothelial cells in vitro. *Biomed. Pharmacother.* 110, 353–361. doi: 10.1016/j.biopha.2018.11.107

Decrem, Y., Rath, G., Blasioli, V., Cauchie, P., Robert, S., Beaufays, J., et al. (2009). Ir-CPI, a coagulation contact phase inhibitor from the tick *Ixodes ricinus*, inhibits thrombus formation without impairing hemostasis. *J. Exp. Med.* 206, 2381–2395. doi: 10.1084/jem.20091007

Deruaz, M., Frauenschuh, A., Alessandri, A. L., Dias, J. M., Coelho, F. M., Russo, R. C., et al. (2008). Ticks produce highly selective chemokine binding proteins with antiinflammatory activity. *J. Exp. Med.* 205, 2019–2031. doi: 10.1084/jem. 20072689

Dinan, T. G. (1996). Serotonin: current understanding and the way forward. *Int. Clin. Psychopharmacol.* 11(Suppl. 1), 19–21.

Drewes, C. C., Dias, R. Y., Branco, V. G., Cavalcante, M. F., Souza, J. G., Abdalla, D. S. P., et al. (2015). Post-transcriptional control of Amblyomin-X on secretion of vascular endothelial growth factor and expression of adhesion molecules in endothelial cells. *Toxicon* 101, 1–10. doi: 10.1016/j.toxicon.2015.04.002

Drewes, C. C., Dias, R. Y., Hebeda, C. B., Simons, S. M., Barreto, S. A., Ferreira Junior, J. M., et al. (2012). Actions of the Kunitz-type serine protease inhibitor amblyomin-X on VEGF-A-induced angiogenesis. *Toxicon* 60, 333–340. doi: 10.1016/j.toxicon.2012.04.349

Duncan, R. C., Wijeyewickrema, L. C., and Pike, R. N. (2007). The initiating proteases of the complement system: controlling the cleavage. *Biochimie* 90, 387–395. doi: 10.1016/j.biochi.2007.07.023

Eaton, J. R. O., Alenazi, Y., Singh, K., Davies, G., Geis-Asteggiante, L., Kessler, B., et al. (2018). The N-terminal domain of a tick evasin is critical for chemokine binding and neutralization and confers specific binding activity to other evasins. *J. Biol. Chem.* 293, 6134–6146. doi: 10.1074/jbc.RA117.000487

Efferth, T., Rauh, R., Kahl, S., Tomicic, M., Bochzelt, H., Tome, M. E., et al. (2005). Molecular modes of action of cantharidin in tumor cells. *Biochem. Pharmacol.* 69, 811–818. doi: 10.1016/j.bcp.2004.12.003

El-behi, M., Rostami, A., and Ciric, B. (2010). Current views on the roles ofTh1 and Th17 cells in experimental autoimmune encephalomyelitis. *J. Neuroimmune Pharmacol.* 5, 189–197. doi: 10.1007/s11481-009-9188-9189

Eldor, A., Orevi, M., and Rigbi, M. (1996). The role of the leech in medical therapeutics. *Blood Rev.* 10, 201–209. doi: 10.1016/s0268-960x(96)90000-4

Esteves, E., Maruyama, S. R., Kawahara, R., Fujita, A., Martins, L. A., Righi, A. A., et al. (2017). Analysis of the salivary gland transcriptome of unfed, and partially fed *Amblyomma sculptum* ticks, and descriptive proteome of the saliva. *Front. Cell Infect. Microbiol.* 7:476. doi: 10.3389/fcimb.2017.00476

Ferrara, J. L., and Deeg, H. J. (1991). Graft-versus-host disease. *N. Engl. J. Med.* 324, 667–674.

Figueiredo, A. C., de Sanctis, D., and Pereira, P. J. B. (2013). The tick-derived anticoagulant madanin is processed by thrombin and factor Xa. *PLoS One* 8:e71866. doi: 10.1371/journal.pone.0071866

Francischetti, I. M. B. (2010). Platelet aggregation inhibitors from hematophagous animals. *Toxicon* 56, 1130–1144. doi: 10.1016/j.toxicon.2009.12.003

Francischetti, I. M. B., Anderson, J. M., Manoukis, N., Pham, V. M., and Ribeiro, J. M. C. (2011). An insight into the sialotranscriptome and proteome of the coarse bontlegged tick, *Hyalomma marginatum rufipes*. *J. Proteomics* 74, 2892–2908. doi: 10.1016/j.jprot.2011.07.015

Francischetti, I. M. B., Mather, T. N., and Ribeiro, J. M. C. (2004). Penthalaris, a novel recombinant five-Kunitz tissue factor pathway inhibitor (TFPI) from the salivary gland of the tick vector of Lyme disease, *Ixodes scapularis*. *Thromb. Haemost.* 91, 886–898. doi: 10.1160/TH03-11-0715

Francischetti, I. M. B., Pham, V. M., Mans, B. J., Andersen, J. F., Mather, T. N., Lane, R. S., et al. (2005). The transcriptome of the salivary glands of the female western black-legged tick *Ixodes pacificus* (Acari: Ixodidae). *Insect Biochem. Mol. Biol.* 35, 1142–1161. doi: 10.1016/j.ibmb.2005.05.007

Francischetti, I. M. B., Sa-Nunes, A., Mans, B. J., Santos, I. M., and Ribeiro, J. M. C. (2009). The role of saliva in tick feeding. *Front. Biosci.* 14, 2051–2088.

Francischetti, I. M. B., Valenzuela, J. G., Andersen, J. F., Mather, T. N., and Ribeiro, J. M. C. (2002). Ixolaris, a novel recombinant tissue factor pathway inhibitor (TFPI) from the salivary gland of the tick, *Ixodes scapularis*: identification of factor X and factor Xa as scaffolds for the inhibition of factor VIIa/tissue factor complex. *Blood* 99, 3602–3612. doi: 10.1182/blood-2001-12-0237

Frauenschuh, A., Power, C. A., Deruaz, M., Ferreira, B. R., Silva, J. S., Teixeira, M. M., et al. (2007). Molecular cloning and characterization of a highly selective chemokine-binding protein from the tick *Rhipicephalus sanguineus*. *J. Biol. Chem.* 282, 27250–27258. doi: 10.1074/jbc.m704706200

Fredslund, F., Laursen, N. S., Roversi, P., Jenner, L., Oliveira, C. L., Pedersen, J. S., et al. (2008). Structure of and influence of a tick complement inhibitor on human complement component 5. *Nat. Immunol.* 9, 753–760. doi: 10.1038/ni.1625

Funderburg, N. T., and Lederman, M. M. (2014). Coagulation and morbidity in treated HIV infection. *Thromb. Res.* 133(Suppl. 1), S21–S24. doi: 10.1016/j.thromres.2014.03.012

Garcia, G. R., Gardinassi, L. G., Ribeiro, J. M. C., Anatriello, E., Ferreira, B. R., Moreira, H. N. S., et al. (2014). The sialotranscriptome of *Amblyomma triste*, *Amblyomma parvum* and *Amblyomma cajennense* ticks, uncovered by 454-based RNA-seq. *Parasit. Vectors* 7:430. doi: 10.1186/1756-3305-7-430

Garg, R., Juncadella, I. J., Ramamoorthi, N., Ashish, Ananthanarayanan, S. K., Thomas, V., et al. (2014). Cutting edge: CD4 is the receptor for the tick saliva immunosuppressor, Salp15. *J. Immunol.* 177, 6579–6583. doi: 10.4049/jimmunol.177.10.6579

Gradowski do Nascimento, T., Santos Vieira, P., Campos Cogo, S., Ferreira Dias-Netipanyj, M., de França, F., Dias Câmara, D. A., et al. (2019). Antitumoral effects of *Amblyomma sculptum* berlese saliva in neuroblastoma cell lines involve cytoskeletal deconstruction and cell cycle arrest. *Braz. J. Vet. Parasitol.* 28, 126–133. doi: 10.1590/S1984-296120180098

Hajnická, V., Kocáková, P., Slávíková, M., Slovák, M., Gašperík, J., Fuchsberger, N., et al. (2001). Anti-interleukin-8 activity of tick salivary gland extracts. *Parasite Immunol.* 23, 483–489. doi: 10.1046/j.1365-3024.2001.00403.x

Hajnicka, V., Vancova, I., Kocakova, P., Slovak, M., Gasperik, J., Slavikova, M., et al. (2005). Manipulation of host cytokine network by ticks: a potential gateway for pathogen transmission. *Parasitology* 130, 333–342. doi: 10.1017/s0031182004006535

Hajnicka, V., Vancova-Stibraniova, I., Slovak, M., Kocakova, P., and Nuttall, P. A. (2011). Ixodid tick salivary gland products target host wound healing growth factors. *Int. J. Parasitol.* 41, 213–223. doi: 10.1016/j.ijpara.2010.09.005

Harris, C. L. (2018). Expanding horizons in complement drug discovery: challenges and emerging strategies. *Semin. Immunopathol.* 40, 125–140. doi: 10.1007/s00281-017-0655-658

Hashemzadeh, M., Furukawa, M., Goldsberry, S., and Movahed, M. R. (2008). Chemical structures and mode of action of intravenous glycoprotein IIb/IIIa receptor blockers: a review. *Exp. Clin. Cardiol.* 13, 192–197.

Hayward, J., Sanchez, J., Perry, A., Huang, C., Rodriguez Valle, M., Canals, M., et al. (2017). Ticks from diverse genera encode chemokine-inhibitory evasin proteins. *J. Biol. Chem.* 292, 15670–15680. doi: 10.1074/jbc.M117.807255

Hepburn, N. J., Williams, A. S., Nunn, M. A., Chamberlain-Banoub, J. C., Hamer, J., Morgan, B. P., et al. (2007). *In Vivo* characterization and therapeutic efficacy of a C5-specific inhibitor from the soft tick *Ornithodoros moubata*. J. Biol. Chem. 282, 8292–8299. doi: 10.1074/jbc.m609858200

Hesketh, P. J. (2004). Understanding the pathobiology of chemotherapy induced nausea and vomiting. Providing a basis for therapeutic progress. *Oncology* 18(10 Suppl. 6), 9–14.

Hoffman, R., Benz, E. J., Furie, B., and Shattil, S. J. (2009). *Hematology: Basic Principles and Practice*. California, CA: Churchill Livingstone.

Holíková, V., Štibrániová, I., Bartíková, P., Slovák, M., and Kazimírová, M. (2018). Ixodid tick salivary gland extracts suppress human transforming growth factor-β1 triggered signalling pathways in cervical carcinoma cells. *Biologia* 73, 1109–1122. doi: 10.2478/s11756-018-0129-z

Horka, H., Staudt, V., Klein, M., Taube, C., Reuter, S., Dehzad, N., et al. (2012). The tick salivary protein sialostatin L inhibits the Th9-derived production of the asthma-promoting cytokine IL-9 and is effective in the prevention of experimental asthma. *J. Immunol.* 188, 2669–2676. doi: 10.4049/jimmunol.1100529

Hourcade, D. E., Akk, A. M., Mitchell, L. M., Zhou, H. F., Hauhart, R., and Pham, C. T. (2016). Anti-complement activity of the *Ixodes scapularis* salivary protein Salp20. *Mol. Immunol.* 69, 62–69. doi: 10.1016/j.molimm.2015.11.008

Hovius, J. W. R., Levi, M., and Fikrig, E. (2008). Salivating for knowledge: potential pharmacological agents in tick saliva. *PLoS Med.* 5:e43. doi: 10.1371/journal.pmed.0050043

Iqbal, A., Goldfeder, M. B., Marques-Porto, R., Asif, H., de Souza, J. G., Faria, F., et al. (2017). Revisiting antithrombotic therapeutics; sculptin, a novel specific, competitive, reversible, scissile and tight binding inhibitor of thrombin. *Sci. Rep.* 7:1431. doi: 10.1038/s41598-017-01486-w

Islam, M. K., Tsuji, N., Miyoshi, T., Alim, M. A., Huang, X., Hatta, T., et al. (2009). The Kunitz-like modulatory protein haemangin is vital for hard tick blood-feeding success. *PLoS Pathog.* 5:e1000497. doi: 10.1371/journal.ppat.1000497

Iwanaga, S., Okada, M., Isawa, H., Morita, A., Yuda, M., and Chinzei, Y. (2003). Identification and characterization of novel salivary thrombin inhibitors from the ixodidae tick, *Haemaphysalis longicornis*. *Eur. J. Biochem.* 270, 1926–1934. doi: 10.1046/j.1432-1033.2003.03560.x

Iyer, J. K., Koh, C. Y., Kazimirova, M., Roller, L., Jobichen, C., Swaminathan, K., et al. (2017). Avathrin: a novel thrombin inhibitor derived from a multicopy precursor in the salivary glands of the ixodid tick, *Amblyomma variegatum*. *FASEB J.* 31, 2981–2995. doi: 10.1096/fj.201601216R

Iyer, J. K., Koh, C. Y., Kini, R. M., Kazimirova, M., and Roller, L. (2019). *Novel Thrombin Inhibitors*. U.S. Patent No 15/737,266. Washington, DC: U.S. Patent and Trademark Office.

Jablonka, W., Kotsyfakis, M., Mizurini, D. M., Monteiro, R. Q., Lukszo, J., Drake, S. K., et al. (2015). Identification and mechanistic analysis of a novel tick-derived inhibitor of thrombin. *PLoS One* 10:e0133991. doi: 10.1371/journal.pone.0133991

Juncadella, I. J., Bates, T. C., Suleiman, R., Monteagudo-Mera, A., Olson, C. M., Navasa, N., et al. (2010). The tick saliva immunosuppressor, Salp15, contributes to Th17-induced pathology during experimental autoimmune encephalomyelitis. *Biochem. Biophys. Res. Commun.* 402, 105–109. doi: 10.1016/j.bbrc.2010.09.125

Juncadella, I. C., Garg, R., Ananthnarayanan, S. K., Yengo, C. M., and Anguita, J. (2007). T-cell signaling pathways inhibited by the tick saliva immunosuppressor, Salp15. *FEMS Immunol. Med. Microbiol.* 49, 433–438. doi: 10.1111/j.1574-695X.2007.00223.x

Karczewski, J., Endris, R., and Connolly, T. M. (1994). Disagregin is a fibrinogen receptor antagonist lacking the Arg-Gly-Asp sequence from the tick, *Ornithodoros moubata*. *J. Biol. Chem.* 269, 6702–6708.

Kazimírová, M. (2011). "Pharmacologically active compounds from ticks and other arthropods and their potential use in anticancer therapy" Chapter 3," in *Natural Compounds as Inducers of Cell Death*, Vol. 1, eds M. Diederich and K. Noworyta (Dordrecht: Springer Science+Business Media), 163–182. doi: 10.1007/978-94-007-4575-9_7

Kazimirova, M., Dovinova, I., Rolnikova, T., Tothova, L., and Hunakova, L. (2006). Antiproliferative activity and apoptotic effect of tick salivary gland extracts on human HeLa cells. *Neuro Endocrinol. Lett.* 27(Suppl. 2), 48–52.

Kazimírová, M., Kini, M., and Koh, Y. (2015). *Thrombin Inhibitor*. U.S. Patent No 9,217,027 B2. Washington, DC: U.S. Patent and Trademark Office.

Kazimírová, M., Koh, C. Y., and Kini, R. M. (2010). "Tiny ticks are vast sources of antihaemostatic factors," in *Toxins and Hemostasis*, eds R. Kini, K. Clemetson, F. Markland, M. McLane, and T. Morita (Dordrecht: Springer), 113–130. doi: 10.1007/978-90-481-9295-3_8

Kazimírová, M., and Štibrániová, I. (2013). Tick salivary compounds: their role in modulation of host defences and pathogen transmission. *Front. Cell Infect. Microbiol.* 3:43. doi: 10.3389/fcimb.2013.00043

Keller, P. M., Waxman, L., Arnold, B. A., Schultz, L. D., Condra, C., and Connolly, T. M. (1993). Cloning of the cDNA and expression of moubatin, an inhibitor of platelet-aggregation. *J. Biol. Chem.* 268, 5445–5449.

Klein, M., Brühl, T. J., Staudt, V., Reuter, S., Grebe, N., Gerlitzki, B., et al. (2015). Tick salivary sialostatin L represses the initiation of immune responses by targeting IRF4-dependent transcription in murine mast cells. *J. Immunol.* 195, 621–631. doi: 10.4049/jimmunol.1401823

Koh, C. Y., Kazimirova, M., Nuttall, P. A., and Kini, R. M. (2009). Noncompetitive inhibitor of thrombin. *Chem. Biol. Chem.* 10, 2155–2158. doi: 10.1002/cbic.200900371

Koh, C. Y., Kazimirova, M., Trimnell, A., Takac, P., Labuda, M., Nuttall, P. A., et al. (2007). Variegin, a novel fast and tight binding thrombin inhibitor from the tropical bont tick. *J. Biol. Chem.* 282, 29101–29113. doi: 10.1074/jbc.M705600200

Koh, C. Y., Kumar, S., Kazimirova, M., Nuttall, P. A., Radhakrishnan, U. P., Kim, S., et al. (2011). Crystal structure of thrombin in complex with S-variegin: insights of a novel mechanism of inhibition and design of tunable thrombin inhibitors. *PLoS One* 6:e26367. doi: 10.1371/journal.pone.0026367

Koh, C. Y., Modahl, C. M., Kulkarni, N., and Kini, R. (2018). Toxins are an excellent source of therapeutic agents against cardiovascular diseases. *Semin. Thromb. Hemost.* 44, 691–706. doi: 10.1055/s-0038-1661384

Kotal, J., Langhansova, H., Lieskovska, J., Andersen, J. F., Francischetti, I. M., Chavakis, T., et al. (2015). Modulation of host immunity by tick saliva. *J. Proteomics* 128, 58–68. doi: 10.1016/j.jprot.2015.07.005

Kotál, J., Stergiou, N., Buša, M., Chlastáková, A., Beránková, Z., Řezáčová, P., et al. (2019). The structure and function of Iristatin, a novel immunosuppressive tick salivary cystatin. *Cell Mol. Life Sci.* 76, 2003–2013. doi: 10.1007/s00018-019-03034-3033

Kotsyfakis, M., Horka, H., Salat, J., and Andersen, J. F. (2010). The crystal structures of two salivary cystatins from the tick *Ixodes scapularis* and the effect of these inhibitors on the establishment of *Borrelia burgdorferi* infection in a murine model. *Mol. Microbiol.* 77, 456–470. doi: 10.1111/j.1365-2958.2010.07220.x

Kotsyfakis, M., Karim, S., Andersen, J. F., Mather, T. N., and Ribeiro, J. M. C. (2007). Selective cysteine protease inhibition contributes to blood-feeding success of the tick *Ixodes scapularis*. *J. Biol. Chem.* 282, 29256–29263. doi: 10.1074/jbc.M703143200

Kotsyfakis, M., Sa-Nunes, A., Francischetti, I. M. B., Mather, T. N., Andersen, J. F., and Ribeiro, J. M. C. (2006). Antiinflammatory and immunosuppressive activity of sialostatin L, a salivary cystatin from the tick *Ixodes scapularis*. *J. Biol. Chem.* 281, 26298–26307. doi: 10.1074/jbc.M513010200

Kotsyfakis, M., Schwarz, A., Erhart, J., and Ribeiro, J. M. C. (2015). Tissue- and time-dependent transcription in *Ixodes ricinus* salivary glands and midguts when blood feeding on the vertebrate host. *Sci. Rep.* 5:9103. doi: 10.1038/srep09103

Kuhn, N., Schmidt, C. Q., Schlapschy, M., and Skerra, A. (2016). PASylated Coversin, a C5-specific complement inhibitor with extended pharmacokinetics, shows enhanced anti-hemolytic activity *in vitro*. *Bioconjugate Chem.* 27, 2359–2371. doi: 10.1021/acs.bioconjchem.6b00369

Leboulle, G., Crippa, M., Decrem, Y., Mejri, N., Brossard, M., Bollen, A., et al. (2002). Characterization of a novel salivary immunosuppressive protein from *Ixodes ricinus* ticks. *J. Biol. Chem.* 277, 10083–10089.

Lieskovská, J., Páleníková, J., Langhansová, H., Campos Chagas, A., Calvo, E., Kotsyfakis, M., et al. (2015a). Tick sialostatins L and L2 differentially influence dendritic cell responses to *Borrelia* spirochetes. *Parasit. Vectors* 8:275. doi: 10.1186/s13071-015-0887-1

Lieskovská, J., Palenikova, J., Sirmarová, J., Elsterová, J., Kotsyfakis, M., Campos Chagas, A., et al. (2015b). Tick salivary cystatin sialostatin L2 suppresses IFN responses in mouse dendritic cells. *Parasite Immunol.* 37, 70–78. doi: 10.1111/pim.12162

Lincoff, A. M., Bittl, J. A., Kleiman, N. S., Sarembock, I. J., Jackman, J. D., Mehta, S., et al. (2004). Comparison of bivalirudin versus heparin during percutaneous coronary intervention (the randomized evaluation of PCI linking angiomax to reduced clinical events [REPLACE]-1 trial). *Am. J. Cardiol.* 93, 1092–1096. doi: 10.1016/j.amjcard.2004.01.033

Liu, D., and Chen, Z. (2009). The effects of cantharidin and cantharidin derivates on tumour cells. *Anticancer Agents Med. Chem.* 9, 392–396. doi: 10.2174/187152061090904392

Liu, X. Y., and Bonnet, S. I. (2014). Hard tick factors implicated in pathogen transmission. *PLoS Negl. Trop. Dis.* 8:e2566. doi: 10.1371/journal.pntd.0002566

Liu, X. Y., de la Fuente, J., Cote, M., Galindo, R. C., Moutailler, S., Vayssier-Taussat, M., et al. (2014). IrSPI, a tick serine protease inhibitor involved in tick feeding and *Bartonella henselae* infection. *PLoS Negl. Trop. Dis.* 8:e2993. doi: 10.1371/journal.pntd.0002993

Lourenço, J. D., Neves, L. P., Olivo, C. R., Duran, A., Almeida, F. M., Arantes, P. M., et al. (2014). A treatment with a protease inhibitor recombinant from the cattle tick *Rhipicephalus (Boophilus) microplus* ameliorates emphysema in mice. *PLoS One* 9:e98216. doi: 10.1371/journal.pone.0098216

Mans, B. J. (2005). Tick histamine-binding proteins and related lipocalins: potential as therapeutic agents. *Curr. Opin. Investig. Drugs* 6, 1131–1135.

Mans, B. J. (2016). "Glandular matrices and secretions: Blood-feeding arthropods," in *Extracellular Composite Matrices in Arthropods*, eds E. Cohen and B. Moussian (Cham: Springer), 625–688. doi: 10.1007/978-3-319-40740-1_17

Mans, B. J., Louw, A. I., and Neitz, A. W. (2003). The major tick salivary gland proteins and toxins from the soft tick, *Ornithodoros savignyi*, are part of the tick lipocalin family: implications for the origins of tick toxicoses. *Mol. Biol. Evol.* 20, 1158–1167. doi: 10.1093/molbev/msg126

Mans, B. J., and Ribeiro, J. M. C. (2008). Function, mechanism and evolution of the moubatin-clade of soft tick lipocalins. *Insect Biochem. Mol. Biol.* 38, 841–852. doi: 10.1016/j.ibmb.2008.06.007

Mans, B. J., Ribeiro, J. M. C., and Andersen, J. F. (2008). Structure, function, and evolution of biogenic amine-binding proteins in soft ticks. *J. Biol. Chem.* 283, 18721–18733. doi: 10.1074/jbc.M800188200

Maria, D. A., de Souza, J. G., Morais, K. L. P., Berra, C. M., de Campos Zampoli, H., Demasi, M., et al. (2013). A novel proteasome inhibitor acting in mitochondrial dysfunction, ER stress and ROS production. *Invest. New Drugs* 31, 493–505. doi: 10.1007/s10637-012-9871-1

Maria, D. A., Will, S. E. A. L., Bosch, R. V., Souza, J. G., Sciani, J. M., Goldfeder, M. B., et al. (2019). Preclinical evaluation of Amblyomin-X, a Kunitz-type protease inhibitor with antitumor activity. *Toxicol. Rep.* 6, 51–63. doi: 10.1016/j.toxrep.2018.11.014

Maritz-Olivier, C., Stutzer, C., Jongejan, F., Neitz, A. W. H., and Gaspar, A. R. M. (2007). Tick anti-hemostatics: targets for future vaccines and therapeutics. *Trends Parasitol.* 23, 397–407. doi: 10.1016/j.pt.2007.07.005

Markwardt, F. (2002). Hirudin as alternative anticoagulant – a historical review. *Semin. Thromb. Hemost.* 28, 405–414. doi: 10.1055/s-2002-35292

Matthijs, M. J., Johnson, S., Sheppard, D., Barber, N. M., Li, Y. I., Nunn, M. A., et al. (2016). Structural basis for therapeutic inhibition of complement C5. *Nat. Struct. Mol. Biol.* 23, 378–386. doi: 10.1038/nsmb.3196

Michalsen, A., Moebus, S., Spahn, G., Esch, T., Langhorst, J., and Dobos, G. J. (2002). Leech therapy for symptomatic treatment of knee osteoarthritis: results and implications of a pilot study. *Altern. Ther. Health Med.* 8, 84–88.

Moed, L., Shwayder, T. A., and Chang, M. W. (2001). Cantharidin revisited: a blistering defense of an ancient medicine. *Arch. Dermatol.* 137, 1357–1360.

Mollnes, T. E., Song, W. C., and Lambris, J. D. (2002). Complement in inflammatory tissue damage and disease. *Trends Immunol.* 23, 61–64. doi: 10.1016/S1471-4906(01)02129-9

Montecucco, F., Mach, F., Lenglet, S., Vonlaufen, A., Gomes Quinderé, A. L., Pelli, G., et al. (2014). Treatment with evasin-3 abrogates neutrophil-mediated inflammation in mouse acute pancreatitis. *Eur. J. Clin. Invest.* 44, 940–950. doi: 10.1111/eci.12327

Monteiro, R. Q., Rezaie, A. R., Ribeiro, J. M. C., and Francischetti, I. M. B. (2005). Ixolaris: a factor Xa heparin-binding exosite inhibitor. *Biochem. J.* 387, 871–877. doi: 10.1042/BJ20041738

Morais, K. L. P., Pasqualoto, K. F. M., Pacheco, M. T. F., Berra, C. M., Alvarez-Flores, M. P., and Chudzinski-Tavassi, A. M. (2014). Rational development of a novel TFPI-like inhibitor from *Amblyomma cajennense* tick. *Toxin Rev.* 33, 48–52. doi: 10.3109/15569543.2013.845217

Murfin, K. E., and Fikrig, E. (2017). Tick bioactive molecules as novel therapeutics: beyond vaccine targets. *Front. Cell Infect. Microbiol.* 7:222. doi: 10.3389/fcimb.2017.00222

Narasimhan, S., Koski, R. A., Beaulieu, B., Anderson, J. F., Ramamoorthi, N., Kantor, F., et al. (2002). A novel family of anticoagulants from the saliva of *Ixodes scapularis*. *Insect Mol. Biol.* 11, 641–650. doi: 10.1046/j.1365-2583.2002.00375.x

Nazareth, R. A., Tomaz, L. S., Ortiz-Costa, S., Atella, G. C., Ribeiro, J. M. C., Francischetti, I. M., et al. (2006). Antithrombotic properties of Ixolaris, a potent inhibitor of the extrinsic pathway of the coagulation cascade. *Thromb. Haemost.* 96, 7–13. doi: 10.1160/TH06-02-0105

Neeper, M. P., Waxman, L., Smith, D. E., Schulman, C. A., Sardana, M., Ellis, R. W., et al. (1990). Characterization of recombinant tick anticoagulant peptide. A highly selective inhibitor of blood coagulation factor Xa. *J. Biol. Chem.* 265, 17746–17752.

Nunn, M. A., Sharma, A., Paesen, G. C., Adamson, S., Lissina, O., Willis, A. C., et al. (2005). Complement inhibitor of C5 activation from the soft tick *Ornithodoros moubata*. *J. Immunol.* 174, 2084–2091. doi: 10.4049/jimmunol.174.4.2084

Nuttall, P. A. (2018). Wonders of tick saliva. *Ticks Tick Borne Dis.* 10, 470–481. doi: 10.1016/j.ttbdis.2018.11.005

Nuttall, P. A., and Paesen, G. C. (2001a). *Treatment of Allergic Rhinitis. WO-*00116164 (2001). South Oak Way Green Park: Evolutec LTD.

Nuttall, P. A., and Paesen, G. C. (2001b). *Treatment of Conjunctivitis. WO-*00115719 (2001). South Oak Way Green Park: Evolutec LTD.

Pacheco, M. T., Berra, C. M., Morais, K. L., Sciani, J. M., Branco, V. G., Bosch, R. V., et al. (2014). Dynein function and protein clearance changes in tumor cells induced by a Kunitz-type molecule, Amblyomin-X. *PLoS One* 9:e111907. doi: 10.1371/journal.pone.0111907

Paesen, G. C., Adams, P. L., Harlos, K., Nuttall, P. A., and Stuart, D. I. (1999). Tick histamine-binding proteins: isolation, cloning, and three-dimensional structure. *Mol. Cell* 3, 661–671. doi: 10.1016/S1097-2765(00)80359-80357

Paesen, G. C., Adams, P. L., Nuttall, P. A., and Stuart, D. I. (2000). Tick histamine-binding proteins: lipocalins with a second binding cavity. *Biochim. Biophys. Acta* 1482, 92–101. doi: 10.1016/s0167-4838(00)00168-0

Paesen, G. C., Siebold, C., Harlos, K., Peacey, M. F., Nuttall, P. A., and Stuart, D. I. (2007). A tick protein with a modified Kunitz fold inhibits human tryptase. *J. Mol. Biol.* 368, 1172–1186. doi: 10.1016/j.jmb.2007.03.011

Palenikova, J., Lieskovska, J., Langhansova, H., Kotsyfakis, M., Chmelar, J., and Kopecky, J. (2015). *Ixodes ricinus* salivary serpin IRS-2 affects Th17 differentiation via inhibition of the interleukin-6/STAT-3 signaling pathway. *Infect Immun.* 83, 1949–1956. doi: 10.1128/IAI.03065-14

Parizi, L. F., Ali, A., Tirloni, L., Oldiges, D. P., Sabadin, G. A., Coutinho, M. L., et al. (2018). Peptidase inhibitors in tick physiology. *Med. Vet. Entomol.* 32, 129–144. doi: 10.1111/mve.12276

Paveglio, S. A., Allard, J., Mayette, J., Whittaker, L. A., Juncadella, I., Anguita, J., et al. (2007). The tick salivary protein, Salp15, inhibits the development of experimental asthma. *J. Immunol.* 178, 7064–7071. doi: 10.4049/jimmunol.178.11.7064

Pemberton, R. W. (1999). Insects and other arthropods used as drugs in Korean traditional medicine. *J. Ethnopharmacol.* 65, 207–216. doi: 10.1016/s0378-8741(98)00209-8

Peterková, K., Vančová, I., Hajnická, V., Slovák, M., Šimo, L., and Nuttall, P. A. (2008). Immunomodulatory arsenal of nymphal ticks. *Med. Vet. Entomol.* 22, 167–171. doi: 10.1111/j.1365-2915.2008.00726.x

Poole, N. M., Nyindodo-Ogari, L., Kramer, C., Coons, L. B., and Cole, J. A. (2013). Effects of tick saliva on the migratory and invasive activity of Saos-2 osteosarcoma and MDAMB-231 breast cancer cells. *Ticks Tick Borne Dis.* 4, 120–127. doi: 10.1016/j.ttbdis.2012.09.003

Preston, S. G., Majtán, J., Kouremenou, C., Rysnik, O., Burger, L. F., Cabezas Cruz, A., et al. (2013). Novel immunomodulators from hard ticks selectively reprogramme human dendritic cell Responses. *PLoS Pathog.* 9:e1003450. doi: 10.1371/journal.ppat.1003450

Prevot, P. P., Adam, B., Boudjeltia, K. Z., Brossard, M., Lins, L., Cauchie, P., et al. (2006). Anti-hemostatic effects of a serpin from the saliva of the tick *Ixodes ricinus*. *J. Biol. Chem.* 281, 26361–26369. doi: 10.1074/jbc.M604197200

Prevot, P. P., Beschin, A., Lins, L., Beaufays, J., Grosjean, A., Bruys, L., et al. (2009). Exosites mediate the anti-inflammatory effects of a multifunctional serpin from the saliva of the tick ixodes ricinus. *FEBS J.* 276, 3235–3246. doi: 10.1111/j.1742-4658.2009.07038.x

Radulovič, Ž. M., Kim, T. K., Porter, L. M., Sze, S.-H., Lewis, L., and Mulenga, A. (2014). A 24-48 h fed *Amblyomma americanum* tick saliva immuno-proteome. *BMC Genomics* 15:518. doi: 10.1186/1471-2164-15-518

Ratcliffe, N., Azambuja, P., and Mello, C. B. (2014). Recent advances in developing insect natural products as potential modern day medicines. *Evid. Based Complement. Alternat. Med.* 2014:904958. doi: 10.1155/2014/904958

Ribeiro, J. M. C., Alarcon-Chaidez, F., Francischetti, I. M., Mans, B. J., Mather, T. N., Valenzuela, J. G., et al. (2006). An annotated catalog of salivary gland transcripts from *Ixodes scapularis* ticks. *Insect Biochem. Mol. Biol.* 36, 111–129. doi: 10.1016/j.ibmb.2005.11.005

Roversi, P., Johnson, S., Preston, S. G., Nunn, M. A., Paesen, G. C., Austyn, J. M., et al. (2017). Structural basis of cholesterol binding by a novel clade of dendritic cell modulators from ticks. *Sci. Rep.* 7:16057. doi: 10.1038/s41598-017-16413-2

Roversi, P., Lissina, O., Johnson, S., Ahmat, N., Paesen, G. C., Ploss, K., et al. (2007). The structure of OMCI, a novel lipocalin inhibitor of the complement system. *J. Mol. Biol.* 369, 784–793. doi: 10.1016/j.jmb.2007.03.064

Russo, R. C., Alessandri, A. L., Garcia, C. C., Cordeiro, B. F., Pinho, V., Cassali, G. D., et al. (2011). Therapeutic effects of evasin-1, a chemokine binding protein, in bleomy-cin-induced pulmonary fibrosis. *Am. J. Respir. Cell. Mol. Biol.* 45, 72–80. doi: 10.1165/rcmb.2009-0406OC

Sangamnatdej, S., Paesen, G. C., and Slovak, M. (2002). A high affinity serotonin- and histamine-binding lipocalin from tick saliva. *Insect Mol. Biol.* 11, 79–86. doi: 10.1046/j.0962-1075.2001.00311.x

Sa-Nunes, A., Bafica, A., Antonelli, L. R., Choi, E. Y., Francischetti, I. M. B., Andersen, J. F., et al. (2009). The immunomodulatory action of sialostatin L on dendritic cells reveals its potential to interfere with autoimmunity. *J. Immunol.* 182, 7422–7429. doi: 10.4049/jimmunol.0900075

Schaffer, L. W., Davidson, J. T., Vlasuk, G. P., and Siegl, P. K. S. (1991). Antithrombotic efficacy of recombinant tick anticoagulant peptide. A potent inhibitor of coagulation factor Xa in a primate model of arterial thrombosis. *Circulation* 84, 1741–1748. doi: 10.1161/01.CIR.84.4.1741

Schechter, M. E., Andrade, B. B., He, T., Richter, G. H., Tosh, K. W., Policicchio, B. B., et al. (2017). Inflammatory monocytes expressing tissue factor drive SIV and HIV coagulopathy. *Sci. Transl. Med.* 9, 1–14. doi: 10.1126/scitranslmed.aam5441

Schlehuber, S., and Skerra, A. (2005). Lipocalins in drug discovery: from natural ligand-binding proteins to "anticalins". *Drug Discov. Today* 10, 23–33. doi: 10.1016/S1359-6446(04)03294-3295

Schmidt, M. C. B., Morais, K. L. P., Almeida, M. E. S., Iqbal, A., Goldfeder, M. B., and Chudzinski-Tavassi, A. M. (2018). Amblyomin-X, a recombinant Kunitz-type inhibitor, regulates cell adhesion and migration of human tumor cells. *Cell Adh. Migr.* 25, 1–10. doi: 10.1080/19336918.2018.1516982

Schnirer, I. I., Yao, J. C., and Ajani, J. A. (2003). Carcinoid - a comprehensive review. *Acta Oncol.* 42, 672–692. doi: 10.1080/02841860310010547

Schuijt, T. J., Bakhtiari, K., Daffre, S., Deponte, K., Wielders, S. J. H., Marquart, J. A., et al. (2013). Factor XA activation of factor V is of paramount importance in initiating the coagulation system: lessons from a tick salivary protein. *Circulation* 128, 254–266. doi: 10.1161/CIRCULATIONAHA.113.003191

Schuijt, T. J., Narasimhan, S., Daffre, S., Deponte, K., Hovius, J. W., Veer, C. V., et al. (2011). Identification and characterization of *Ixodes scapularis* antigens that elicit tick immunity using yeast surface display. *PLoS One* 6:e15926. doi: 0.1371/journal.pone.0015926

Schwarz, A., Valdés, J. J., and Kotsyfakis, M. (2012). The role of cystatins in tick physiology and blood feeding. *Ticks Tick Borne Dis.* 3, 117–127. doi: 10.1016/j.ttbdis.2012.03.004

Šimo, L., Kazimirova, M., Richardson, J., and Bonnet, S. I. (2017). The essential role of tick salivary glands and saliva in tick feeding and pathogen transmission. *Front. Cell Infect. Microbiol.* 7:281. doi: 10.3389/fcimb.2017.00281

Simons, S. M., de Júnior, P. L., Faria, F., Batista, I. D., Barros-Battesti, D. M., Labruna, M. B., et al. (2011). The action of *Amblyomma cajennense* tick saliva in compounds of the hemostatic system and cytotoxicity in tumor cell lines. *Biomed. Pharmacother.* 65, 443–450. doi: 10.1016/j.biopha.2011.04.030

Singh, K., Davies, G., Alenazi, Y., Eaton, J. R. O., Kawamura, A., and Bhattacharya, S. (2017). Yeast surface display identifies a family of evasins from ticks with novel polyvalent CC chemokine-binding activities. *Sci. Rep.* 7:4267. doi: 10.1038/s41598-017-04378-4371

Slovák, M., Štibrániová, I., Hajnická, V., and Nuttall, P. A. (2014). Antiplatelet-derived growth factor (PDGF) activity in the saliva of ixodid ticks is linked with their long mouthparts. *Parasite Immunol.* 36, 32–42. doi: 10.1111/pim.12075

Soares, T. S., Oliveira, F., Torquato, R. J. S., Sasaki, S. D., Araujo, M. S., Paschoalin, T., et al. (2016). BmTI-A, a Kunitz type inhibitor from *Rhipicephalus microplus* able to interfere in vessel formation. *Vet. Parasitol.* 219, 44–52. doi: 10.1016/j.vetpar.2016.01.021

Soltys, J., Kusner, L. L., Young, A., Richmonds, C., Hatala, D., Gong, B., et al. (2009). Novel complement inhibitor limits severity of experimentally myasthenia gravis. *Ann. Neurol.* 65, 67–75. doi: 10.1002/ana.21536

Sommerhoff, C. P., and Schaschke, N. (2007). Mast cell tryptase beta as a target in allergic inflammation: an evolving story. *Curr. Pharm. Des.* 13, 313–332. doi: 10.2174/138161207779313579

Sousa, A. C. P., Oliviera, C. J. F., Szabó, M. P. J., and Silva, M. J. B. (2018). Anti-neoplastic activity of *Amblyomma sculptum*, *Amblyomma parvum* and *Rhipicephalus sanguineus* tick saliva on brest tumor cell lines. *Toxicon* 148, 165–171. doi: 10.1016/j.toxicon.2018.04.024

Sousa, A. C. P., Szabó, M. P. J., Oliveira, C. J. F., and Silva, M. J. B. (2015). Exploring the anti-tumoral effects of tick saliva and derived components. *Toxicon.* 102, 69–73. doi: 10.1016/j.toxicon.2015.06.001

Spronk, H. M. H., de Jong, A. M., Crijns, H. J., Schotten, U., Van Gelder, I. C., and Ten Cate, H. (2014). Pleiotropic effects of factor Xa and thrombin: what to expect from novel anticoagulants. *Cardiovasc. Res.* 101, 344–351. doi: 10.1093/cvr/cvt343

Štibrániová, I., Lahová, M., and Bartíková, P. (2013). Immunomodulators in tick saliva and their benefits. *Acta Virol.* 57, 200–216. doi: 10.4149/av_2013_02_200

Stoll, P., Bassler, N., Hagemeyer, C. E., Eisenhardt, S. U., Chen, Y. C., Schmidt, R., et al. (2007). Targeting ligand-induced binding sites on GPIIb/IIIa via single-chain antibody allows effective anticoagulation without bleeding time prolongation. *Arterioscler. Thromb. Vasc. Biol.* 27, 1206–1212. doi: 10.1161/ATVBAHA.106.138875

Stone, G. W., McLaurin, B. T., Cox, D. A., Bertrand, M. E., Lincoff, A. M., Moses, J. W., et al. (2006). Bivalirudin for patients with acute coronary syndromes. *New Engl. J. Med.* 355, 2203–2216. doi: 10.1056/NEJMoa062437

Sun, T., Wang, F., Pan, W., Wu, Q., Wang, J., and Dai, J. (2018). An immunosuppressive tick salivary gland protein DsCystatin interferes with toll-like receptor signaling by downregulating TRAF6. *Front. Immunol.* 9:1245. doi: 10.3389/fimmu.2018.01245

Suppan, J., Engel, B., Marchetti-Deschmann, M., and Nürnberger, S. (2018). Tick attachment cement - reviewing the mysteries of a biological skin plug system. *Biol. Rev.* 93, 1056–1076. doi: 10.1111/brv.12384

Tambourgi, D. V., and van den Berg, C. W. (2014). Animal venoms/toxins and the complement system. *Mol. Immunol.* 61, 153–162. doi: 10.1016/j.molimm.2014.06.020

Tan, A. W. L., Francischetti, I. M. B., Slovak, M., Kini, R. M., and Ribeiro, J. M. C. (2015). Sexual differences in the sialomes of the zebra tick, *Rhipicephalus pulchellus*. *J. Proteomics* 117, 120–144. doi: 10.1016/j.jprot.2014.12.014

Tanaka, A. S., Andreotti, R., Gomes, A., Torquato, R. J., Sampaio, M. U., and Sampaio, C. A. (1999). A double headed serine proteinase inhibitor–human plasma kallikrein and elastase inhibitor–from *Boophilus microplus* larvae. *Immunopharmacology* 45, 171–177. doi: 10.1016/s0162-3109(99)00074-0

Tang, J., Fang, Y. Q., Han, Y. J., Bai, X. W., Yan, X. W., Zhang, Y., et al. (2015). YY-39, a tick anti-thrombosis peptide containing RGD domain. *Peptides* 68, 99–104. doi: 10.1016/j.peptides.2014.08.008

Thiel, S. (2007). Complement activating soluble pattern recognition molecules with collagen-like regions, mannan-binding lectin, ficolins and associated proteins. *Mol. Immunol.* 44, 3875–3888. doi: 10.1016/j.molimm.2007.06.005

Thompson, R. E., Liu, X., Ripoll-Rozada, J., Alonso-García, N., Parker, B. L., Pereira, P. J. B., et al. (2017). Tyrosine sulfation modulates activity of tick-derived thrombin inhibitors. *Nat. Chem.* 9, 909–917. doi: 10.1038/NCHEM.2744

Tian, Y., Yedid, G., Yan, X., Fang, M., Mo, G., Chen, R., et al. (2016). An immunosuppressant peptide from the hard tick *Amblyomma variegatum*. *Toxins* 8:133. doi: 10.3390/toxins8050133

Timp, J. F., Braekkan, S. K., Versteeg, H. H., and Cannegieter, S. C. (2013). Epidemiology of cancer-associated venous thrombosis. *Blood* 122, 1712–1723. doi: 10.1182/blood-2013-04-460121

Tomás-Cortázar, J., Martín-Ruiz, I., Barriales, D., Pascual-Itoiz, M. A., Gutiérrez de Juan, V., Caro-Maldonado, A., et al. (2017). The immunosuppressive effect of the tick protein, Salp15, is long-lasting and persists in a murine model of hematopoietic transplant. *Sci. Rep.* 7:10740. doi: 10.1038/s41598-017-11354-2

Tyson, K., Elkins, C., Patterson, H., Fikrig, E., and de Silva, A. (2007). Biochemical and functional characterization of Salp20, an *Ixodes scapularis* tick salivary protein that inhibits the complement pathway. *Insect Mol. Biol.* 16, 469–479. doi: 10.1111/j.1365-2583.2007.00742.x

Tyson, K. R., Elkins, C., and de Silva, A. M. (2008). A novel mechanism of complement inhi-bition unmasked by a tick salivary protein that binds to properdin. *J. Immunol.* 180, 3964–3968. doi: 10.4049/jimmunol.180.6.3964

Valdés, J. J., Schwarz, A., Cabeza de Vaca, I., Calvo, E., Pedra, J. H. F., Guallar, V., et al. (2013). Tryptogalinin is a tick kunitz serine protease inhibitor with a unique intrinsic disorder. *PLoS One* 8:e62562. doi: 10.1371/journal.pone.0062562

Vančová, I., Hajnická, V., Slovák, M., and Nuttall, P. A. (2010). Anti-chemokine activities of ixodid ticks depend on tick species, developmental stage, and duration of feeding. *Vet. Parasitol.* 167, 274–278. doi: 10.1016/j.vetpar.2009.09.029

Vančová, I., Slovák, M., Hajnická, V., Labuda, M., Simo, L., Peterková, K., et al. (2007). Differential anti-chemokine activity of *Amblyomma variegatum* adult ticks during blood-feeding. *Parasite Immunol.* 29, 169–177. doi: 10.1111/j.1365-3024.2006.00931.x

Valenzuela, J. G. (2002). High-throughput approaches to study salivary proteins and genes from vectors of disease. *Insect Biochem. Mol. Biol.* 32, 1199–1209. doi: 10.1016/S0965-1748(02)00083-88

Valenzuela, J. G., Charlab, R., Mather, T. N., and Ribeiro, J. M. C. (2000). Purification, cloning, and expression of a novel salivary anticomplement protein from the tick, Ixodes scapularis. *J. Biol. Chem.* 275, 18717–18723. doi: 10.1074/jbc.m001486200

van der Locht, A., Stubbs, M. T., Bode, W., Friedrich, T., Bollschweiler, C., Höffken, W., et al. (1996). The ornithodorin thrombin crystal structure, a key to the TAP enigma? *EMBO J.* 15, 6011–6017. doi: 10.1002/j.1460-2075.1996.tb00989.x

Ventura, J. S., Faria, F., Batista, I. F., Simons, S. M., Oliveira, D. G., Morais, K. L., et al. (2013). A Kunitz-type FXa inhibitor affects tumor progression, hypercoagulable state and triggers apoptosis. *Biomed. Pharmacother.* 67, 192–196. doi: 10.1016/j.biopha.2012.11.009

Vieira, A. T., Fagundes, C. T., Alessandri, A. L., Castor, M. G., Guabiraba, R., Borges, V. O., et al. (2009). Treatment with a novel chemokine-binding protein or eosinophil lineage-ablation protects mice from experimental colitis. *Am. J. Pathol.* 175, 2382–2391. doi: 10.2353/ajpath.2009.090093

Wang, X., Coons, L. B., Taylor, D. B., Stevens, S. E., and Gartner, T. K. (1996). Variabilin, a novel RGD-containing antagonist of glycoprotein IIb-IIIa and platelet aggregation inhibitor from the hard tick *Dermacentor variabilis*. *J. Biol. Chem.* 271, 17785–17790. doi: 10.1074/jbc.271.30.17785

Wang, Y., Li, Z., Zhou, Y., Cao, J., Zhang, H., Gong, H., et al. (2016). Specific histamine binding activity of a new lipocalin from *Hyalomma asiaticum* (Ixodidae) and therapeutic effects on allergic asthma in mice. *Parasit. Vectors* 9:506. doi: 10.1186/s13071-016-1790-0

Waxman, L., and Connolly, T. M. (1993). Isolation of an inhibitor selective for collagen-stimulated platelet aggregation from the soft tick *Ornithodoros moubata*. *J. Biol. Chem.* 268, 5445–5449.

Waxman, L., Smith, D. E., Arcuri, K. E., and Vlasuk, G. P. (1990). Tick anticoagulant peptide (TAP) is a novel inhibitor of blood coagulation factor Xa. *Science* 248, 593–596. doi: 10.1126/science.2333510

Wei, A., Alexander, R. S., Duke, J., Ross, H., Rosenfeld, S. A., and Chang, C.-H. (1998). Unexpected binding mode of tick anticoagulant peptide complexed to bovine factor Xa. *J. Mol. Biol.* 283, 147–154. doi: 10.1006/jmbi.1998.2069

Weston-Davies, W. (2004). *Histamine Binding Compounds for Treatment Method for Disease Conditions Mediated by Neutrophils. WO*-2004087188 (2004). South Oak Way Green Park: Evolutec LTD.

Wikel, S. (2013). Ticks and tick-borne pathogens at the cutaneous interface: host defenses, tick countermeasures, and a suitable environment for pathogen establishment. *Front. Microbiol.* 4:337. doi: 10.3389/fmicb.2013.00337

Wikel, S. K. (2018). Tick-host-pathogen systems immunobiology: an interactive trio. *Front. Biosci.* 23, 265–283. doi: 10.2741/4590

Wolf, H., and Hansson, C. (2003). Larval therapy – an effective method of ulcer debridement. *Clin. Exp. Dermatol.* 28, 134–137. doi: 10.1046/j.1365-2230.2003.01226.x

Wu, J., Wang, Y., Liu, H., Yang, H., Ma, D., Li, J., et al. (2010). Two immunoregulatory peptides with antioxidant activity from tick salivary glands. *J. Biol. Chem.* 285, 16606–16613. doi: 10.1074/jbc.M109.094615

Xu, X.-L., Cheng, T.-Y., Yang, H., Yan, F., and Yang, Y. (2015). De novo sequencing, assembly and analysis of salivary gland transcriptome of *Haemaphysalis flava* and identification os sialoprotein genes. *Infect. Genet. Evol.* 32, 135–142. doi: 10.1016/j.meegid.2015.03.010

Yanan, W., Zhuang, L., Yongzhi, Z., Jie, C., Houshuang, Z., Haiyan, G., et al. (2016). Specific histamine binding activity of a new lipocalin from *Hyalomma asiaticum* (Ixodidae) and therapeutic effects on allergic asthma in mice. *Parasit. Vectors* 9:506. doi: 10.1186/s13071-016-1790-0

Yeh, C. H., Fredenburgh, J. C., and Weitz, J. I. (2012). Oral direct factor Xa inhibitors. *Circ. Res.* 111, 1069–1078. doi: 10.1161/CIRCRESAHA.112.276741

Yoshikai, Y. (2001). Roles of prostaglandins and leukotrienes in acute inflammation caused by bacterial infection. *Curr. Opin. Infect. Dis.* 14, 257–263. doi: 10.1097/00001432-200106000-00003

Yu, X., Gong, H., Zhou, Y., Zhang, H., Cao, J., and Zhou, J. (2015). Differential sialotranscriptomes of unfed and fed *Rhipicephalus haemaphysaloides*, with particular regard to differentially expressed genes of cysteine proteases. *Parasit. Vectors.* 8:597. doi: 10.1186/s13071-015-1213-7

Zipfel, P. F., Mihlan, M., and Skerka, C. (2007a). The alternative pathway of complement: a pattern recognition system. *Adv. Exp. Med. Biol.* 598, 80–92. doi: 10.1007/978-0-387-71767-8_7

Zipfel, P. F., Wurzner, R., and Skerka, C. (2007b). Complement evasion of pathogens: common strategies are shared by diverse organisms. *Mol. Immunol.* 44, 3850–3857. doi: 10.1016/j.molimm.2007.06.149

3

Tick Genome Assembled: New Opportunities for Research on Tick-Host-Pathogen Interactions

José de la Fuente[1,2]*, *Robert M. Waterhouse*[3,4,5,6], *Daniel E. Sonenshine*[7], *R. Michael Roe*[8], *Jose M. Ribeiro*[9], *David B. Sattelle*[10] *and Catherine A. Hill*[11]

[1] SaBio, Instituto de Investigación en Recursos Cinegéticos IREC-CSIC-UCLM-JCCM, Ciudad Real, Spain, [2] Department of Veterinary Pathobiology, Center for Veterinary Health Sciences, Oklahoma State University, Stillwater, OK, USA, [3] Department of Genetic Medicine and Development, University of Geneva Medical School, Geneva, Switzerland, [4] Swiss Institute of Bioinformatics, Geneva, Switzerland, [5] Computer Science and Artificial Intelligence Laboratory, Massachusetts Institute of Technology, Cambridge, MA, USA, [6] Broad Institute of MIT and Harvard, Cambridge, MA, USA, [7] Department of Biological Sciences, Old Dominion University, Norfolk, VA, USA, [8] Department of Entomology, North Carolina State University, Raleigh, NC, USA, [9] Laboratory of Malaria and Vector Research, National Institute of Allergy and Infectious Diseases, Rockville, MD, USA, [10] Division of Medicine, University College London, London, UK, [11] Department of Entomology, Purdue University, West Lafayette, IN, USA

***Correspondence:**
José de la Fuente
jose_delafuente@yahoo.com

As tick-borne diseases are on the rise, an international effort resulted in the sequence and assembly of the first genome of a tick vector. This result promotes research on comparative, functional and evolutionary genomics and the study of tick-host-pathogen interactions to improve human, animal and ecosystem health on a global scale.

Keywords: tick, *Ixodes scapularis*, genomics, proteomics, *Borrelia*, *Anaplasma*, evolution

TICK-BORNE DISEASES: A GROWING BURDEN FOR HUMAN AND ANIMAL HEALTH WORLDWIDE

Ticks are obligate blood-feeding arthropod ectoparasites that are distributed worldwide and one of the most important vectors of pathogens affecting humans and animals (Jongejan and Uilenberg, 2004; de la Fuente et al., 2008). Globally, emerging and re-emerging tick-borne diseases exert an enormous impact on public health (Jones et al., 2008). Urbanization, exploitation of environmental resources and outdoor recreational activities increase human contact with ticks and the transmission of tick-borne pathogens (Gortazar et al., 2014). In addition, tick populations are expanding due to changes in climate (Estrada-Peña et al., 2014) and new tick-borne diseases are emerging (Kosoy et al., 2015; Kernif et al., 2016). However, despite the growing burden that tick-borne diseases represent for human and animal health worldwide, the pace of research in this area has been restricted by the lack of access to a completed tick genome. The recent description of the first tick genome is therefore timely and a spur to future research (Gulia-Nuss et al., 2016).

THE FIRST TICK GENOME SEQUENCED AND ASSEMBLED: RESULTS AND POSSIBILITIES

More recently, a global consortium of 93 scientists described the 2.1 Gbp nuclear genome of the black-legged tick, *Ixodes scapularis* (Say) (Gulia-Nuss et al., 2016). This tick species is a vector of pathogens that cause, among others, the emerging diseases Lyme disease [Lyme borreliosis is the most common tick-borne disease in Europe and the U.S. (Centers for Disease Control and Prevention (CDC), 2016; European Centre for Disease Prevention and Control (ECDC), 2016)], human granulocytic anaplasmosis (HGA), babesiosis and tick-borne encephalitis (TBE)

(Wormser et al., 2006). The genome of *I. scapularis* Wikel strain was sequenced in a joint effort by the Broad Institute of MIT and Harvard and The J. Craig Venter Institute (JCVI) and funded by the National Institute of Allergy and Infectious Diseases, National Institutes of Health. Annotation for this assembly was produced in a joint effort between JCVI and VectorBase (https://www.vectorbase.org/) with support from The Broad Institute (Gulia-Nuss et al., 2016).

The *I. scapularis* project proved challenging due to the large size and high repeat content of the genome. However, the results show the assembly and description of features associated with ~57% of the genome. As the only assembly available for a tick, the *I. scapularis* genome constitutes an invaluable reference for comparative genomic analyses, including resolution of phylogenetic relationships within the diverse phylum Arthropoda. Analysis of the *I. scapularis* genome revealed new features that may be unique to this organism and with important implications for future research. Highlights include the identification of two new repeat elements, a large-scale gene duplication event that likely occurred ~40 MYA coinciding with tick radiation, gene exon-intron structures more closely resembling that of an ancient protostome/deuterostome ancestor than of extant arthropods examined to date, an expansion of Kunitz domain proteins and other proteins implicated in tick blood feeding, possible remnants of a heme synthesis pathway contrasting with an expansion of heme carrier and storage proteins. Also identified were orthologs for at least 39 invertebrate neuropeptides and neuropeptide receptor genes that are believed or known to regulate tick diuresis, ecdysis, cuticle synthesis, blood feeding and reproduction. The genome contains one of the largest expansions of cytochrome P450 genes known for sequenced arthropods, suggesting potential for rapid development of acaricide resistance in ticks, and it will be important to explore the families of candidate acaricide targets uncovered by genome analyses, the de-orphanisation of which is underway.

The first genome-wide population genomics study suggested genetic variation between ticks from Lyme prevalent northern and mid-western states compared with southern states in the U.S., paving the way for identification of genes tied to vector competence (Gulia-Nuss et al., 2016). The *I. scapularis* genome sequence and annotation also contributed to the characterization of the transcriptome in related tick species such as *I. ricinus* (Genomic Resources Development Consortium et al., 2014; Kotsyfakis et al., 2015), the main vector for tick-borne pathogens of public health importance in Europe. Additional studies that explore the biology of *I. scapularis* and other tick species, and extend genome analyses were described based on the publication

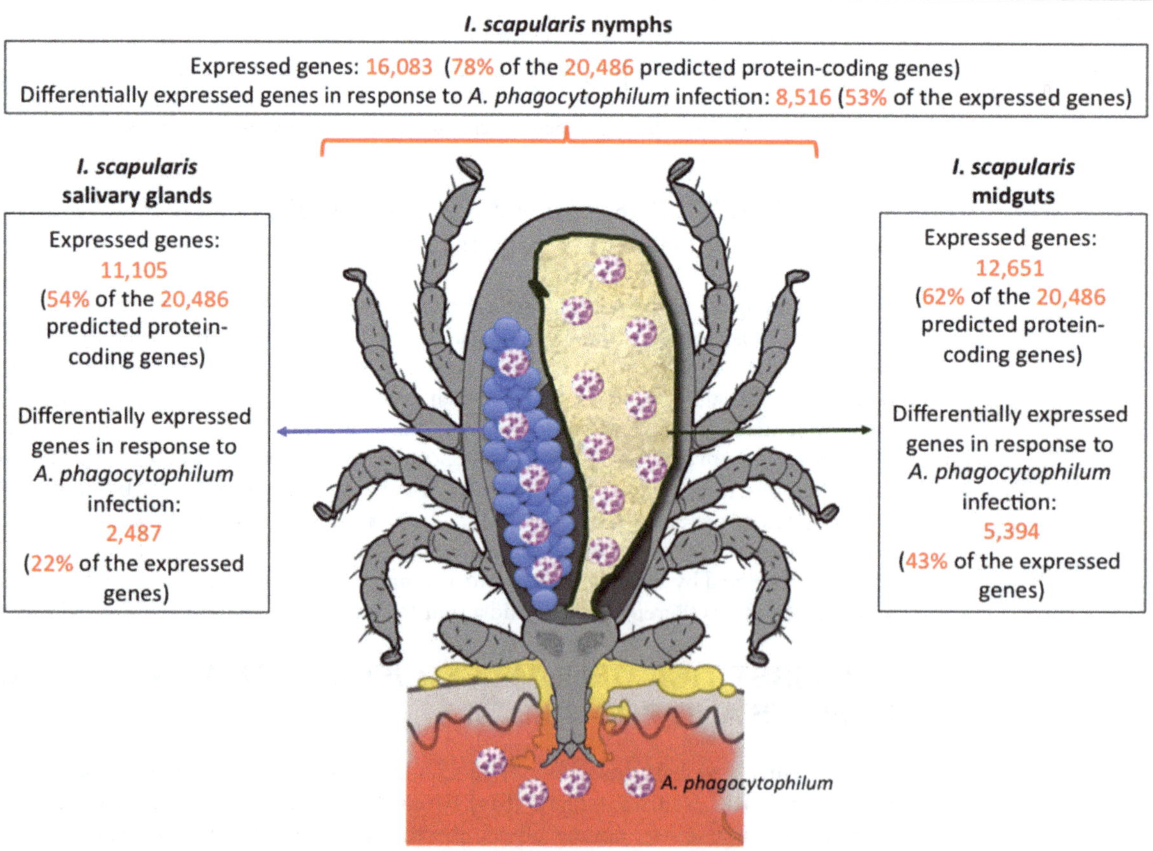

FIGURE 1 | Example of the advance in the characterization of tick-pathogen interactions based on the sequence and assembly of the *I. scapularis* genome. Transcriptomics data was obtained from Ayllón et al. (2015).

of the *I. scapularis* genome sequence (e.g., Cabezas-Cruz et al., 2016; Carr et al., 2016; Egekwu et al., 2016; Grabowski et al., 2016; Van Zee et al., 2016; Zhu et al., 2016). The *I. scapularis* genome also provides a key reference for comparative genomics with other Parasitiformes like the western orchard predatory mite (Hoy et al., 2016), as well as across Chelicerata where large genome sizes often make sequencing and assembly a very challenging undertaking.

Recent results on the characterization of tick-host and tick-pathogen interactions highlighted the impact of *I. scapularis* genome sequence and assembly on these studies (**Figure 1**). Transcriptomics, proteomics and metabolomics studies showed the tissue-specific tick response to infection with *Anaplasma phagocytophilum*, the causative agent of HGA (Ayllón et al., 2015; Villar et al., 2015; Alberdi et al., 2016). Complementary proteomics analyses also revealed proteins associated with transmission of *A. phagocytophilum* and the encephalitis-causing Langat virus (Grabowski et al., 2016; Gulia-Nuss et al., 2016). New advances in experimental approaches using omics technologies also boost our knowledge of the tick-host interface (Sojka et al., 2013; Schwarz et al., 2014; Chmelař et al., 2016a,b). Finally, the analysis of the evolution of tick-host-pathogen interactions suggested conflict and cooperation between hosts, vectors and pathogens (de la Fuente et al., 2016a).

CONCLUSIONS AND FUTURE DIRECTIONS

The features discovered in the *I. scapularis* genome provide insights into parasitic processes unique to ticks, including host "questing," prolonged feeding, cuticle synthesis, blood meal concentration, novel methods of hemoglobin digestion, heme detoxification, vitellogenesis, reproduction, oviposition, prolonged off-host survival and host-tick-pathogen interactions. The *I. scapularis* gene models will advance research on comparative and functional genomics, while the assembly and physical map will underpin much needed studies of tick genetics. Recent efforts addressed the need for additional tick genomic resources by focusing on tick species relevant for human and animal health (Guerrero et al., 2010; Cramaro et al., 2015). Advances in tick genomics have also facilitated the characterization of the impact of co-infections and microbiome composition on tick vector capacity (Narasimhan and Fikrig, 2015; Vayssier-Taussat et al., 2015). These results greatly improve our understanding of tick biology and will advance research on tick-host-pathogen interactions to develop effective and environmentally friendly measures to control ticks and the many pathogens and parasites they transmit (de la Fuente and Contreras, 2015; Benelli et al., 2016; Carr and Roe, 2016; de la Fuente et al., 2016b; Esteve-Gassent et al., 2016; Kuleš et al., 2016).

AUTHOR CONTRIBUTIONS

All authors listed, have made substantial, direct and intellectual contribution to the work, and approved it for publication.

FUNDING

The National Institutes of Health, the National Institute of Allergy and Infectious Diseases and the U.S. Department of Health and Human Services provided principle funding for the sequence and assembly of the *I. scapularis* genome.

REFERENCES

Alberdi, P., Mansfield, K. L., Manzano-Román, R., Cook, C., Ayllón, N., Villar, M., et al. (2016). Tissue-specific signatures in the transcriptional response to *Anaplasma phagocytophilum* infection of *Ixodes scapularis* and *Ixodes ricinus* tick cell lines. *Front. Cell. Infect. Microbiol.* 6:20. doi: 10.3389/fcimb.2016.00020

Ayllón, N., Villar, M., Galindo, R. C., Kocan, K. M., Šíma, R., López, J. A., et al. (2015). Systems biology of tissue-specific response to *Anaplasma phagocytophilum* reveals differentiated apoptosis in the tick vector *Ixodes scapularis*. *PLoS Genet.* 11:e1005120. doi: 10.1371/journal.pgen.1005120

Benelli, G., Pavela, R., Canale, A., and Mehlhorn, H. (2016). Tick repellents and acaricides of botanical origin: a green roadmap to control tick-borne diseases? *Parasitol. Res.* 115, 2545–2560. doi: 10.1007/s00436-016-5095-1

Cabezas-Cruz, A., Alberdi, P., Ayllón, N., Valdés, J. J., Pierce, R., Villar, M., et al. (2016). *Anaplasma phagocytophilum* increases the levels of histone modifying enzymes to inhibit cell apoptosis and facilitate pathogen infection in the tick vector *Ixodes scapularis*. *Epigenetics* 11, 303–319. doi: 10.1080/15592294.2016.1163460

Carr, A. L., and Roe, M. (2016). Acarine attractants: chemoreception, bioassay, chemistry and control. *Pestic. Biochem. Physiol.* 131, 60–79. doi: 10.1016/j.pestbp.2015.12.009

Carr, A. L., Sonenshine, D. E., Strider, J. B. Jr., and Roe, R. M. (2016). Evidence of female sex pheromones and characterization of the cuticular lipids of unfed, adult male versus female blacklegged ticks, *Ixodes scapularis*. *Exp. Appl. Acarol.* 68, 519–538. doi: 10.1007/s10493-015-0009-y

Centers for Disease Control and Prevention (CDC) (2016). *Tick-borne diseases of the United States*. Available online at: http://www.cdc.gov/ticks/diseases/

Chmelař, J., Kotál, J., Kopecký, J., Pedra, J. H., and Kotsyfakis, M. (2016b). All for one and one for all on the tick-host battlefield. *Trends Parasitol.* 32, 368–377. doi: 10.1016/j.pt.2016.01.004

Chmelař, J., Kotál, J., Karim, S., Kopacek, P., Francischetti, I. M., Pedra, J. H., et al. (2016a). Sialomes and mialomes: a systems-biology view of tick tissues and tick-host interactions. *Trends Parasitol.* 32, 242–254. doi: 10.1016/j.pt.2015.10.002

Cramaro, W. J., Revets, D., Hunewald, O. E., Sinner, R., Reye, A. L., and Muller, C. P. (2015). Integration of *Ixodes ricinus* genome sequencing with transcriptome and proteome annotation of the naïve midgut. *BMC Genomics* 16:871. doi: 10.1186/s12864-015-1981-7

de la Fuente, J., and Contreras, M. (2015). Tick vaccines: current status and future directions. *Expert Rev. Vaccines* 14, 1367–1376. doi: 10.1586/14760584.2015.1076339

de la Fuente, J., Estrada-Peña, A., Venzal, J. M., Kocan, K. M., and Sonenshine, D. E. (2008). Overview: ticks as vectors of pathogens that cause disease in humans and animals. *Front. Biosci.* 13, 6938–6946. doi: 10.2741/3200

de la Fuente, J., Kopáček, P., Lew-Tabor, A., and Maritz-Olivier, C. (2016b). Strategies for new and improved vaccines against ticks and tick-borne diseases. *Parasite Immunol.* doi: 10.1111/pim.12339. [Epub ahead of print].

de la Fuente, J., Villar, M., Cabezas-Cruz, A., Estrada-Peña, A., Ayllón, N., and Alberdi, P. (2016a). Tick-host-pathogen interactions: conflict and cooperation. *PLoS Pathog.* 12:e1005488. doi: 10.1371/journal.ppat.1005488

Egekwu, N., Sonenshine, D. E., Garman, H., Barshis, D. J., Cox, N., Bissinger, B. W., et al. (2016). Comparison of synganglion neuropeptides, neuropeptide receptors and neurotransmitter receptors and their gene expression in response to feeding in *Ixodes scapularis* (Ixodidae) vs. *Ornithodoros turicata* (Argasidae). *Insect Mol. Biol.* 25, 72–92. doi: 10.1111/imb.12202

Esteve-Gassent, M. D., Castro-Arellano, I., Feria-Arroyo, T. P., Patino, R., Li, A. Y., Medina, R. F., et al. (2016). Translating ecology, physiology, biochemistry, and population genetics research to meet the challenge of tick and tick-borne diseases in north America. *Arch. Insect Biochem. Physiol.* 92, 38–64. doi: 10.1002/arch.21327

Estrada-Peña, A., Ostfeld, R. S., Peterson, A. T., Poulin, R., and de la Fuente, J. (2014). Effects of environmental change on zoonotic disease risk: an ecological primer. *Trends Parasitol.* 30, 205–214. doi: 10.1016/j.pt.2014.02.003

European Centre for Disease Prevention and Control (ECDC) (2016). *Tick-borne diseases.* Available online at: http://ecdc.europa.eu/en/healthtopics/emerging_and_vector-borne_diseases/tick_borne_diseases/pages/index.aspx

Genomic Resources Development Consortium, Contreras, M., de la Fuente, J., Estrada-Peña, A., Grubhoffer, L., and Tobes, R. (2014). Genomic resources notes accepted 1 April 2014 - 31 May 2014. *Mol. Ecol. Resour.* 14, 1095. doi: 10.1111/1755-0998.12298

Gortazar, C., Reperant, L. A., Kuiken, T., de la Fuente, J., Boadella, M., Martínez-Lopez, B., et al. (2014). Crossing the interspecies barrier: opening the door to zoonotic pathogens. *PLoS Pathog.* 10:e1004129. doi: 10.1371/journal.ppat.1004129

Grabowski, J. M., Perera, R., Roumani, A. M., Hedrick, V. E., Inerowicz, H. D., Hill, C. A., et al. (2016). Changes in the proteome of Langat-Infected *Ixodes scapularis* ISE6 cells: metabolic pathways associated with Flavivirus infection. *PLoS Negl. Trop. Dis.* 10:e0004180. doi: 10.1371/journal.pntd.0004180

Guerrero, F. D., Moolhuijzen, P., Peterson, D. G., Bidwell, S., Caler, E., Bellgard, M., et al. (2010). Reassociation kinetics-based approach for partial genome sequencing of the cattle tick, *Rhipicephalus (Boophilus) microplus*. *BMC Genomics* 11:374. doi: 10.1186/1471-2164-11-374

Gulia-Nuss, M., Nuss, A. B., Meyer, J. M., Sonenshine, D. E., Roe, R. M., Waterhouse, R. M., et al. (2016). Genomic insights into the *Ixodes scapularis* tick vector of Lyme disease. *Nat. Commun.* 7:10507. doi: 10.1038/ncomms10507

Hoy, M. A., Waterhouse, R. M., Wu, K., Estep, A. S., Ioannidis, P., Palmer, W. J., et al. (2016). Genome sequencing of the phytoseiid predatory mite *Metaseiulus occidentalis* reveals completely atomized *Hox* genes and superdynamic intron evolution. *Genome Biol. Evol.* 8, 1762–1775. doi: 10.1093/gbe/evw048

Jones, K. E., Patel, N. G., Levy, M. A., Storeygard, A., Balk, D., Gittleman, J. L., et al. (2008). Global trends in emerging infectious diseases. *Nature* 451, 990–993. doi: 10.1038/nature06536

Jongejan, F., and Uilenberg, G. (2004). The global importance of ticks. *Parasitol.* 129, S3–S14. doi: 10.1017/S0031182004005967

Kernif, T., Leulmi, H., Raoult, D., and Parola, P. (2016). Emerging tick-borne bacterial pathogens. *Microbiol. Spectr.* 4:EI10-0012-2016. doi: 10.1128/microbiolspec.ei10-0012-2016

Kosoy, O. I., Lambert, A. J., Hawkinson, D. J., Pastula, D. M., Goldsmith, C. S., Hunt, D. C., et al. (2015). Novel thogotovirus associated with febrile illness and death, United States, 2014. *Emerg. Infect. Dis.* 21, 760–764. doi: 10.3201/eid2105.150150

Kotsyfakis, M., Schwarz, A., Erhart, J., and Ribeiro, J. M. (2015). Tissue- and time-dependent transcription in *Ixodes ricinus* salivary glands and midguts when blood feeding on the vertebrate host. *Sci. Rep.* 5:9103. doi: 10.1038/srep09103

Kuleš, J., Horvatić, A., Guillemin, N., Galan, A., Mrljak, V., and Bhide, M. (2016). New approaches and omics tools for mining of vaccine candidates against vector-borne diseases. *Mol. Biosyst.* 12, 2680–2694. doi: 10.1039/c6mb00268d

Narasimhan, S., and Fikrig, E. (2015). Tick microbiome: the force within. *Trends Parasitol.* 31, 315–323. doi: 10.1016/j.pt.2015.03.010

Schwarz, A., Tenzer, S., Hackenberg, M., Erhart, J., Gerhold-Ay, A., Mazur, J., et al. (2014). A systems level analysis reveals transcriptomic and proteomic complexity in *Ixodes ricinus* midgut and salivary glands during early attachment and feeding. *Mol. Cell. Proteomics* 13, 2725–2735. doi: 10.1074/mcp.M114.039289

Sojka, D., Franta, Z., Horn, M., Caffrey, C. R., Mareš, M., and Kopáček, P. (2013). New insights into the machinery of blood digestion by ticks. *Trends Parasitol.* 29, 276–285. doi: 10.1016/j.pt.2013.04.002

Van Zee, J. P., Schlueter, J. A., Schlueter, S., Dixon, P., Sierra, C. A., and Hill, C. A. (2016). Paralog analyses reveal gene duplication events and genes under positive selection in *Ixodes scapularis* and other ixodid ticks. *BMC Genomics* 17:241. doi: 10.1186/s12864-015-2350-2

Vayssier-Taussat, M., Kazimirova, M., Hubalek, Z., Hornok, S., Farkas, R., Cosson, J. F., et al. (2015). Emerging horizons for tick-borne pathogens: from the 'one pathogen-one disease' vision to the pathobiome paradigm. *Future Microbiol.* 10, 2033–2043. doi: 10.2217/fmb.15.114

Villar, M., Ayllón, N., Alberdi, P., Moreno, A., Moreno, M., Tobes, R., et al. (2015). Integrated metabolomics, transcriptomics and proteomics identifies metabolic pathways affected by *Anaplasma phagocytophilum* infection in tick cells. *Mol. Cell. Proteomics* 14, 3154–3172. doi: 10.1074/mcp.M115.051938

Wormser, G. P., Dattwyler, R. J., Shapiro, E. D., Halperin, J. J., Steere, A. C., Klempner, M. S., et al. (2006). The clinical assessment, treatment, and prevention of lyme disease, human granulocytic anaplasmosis, and babesiosis: clinical practice guidelines by the Infectious Diseases Society of America. *Clin. Infect. Dis.* 43, 1089–1134. doi: 10.1086/508667

Zhu, J., Khalil, S. M., Mitchell, R. D., Bissinger, B. W., Egekwu, N., Sonenshine, D. E., et al. (2016). Mevalonate-farnesal biosynthesis in ticks: comparative synganglion transcriptomics and a new perspective. *PLoS ONE* 11:e0141084. doi: 10.1371/journal.pone.0141084

4

Anaplasma phagocytophilum Infection Subverts Carbohydrate Metabolic Pathways in the Tick Vector, *Ixodes scapularis*

Alejandro Cabezas-Cruz[1,2*†], *Pilar Alberdi*[3†], *James J. Valdés*[1,4], *Margarita Villar*[3] and *José de la Fuente*[3,5*]

[1] *Institute of Parasitology, Biology Center, Czech Academy of Sciences, Ceské Budejovice, Czechia,* [2] *Faculty of Science, University of South Bohemia, Ceské Budejovice, Czechia,* [3] *SaBio. Instituto de Investigación en Recursos Cinegéticos (CSIC-UCLM-JCCM), Ciudad Real, Spain,* [4] *Department of Virology, Veterinary Research Institute, Brno, Czechia,* [5] *Department of Veterinary Pathobiology, Center for Veterinary Health Sciences, Oklahoma State University, Stillwater, OK, USA*

Correspondence:
Alejandro Cabezas-Cruz
cabezasalejandrocruz@gmail.com
José de la Fuente
jose_delafuente@yahoo.com

† These authors have contributed equally to this work.

The obligate intracellular pathogen, *Anaplasma phagocytophilum*, is the causative agent of human, equine, and canine granulocytic anaplasmosis and tick-borne fever (TBF) in ruminants. *A. phagocytophilum* has become an emerging tick-borne pathogen in the United States, Europe, Africa, and Asia, with increasing numbers of infected people and animals every year. It has been recognized that intracellular pathogens manipulate host cell metabolic pathways to increase infection and transmission in both vertebrate and invertebrate hosts. However, our current knowledge on how *A. phagocytophilum* affect these processes in the tick vector, *Ixodes scapularis* is limited. In this study, a genome-wide search for components of major carbohydrate metabolic pathways was performed in *I. scapularis* ticks for which the genome was recently published. The enzymes involved in the seven major carbohydrate metabolic pathways glycolysis, gluconeogenesis, pentose phosphate, tricarboxylic acid cycle (TCA), glyceroneogenesis, and mitochondrial oxidative phosphorylation and β-oxidation were identified. Then, the available transcriptomics and proteomics data was used to characterize the mRNA and protein levels of *I. scapularis* major carbohydrate metabolic pathway components in response to *A. phagocytophilum* infection of tick tissues and cultured cells. The results showed that major carbohydrate metabolic pathways are conserved in ticks. *A. phagocytophilum* infection inhibits gluconeogenesis and mitochondrial metabolism, but increases the expression of glycolytic genes. A model was proposed to explain how *A. phagocytophilum* could simultaneously control tick cell glucose metabolism and cytoskeleton organization, which may be achieved in part by up-regulating and stabilizing hypoxia inducible factor 1 alpha in a hypoxia-independent manner. The present work provides a more comprehensive view of the major carbohydrate metabolic pathways involved in the response to *A. phagocytophilum* infection in ticks, and provides the basis for further studies to develop novel strategies for the control of granulocytic anaplasmosis.

Keywords: proteomics, transcriptomics, glucose metabolism, *Ixodes scapularis*, *Anaplasma phagocytophilum*

INTRODUCTION

Anaplasma phagocytophilum (Rickettsiales: Anaplasmataceae) is an obligate intracellular bacterium mainly transmitted by *Ixodes* spp. ticks. This emerging pathogen has been reported in the United States, Europe, Africa, and Asia (de la Fuente et al., 2008; Stuen et al., 2013; Kocan et al., 2015), causing human granulocytic anaplasmosis (HGA), equine and canine granulocytic anaplasmosis and tick-borne fever (TBF) of ruminants (de la Fuente et al., 2008; Stuen et al., 2013; Kocan et al., 2015).

The development of *A. phagocytophilum* is complex and coordinated with the tick feeding cycle. Infection and multiplication in ticks occurs first in midgut cells during blood feeding, and then subsequently in other tissues including hemocytes and salivary glands from where transmission occurs to susceptible hosts (Kocan et al., 2015). To establish infection, *A. phagocytophilum* affect mechanisms that appear to be common to ticks and vertebrate hosts (de la Fuente et al., 2016a). These mechanisms include but are not limited to remodeling of the cytoskeleton, inhibition of cell apoptosis, manipulation of the immune response, and modification of cell epigenetics and metabolism (de la Fuente et al., 2016a).

Recently, transcriptomics, proteomics and metabolomics analyses of infected *I. scapularis* ISE6 cells showed that *A. phagocytophilum* infection affects glucose metabolic pathways (Villar et al., 2015). These results suggested that *A. phagocytophilum* manipulate carbohydrate metabolism to facilitate infection and multiplication in tick cells. However, the mechanisms used by *A. phagocytophilum* for the manipulation of carbohydrate metabolic pathways have not been fully characterized.

To better characterize the mechanisms used by *A. phagocytophilum* to manipulate carbohydrate metabolic pathways during infection of tick cells, the dynamics of the carbohydrate metabolism was characterized in the tick vector, *I. scapularis* in response to pathogen infection. First, the composition of major carbohydrate metabolic pathways was annotated using the recently published genome of *I. scapularis* (Gulia-Nuss et al., 2016). Then, previously published transcriptomics and proteomics data (Ayllón et al., 2015; Villar et al., 2015) was used to characterize the mRNA and protein levels of carbohydrate metabolic pathway components in response to *A. phagocytophilum* infection of *I. scapularis* nymphs, female midguts and salivary glands, and ISE6 cultured tick cells. Finally, functional studies were conducted in ISE6 tick cells to provide additional support for the role of these components during pathogen infection. These results expanded our knowledge of the different pathways affected by *A. phagocytophilum* infection in ticks, and provided new potential targets for the development of therapeutic and prevention strategies for the control of granulocytic anaplasmosis and other tick-borne diseases.

MATERIALS AND METHODS

Annotation of the Major Carbohydrate Metabolic Pathway Components in the *I. scapularis* Genome

The *I. scapularis* genome (Gulia-Nuss et al., 2016) was searched with the specific names of genes encoding for enzymes involved in the major carbohydrate metabolic pathways, glycolysis, gluconeogenesis, pentose phosphate, tricarboxylic acid cycle (TCA), glyceroneogenesis, and mitochondrial oxidative phosphorylation and β-oxidation. When records were not obtained using specific enzyme names, then the *I. scapularis* genome was searched with the Blastp tool from the Basic Local Alignment Search Tool (BLAST) using the human ortholog as "query" (Altschul et al., 1990; Madden et al., 1996). The sequences with the lowest *E*-value were selected. The conserved domains of identified protein sequences were classified using the protein families database Pfam (Finn et al., 2014). The *I. scapularis* orthologs found in the genome were double-checked by searching the *Homo sapiens* genome database using as queries the tick homologs identified in the previous step.

Characterization of the *I. scapularis* mRNA and Protein Levels in Response to *A. phagocytophilum* Infection

The quantitative transcriptomics and proteomics data for uninfected and *A. phagocytophilum*-infected *I. scapularis* nymphs, female midguts and salivary glands, and ISE6 cultured cells were obtained from previously published results (Ayllón et al., 2015; Villar et al., 2015) and deposited at the Dryad repository database, NCBI's Gene Expression Omnibus database and ProteomeXchange Consortium via the PRIDE partner repository with the dataset identifier PXD002181 and doi: 10.6019/PXD002181. For transcriptomics and proteomics analysis in *I. scapularis* nymphs, female midguts and salivary glands, the procedures were described in Ayllón et al. (2015). Briefly, nymphs and adult female *I. scapularis* were infected with *A. phagocytophilum* by feeding on a sheep inoculated intravenously with $\sim 1 \times 10^7$ *A. phagocytophilum* (NY18 isolate)-infected HL-60 cells (90–100% infected cells). In this model, over 85% of ticks become infected with *A. phagocytophilum* in nymphs, midguts and salivary glands. Ticks (200 nymphs and 100 female adults) were removed from the sheep 7 days after infestation, held in the humidity chamber for 4 days and dissected for DNA, RNA, and protein extraction from whole internal tissues (nymphs) or midguts and salivary glands (adult females). Adult midguts and salivary glands were washed in PBS after collection to remove hemolymphs-related cells. Uninfected ticks were prepared in a similar way but feeding on an uninfected sheep. Two independent samples were collected and processed for each tick developmental stage and tissue. After RNA sequencing on an Illumina Hiseq 2000, TopHat was used to align the reads to the *I. scapularis* (assembly JCVI_ISG_i3_1.0; http://www.ncbi.nlm.nih.gov/

nuccore/NZ_ABJB000000000) reference genome. Raw counts per gene were estimated by the Python script HTSeq count [http://www-huber.embl.de/users/anders/HTSeq/] using the reference genome. The raw counts per gene were used by DEGseq to estimate differential expression at $P < 0.05$. For peptide identification by liquid chromatography-tandem mass spectrometry (LC-MS/MS) using iTRAQ labeled peptides, all spectra were analyzed with Proteome Discoverer (version 1.4.0.29, Thermo Fisher Scientific) using a Uniprot database (http://www.uniprot.org) containing all sequences from Ixodida, Anaplasmataceae and Ruminantia. Peptide identification was validated using the probability ratio method and false discovery rate (FDR) was calculated using inverted databases and the refined method with an additional filtering for precursor mass tolerance of 12 ppm. Only peptides with a confidence of at least 95% were used to quantify the relative abundance of each peptide. Outliers at the scan and peptide levels and significant protein-abundance changes were detected from the *z*-values (the standardized variable used by the model that expresses the quantitative values in units of standard deviation) by using a FDR threshold of 5%. Results were the mean of two replicates. For transcriptomics and proteomics analysis in tick cells, the *I. scapularis* embryo-derived tick cell line ISE6, provided by Ulrike Munderloh, University of Minnesota, USA, was cultured in L-15B300 medium (Munderloh et al., 1999), except that the osmotic pressure was lowered by the addition of one-fourth sterile water by volume. The ISE6 cells were first inoculated with *A. phagocytophilum* (human NY18 isolate; Asanovich et al., 1997)-infected HL-60 cells and maintained until infection was established and routinely passaged. Uninfected and infected cultures ($N = 3$ independent cultures with $\sim 10^7$ cells each) were sampled at 7 days post-infection (dpi; percent infected cells 71–77%; Ave $\pm$ *SD*, 74 $\pm$ 3). Transcriptomics data was obtained as described above for nymphs and adult female ticks. Two biological replicates were used for each of uninfected and infected tick cells and genes differentially expressed in response to *A. phagocytophilum* infection were selected with $P \leq 0.05$. The proteomics analysis followed the same pipeline describe above in ticks and the MS/MS raw files generated with Xcalibur (version 2.1, Thermo Fisher Scientific) were searched against a compiled database containing all sequences from Ixodida and Anaplasmataceae (http://www.uniprot.org). Three biological replicates were used for each of uninfected and infected tick cells. For the quantitative analysis of tick proteins, after discarding *Anaplasma* proteins in infected cells, the total number of peptide-spectrum matches (PSMs) for each tick protein were normalized against the total number of PSMs in tick cells and compared between control and infected cells by Chi2-test ($P \leq 0.05$). Although the percent of infected ticks and cultured cells was determined as described above, the bacterial load on these samples was not considered in the analysis.

The identified genes in the carbohydrate metabolic pathways were searched against the transcriptomics and proteomics data to characterize their mRNA and protein levels in response to *A. phagocytophilum* infection.

Tertiary Structure Modeling and Optimization

The tertiary structures of the partial protein sequences of *I. scapularis* hypoxia-inducible factor 1 alpha HIF-1α (XP_002414889) and HIF-1β (XP_002416629) proteins, which are the DNA binding N-terminus domains, were modeled using the Swiss-Model server (Biasini et al., 2014). The tertiary models were optimized using the Protein Preparation Wizard (Li et al., 2007) in the Schrödinger's Maestro software package. The Protein Preparation Wizard clusters at the highest degree of hydrogen bonding in equilibrium. Monte Carlo orientations are performed (100,000) for each cluster. The optimized structure is based on electrostatic and geometric scoring functions. Any remaining steric clashes were eliminated by minimization of the entire system with the default settings in the Schrodinger's Maestro package. The ternary structure that includes the hypoxia response element (HRE) was constructed via superimposition by using the Swiss-Model server used the mouse HIF-1α, HIF-1β, and the HRE (Dalei et al., 2015) as a template for both *I. scapularis* hypoxia-inducible protein sequences. As a final optimization step, the ternary structure (HIF-1α/HIF-1β/HRE) was processed using the normal mode ready-made script in the Metropolis Monte Carlo-based Protein Energy Landscape Exploration (PELE) server (Borrelli et al., 2005). The PELE software implements an anisotropic network model (Atilgan et al., 2001) for perturbations of the alpha-carbon backbone causing structural conformational changes. The PELE server can be accessed at https://pele.bsc.es/.

Immunofluorescence Assay in *I. scapularis* Midguts and Salivary Glands

Female ticks fed on *A. phagocytophilum*-infected and uninfected sheep and fixed with 4% paraformaldehyde in 0.2 M sodium cacodylate buffer were embedded in paraffin and used to prepare sections on glass slides as previously described (Ayllón et al., 2015). The paraffin was removed from the sections through two washes in xylene and the sections were hydrated by successive 5 min washes with a graded series of 100, 96, and 65% ethanol and finally with distilled water. Next, the slides were treated with Proteinase K (Dako, Barcelona, Spain) for 7 min, washed with 0,1% PBS-Tween 20 (Sigma-Aldrich, St. Louis, MI, USA) and blocked with 2% bovine serum albumin (BSA; Sigma-Aldrich) in PBS-Tween 20 during 1 h at room temperature. The slides were then incubated overnight at 4°C with mouse anti-Glyceraldehyde 3-phosphate dehydrogenase (GAPDH) monoclonal antibodies (ab50567; Abcam, Cambridge, UK) diluted 1:100 in 2% BSA/PBS-Tween 20. Preimmune serum was used as control. After 3 washes with PBS-Tween 20, the slides were incubated for 1 h with rabbit anti-mouse IgG conjugated with FITC (Sigma-Aldrich) diluted 1:160 in 2% BSA/PBS-Tween 20. Finally, after two washes with PBS the slides were mounted on ProLong Diamond Antifade Mountant with DAPI reagent (Thermo Scientific, Madrid, Spain). The sections were examined using a Zeiss LSM 800 with Airyscan (Carl Zeiss, Oberkochen, Germany).

Infected and Uninfected Cultured ISE6 Tick Cells

The *I. scapularis* embryo-derived tick cell line ISE6 were cultured as described above, infected with *A. phagocytophilum* (human NY18 isolate; Asanovich et al., 1997) or mock-infected and maintained according to Munderloh et al. (1999).

Pharmacological Studies in Cultured ISE6 Tick Cells

A. phagocytophilum-infected ISE6 cells were left untreated or treated for 24 or 48 h with 5 mM 2-Deoxy-D-Glucose (ab142242, Abcam) to inhibit glycolysis (Wang et al., 2011), 100 μM LY294002 (ab120243, Abcam) to inhibit the phosphatidylinositol 3-kinase (PI3K; Sultana et al., 2010), 100 nM Chetomin (ab144222, Abcam) to inhibit the activity of HIF-1α (Misra et al., 2012) or 0.5 mM Deferoxamine mesylate (Sigma-Aldrich) to activate HIF-1α (Choi et al., 2004). After treatment, cells were harvested for the preparation of whole cell lysates to determine HIF-1α activity and for DNA extraction. Tick cell lysates were prepared by adding to cell pellets the RIPA lysis buffer (Thermo Scientific) supplemented with a protease inhibitor cocktail (cOmplete Mini, EDTA-free, Roche, Sigma-Aldrich). HIF-1α activity was determined in the cell lysate supernatants with the HIF-1 alpha Transcription Factor Assay Kit (ab133104, Abcam) following manufacturer's recommendations. *A. phagocytophilum* DNA levels were characterized by *msp4* real-time PCR normalizing against tick *16S rDNA* as described previously (Ayllón et al., 2013). Optical density values (O.D. 450 nm) for HIF-1α activity and normalized Ct values for *A. phagocytophilum* DNA levels were compared between treated and untreated control cells by Student's *t*-test with unequal variance ($P = 0.05$; $N = 4$ biological replicates).

RESULTS

Major Carbohydrate Metabolic Pathways Described in Other Organisms Are Present in *I. scapularis* and Are Affected by *A. phagocytophilum* Infection

Seven major pathways involved in carbohydrate metabolism were selected for characterization (**Table 1**). A total of 79 genes coding for the proteins involved in glycolysis, gluconeogenesis, pentose phosphate pathway (PPP), glyceroneogenesis, TCA, mitochondrial oxidative phosphorylation (OXPHOS) and β-oxidation were identified in the *I. scapularis* genome (**Table 1**). Based on these results, a model for glucose metabolism in ticks was proposed (**Figure 1**). At least in humans, pyruvate carboxylase (PC) catalyzes the irreversible carboxylation of pyruvate to form oxaloacetate, which is then transformed in phosphoenolpyruvate by the cytoplasmic enzyme phosphoenolpyruvate carboxykinase (PEPCK-C; Berg et al., 2002). However, the PC orthologue was not identified in the *I. scapularis* genome.

The carbohydrate metabolic response to *A. phagocytophilum* infection was then characterized using the quantitative transcriptomics and proteomics data generated from uninfected and *A. phagocytophilum*-infected *I. scapularis* ticks and ISE6 cultured cells (Ayllón et al., 2015; Villar et al., 2015). Most of the identified carbohydrate metabolism genes were differentially regulated in response to *A. phagocytophilum* infection in at least one of the analyzed tick tissues (**Figure 2**). Twenty-eight (35%), 23 (29%), 62 (78%), and 64 (81%) carbohydrate metabolism components were identified in both transcriptome and proteome of ISE6 cells, nymphs, adult female midguts, and salivary glands, respectively (**Figure 2**). Of these genes, 59 (75%), 14 (18%), 60 (76%), and 41 (52%) were up-regulated, while 20 (25%), 65 (82%), 16 (20%), and 35 (44%) were down-regulated in response to infection in ISE6 cells, nymphs, adult female midguts, and salivary glands, respectively (**Figure 2**). Many of the carbohydrate metabolism proteins were not identified by mass spectrometry (**Figure 2**), but the results showed similar differential regulation at the mRNA and protein levels for 50% of the identified proteins.

Glucose transporters, and mainly facilitative glucose transporters (GLUT) are an important component of the glycolytic pathway because they transport glucose from the extracellular space to the cellular cytoplasm, which makes the glucose accessible to hexokinase (HXK; Augustin, 2010; Li et al., 2015). We found 11 putative glucose transporters in the genome of *I. scapularis*, 2 members (*sglt1* and *sglt2*) of the sodium-glucose linked transporter family (SGLT), and 9 members (2 isoforms of *glut1*, *glut3*, 4 isoforms of *glut8*, *glut10*, and *glut12*) of the GLUT family. In response to *A. phagocytophilum* infection, *glut1B*, *glut3*, *glut8C*, *glut10*, *glut12*, and *sglt1* genes were up-regulated in tick midguts, and the GLUT1A and SGLT2 proteins were over-represented in infected midguts when compared to uninfected controls (**Figure 3**).

As in previous experiments (Villar et al., 2015), these results supported a role for carbohydrate metabolism during *A. phagocytophilum* infection in *I. scapularis*, and suggested tissue-specific differences in response to infection.

A. phagocytophilum Infection Activates the Glycolysis Pathway, but Reduces Gluconeogenesis and the TCA Cycle in Tick Midguts

Based on these results, the putative glucose metabolic pathways affected by *A. phagocytophilum* infection in different *I. scapularis* tissues and ISE6 cells were proposed (**Figures 4, 5**). The results showed that the genes involved in glycolysis were all up-regulated in tick midguts after *A. phagocytophilum* infection, except for phosphofructokinase (*pfk*) and *hxk* genes that did not change in response to infection (**Figure 2**). The up-regulation of glycolytic genes correlated with protein over-representation in tick midguts, except for the cofactor-independent phosphoglycerate mutase (*ipgm*) and pyruvate kinase (*pk*) that despite gene up-regulation in infected midguts, protein was under-represented in response to infection (**Figure 2**). However, since iPGM catalyzes a reversible reaction, it is not a site of major regulatory mechanisms for the glycolytic pathway. In contrast, HXK and PFK proteins, which catalyze irreversible steps of glucose glycolysis and therefore constitute major regulatory

TABLE 1 | Annotation of carbohydrate metabolic enzymes identified in the *I. scapularis* genome.

Enzymes	Abbreviation	Genome accession	GenBank ID	Length (amino acids)
GLYCOLYSIS (GLY)				
Hexokinase	HXK	ISCW012387	EEC16047	454
Phosphoglucose isomerase	PGI	ISCW014868	EEC19698	543
Phosphofructokinase	PFK	ISCW014412	EEC18711	55
Fructose-bisphosphate aldolase A	ALDA	ISCW011371	EEC14101	364
Glyceraldehyde 3-phosphate dehydrogenase	GAPDH	ISCW018700	EEC07171	334
Phosphoglycerate kinase 1	PGK1	ISCW015616	EEC01763	415
Phosphoglycerate mutase (cofactor-independent)	iPGM	ISCW020443	EEC12432	510
Enolase	ENOL	ISCW017666	EEC06821	199
Pyruvate kinase	PK	ISCW020197	EEC12307	538
GLUCONEOGENESIS (GLN)				
Glucose 6-phosphatase (1)	G6Pase (1)	ISCW017459	EEC03691	356
Glucose 6-phosphatase (2)	G6Pase (2)	ISCW018612	EEC07273	282
Fructose-1,6-bisphosphatase	FBP	ISCW005292	EEC07486	338
Phosphoenolpyruvate carboxykinase mitochondrial (1)	PEPCK-M (1)	ISCW001902	EEC03297	503
Phosphoenolpyruvate carboxykinase mitochondrial (2)	PEPCK-M (2)	ISCW000524	EEC01808	288
Phosphoenolpyruvate carboxykinase 1 cytoplasmatic	PEPCK-C	ISCW001905	EEC03300	165
Phosphoenolpyruvate carboxykinase	PEPCK	ISCW008211	EEC10279	192
Pyruvate carboxylase	PC	Not found	Not found	...
PENTOSE PHOSPHATE PATHWAY (PPP)				
Glucose 6-phosphate dehydrogenase	G6PD	ISCW010043	EEC13253	523
6-phosphogluconolactonase	PGLS	ISCW002068	EEC04321	101
6-phosphogluconate dehydrogenase	6PGD	ISCW010101	EEC12854	507
Ribose 5-Phosphate Isomerase	RPI	ISCW012092	EEC16597	172
Ribulose 5-Phosphate 3-Epimerase	RPPE	ISCW001125	EEC01731	236
Transketolase	TKT	Not found	Not found	...
Transaldolase	TALDO	ISCW023506	EEC20008	219
TRICARBOXYLIC ACID CYCLE (TCA CYCLE)				
Pyruvate dehydrogenase E1	PDE1	ISCW019126	EEC09108	393
Citrate synthase	CS	ISCW009586	EEC13404	471
Aconitase	ACON	ISCW010818	EEC15463	65
Isocitrate dehydrogenase 3 α subunit	IDH3A	ISCW004116	EEC06101	362
Isocitrate dehydrogenase 3 β subunit	IDH3B	ISCW018585	EEC07698	207
Isocitrate dehydrogenase 3 γ-subunit (I)	IDH3G1	ISCW022614	EEC16834	132
Isocitrate dehydrogenase 3 γ-subunit (II)	IDH3G2	ISCW017423	EEC04192	365
2-oxoglutarate dehydrogenase E1	OXOE1	ISCW021407	EEC14367	831
GTP/ATP-specific Succinyl-CoA synthetase—α subunit	B/A-SCS-α	ISCW020686	EEC11198	217
ATP-specific Succinyl-CoA synthetase—β subunit	A-SCS-β	ISCW011750	EEC14163	425
GTP-specific Succinyl-CoA synthetase—β subunit	G-SCS-β	ISCW015999	EEC00562	422
Succinate dehydrogenase flavoprotein subunit	SDHA	ISCW000555	EEC02042	608
Succinate dehydrogenase iron-sulfur subunit	SDHB	ISCW018067	EEC06202	286
Succinate dehydrogenase cytochrome b560 subunit	SDHC	ISCW020744	EEC12476	132
Succinate dehydrogenase cytochrome b small subunit	SDHD	ISCW012012	EEC15988	208
Fumarase hydratase mitochondrial	FH	ISCW020593	EEC13182	481
Malate dehydrogenase 1 cytoplasmatic	MDH1	ISCW007624	EEC09194	302
Malate dehydrogenase 2 mitochondrial	MDH2	ISCW003528	EEC05916	340
REGULATORY PROTEINS OF TCA CYCLE				
Pyruvate dehydrogenase kinase	PDK	ISCW013649	EEC19175	344
Pyruvate dehyrogenase phosphatase catalytic subunit 1	PDPC1	ISCW014874	EEC19704	401

(Continued)

TABLE 1 | Continued

Enzymes	Abbreviation	Genome accession	GenBank ID	Length (amino acids)
OXIDATIVE PHOSPHORYLATION (OXPHOS) COMPLEX I (CORE SUBUNITS)				
NADH dehydrogenase (ubiquinone) iron-sulfur protein 7	NDUS7	ISCW013042	EEC17810	162
NADH dehydrogenase (ubiquinone) iron-sulfur protein 8	NDUS8	ISCW010554	EEC13775	210
NADH dehydrogenase (ubiquinone) flavoprotein 2	NDUV2	ISCW014272	EEC18480	244
NADH dehydrogenase (ubiquinone) iron-sulfur protein 3	NDUS3	ISCW012366	EEC17298	268
NADH dehydrogenase (ubiquinone) iron-sulfur protein 2	NDUS2	ISCW017643	EEC06293	462
NADH dehydrogenase (ubiquinone) flavoprotein 1	NDUV1	ISCW005985	EEC08296	477
NADH-ubiquinone oxidoreductase 75 kDa subunit	NDUS1	ISCW003299	EEC03949	729
NADH-ubiquinone oxidoreductase chain 1	ND1	ISCW016073	EEC02134	339
NADH-ubiquinone oxidoreductase chain 2	ND2	Not found	Not found	...
NADH-ubiquinone oxidoreductase chain 3	ND3	Not found	Not found	...
NADH-ubiquinone oxidoreductase chain 4	ND4	Not found	Not found	...
NADH-ubiquinone oxidoreductase chain 4L	ND4L	Not found	Not found	...
NADH-ubiquinone oxidoreductase chain 5	ND5	ISCW016735	EEC02838	385
NADH-ubiquinone oxidoreductase chain 6	ND6	Not found	Not found	...
OXPHOS COMPLEX II				
Succinate dehydrogenase flavoprotein subunit	SDHA	ISCW000555	EEC02042	608
Succinate dehydrogenase iron-sulfur subunit	SDHB	ISCW018067	EEC06202	286
Succinate dehydrogenase cytochrome b560 subunit	SDHC	ISCW020744	EEC12476	132
Succinate dehydrogenase cytochrome b small subunit	SDHD	ISCW012012	EEC15988	208
OXPHOS COMPLEX III				
Cytochrome b-c1 complex subunit 1	QCR1	Not found	Not found	...
Cytochrome b-c1 complex subunit 2	QCR2	Not found	Not found	...
Cytochrome b	CYTB	ISCW016730	EEC02834	385
Cytochrome c1	CYTC1	ISCW016731	EEC02835	251
Cytochrome b-c1 complex subunit Rieske	RIESKE	ISCW014071	EEC19414	229
Cytochrome b-c1 complex subunit 6	QCR6	ISCW017835	EEC05133	80
Cytochrome b-c1 complex subunit 7	QCR7	ISCW012532	EEC17642	81
Cytochrome b-c1 complex subunit 8	QCR8	ISCW019560	EEC09147	82
Cytochrome b-c1 complex subunit 9	QCR9	ISCW008376	EEC10144	59
Cytochrome b-c1 complex subunit 10	QCR10	Not found	Not found	...
Cytochrome b-c1 complex subunit 11	QCR11	Not found	Not found	...
OXPHOS COMPLEX IV				
Cytochrome c oxidase subunit 1	COX1	Not found	ADO64507	276
Cytochrome c oxidase subunit 2	COX2	ISCW016021	EEC02091	244
Cytochrome c oxidase subunit 3	COX3	ISCW020757	EEC11360	278
Cytochrome c oxidase subunit 4	COX4	Not found	AAY66918	179
Cytochrome c oxidase subunit 5A	COX5A	ISCW008682	EEC12772	153
Cytochrome c oxidase subunit 5B	COX5B	ISCW019526	EEC10693	124
Cytochrome c oxidase subunit 6A	COX6A	ISCW019235	EEC08541	111
Cytochrome c oxidase subunit 6B	COX6B	ISCW015139	EEC20473	82
Cytochrome c oxidase subunit 6C	COX6C	ISCW016559	EEC02407	76
Cytochrome c oxidase subunit 7	COX7	Not found	Not found	...
Cytochrome c oxidase subunit 8	COX8	ISCW024928	EEC20083	68
OXPHOS COMPLEX V (ATP SYNTHASE: F1-ATP SYNTHASE STRUCTURE/F0-ATP SYNTHASE STRUCTURE)				
ATP synthase subunit α 1 (F1)	ATPSA1	ISCW011988	EEC16574	555
ATP synthase subunit α 2 (F1)	ATPSA2	ISCW019217	EEC08626	355
ATP synthase subunit β (F1)	ATPSB	ISCW012509	EEC17118	563
ATP synthase subunit γ (F1)	ATPSG	ISCW023477	EEC19169	314
ATP synthase subunit δ (F1)	ATPSD	ISCW018418	EEC06183	168

(Continued)

TABLE 1 | Continued

Enzymes	Abbreviation	Genome accession	GenBank ID	Length (amino acids)
ATP synthase subunit ϵ (F1)	ATPSE	ISCW022265	EEC17228	55
ATP synthase subunit A (F0)	ATPA	Not found	Not found	...
ATP synthase subunit B (F0)	ATPB	ISCW012060	EEC15991	264
ATP synthase subunit C (F0)	ATPC	ISCW010495	EEC14551	152
β-OXIDATION				
Acyl-CoA dehydrogenase family member 9	ACAD9	ISCW010038	EEC13248	433
Short-chain specific acyl-CoA dehydrogenase (1)	SCAD1	ISCW013995	EEC19715	76
Short-chain specific acyl-CoA dehydrogenase (2)	SCAD2	ISCW002863	EEC02614	410
Medium-chain acyl-CoA dehydrogenase	MCAD	ISCW001274	EEC01138	275
Very long-chain acyl-CoA dehydrogenase	VLCAD	ISCW024772	EEC16420	254
Enoyl-CoA hydratase	ECHD	ISCW012475	EEC16250	290
3-hydroxyacyl CoA dehydrogenase	3HCD	ISCW014460	EEC18745	310
3-ketoacyl-CoA thiolase (Thiolase I)	THIOL	ISCW022661	EEC17467	406
GLYCERONEOGENESIS				
Triosephosphate isomerase	TPI	ISCW008869	EEC13429	247
Glycerol-3-phosphate dehydrogenase cytoplasmic	GPDHc	ISCW005254	EEC07468	340

steps of this pathway, were over-represented and did not change, respectively in response to infection of tick midguts (**Figure 4**). The expression of the p53 target TP53-inducible glycolysis and apoptosis regulator (*tigar*, ISCW020485), which was recently shown to inhibit glycolysis (Bensaad et al., 2006), was down-regulated in tick nymphs, midguts, salivary glands, and ISE6 cells. The over-representation of all glycolytic enzymes correlated with up-regulation of their respective genes, suggesting transcriptional regulation. These data suggested that *A. phagocytophilum* infection activates glucose uptake and degradation in *I. scapularis* midguts. In agreement with an increase in glucose catabolism, the levels of glucose were significantly reduced (0.51 ± 0.06 vs. 0.31 ± 0.05, $p < 0.005$) in infected ISE6 cells when compared to uninfected controls (Villar et al., 2015).

PK catalyzes the final irreversible step of glycolysis, the transfer of a phosphate group from phosphoenolpyruvate to ADP, yielding one molecule of pyruvate and one molecule of adenosine 5′-triphosphate (ATP; Li et al., 2015). This gene was up-regulated, but protein was under-represented in response to infection in tick midguts (**Figures 2**, **4**). Due to the regulatory role of PK, low levels of this enzyme may hamper the flux of pyruvate toward the mitochondrial matrix, decreasing the activity of TCA cycle. PK generates pyruvate, which is transported to the mitochondrial matrix by mitochondrial pyruvate carriers 1 and 2 (MPC1 and MPC2). The homologs for *mpc1* and *mpc2* genes were identified in *I. scapularis* and were up-regulated in tick midguts, but down-regulated in salivary glands in response to *A. phagocytophilum* infection (**Figure 3**). In the mitochondrial matrix, pyruvate is decarboxylated by pyruvate dehydrogenase E1 (PDE1; Berg et al., 2002). The decarboxylation of pyruvate is the first step of a series of enzymatic reactions that transform pyruvate into acetyl coenzyme A (acetyl-Coa), which is oxidized to CO_2 and water in the TCA cycle (Berg et al., 2002). PDE1 is an important regulator of the TCA cycle (Berg et al., 2002). Pyruvate dehydrogenase kinase 1 (PDK1) inhibits, while pyruvate dehydrogenase phosphatase catalytic subunit 1 (PDPC1) activates PDE1 (Berg et al., 2002). We found that in the midguts of infected ticks, PDE1 was under-represented and the genes *pdk1* and *pdpc1* were up-regulated and down-regulated, respectively in response to infection (**Figure 2**). This result strongly suggested that *A. phagocytophilum* infection inhibited the TCA cycle in *I. scapularis* midguts. In agreement with this suggestion, several TCA cycle enzymes such as citrate synthase (CS), aconitase (ACON), isocitrate dehydrogenase [subunits α (IDH3A) and γ (IDH3G1)], 2-oxoglutarate dehydrogenase E1 (OXOE1), succinate dehydrogenase (flavoprotein subunit (SDHA), and iron-sulfur subunit (SDHB) were under-represented in midguts from infected ticks when compared to uninfected controls (**Figures 2, 4**).

The NADH generated by the TCA cycle is fed into the OXPHOS pathway to produce ATP (Li et al., 2015). The mRNA and protein levels of components of the OXPHOS complex I–IV present in *I. scapularis* were examined. Higher mRNA and protein levels were found for most of the respiratory components in infected tick midguts when compared to uninfected controls (**Figure 2**). This result suggested that ticks might have a regulatory mechanism to maintain the levels of ATP in response to the inhibition of the TCA cycle.

Finally, we found that although most genes were up-regulated, all proteins of gluconeogenesis (synthesis of glucose from non-carbohydrate precursors) were under-represented in tick midguts, except for fructose-1,6-bisphosphatase (FBP; **Figure 2**). FBP catalyzes an irreversible reaction in the gluconeogenesis, the conversion of fructose 1,6-bisphosphate into fructose 6-phosphate, and therefore it is a regulatory step of this anabolic pathway. However, the enzyme glucose

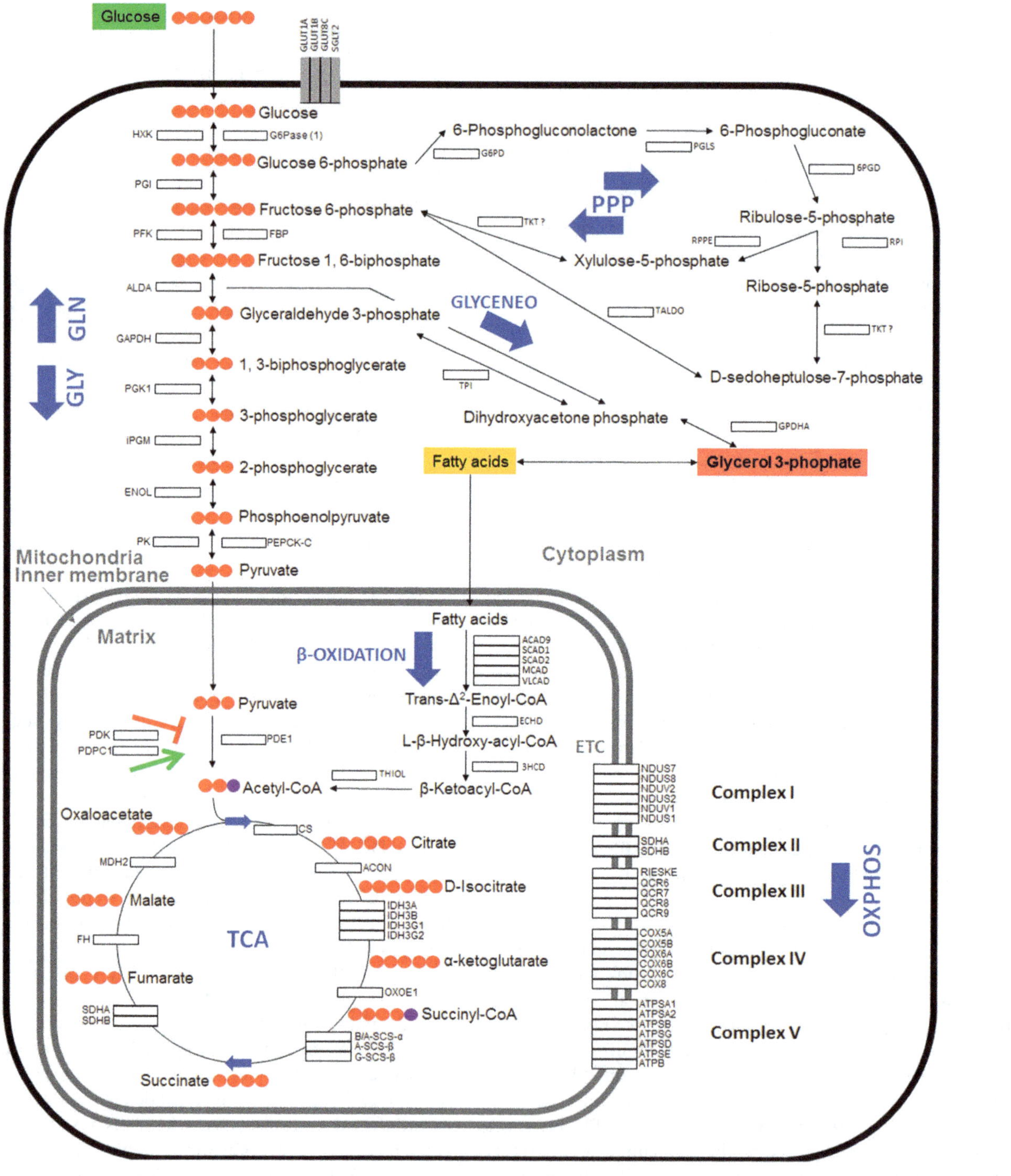

FIGURE 1 | Model of carbohydrate metabolism in *I. scapularis*. The main enzymes involved in Glycolysis (GLY), Gluconeogenesis (GLN), Pentose phosphate pathway (PPP), Tricarboxylic acid cycle (TCA), Oxidative phosphorylation (OXPHOS) complex I to V, β-Oxidation and Glyceroneogenesis (GLYCENEO) and present in the genome of *I. scapularis* (**Table 1**) are shown. The names and number of carbon molecules (Red circles) of the metabolic intermediates of these metabolic pathways are also shown. The names of the enzymes were abbreviated for the different pathways as GLY: Hexokinase (HXK), Phosphoglucose isomerase (PGI), Phosphofructokinase (PFK), Fructose-bisphosphate aldolase A (ALDA), Glyceraldehyde 3-phosphate dehydrogenase (GAPDH), Phosphoglycerate kinase 1 (PGK1), Phosphoglycerate mutase (cofactor-independent) (iPGM), Enolase (ENOL), Pyruvate kinase (PK); GLN: Glucose 6-phosphatase (1) (G6Pase (1)), Fructose-1,6-bisphosphatase (FBP), Phosphoenolpyruvate carboxykinase mitochondrial (1) (PEPCK-M (1)), Phosphoenolpyruvate carboxykinase mitochondrial (2) (PEPCK-M (2)), Phosphoenolpyruvate carboxykinase 1 cytoplasmatic (PEPCK-C), Pyruvate carboxylase (PC); PPP: Glucose 6-phosphate dehydrogenase (G6PD), 6-phosphogluconolactonase (PGLS), 6-phosphogluconate dehydrogenase (6PGD), Ribose 5-Phosphate Isomerase (RPI), Ribulose 5-Phosphate 3-Epimerase (RPPE), Transketolase (TKT), Transaldolase (TALDO); β-Oxidation: Acyl-CoA dehydrogenase family member 9 (ACAD9), Short-chain specific acyl-CoA dehydrogenase

(Continued)

FIGURE 1 | Continued
(1) (SCAD1), Short-chain specific acyl-CoA dehydrogenase (2) (SCAD2), Medium-chain acyl-CoA dehydrogenase (MCAD), Very long-chain acyl-CoA dehydrogenase (VLCAD), Enoyl-CoA hydratase (ECHD), 3-hydroxyacyl CoA dehydrogenase (3HCD), 3-ketoacyl-CoA thiolase (Thiolase I) (THIOL); GLYCENEO: Triosephosphate isomerase (TPI), Glycerol-3-phosphate dehydrogenase cytoplasmic (GPDHc); OXPHOS: Complex I: NADH dehydrogenases (NDUS7, NDUS8, NDUV2, NDUS3, NDUS2 and NDUV1), NADH-ubiquinone oxidoreductases (NDUS1, ND1 and ND5); Complex II: Succinate dehydrogenases (SDHA, SDHB, SDHC, SDHD); Complex III: Cytochrome b and b-c1 complexe subunits (QCR1, QCR2, CYTB, RIESKE, QCR6, QCR7, QCR8, QCR9, QCR10, QCR11), Cytochrome c1 (CYTC1); Complex IV: Cytochrome c oxidase subunits (COX1, COX2, COX3, COX5A, COX5B, COX6A, COX6B, COX6C, COX8); Complex V: ATP synthase subunits (ATPSA1, ATPSA2, ATPSB, ATPSG, ATPSD, ATPSE, ATPB, ATPC).

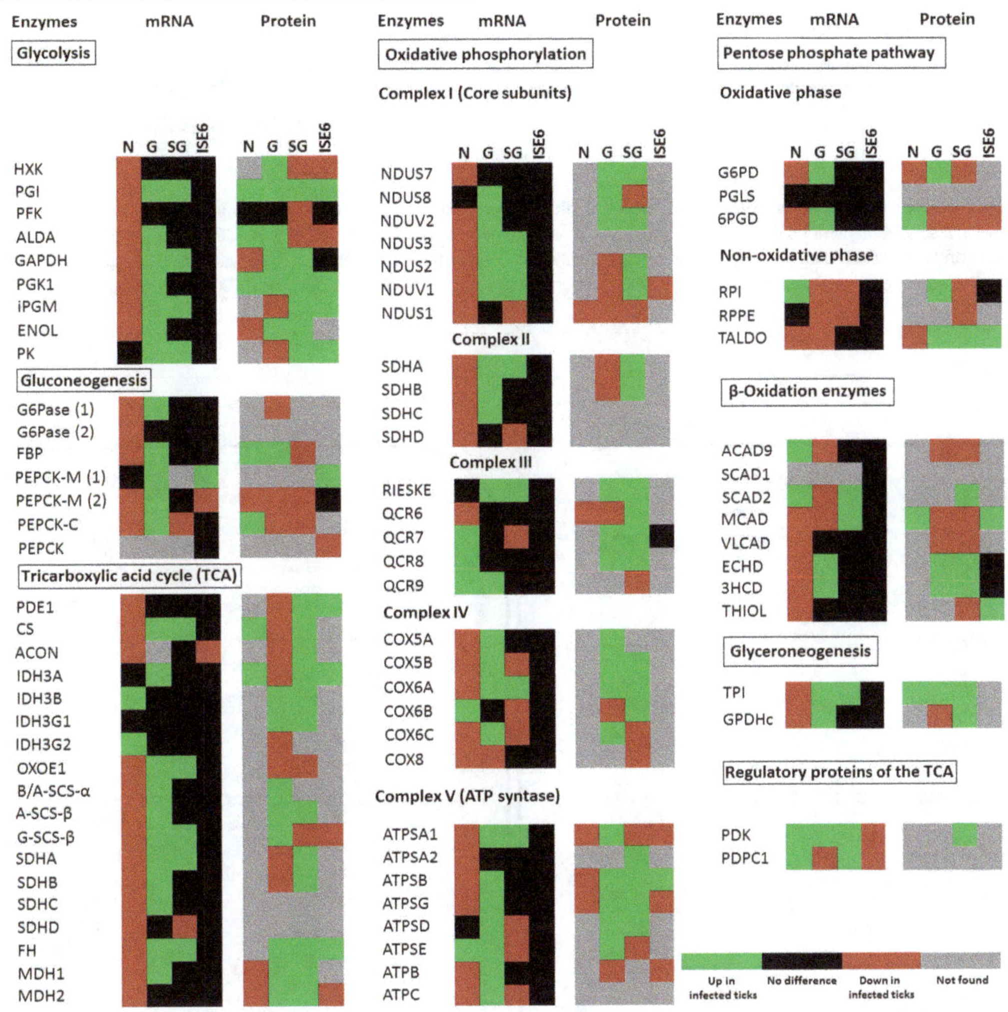

FIGURE 2 | *I. scapularis* carbohydrate metabolism enzymes mRNA and protein levels in response to *A. phagocytophilum* infection. Comparison of carbohydrate metabolism enzymes mRNA and protein levels in *I. scapularis* nymphs (N), female midguts (G), female salivary glands (SG), and ISE6 cells (ISE6) in response to *A. phagocytophilum* infection. Transcriptomics and proteomics data were obtained from previously published datasets available on the Dryad repository database, NCBI's Gene Expression Omnibus database and ProteomeXchange Consortium via the PRIDE partner repository with the dataset identifier PXD002181 and doi: 10.6019/PXD002181 (Ayllón et al., 2015; Villar et al., 2015). Name of enzymes are abbreviated as in **Table 1** and **Figure 1**.

6-phosphatase that catalyzes the last step of gluconeogenesis, the transformation of glucose 6-phosphate into free glucose was under-represented. These results suggested that midgut cells in *A. phagocytophilum*-infected ticks tend to keep glucose 6-phosphate within the cells for other metabolic processes (e.g., glycogen synthesis).

HIF-1 Components Are Up-Regulated in *I. scapularis* Infected with *A. phagocytophilum*

HIF-1 is a heterodimeric transcription factor consisting of a constitutively expressed β-subunit (HIF-1β) and an oxygen-regulated α-subunit (HIF-1α; Pagé et al., 2002; Déry et al., 2005;

Glucose transporters	Abbreviation	Genome accession	GenBank ID	Length (aa)
Facilitated glucose transporter 1 A	GLUT1A	ISCW013894	EEC19934	479
Facilitated glucose transporter 1 B	GLUT1B	ISCW002239	EEC04592	355
Facilitated glucose transporter 3	GLUT3	ISCW004700	EEC06442	512
Facilitated glucose transporter 8 C	GLUT8C	ISCW010927	EEC14072	512
Facilitated glucose transporter 8 D	GLUT8D	ISCW024591	EEC11630	273
Facilitated glucose transporter 10	GLUT10	ISCW000394	EEC02475	149
Facilitated glucose transporter 12	GLUT12	ISCW024255	EEC06363	165
Sodium-dependent glucose transporter 1	SGLT1	ISCW019840	EEC09410	383
Sodium-dependent glucose transporter 2	SGLT2	ISCW019037	EEC07109	462
Mitochondrial pyruvate carriers				
Mitochondrial pyruvate carrier 1	MPC1	ISCW015574	EEC00490	108
Mitochondrial pyruvate carrier 2	MPC2	ISCW019127	EEC09109	115

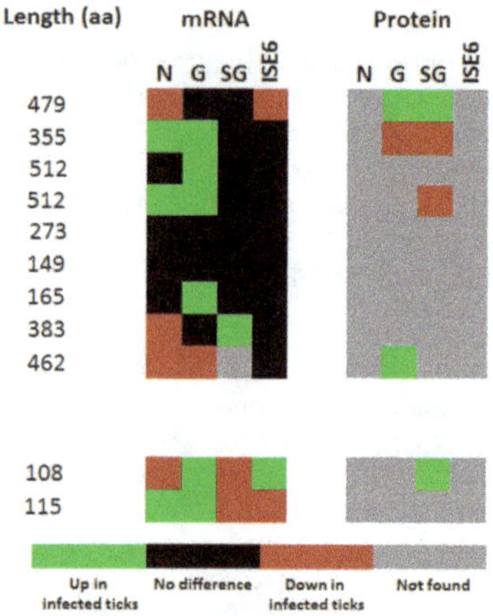

FIGURE 3 | *I. scapularis* glucose transporters mRNA and protein levels in response to *A. phagocytophilum* infection. Comparison of glucose transporters mRNA and protein levels in *I. scapularis* nymphs (N), female midguts (G), female salivary glands (SG) and ISE6 cells (ISE6) in response to *A. phagocytophilum* infection. Transcriptomics and proteomics data were obtained from previously published datasets available on the Dryad repository database, NCBI' Gene Expression Omnibus database and ProteomeXchange Consortium via the PRIDE partner repository with the dataset identifier PXD002181 and doi: 10.6019/PXD002181 (Ayllón et al., 2015; Villar et al., 2015).

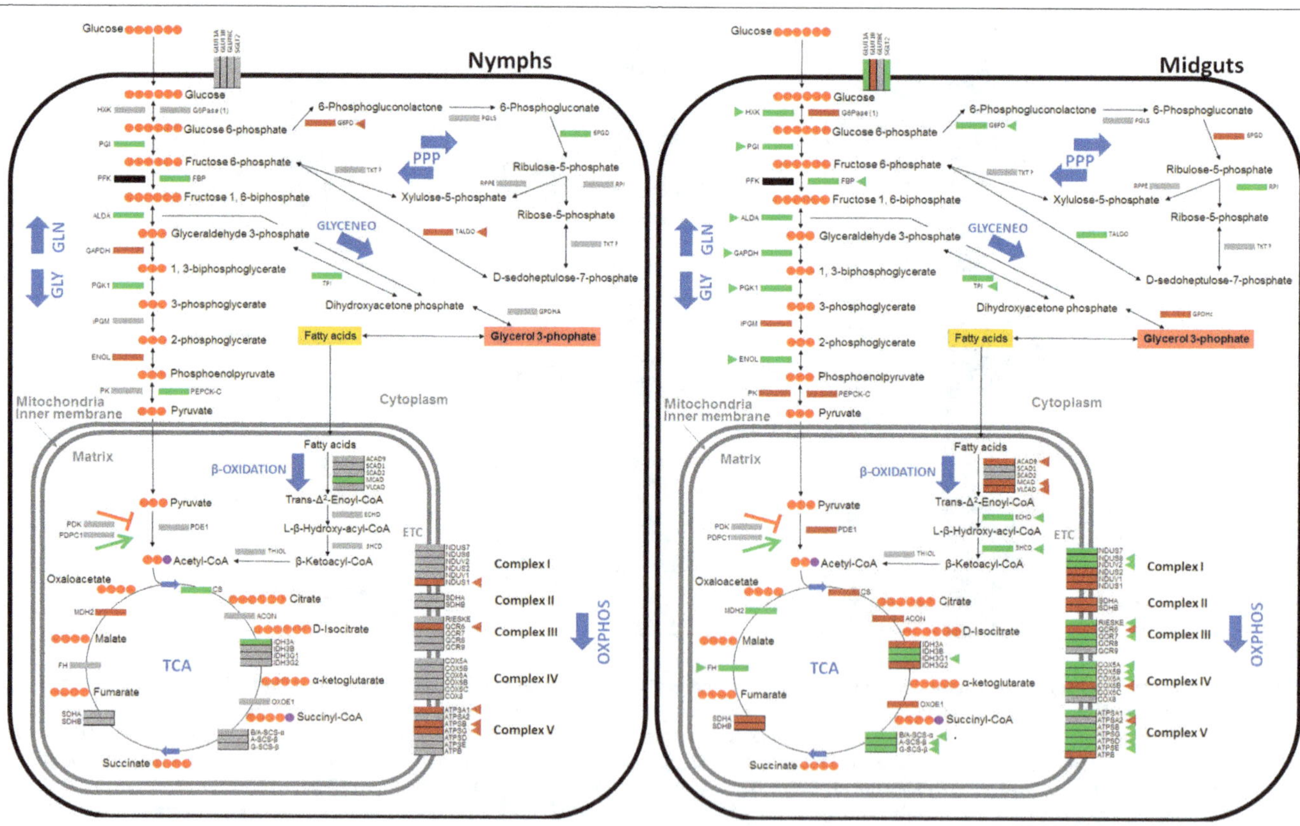

FIGURE 4 | Carbohydrate metabolic pathways in response to *A. phagocytophilum* infection in *I. scapularis* nymphs and female midguts. Protein representation of enzymes of the *I. scapularis* carbohydrate metabolic pathways in response to *A. phagocytophilum* infection is shown. Similar changes in mRNA and protein levels are highlighted (triangles). Code: green, up-regulated/over-represented; red, down-regulated/under-represented.

Ziello et al., 2007; Badeaux and Shi, 2013). The gene encoding for HIF-1α (ISCW023657), which is a major transcriptional activator of glycolytic genes (Hu et al., 2006), was significantly up-regulated in tick midguts, but not in nymphs, salivary glands or ISE6 cells in response to *A. phagocytophilum* infection (Ayllón et al., 2015; Villar et al., 2015). The expression of the gene

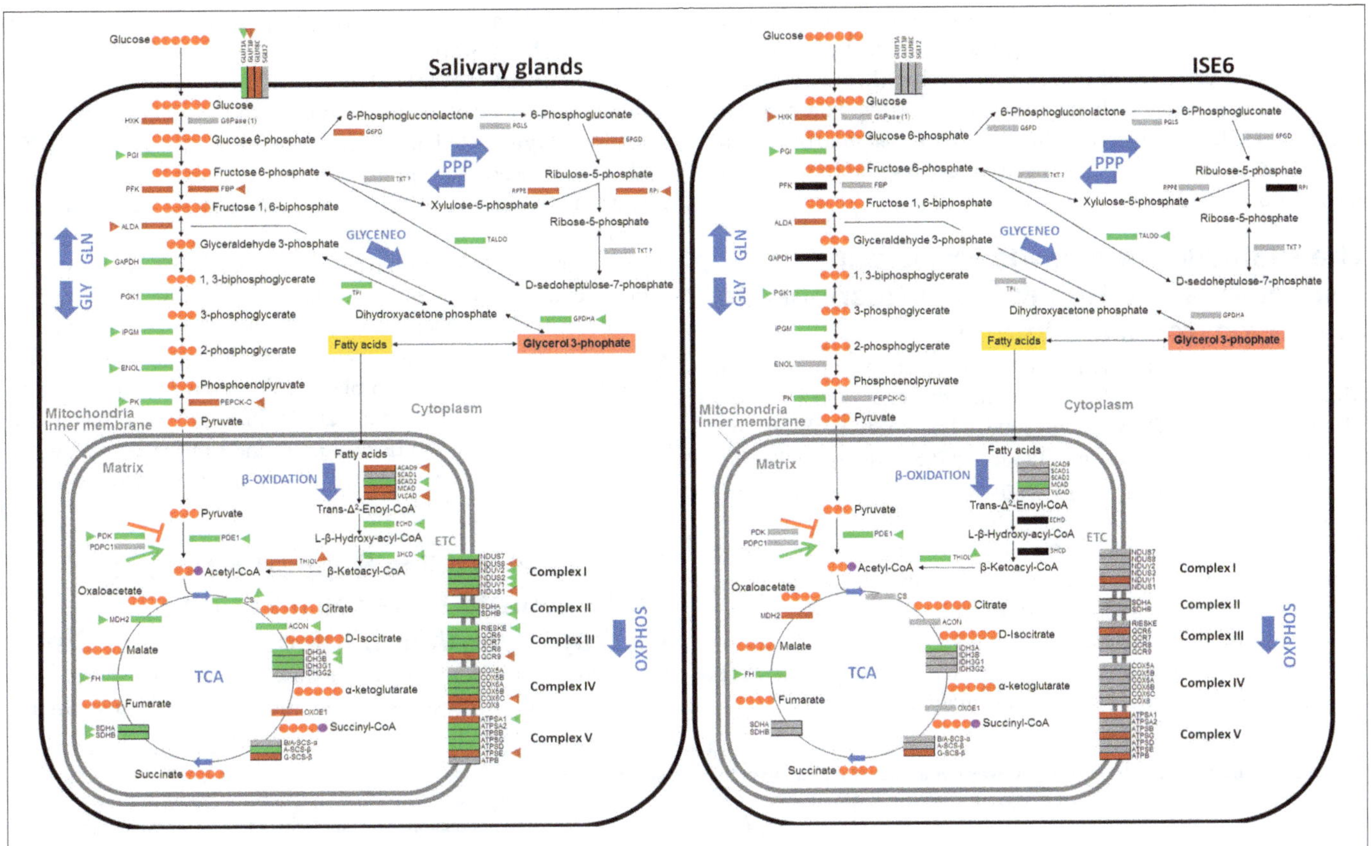

FIGURE 5 | Carbohydrate metabolic pathways in response to *A. phagocytophilum* infection in *I. scapularis* salivary glands and ISE6 cells. Protein representation of enzymes of the *I. scapularis* carbohydrate metabolic pathways in response to *A. phagocytophilum* infection is shown. Similar changes in mRNA and protein levels are highlighted (triangles). Code: green, up-regulated/over-represented; red, down-regulated/under-represented.

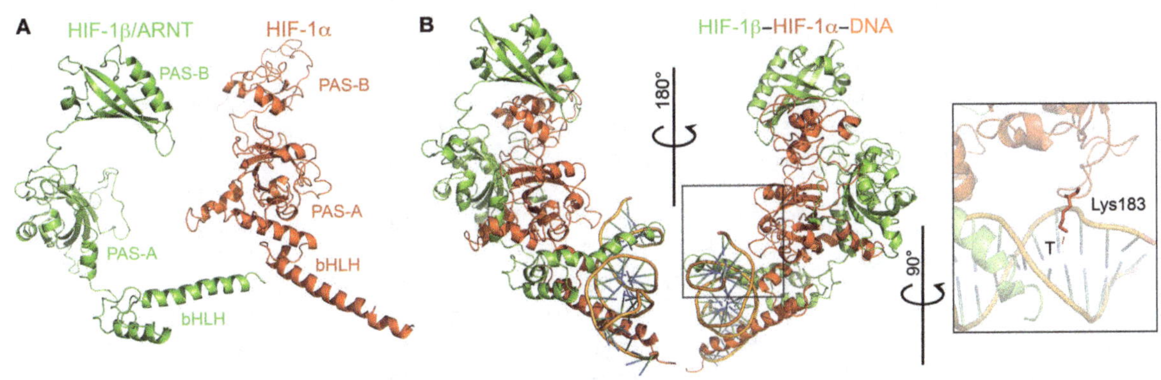

FIGURE 6 | Modeling of the HIF-1α-HIF-1β-HRE complex. (A) HIF-1α (red) and HIF-1β (green) monomers with their respective domains labeled. **(B)** Ternary complex of both monomers plus the hypoxia response element (HRE; orange). The inset shows the conserved Lys residue that interacts with the thymine (T) of HRE.

encoding for the HIF-1β (ISCW023999), which is a molecular partner of HIF-1α, was up-regulated in midguts from infected ticks, but was down-regulated in nymphs and did not change in salivary glands and ISE6 cells in response to infection (Ayllón et al., 2015; Villar et al., 2015).

Both *I. scapularis* HIF-1α and HIF-1β (a.k.a, aryl hydrocarbon receptor nuclear translocator or ARNT) possess the conserved basic helix-loop-helix (bHLH) domain and two PAS domains (**Figures 6A,B**). The bHLH domain of HIF-1α and HIF-1β were highly conserved with identical interacting residues as those previously identified (Dalei et al., 2015). The PAS-B domain of HIF-1α was disordered due to its low conservation and the presence of small insertions and deletions when compared to the mouse HIF-1α (Dalei et al., 2015). The PAS-B of HIF-1α interacts with both the PAS domain of HIF-1β, thereby making it difficult to determine interacting residues. One key feature of HIF-1α is the presence of two residues lysine (Lys) and glycine (Gly), which interact with the nucleotides of hypoxia response element (HRE; Dalei et al., 2015). The *I. scapularis* HIF-1α had the conserved Lys, but showed an asparagine (Asn) to Gly substitution (**Figure 6**).

The PI3K/Akt Pathway Is Present in *I. scapularis* and Regulated in Response to *A. phagocytophilum* Infection

It has been demonstrated that a number of non-hypoxic stimuli are highly capable of inducing the expression of *hif-1* (Pagé et al., 2002; Déry et al., 2005). The PI3K pathway and its downstream effectors, mTOR and p70S6 kinase (p70S6K), may induce a hypoxia-independent increase in HIF-1α levels (Déry et al., 2005). In addition, diacylglycerol (DAG)-sensitive protein kinases C (PKC) were shown to up-regulate *hif-1α* gene expression in a hypoxia-independent manner (Pagé et al., 2002; Déry et al., 2005). Infection with *A. phagocytophilum* activates PI3K in *I. scapularis* (Sultana et al., 2010). Therefore, we characterized the mRNA and protein levels of tick PI3K components in response to *A. phagocytophilum* infection.

Most PI3K-mTOR pathway components found in other organisms (Pilot-Storck et al., 2010) were identified in the *I. scapularis* genome (**Table 2**). The tick PI3K components were differentially regulated in response to *A. phagocytophilum* infection (**Figure 7**). The *p70S6K* and PI3K components (*p85α* and *p110α*) were up-regulated in tick midguts and salivary glands in response to infection. Additionally, p70S6K and p85α proteins were over-represented in midguts from infected ticks when compared to uninfected controls (**Figure 7**). Oxygen-independent activation of *hif-1α* may involve PI3K components, p70S6K and mTOR (Déry et al., 2005). However, we did not find an mTOR ortholog in the *I. scapularis* genome. DAG-sensitive PKCs were also suggested to play a role in oxygen-independent activation of *hif-1α* (Pagé et al., 2002). Protein PKCα was found to be over-represented in tick midguts and salivary glands, while the *PKCε* gene was up-regulated in tick midguts in response to infection.

Functional Studies Support a Role for Carbohydrate Metabolism during *A. phagocytophilum* Infection of Tick Cells

Functional studies were focused on glycolysis by targeting the process at different levels (**Figures 8A,B**).

TABLE 2 | Annotation of PI3K-mTOR pathway components identified in the *I. scapularis* genome.

Proteins	Abbreviation	Genome accession	GenBank ID	Length (amino acids)
RAC-alpha serine/threonine-protein kinase	AKT2	ISCW018284	EEC06033	371
Phosphatidylinositol 4,5-bisphosphate 3-kinase catalytic subunit α	p110α	ISCW014229	EEC18977	617
Phosphatidylinositol 4,5-bisphosphate 3-kinase catalytic subunit β	p110β	ISCW010469	EEC14480	491
Phosphatidylinositol-4-phosphate 3-kinase C2 domain-containing α (1)	PI3K-C2α1	ISCW022811	EEC17358	1638
Phosphatidylinositol-4-phosphate 3-kinase C2 domain-containing α (2)	PI3K-C2α2	ISCW004026	EEC06376	1142
Phosphatidylinositol 3-kinase regulatory subunit α	p85α	ISCW011707	EEC13970	427
3- phosphoinositide-dependent protein kinase 1	PDK1	ISCW021115	EEC15400	521
Phosphatidylinositol 3,4,5-trisphosphate 5-phosphatase 1	SHIP1	ISCW000015	EEC00572	535
Phosphatidylinositol 3,4,5-trisphosphate 3-phosphatase PTEN	PTEN	ISCW021211	EEC15363	363
Arf-GAP with GTPase, ANK repeat and PH domain-containing protein	PIKE	ISCW014072	EEC18950	558
Glycogen synthase kinase 3 β (2)	GSK3β2	ISCW009451	EEC11886	588
Hamartin	TSC1	ISCW023319	EEC19233	874
Tuberin	TSC2	ISCW012320	EEC16560	429
Serine/threonine kinase 11 (1)	LKB1/STK11A	ISCW024898	EEC19357	170
Serine/threonine kinase 11 (2)	LKB1/STK11B	ISCW015294	EEC20092	293
AMP-activated protein kinase α	AMPKα	ISCW020637	EEC13103	510
AMP-activated protein kinase β	AMPKβ	ISCW021036	EEC15614	183
AMP-activated protein kinase γ	AMPKγ	ISCW010164	EEC13342	154
Ras homolog enriched in brain	RHEB	ISCW018020	EEC05182	182
Regulatory-associated protein of mTOR	RAPTOR	ISCW018753	EEC07385	995
G protein β subunit-like	GβL	ISCW002765	EEC03813	324
Rapamycin-insensitive companion of mTOR	RICTOR	ISCW018420	EEC06185	987
Phosphatidylinositol 3-kinase catalytic subunit type 3	Vps34	ISCW008679	EEC12769	864
Serine/threonine-protein kinase VPS15	Vps15	ISCW017661	EEC06819	1351
Pleckstrin homology domain-containing, family O member 1	CKIP1	ISCW021605	EEC15223	359
Casein kinase 2 subunit α	CK2α	ISCW007259	EEC10594	436
Casein kinase 2 subunit β	CK2β	ISCW014459	EEC18744	222
Ribosomal protein S6 kinase beta-1 (p70s6 kinase)	S6K1/p70s6K	ISCW017390	EEC03348	344

A. phagocytophilum-infected ISE6 cells were left untreated or treated for 24 or 48 h with 2-Deoxy-D-Glucose to inhibit glycolysis (Wang et al., 2011), LY294002 to inhibit the PI3K (Sultana et al., 2010), Chetomin to inhibit the activity of HIF-1α (Misra et al., 2012) or Deferoxamine mesylate to activate HIF-1α (**Figures 8A,B**). Both HIF-1α (Ayllón et al., 2015; Villar et al., 2015), which is a major transcriptional activator of glycolytic genes (Hu et al., 2006), and most PI3K components (**Figure 7**) were affected in response to *A. phagocytophilum* infection. The results showed that LY294002 was the only compound active in ISE6 tick cells (**Figure 8A**). The lack of effect of chetomin and Deferoxamine mesylate on tick HIF-1α activity may be due to structural differences between tick and mammalian HIF-1α. The treatment of tick cells with LY294002 for 48 h resulted in lower HIF-1α activity when compared to untreated control cells (**Figure 8A**). Treatment with LY294002 has been shown in *I. scapularis* and other organisms to inhibit the PI3K pathway (Sultana et al., 2010), which is involved in the induction of HIF-1α to activate the glycolysis (Déry et al., 2005). Therefore, the results obtained in tick cells supported a role for PI3K in HIF-1α induction in tick cells. The decrease in *A. phagocytophilum* infection after LY294002 treatment for 24 and 48 h (**Figure 8B**) provided additional support to these results. As expected from the lack of effect on HIF-1α activity after incubation of tick cells with the other compounds, treatment did not affect *A. phagocytophilum* infection in these cells. Additionally, the immunofluorescence assay of GAPDH, which was over-represented in *I. scapularis* midguts and salivary glands in response to *A. phagocytophilum* infection (**Figures 4, 5**), corroborated the results of the proteomics analysis in tick salivary glands (**Figure 8C**).

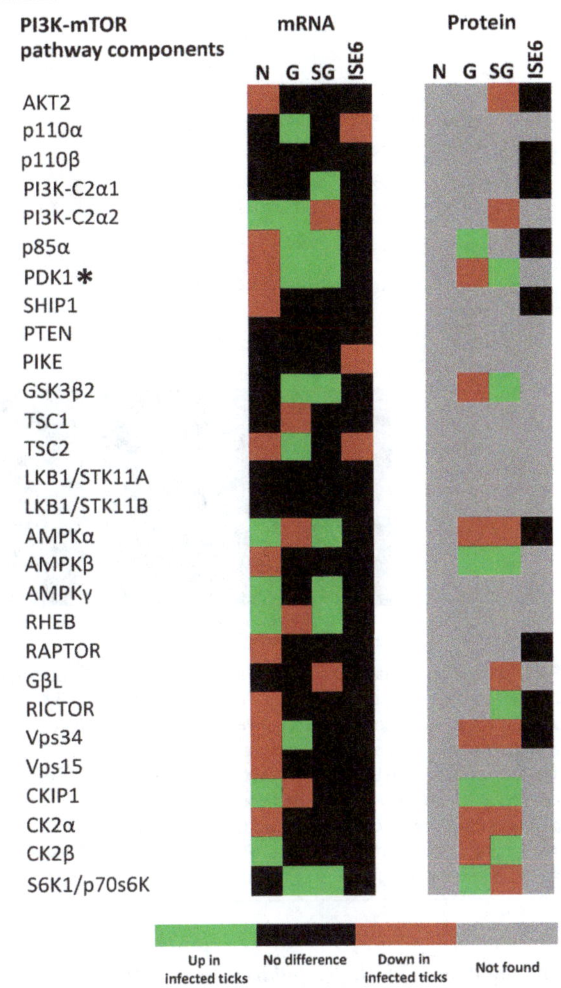

FIGURE 7 | *I. scapularis* PI3K-mTOR pathway components mRNA and protein levels in response to *A. phagocytophilum* infection. Comparison of PI3K-mTOR pathway components mRNA and protein levels in *I. scapularis* nymphs (N), female midguts (G), female salivary glands (SG) and ISE6 cells (ISE6) in response to *A. phagocytophilum* infection. Transcriptomics and proteomics data were obtained from previously published datasets available on the Dryad repository database, NCBI's Gene Expression Omnibus database and ProteomeXchange Consortium via the PRIDE partner repository with the dataset identifier PXD002181 and doi: 10.6019/PXD002181 (Ayllón et al., 2015; Villar et al., 2015). Name of enzymes are abbreviated as in **Table 2**. (*) In this figure, PDK1 stands for 3- phosphoinositide-dependent protein kinase 1, and not Pyruvate dehydrogenase kinase 1, which is also abbreviated as PDK1.

DISCUSSION

Recently, Villar et al. (2015) showed modifications in tick cell glucose metabolism during *A. phagocytophilum* infection. The results evidenced that infection affected the glucose metabolic pathway in tick cells through phosphoenolpyruvate carboxykinase (PEPCK) inhibition leading to decreased gluconeogenesis, which also results in the inhibition of cell apoptosis that increases pathogen infection of tick cells (Villar et al., 2015). Furthermore, these results provided evidence that other carbohydrate metabolic pathways are also affected by pathogen infection. Therefore, the objective of this study was the characterization of the dynamics of major carbohydrate pathways during *A. phagocytophilum* infection of *I. scapularis*.

Cellular glycolysis converts glucose to pyruvate, which enters the mitochondria where it is converted into acetyl-CoA, and is metabolized via the TCA cycle yielding reducing equivalents that are used for OXPHOS to generate ATP (Eisenreich et al., 2013, 2015). TCA cycle can be also fueled by the acetyl-CoA produced via degradation of fatty acids after β-Oxidation (Eisenreich et al., 2013). Alternatively, glucose can be used to produce Ribose 5-phosphate, a precursor for the synthesis of nucleotides through the PPP (Berg et al., 2002; **Figure 1**). In addition, glyceroneogenesis uses glycerol 3-phophate, obtained from the reduction of dihydroxyacetone phosphate (glycolytic intermediate) to synthetize fatty acids, and therefore is a major link between carbohydrate metabolism and lipid metabolism (Berg et al., 2002; **Figure 1**).

In this study, orthologs for 79 components of major carbohydrate metabolic pathways were identified in *I. scapularis*, and their role was characterized in response to *A. phagocytophilum* infection. The analysis was focused on seven pathways including glycolysis, gluconeogenesis, PPP, glyceroneogenesis, β-Oxidation, TCA cycle, and OXPHOS. The results showed that genes involved in glycolysis

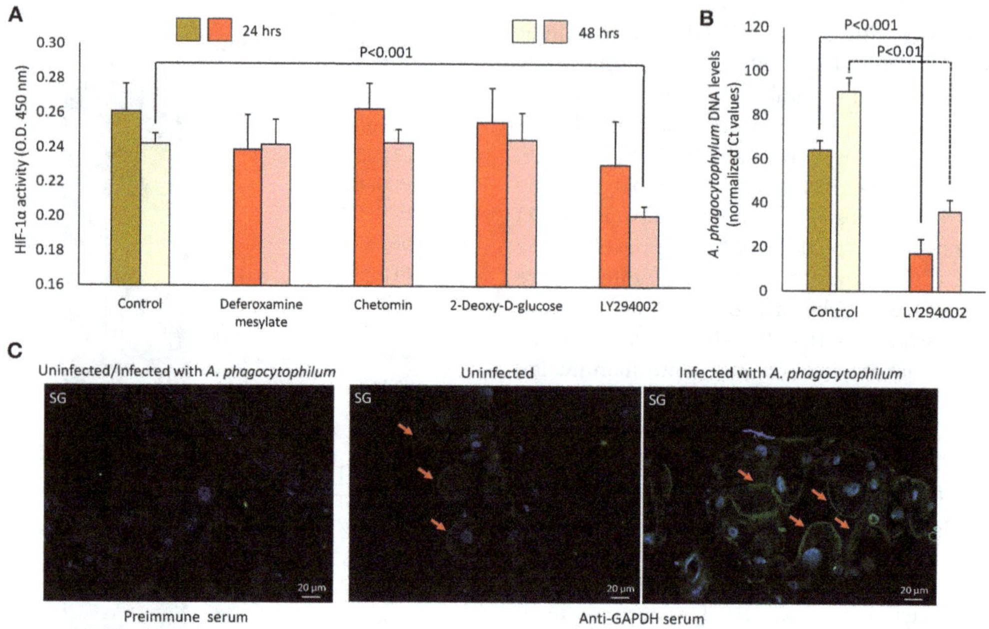

FIGURE 8 | Functional analysis supports a role for glycolysis during *A. phagocytophilum* infection of tick cells. (A) *A. phagocytophilum*-infected ISE6 cells were left untreated (Control) or treated for 24 or 48 h with 2-Deoxy-D-Glucose to inhibit glycolysis, LY294002 to inhibit the PI3K, Chetomin to inhibit the activity of HIF-1α or Deferoxamine mesylate to activate HIF-1α. HIF-1α activity was determined in cell lysates, and O.D. 450 nm values were shown as average + *SD* and compared between treated and untreated control cells by Student's *t*-test with unequal variance ($P = 0.05$; $N = 4$ biological replicates). **(B)** *A. phagocytophilum* DNA levels were characterized in LY294002-treated and untreated control cells by *msp4* real-time PCR normalizing against tick *16S rDNA*. Normalized Ct values were compared between treated and untreated control cells by Student's *t*-test with unequal variance ($P < 0.01$; $N = 4$ biological replicates). **(C)** Representative images of imunofluorescence analysis of uninfected and *A. phagocytophilum*-infected adult female *I. scapularis* salivary gland acini (SG). Tick tissues were stained with preimmune control serum or mouse anti-GAPDH monoclonal antibodies (green, FITC) or DAPI (blue) and superimposed (FITC+DAPI). Bars, 20 μm. Red arrows illustrate the positive staining for GAPDH in tick SG.

were up-regulated in *I. scapularis* ticks infected with *A. phagocytophilum*. In contrast, PEPCK, which is the enzyme that catalyzes the first step of gluconeogenesis (after this step the molecules are "committed" to the pathway and will ultimately end up in the pathway's final product) was under-represented (**Figure 2**). However, in addition to low levels of PEPCK, low TCA cycle activity might be also necessary to control gluconeogenesis (Burgess et al., 2007). Interestingly, we found that several enzymes and intermediates such as succinate of the TCA cycle are also under-represented in infected tick ISE6 cells and midguts (**Figures 4, 5**; Villar et al., 2015). These results strongly suggested that upon *A. phagocytophilum* infection, glycolysis is enhanced, TCA cycle inhibited and in agreement with our previous results (Villar et al., 2015), gluconeogenesis is inhibited. These findings supported the idea that *A. phagocytophilum* infection might be an energy-demanding process for the tick cells and that the pathogen may benefit from glycolytic intermediates.

Intracellular bacteria trigger diverse host metabolic responses (Eisenreich et al., 2013, 2015). Numerous transcriptome studies have identified some of these metabolic responses as unspecific (triggered by extracellular/intracellular and pathogenic/non-pathogenic bacteria) and are therefore called "core host responses" (Boldrick et al., 2002). These "core host responses" are modulated in different ways by virulence mechanisms of different bacteria species (Boldrick et al., 2002). For example, *in vivo* studies in mice showed that the facultative intracellular pathogen *Mycobacterium tuberculosis* induces a reduction in the levels of glucose and the TCA cycle intermediates oxaloacetate and fumarate, but also an increase in lactate and succinate concentration (Shin et al., 2011; Somashekar et al., 2011). In *Listeria monocytogenes*, Lecuit et al. (2007) found that the transcription of most glycolytic genes was enhanced after infection in mice, particularly *hxk II*. The upregulation of glycolytic genes was linked to enhanced *hif-1α* expression and downregulation of the gluconeogenic gene *fbp* (Lecuit et al., 2007). The above examples illustrate commonalities among the host metabolic responses to *M. tuberculosis*, *L. monocytogenes* and *A. phagocytophilum* infection.

Based on the results of this study, a model was proposed in which *A. phagocytophilum* induces transcriptional activation of *hif-1α* through PI3K (p85α, p110α, and p70S6K) and PKC to activate the glycolytic pathway and inhibit the TCA cycle in infected ticks (**Figure 9**). This model was partially supported by functional studies using a PI3K inhibitor to monitor the effect on HIF-1α activity and pathogen infection (**Figures 8A,B**). In normoxia, HIF-1α is rapidly degraded. Therefore, *A. phagocytophilum* may have additional mechanisms to stabilize HIF-1α at normal oxygen concentrations. The increase in the levels of heat shock proteins HSP70 and HSP90

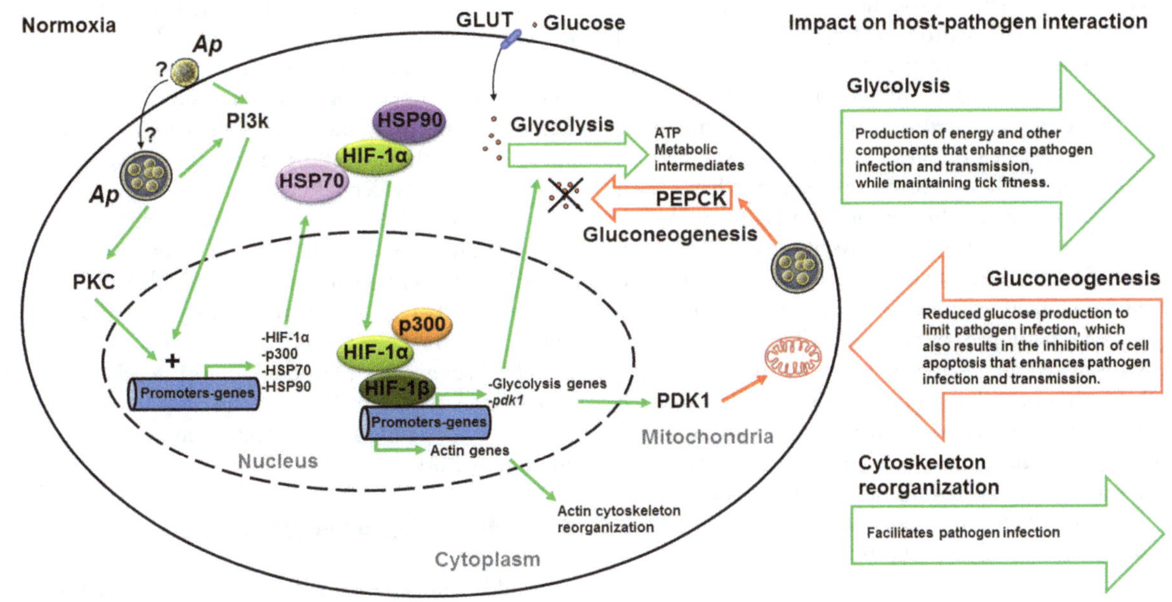

FIGURE 9 | Mechanistic model of carbohydrate metabolism manipulation by *A. phagocytophilum*. We propose a mechanism by which *A. phagocytophilum* enhances glycolysis through HIF activation under normoxic conditions. Upon contact with the host membrane or once inside the parasitophorous vacuole, *A. phagocytophilum* induces the activation of PI3K and PKC that ultimately induce the expression of heat shock proteins HSP70 and HSP90, the acetyltransferase p300 and *hif-1α*. In normoxia, HSP70 and HSP90 stabilize HIF-1α, making possible the recruitment of p300 and HIF-1α to form a complex with HIF-1β in the nucleus. This complex activates the expression of HIF-1α target genes, which include glycolytic genes and *pdk1*. This mechanism will result in the increase in glycolysis and inhibition of gluconeogenesis. Furthermore, HIF activation can also leads to actin cytoskeleton reorganization. Therefore, by activating the HIF system *A. phagocytophilum* may regulate at the same time the tick cell carbohydrate metabolism and cytoskeleton organization. Green and red lines indicate induction/activation and inhibition, respectively. Question marks indicate that we do not know whether *A. phagocytophilum* induces the activation of PI3K and PKC upon contact with the host membrane or once inside the parasitophorous vacuole. Ap, *A. phagocytophilum*; PI3K, phosphatidylinositol 3-kinase pathway; diacylglycerol (DAG)-sensitive protein kinases C (PKC); HIF, hypoxia-inducible factor; PDK1, pyruvate dehydrogenase kinase 1; GLUT, facilitative glucose transporters; PEPCK, phosphoenolpyruvate carboxykinase.

may contribute to the stabilization of HIF-1α in normoxia (Zhou et al., 2004). Previously, we showed that HSP70 and HSP90 were over-represented in *A. phagocytophilum*-infected ISE6 tick cells when compared to uninfected cells (Villar et al., 2015). Furthermore, mobilization of p300 at HIF target genes may be an additional requirement of HIF-mediated transcriptional activation (Badeaux and Shi, 2013). In agreement with this model, recently we showed that *A. phagocytophilum* induces the production of p300 to inhibit cell apoptosis and increase bacterial multiplication in tick cells (Cabezas-Cruz et al., 2016). By inhibiting the TCA cycle in host cells, *A. phagocytophilum* may inhibit the entrance of glutamine and glutamate to the TCA cycle via α-ketoglutarate, which is one of the intermediates in the TCA cycle. This process may increase the cytoplasmic concentration of glutamine and glutamate that can then be used by *A. phagocytophilum*. The TCA cycle of *A. phagocytophilum* is incomplete (because one gene for isocitrate dehydrogenase is missing from the genome) and requires the exogenous acquisition of glutamine and glutamate (Huang et al., 2007), which the pathogen may obtain from the host cell cytoplasm. *A. phagocytophilum* has the enzyme that converts glutamine to glutamate and glutamate can be then transformed to α-ketoglutarate that may fuel the bacterial TCA cycle.

Interestingly, it was recently shown that inhibition of prolyl hydroxylases, which are involved in the regulation of HIF-1α activity, induces HIF-1α-dependent cytoskeletal remodeling in endothelial cells (Weidemann et al., 2013). Therefore, it is possible that *A. phagocytophilum* activates HIF-1α through PI3K to regulate simultaneously the carbohydrate metabolism and cytoskeleton organization to facilitate infection and multiplication in tick cells (**Figure 9**).

The comparison of metabolic pathways between selected Anaplasmataceae showed that *Rickettsia prowazekii*, *Ehrlichia chaffeensis*, *Neorickettsia sennetsu*, *Wolbachia pipientis*, and *A. phagocytophilum* might not be able to actively carry out glycolysis. Therefore, glycolytic metabolic intermediates produced by host cells may be necessary for the development of these bacteria. Only those glycolysis enzymes necessary to produce glyceraldehyde-3-phosphate and dihydroxyacetone phosphate from phosphoenolpyruvate are present in the genome of these *Rickettsia* spp. (Dunning Hotopp et al., 2006). Therefore, phosphoenolpyruvate may be one of the glycolytic intermediates that *A. phagocytophilum* hijacks from the host cell cytoplasm. Additionally, glycerol-3-phosphate, which is a product of glyceroneogenesis, was proposed as another metabolite taken from the host by *Rickettsia* spp. (Dunning Hotopp et al., 2006). In agreement with this proposed model, the glyceroneogenesis enzymes triosephosphate isomerase (TPI) and glycerol-3-phosphate dehydrogenase cytoplasmic (GPDHc) were over-represented in infected tick nymphs, midguts and/or salivary glands when compared to uninfected controls.

The failure to identify *I. scapularis* orthologs for some genes may be due to the absence of these pathway components in ticks or the fact that only ~57% of the genome have been sequenced and assembled for this species (de la Fuente et al., 2016b; Gulia-Nuss et al., 2016). These results were similar to those obtained before for other genes and proteins in response to *A. phagocytophilum* infection, showing tissue-specific differences in the response to pathogen infection (Ayllón et al., 2015). As previously discussed, these results suggested that differences between mRNA and protein levels could be due to delay between mRNA and protein accumulation which requires sampling at different time points and/or the role for post-transcriptional and post-translational modifications in the tick tissue-specific response to *A. phagocytophilum* infection (Ayllón et al., 2015; Villar et al., 2015; Cabezas-Cruz et al., 2016).

CONCLUSIONS

These results support that major carbohydrate metabolic pathways are conserved in ticks. *A. phagocytophilum* infection has a major impact on the regulation of carbohydrate metabolic pathways in tick cells. As a result of the studies reported here, a mechanism was proposed by which this pathogen might induce the expression and stabilization of HIF-1α to increase glycolysis, suppress TCA cycle to reduce gluconeogenesis, and regulate cytoskeleton organization (**Figure 9**). This may be achieved by a coordinated action of PI3K/PKC pathway, for induction of *hif-1α* expression, and HSP70/90 and p300, for HIF-1α stabilization. The increase in glycolysis results in the production of energy and other components that enhance pathogen infection and transmission while preserving tick fitness. The reduction in gluconeogenesis may be a cell response to limit pathogen infection, but also results in the inhibition of cell apoptosis to enhance pathogen infection and transmission. These mechanisms provided additional support for the co-evolution of tick-pathogen interactions that can produce both conflict and cooperation between them (de la Fuente et al., 2016c). The identification of these mechanisms provided additional evidences to support that *A. phagocytophilum* uses similar strategies to infect vertebrate hosts and ticks (de la Fuente et al., 2016a), therefore suggesting the possibility of developing strategies for a more effective control of *A. phagocytophilum* and its associated diseases by targeting similar mechanisms in both vertebrate hosts and tick vectors.

AUTHOR CONTRIBUTIONS

AC and JF conceived the study. PA performed the experiments. AC, PA, JV, MV, and JF performed data analyses. AC and JF wrote the paper, and other co-authors made additional suggestions and approved the manuscript.

FUNDING

This research was supported by the Ministerio de Economia y Competitividad (Spain) grant BFU2016-79892-P and the European Union (EU) Seventh Framework Programme (FP7) ANTIGONE project number 278976. MV was supported by the Research Plan of the University of Castilla-La Mancha (UCLM), Spain.

REFERENCES

Altschul, S. F., Gish, W., Miller, W., Myers, E. W., and Lipman, D. J. (1990). Basic local alignment search tool. *J. Mol. Biol.* 215, 403–410. doi: 10.1016/S0022-2836(05)80360-2

Asanovich, K. M., Bakken, J. S., Madigan, J. E., Aguero-Rosenfeld, M., Wormser, G. P., and Dumler, J. S. (1997). Antigenic diversity of granulocytic Ehrlichia isolates from humans in Wisconsin and New York and a horse in California. *J. Infect. Dis.* 176, 1029–1034. doi: 10.1086/516529

Atilgan, A. R., Durell, S. R., Jernigan, R. L., Demirel, M. C., Keskin, O., and Bahar, I. (2001). Anisotropy of fluctuation dynamics of proteins with an elastic network model. *Biophys. J.* 80, 505–515. doi: 10.1016/S0006-3495(01)76033-X

Augustin, R. (2010). The protein family of glucose transport facilitators: it's not only about glucose after all. *IUBMB Life* 62, 315–333. doi: 10.1002/iub.315

Ayllón, N., Villar, M., Busby, A. T., Kocan, K. M., Blouin, E. F., Bonzón-Kulichenko, E., et al. (2013). *Anaplasma phagocytophilum* inhibits apoptosis and promotes cytoskeleton rearrangement for infection of tick cells. *Infect. Immun.* 81, 2415–2425. doi: 10.1128/IAI.00194-13

Ayllón, N., Villar, M., Galindo, R. C., Kocan, K. M., Šíma, R., López, J. A., et al. (2015). Systems biology of tissue-specific response to *Anaplasma phagocytophilum* reveals differentiated apoptosis in the tick vector *Ixodes scapularis*. *PLoS Genet.* 11:e1005120. doi: 10.1371/journal.pgen.1005120

Badeaux, A. I., and Shi, Y. (2013). Emerging roles for chromatin as a signal integration and storage platform. *Nat. Rev. Mol. Cell. Biol.* 14, 211–224. doi: 10.1038/nrm3545

Bensaad, K., Tsuruta, A., Selak, M. A., Vidal, M. N., Nakano, K., Bartrons, R., et al. (2006). TIGAR, a p53-inducible regulator of glycolysis and apoptosis. *Cell* 126, 107–120. doi: 10.1016/j.cell.2006.05.036

Berg, J. M., Tymoczko, J. L., and Stryer, L. (2002). *Biochemistry, 5th Edn.* New York, NY: W H Freeman Press.

Biasini, M., Bienert, S., Waterhouse, A., Arnold, K., Studer, G., Schmidt, T., et al. (2014). SWISS-MODEL: modelling protein tertiary and quaternary structure using evolutionary information. *Nucleic. Acids. Res.* 42, W252–W258. doi: 10.1093/nar/gku340

Boldrick, J. C., Alizadeh, A. A., Diehn, M., Dudoit, S., Liu, C. L., Belcher, C. E., et al. (2002). Stereotyped and specific gene expression programs in human innate immune responses to bacteria. *Proc. Natl. Acad. Sci. U.S.A.* 99, 972–977. doi: 10.1073/pnas.231625398

Borrelli, K. W., Vitalis, A., Alcantara, R., and Guallar, V. (2005). PELE: protein energy landscape exploration. A novel Monte Carlo based technique. *J. Chem. Theor. Comput.* 1, 1304–1311. doi: 10.1021/ct0501811

Burgess, S. C., He, T., Yan, Z., Lindner, J., Sherry, A. D., Malloy, C. R., et al. (2007). Cytosolic phosphoenolpyruvate carboxykinase does not solely control the rate of hepatic gluconeogenesis in the intact mouse liver. *Cell Metab.* 5, 313–320. doi: 10.1016/j.cmet.2007.03.004

Cabezas-Cruz, A., Alberdi, P., Ayllón, N., Valdés, J. J., Pierce, R., Villar, M., et al. (2016). *Anaplasma phagocytophilum* increases the levels of histone modifying enzymes to inhibit cell apoptosis and facilitate pathogen infection in the tick vector *Ixodes scapularis*. *Epigenetics* 11, 303–319. doi: 10.1080/15592294.2016.1163460

Choi, E. Y., Kim, E. C., Oh, H. M., Kim, S., Lee, H. J., Cho, E. Y., et al. (2004). Iron chelator triggers inflammatory signals in human intestinal epithelial cells: involvement of p38 and extracellular signal-regulated kinase signaling pathways. *J. Immunol.* 172, 7069–7077. doi: 10.4049/jimmunol.172.11.7069

Dalei, W., Nalini, P., Jingping, L., Youngchang, K., and Fraydoon, R. (2015). Structural integration in hypoxia-inducible factors. *Nature* 524, 303–308. doi: 10.1038/nature14883

de la Fuente, J., Estrada-Peña, A., Cabezas-Cruz, A., and Kocan, K. M. (2016a). *Anaplasma phagocytophilum* uses common strategies for infection of ticks and vertebrate hosts. *Trends Microbiol.* 24, 173–180. doi: 10.1016/j.tim.2015.12.001

de la Fuente, J., Estrada-Pena, A., Venzal, J. M., Kocan, K. M., and Sonenshine, D. E. (2008). Overview: ticks as vectors of pathogens that cause disease in humans and animals. *Front. Biosci.* 13, 6938–6946. doi: 10.2741/3200

de la Fuente, J., Villar, M., Cabezas-Cruz, A., Estrada-Peña, A., Ayllón, N., and Alberdi, P. (2016c). Tick-host-pathogen interactions: conflict and cooperation. *PLoS Pathog.* 12:e1005488. doi: 10.1371/journal.ppat.1005488

de la Fuente, J., Waterhouse, R. M., Sonenshine, D. E., Roe, R. M., Ribeiro, J. M., and Sattelle, D. B. (2016b). Tick genome assembled: new opportunities for research on tick-host-pathogen interactions. *Front. Cell. Infect. Microbiol.* 6:103. doi: 10.3389/fcimb.2016.00103

Déry, M. A., Michaud, M. D., and Richard, D. E. (2005). Hypoxia-inducible factor 1: regulation by hypoxic and non-hypoxic activators. *Int. J. Biochem. Cell. Biol.* 37, 535–540. doi: 10.1016/j.biocel.2004.08.012

Dunning Hotopp, J. C., Lin, M., Madupu, R., Crabtree, J., Angiuoli, S. V., Eisen, J. A., et al. (2006). Comparative genomics of emerging human ehrlichiosis agents. *PLoS Genet.* 2:e21. doi: 10.1371/journal.pgen.0020021

Eisenreich, W., Heesemann, J., Rudel, T., and Goebel, W. (2013). Metabolic host responses to infection by intracellular bacterial pathogens. *Front. Cell. Infect. Microbiol.* 3:24. doi: 10.3389/fcimb.2013.00024

Eisenreich, W., Heesemann, J., Rudel, T., and Goebel, W. (2015). Metabolic adaptations of intracellullar bacterial pathogens and their mammalian host cells during infection ("Pathometabolism"). *Microbiol. Spectr.* 3, 27–58. doi: 10.1128/microbiolspec.MBP-0002-2014

Finn, R. D., Bateman, A., Clements, J., Coggill, P., Eberhardt, R. Y., Eddy, S. R., et al. (2014). Pfam: the protein families database. *Nucleic Acids Res.* 42, D222–D230. doi: 10.1093/nar/gkt1223

Gulia-Nuss, M., Nuss, A. B., Meyer, J. M., Sonenshine, D. E., Roe, R. M., Waterhouse, R. M., et al. (2016). Genomic insights into the *Ixodes scapularis* tick vector of Lyme disease. *Nat. Commun.* 7:10507. doi: 10.1038/ncomms10507

Hu, C. J., Iyer, S., Sataur, A., Covello, K. L., Chodosh, L. A., and Simon, M. C. (2006). Differential regulation of the transcriptional activities of hypoxia-inducible factor 1 α (HIF-1α) and HIF-2α in stem cells. *Mol. Cell. Biol.* 26, 3514–3526. doi: 10.1128/MCB.26.9.3514-3526.2006

Huang, H., Wang, X., Kikuchi, T., Kumagai, Y., and Rikihisa, Y. (2007). Porin activity of *Anaplasma phagocytophilum* outer membrane fraction and purified P44. *J. Bacteriol.* 189, 1998–2006. doi: 10.1128/JB.01548-06

Kocan, K. M., de la Fuente, J., and Cabezas-Cruz, A. (2015). The genus Anaplasma: new challenges after reclassification. *Rev. Sci. Technol.* 34, 577–586. doi: 10.20506/rst.34.2.2381

Lecuit, M., Sonnenburg, J. L., Cossart, P., and Gordon, J. I. (2007). Functional genomic studies of the intestinal response to a foodborne enteropathogen in a humanized gnotobiotic mouse model. *J. Biol. Chem.* 282, 15065–15072. doi: 10.1074/jbc.M610926200

Li, X. B., Gu, J. D., and Zhou, Q. H. (2015). Review of aerobic glycolysis and its key enzymes–new targets for lung cancer therapy. *Thorac. Cancer* 6, 17–24. doi: 10.1111/1759-7714.12148

Li, X., Jacobson, M. P., Zhu, K., Zhao, S., and Friesner, R. A. (2007). Assignment of polar states for protein amino acid residues using an interaction cluster decomposition algorithm and its application to high resolution protein structure modeling. *Proteins* 66, 824–837. doi: 10.1002/prot.21125

Madden, T. L., Tatusov, R. L., and Zhang, J. (1996). Applications of network BLAST server. *Methods Enzymol.* 266, 131–141. doi: 10.1016/S0076-6879(96)66011-X

Misra, R. M., Bajaj, M. S., and Kale, V. P. (2012). Vasculogenic mimicry of HT1080 tumour cells *in vivo*: critical role of HIF-1α-neuropilin-1 axis. *PLoS ONE* 7:e50153. doi: 10.1371/journal.pone.0050153

Munderloh, U. G., Jauron, S. D., Fingerle, V., Leitritz, L., Hayes, S. F., Hautman, J. M., et al. (1999). Invasion and intracellular development of the human granulocytic ehrlichiosis agent in tick cell culture. *J. Clin. Microbiol.* 37, 2518–2524.

Pagé, E. L., Robitaille, G. A., Pouysségur, J., and Richard, D. E. (2002). Induction of hypoxia-inducible factor-1alpha by transcriptional and translational mechanisms. *J. Biol. Chem.* 277, 48403–48409. doi: 10.1074/jbc.M2091 14200

Pilot-Storck, F., Chopin, E., Rual, J. F., Baudot, A., Dobrokhotov, P., Robinson-Rechavi, M., et al. (2010). Interactome mapping of the phosphatidylinositol 3-kinase-mammalian target of rapamycin pathway identifies deformed epidermal autoregulatory factor-1 as a new glycogen synthase kinase-3 interactor. *Mol. Cell. Proteomics* 9, 1578–1593. doi: 10.1074/mcp.M900568-MCP200

Shin, J. H., Yang, J. Y., Jeon, B. Y., Yoon, Y. J., Cho, S. N., Kang, Y. H., et al. (2011). (1)H NMR-based metabolomic profiling in mice infected with *Mycobacterium tuberculosis*. *J. Proteome Res.* 10, 2238–2247. doi: 10.1021/pr1 01054m

Somashekar, B. S., Amin, A. G., Rithner, C. D., Troudt, J., Basaraba, R., Izzo, A., et al. (2011). Metabolic profiling of lung granuloma in *Mycobacterium tuberculosis* infected guinea pigs: *ex vivo* 1H magic angle spinning NMR studies. *J. Proteome Res.* 10, 4186–4195. doi: 10.1021/pr2003352

Stuen, S., Granquist, E. G., and Silaghi, C. (2013). *Anaplasma phagocytophilum*—a widespread multi-host pathogen with highly adaptive strategies. *Front. Cell. Infect. Microbiol.* 3:31. doi: 10.3389/fcimb.2013.00031

Sultana, H., Neelakanta, G., Kantor, F. S., Malawista, S. E., Fish, D., Montgomery, R. R., et al. (2010). *Anaplasma phagocytophilum* induces actin phosphorylation to selectively regulate gene transcription in *Ixodes scapularis* ticks. *J. Exp. Med.* 207, 1727–1743. doi: 10.1084/jem.20100276

Villar, M., Ayllón, N., Alberdi, P., Moreno, A., Moreno, M., Tobes, R., et al. (2015). Integrated metabolomics, transcriptomics and proteomics identifies metabolic pathways affected by *Anaplasma phagocytophilum* infection in tick cells. *Mol. Cell. Proteomics* 14, 3154–3172. doi: 10.1074/mcp.M115.0 51938

Wang, Q., Liang, B., Shirwany, N. A., and Zou, M. H. (2011). 2-Deoxy-D-glucose treatment of endothelial cells induces autophagy by reactive oxygen species-mediated activation of the AMP-activated protein kinase. *PLoS ONE* 6:e17234. doi: 10.1371/journal.pone.0017234

Weidemann, A., Breyer, J., Rehm, M., Eckardt, K. U., Daniel, C., Cicha, I., et al. (2013). HIF-1α activation results in actin cytoskeleton reorganization and modulation of Rac-1 signaling in endothelial cells. *Cell. Commun. Signal.* 11:80. doi: 10.1186/1478-811X-11-80

Zhou, J., Schmid, T., Frank, R., and Brüne, B. (2004). PI3K/Akt is required for heat shock proteins to protect hypoxia-inducible factor 1alpha from pVHL-independent degradation. *J. Biol. Chem.* 279, 13506–13513. doi: 10.1074/jbc.M310164200

Ziello, J. E., Jovin, I. S., and Huang, Y. (2007). Hypoxia-Inducible Factor (HIF)-1 regulatory pathway and its potential for therapeutic intervention in malignancy and ischemia. *Yale J. Biol. Med.* 80, 51–60.

5

Tick Immune System: What is Known, the Interconnections, the Gaps, and the Challenges

Andréa C. Fogaça[1], Géssica Sousa[1], Daniel B. Pavanelo[1], Eliane Esteves[1], Larissa A. Martins[2,3], Veronika Urbanová[2], Petr Kopáček[2] and Sirlei Daffre[1*]*

[1] Department of Parasitology, Institute of Biomedical Sciences, University of São Paulo, São Paulo, Brazil, [2] Institute of Parasitology, Biology Centre, Czech Academy of Sciences, Ceske Budejovice, Czechia, [3] Laboratory of Bacteriology, Tick-Pathogen Transmission Unit, National Institute of Allergy and Infectious Diseases, Hamilton, MT, United States

***Correspondence:**
Andréa C. Fogaça
deafog@usp.br
Sirlei Daffre
sidaffre@icb.usp.br

Ticks are ectoparasitic arthropods that necessarily feed on the blood of their vertebrate hosts. The success of blood acquisition depends on the pharmacological properties of tick saliva, which is injected into the host during tick feeding. Saliva is also used as a vehicle by several types of pathogens to be transmitted to the host, making ticks versatile vectors of several diseases for humans and other animals. When a tick feeds on an infected host, the pathogen reaches the gut of the tick and must migrate to its salivary glands *via* hemolymph to be successfully transmitted to a subsequent host during the next stage of feeding. In addition, some pathogens can colonize the ovaries of the tick and be transovarially transmitted to progeny. The tick immune system, as well as the immune system of other invertebrates, is more rudimentary than the immune system of vertebrates, presenting only innate immune responses. Although simpler, the large number of tick species evidences the efficiency of their immune system. The factors of their immune system act in each tick organ that interacts with pathogens; therefore, these factors are potential targets for the development of new strategies for the control of ticks and tick-borne diseases. The objective of this review is to present the prevailing knowledge on the tick immune system and to discuss the challenges of studying tick immunity, especially regarding the gaps and interconnections. To this end, we use a comparative approach of the tick immune system with the immune system of other invertebrates, focusing on various components of humoral and cellular immunity, such as signaling pathways, antimicrobial peptides, redox metabolism, complement-like molecules and regulated cell death. In addition, the role of tick microbiota in vector competence is also discussed.

Keywords: cell-mediated immunity, immune signaling pathway, immune system, microbiota, tick-borne pathogen

INTRODUCTION

Ticks (Acari: Ixodida) are ectoparasitic arthropods that obligatorily feed on the blood of a diverse list of vertebrate hosts, including mammals, birds, reptiles, and even amphibians. More than 950 tick species have been described to date, which, according to morphological and physiological characteristics, are divided into two main families, Ixodidae (hard ticks), comprising more than

75% of tick species, and Argasidae (soft ticks); a third family, known as Nuttalliellidae, is monospecific (1, 2). As a result of blood spoliation [a single ixodid adult female can ingest more than ~1 mL of blood (3)], the host can suffer from anemia, which negatively impacts the productivity of livestock and causes a huge economic burden worldwide. For example, the estimated annual losses due to reductions in weight gain and milk production caused by the cattle tick *Rhipicephalus microplus* are approximately 3.24 billion dollars in Brazil alone (4).

In addition to ingesting blood, ticks also secrete saliva into the host during feeding. Tick saliva, produced by their salivary glands, returns excess water and ions to the host, thereby concentrating the blood meal (5). Tick saliva contains an arsenal of bioactive molecules that modulate host hemostasis and immune reactions, thus enabling blood acquisition (6, 7). The antihemostatic and immunomodulatory properties of saliva can also facilitate the infection of pathogens that use saliva as a vehicle to be transmitted to the host during tick blood feeding (6, 8). Indeed, ticks are versatile vectors of viruses, bacteria, protozoans and nematodes, which cause life-threatening diseases to humans as well as to other animals, including livestock, pets, and wildlife (9). Among human diseases, we highlight Lyme disease, the most common tick-borne zoonosis, which is caused by spirochetes from the *Borrelia burgdorferi* sensu lato complex. After transmission by the bite of an infected tick, the typical clinical sign of Lyme disease is erythema migrans, but infection can spread and affect joints, heart, and the nervous system (10).

The first organ that a pathogen acquired within the blood meal interacts with is the tick gut (**Figure 1**). Then, the pathogen must colonize the gut epithelial cells and/or cross the gut epithelium to enter the hemocoel, an open body cavity filled with hemolymph, the fluid that irrigates all the tissues and organs in the tick. The pathogen must then reach the salivary glands. In each of these organs, the pathogen must counteract tick immune factors to be successfully transmitted through saliva to the vertebrate host in a subsequent blood-feeding (11). Some pathogens also have the ability to invade tick ovaries and can therefore be transovarially transmitted to progeny (**Figure 1**). Thus, elucidation of the immune factors involved in the interactions between ticks and tick-borne pathogens (TBPs) in each of these steps is essential to understand the biology of tick-transmitted diseases and may help to identify targets for the development of new strategies to block pathogen transmission. In this review, we present an update on humoral and cellular tick immunity components (**Figure 1**), including signaling pathways, antimicrobial peptides (AMPs), redox metabolism, complement-like proteins, and regulated cell death. Using a comparative approach with the immune system of other invertebrates, we highlight the challenges of studying tick immunity, the gaps, such as prophenoloxidase (PPO) and coagulation cascades, and the interconnections, such as immune system signaling pathway crosstalk. In addition, the role of tick microbiota in vector competence is also discussed.

A BRIEF HISTORY OF STUDIES ON THE IMMUNE SYSTEM OF ARTHROPODS

The first records of studies on arthropod disease date to the 19th century, when Louis Pasteur investigated the cause of brown dots on the cuticle of larvae of *Bombyx mori* that predestined larvae to death and affected silk production in France (12). In the 1980s, the isolation of several immune factors from the hemolymph of arthropods that have a large volume of hemolymph, such as larvae of dipteran and lepidopteran insects, horseshoe crabs and crayfish, was achieved. Indeed, the first animal AMP to be characterized was cecropin, isolated from the hemolymph of the moth *Hyalophora cecropia* (13). After that, AMPs were identified as important effectors of mammalian immunity (14, 15). In addition to AMPs, components of the PPO cascade from the hemolymph of *H. cecropia* (16), *B. mori* (17), and the crayfish *Pacifastacus leniusculus* (18) were also elucidated. Some years later, the components of the coagulation cascade, another important arthropod immune reaction, were characterized in *P. leniusculus* (19) and horseshoe crabs (20).

In the 1990s, relevant studies on the immune pathways that regulate AMP production were conducted using the fruit fly *Drosophila melanogaster* (hereafter referred to as *Drosophila*) as a model (21–24). Among them, we highlight the identification of a kappa B (κB)-binding region in the promotor region of certain insect AMP genes (25) and the identification of Toll receptors, posteriorly identified to be homologous to interleukin-1 receptor of mammals (26). Some years later, with the improvement of molecular techniques and funding by major support agencies, such as the MacArthur Foundation, the World Health Organization, and the National Institutes of Health (USA), studies on the arthropod immune system were redirected to vectors of human diseases, principally mosquitoes (27). In this period, Sanger-based technology was largely used to elucidate genomes and generate datasets of expressed sequence tags (ESTs). After the development of next-generation sequencing (NGS) technologies, additional information on arthropod genomes and transcriptomes was added to public databases (28). Indeed, currently, more than 40 arthropod genomes are available in the VectorBase database (https://www.vectorbase.org/organisms).

Knowledge of vector genomes and ESTs allowed *in silico* comparisons of immune factors among species [for example, see (29–33)]. Moreover, studies with diverse approaches, such as transcriptomics, proteomics, and metabolomics analyses, to assess the arthropod response to different microbial stimuli were significantly expanded in the postgenomic era (28). The development and application of RNA interference (RNAi) and CRISPR-Cas9 technologies to arthropods [(34, 35), respectively] were also important to determine the role played by immune factors in the interaction between vectors and vector-borne pathogens.

Despite the importance of ticks as disease vectors, studies on their genomes and the molecular factors involved in their interactions with pathogens are scarce compared to studies on other arthropod vectors. The large size of tick genomes and the

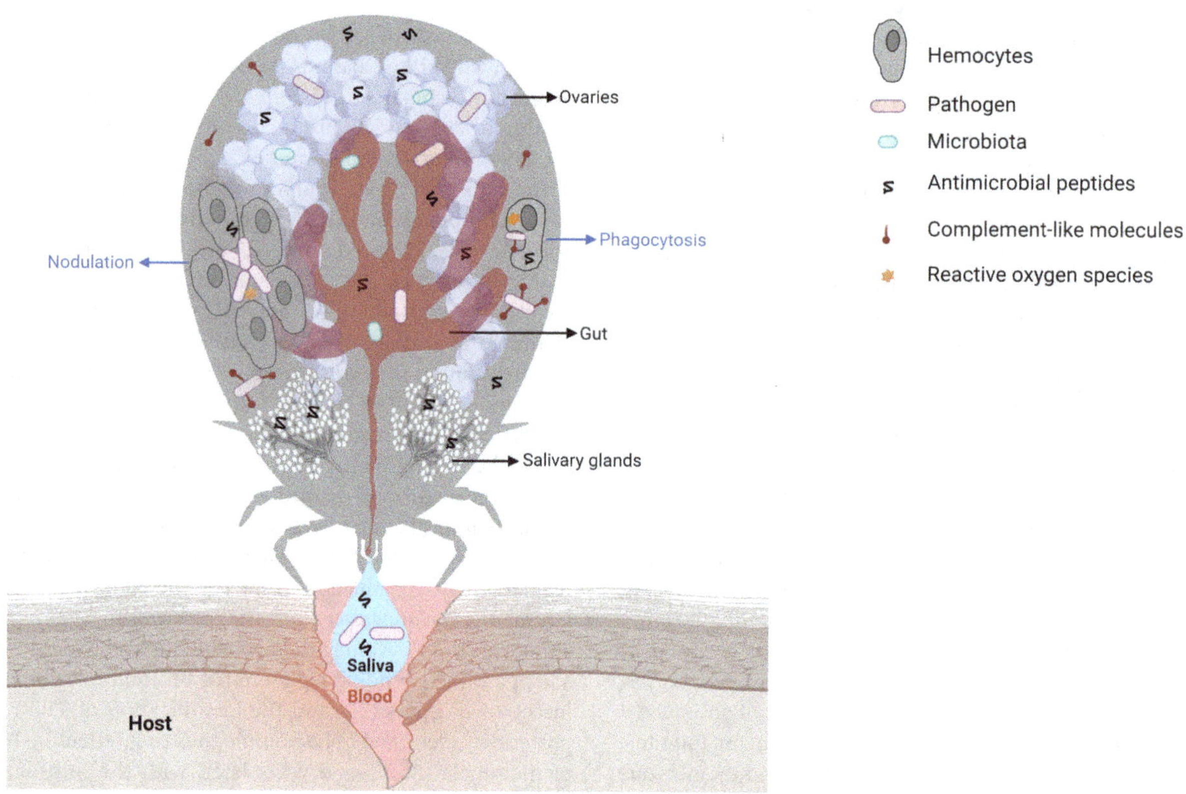

FIGURE 1 | Main interactions among tick immune system components, microbiota, and pathogens. Pathogens ingested within the blood meal initially reach the tick gut, where they interact with components of the gut microbiota and with cytotoxic molecules, such as AMPs (hemocidins and endogenous AMPs) and possibly with factors of redox metabolism, despite not being fully comprised. Pathogens must colonize and/or cross the gut epithelium to reach the hemocoel, which is filled with hemolymph. In hemolymph, complement-like molecules attach to pathogens that can be engulfed or trapped by hemocyte-mediated processes named phagocytosis and nodulation, respectively. Invaders can also be killed by several types of effector molecules, including AMPs, complement-like molecules, and factors of redox metabolism. The tick salivary glands return excess water and ions from the blood meal to the host through saliva, which also contains antihemostatic and immunomodulatory molecules. Pathogens use tick saliva as a vehicle to be transmitted to the host, in which infection can be facilitated by saliva properties. Some pathogens can also colonize the tick ovaries and are transmitted to progeny. In the tick salivary glands and ovaries, as in the gut, pathogens must deal with the members of resident microbiota as well as tick immune reactions. Additional studies are required to elucidate the molecules responsible for hemolymph clotting and melanization in ticks.

high contents of repetitive regions make genome assembly difficult. Indeed, the size of tick genomes is approximately 1.3 Gbp in argasids and 2.6 Gbp in ixodids (36). However, the genome of the cattle tick *R. microplus* is even larger and has been estimated to be approximately 7.1 Gpb, which is more than twice the size of the human genome (37). In addition, approximately 70% of the tick genome includes repetitive regions (37, 38). For this reason, until very recently, only the genome of the tick *Ixodes scapularis* had been annotated (38). Additional genomes were recently assembled by the use of NGS (37, 39). The scarcity of studies on the molecular factors involved in ticks and TBPs is in part due to the need for sophisticated structures to raise vertebrate animals to feed ticks, which is laborious and involves ethical concerns. In the last few years, artificial feeding systems have been successfully used to maintain laboratory tick colonies; however, an animal blood source is still required (40). Finally, the development of continuous cell lines derived from tick embryos, despite representing a mixture of different cell types, has also contributed considerably to studies on tick biology and their interactions with TBPs (41).

TICK IMMUNE SIGNALING PATHWAYS

Blood feeding represents a challenge for hematophagous arthropods due to the large diversity of pathogens to which these animals are exposed. In contrast to other arthropods, hard ticks are strictly hematophagous, feeding on the blood of their host for several days. In addition, some species feed on a different host in each developmental stage (larvae, nymphs, and adults), thereby increasing the chance of either acquiring or transmitting pathogens. Therefore, ticks are important vectors of a large list of disease-causing pathogens (42). In addition to host pathogens, ticks are in close contact with the microbiota of the host skin, which may also be acquired within the blood meal (43). Ticks are also exposed to microorganisms in the environment during the nonparasitic phases of their life cycle. Hence, the immune system of ticks must be activated continuously to protect them from harmful infections.

Most of our knowledge on arthropod immune responses has come from studies on dipteran insects, especially *Drosophila* and the mosquitoes *Aedes* spp. and *Anopheles* spp. In *Drosophila*, invading microorganisms are mainly recognized by the Toll, immune deficiency (IMD), Jun-N-terminal kinase (JNK), Janus kinase/signal transducer and activator of transcription (JAK/STAT) and/or RNAi pathways (44). Nonetheless, the hypothesis that the level of conservation of arthropod immune responses might be high has been rejected by several studies on ticks, mites, lice, hemipterans, and others, and it is now recognized that the immune system displays remarkable diversification across the Arthropoda phylum (30). Tick immunity is, however, still greatly neglected and unexplored (45). Hence, we review the prevailing knowledge on tick immune signaling pathways alongside the connections between them and other equally important factors, such as AMPs, redox metabolism, complement-like proteins, and regulated cell death.

Nuclear Factor-Kappa B Signaling Pathways: Molecular Regulators for Pathogen Recognition

The Unexplored Toll Pathway

The Toll signaling pathway is well studied in *Drosophila*, in which it is preferentially activated in the presence of bacterial [by recognition of lysine-type peptidoglycan (PGN) from the cell

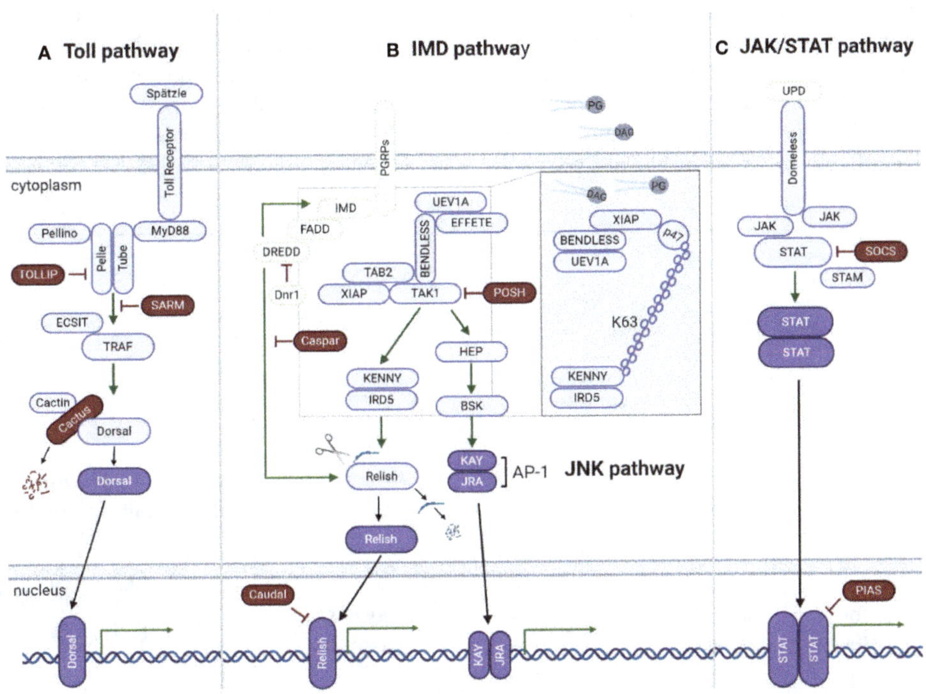

FIGURE 2 | Tick signaling-related genes in the three main immune signaling pathways of arthropods: **(A)** Toll, **(B)** IMD, and **(C)** JAK/STAT. **(A)** A previous *in silico* study (31) showed that components of the Toll signaling pathway of arthropods are conserved in ticks: extracellular cytokine Spatzle (Spz), transmembrane cytokine receptor Toll, Toll-interacting protein (TOLLIP), adaptor protein MyD88, kinases Tube (interleukin-1 receptor-associated kinase 4 or IRAK4), Pelle (interleukin-1 receptor-associated kinase 1 or IRAK1), Pelle-interacting protein Pellino, TNF receptor associated factors (TRAFs), evolutionarily conserved signaling intermediate in toll pathway (ECSIT), sterile alpha- and armadillo-motif-containing protein (SARM), Rel/NF-kappa B transcription factor Dorsal, Dorsal inhibitor protein IkappaB Cactus (IkB), and interacting protein Cactin of the IkB. **(B)** Regarding the IMD pathway, genes encoding downstream members of both the NF-kB/Relish and Jun N-terminal kinase (JNK) branches were identified: peptidoglycan recognition proteins (PGRPs), enzymes involved in ubiquitination (UEV1a, Effete/Ubc13 and Bendless/Ubc5), X-linked inhibitor apoptosis protein (XIAP), negative regulators Caspar (Fas-associating factor 1) and POSH (E3 ligase Plenty of SH3), transforming growth factor-beta activated kinase 1 (TAK1), TAK1-binding protein 2 (TAB2), IRD5 and Kenny/NEMO (IKKγ), and Relish-like Rel/NF-kB transcription factor. The adaptor protein IMD (immune deficiency), its associated molecule FAAD (Fas associated protein with death domain), the caspase DREDD (death related ced-3/Nedd2-like) and Dnr1 (defense repressor 1) have not yet been described in ticks. Components of the JNK branch of the tick IMD pathway include mitogen-activated protein (MAP) kinase hemipterous (HEP), Jun-kinase basket (BSK), activator protein 1 (AP-1) transcription factors JRA (Jun-related antigen) and KAY (Fos-related antigen, Kayak). Some IMD pathway components were functionally characterized by (48) (Insert). The authors showed that the IMD pathway is activated by PODAG (1-palmitoyl-2-oleoyl diacylglycerol) or POPG (1-palmitoyl-2-oleoyl-sn-glycero-3-phosphoglycerol). Once activated, XIAP interacts with the heterodimer Bendless : UEV1a, leading to the ubiquitination of p47 in a K63-dependent manner. Ubiquitylated p47 connects to Kenny (also named NEMO) and induces the phosphorylation of IRD5 and Relish. **(C)** Components of the Janus kinase/signal transducer and activator of transcription (JAK/STAT) signaling pathway are also conserved in ticks: the transmembrane cytokine receptor Domeless, tyrosine kinase JAK (Hopscotch), transcription factor STAT, signal transducing adaptor molecule (STAM) and the inhibitor proteins PIAS (protein inhibitor of activated STAT) and SOCS (suppressor of cytokine signaling). The ligand of the Domeless receptor (UPD gene) was not identified in ticks **(C)**. Activated transcription factors are represented in dark blue; the immune signaling pathway components not yet described in ticks are represented in green.

wall of Gram-positive bacteria) and fungal (by recognition of (1,3)-glucan polymers of D-glucose from the cell wall] pathogen-associated molecular patterns (PAMPs) (44, 46). *In silico* and genomic analyses have shown that ticks encode most Toll pathway components (31, 33, 38, 47) (**Figure 2A**), including the NF-κB Dorsal, indicating that conserved mechanisms of Toll pathway activation may exist. Indeed, the NF-κB transcription factor dorsal-related immunity factor (DIF) is the only component of the Toll pathway not yet reported in any tick species.

How the tick Toll pathway operates is largely unclear. Rosa and collaborators showed that the Toll pathway components are differentially expressed in the tick cell line BME26, which is derived from the tick *R. microplus*, in response to live *Anaplasma marginale* and *Rickettsia rickettsii* (two obligate intracellular bacteria) and heat-killed *Saccharomyces cerevisiae* (yeast), *Enterobacter cloacae* (Gram-negative bacterium) and *Micrococcus luteus* (Gram-positive bacterium) (31). Interestingly, heat-killed microorganisms upregulated the gene expression of the majority of the Toll pathway components, *R. rickettsii* upregulated some Toll pathway components and downregulated others, and infection with *A. marginale* (a pathogen naturally transmitted by *R. microplus*) downregulated most of the Toll pathway components. These results suggest that *A. marginale* may downregulate Toll pathway components in an attempt to favor vector colonization, which might correspond to coevolutionary adaptation. Of note, similar results were found for the IMD, JNK, and JAK/STAT signaling pathways (31). However, studies on the mechanisms used by this pathogen to overcome tick immune responses are warranted to confirm the authors' hypothesis. In adult *R. microplus*, only Dorsal was downregulated in both the gut and salivary glands of *A. marginale*-infected ticks, while Relish and STAT remained unmodulated (49). Moreover, Dorsal silencing promoted an increase in the *A. marginale* burden as well as knockdown of Relish and STAT. However, while Relish dsRNA (dsRelish) specifically silenced Relish, this transcription factor was also downregulated in both the dsDorsal and dsSTAT groups, which might explain the increase in the *A. marginale* load in these two groups as well. To determine the pathway responsible for infection control, the gene expression of specific effectors of each immune signaling pathway, which are currently unknown, is warranted. As Dorsal-, Relish-, and STAT-encoding genes do not exhibit significant sequence similarity, the authors suggested the existence of putative crosstalk among the Toll, IMD, and JAK/STAT signaling pathways (49) (**Figure 3C**). Nonetheless, an off-target effect cannot be ruled out. It is also possible that the

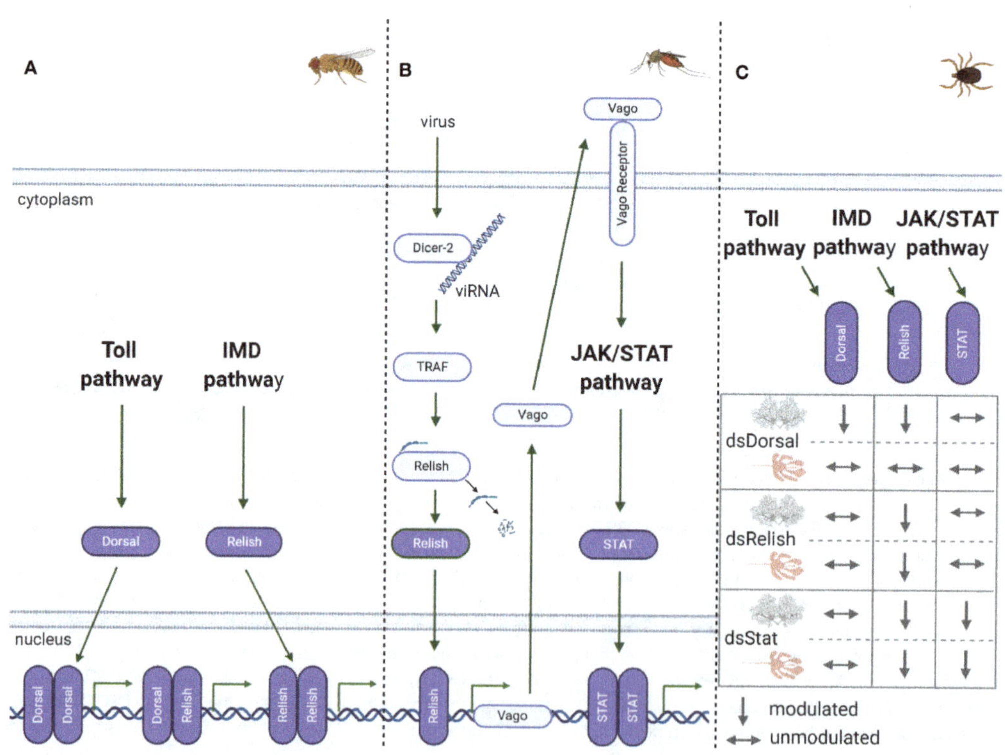

FIGURE 3 | Immune pathway crosstalk. **(A)** In *Drosophila*, the DIF-Relish heterodimer activates the expression of both Toll and IMD pathway effectors, resulting in a stronger response against infection (50). **(B)** In *Culex*, after recognition of West Nile virus (WNV) dsRNA by Dcr-2, TNF receptor-associated factor (TRAF) stimulates Relish, upregulating Vago expression (51, 52). Vago is then secreted by the infected cell and activates the JAK/STAT pathway in adjacent cells, upregulating the expression of antiviral genes. **(C)** In *R. microplus*, knockdown of Dorsal downregulates both Dorsal and Relish expression in salivary glands, while the levels of all the transcription factors remain unaltered in the gut. Relish is also downregulated in the gut and salivary glands of STAT-deficient ticks. Conversely, knockdown of Relish results in the specific silencing of its target gene in both the gut and salivary glands (49).

knockdown of immune signaling transcription factors exerts an effect on the gut microbiota, which, in turn, may modulate their gene expression. In contrast to the results obtained with *R. microplus*, gene silencing of Toll (ISCW018193) did not exhibit any effect on the *Anaplasma phagocytophilum* burden in the salivary glands of *I. scapularis* nymphs (53). However, gut colonization was not evaluated; therefore, it is not possible to guarantee that the Toll pathway is not involved in controlling *A. phagocytophilum* infection in this tick species. In a study carried out with *I. ricinus* cells (IRE/CTVM20), it was shown that the expression of a *Toll* gene (homologous to the *Toll* ISCW022740 of *I. scapularis*) is upregulated after 72 and 120 h of infection with flaviviruses [tick-borne encephalitis virus (TBEV) and louping ill virus (LIV)] but remained unmodulated in response to *A. phagocytophilum* (54). Conversely, infection with these flaviviruses downregulated the expression of three other Toll transcripts (homologous to ISCW017724; ISCW007727; ISCW007724 of *I. scapularis*), while Toll ISCW00727 expression was downregulated by *A. phagocytophilum* (54). The expression of another component of the Toll pathway, MyD88, was also downregulated by infection with these three pathogens, suggesting that they might suppress this pathway to promote vector colonization. To confirm this hypothesis, it is necessary to functionally characterize the role played by Toll components in pathogen proliferation.

The Unconventional Immune Deficiency Pathway

In *Drosophila*, bacterial infections caused by Gram-negative bacteria and certain Gram-positive bacteria, such as *Bacillus* and *Listeria* species, are mainly controlled by the IMD pathway through the recognition of diaminopimelic acid (DAP)-type PGN, which is present in the bacterial cell wall, by PGN-recognition proteins (PGRPs) (44, 55). Genomic and *in silico* studies have shown that ticks lack orthologs of many key elements of the IMD pathway, including the transmembrane PGRP, the Fas-associated protein with death domain (FADD), the adaptor molecule IMD, and the death-related ced-3/Nedd2-like protein (DREDD) (31, 33, 38, 48) (**Figure 2B**). Losses of IMD pathway components are not exclusive to ticks since they have also been described in other arachnids and hemipterans (30, 56). Nevertheless, it is important to highlight that some arthropods have unusual gene architectures, resulting in inaccurate annotation due to the use of software based on standard gene structures, as reported for the kissing bug *Rhodnius prolixus* (57). Gathering data from the genome and transcriptome associated with reciprocal BLAST (Basic Local Alignment Search Tool) and hidden Markov model profile searches, the authors showed that most of the missing IMD pathway components are present in this hemipteran. Therefore, it is possible that the missing IMD pathway components might be a consequence of incorrect annotations due to structural divergences. Indeed, assays showed that the IMD cascade is functional in the insect fat body and is predominantly responsive against Gram-negative bacterial infection (57).

Despite missing several elements, the tick IMD pathway is functional and responsive to distinct pathogens (48, 49, 58). RNAi silencing of several IMD pathway components, including Bendless, ubiquitin E2 variant 1A (UEV1a), Relish, and Caspar (**Figure 2B**, insert), showed that this cascade controls *A. phagocytophilum* and *B. burgdorferi* burden in *I. scapularis* nymphs (48). In contrast to the classical *Drosophila* model of DAP-PGN recognition by PGRPs (44, 55), glycerophospholipids from bacterial membranes, including 1-palmitoyl-2-oleoyl-sn-glycerol-3-phosphoglycerol (POPG) and 1-palmitoyl-2-oleoyl diacylglycerol (PODAG), were reported to act as PAMPs for IMD pathway activation in ticks (48) (**Figure 2B**, insert). However, the mechanisms of POPG and PODAG recognition remain unclear, but it is hypothesized that they are sensed by a yet uncharacterized pattern-recognition receptor. X-linked inhibitor of apoptosis protein (XIAP) is an upstream signaling component of the IMD pathway and, when activated, specifically and directly interacts with the heterodimer E2 conjugating enzyme complex Bendless : UEV1a (48). Upon microbial activation, XIAP, together with Bendless : UEV1a, binds and ubiquitylates its p47 substrate in a K63-dependent manner. Ubiquitylated p47 connects to Kenny (also named NEMO) and induces, by a yet unknown mechanism, phosphorylation of the inhibitor of NF-κB kinase (IKK) β (also known as IRD5) and Relish, the IMD transcription factor. Consequently, Relish is cleaved and translocated to the nucleus (58) (**Figure 2B**, insert). On the other hand, RNAi knockdown of two other components of the IMD pathway, transforming growth factor-β activated kinase 1 (TAK1) and TAK1 adaptor protein 1 (TAB1) (**Figure 2B**), presented no effect on the *A. phagocytophilum* burden in the salivary glands of *I. scapularis* nymphs (53). Therefore, studies carried out by Dr. Pedra's group (48, 58) showed how the IMD pathway is activated in ticks, which is highly relevant since there is a lack of components in this pathway, different from the classic *Drosophila* model (44). However, the effector molecule(s) regulated by the IMD pathway that control(s) infections by pathogens such as *A. phagocytophilum* and *B. burgdorferi* still need to be identified.

In adult *R. microplus*, RNAi silencing of immune signaling of the Toll, IMD, and JAK/STAT pathway transcription factors identified the IMD pathway as the main controller of *A. marginale* infection in the tick gut and salivary glands (49). The expression of the genes encoding the AMPs microplusin, defensin, ixodidin, and lysozyme was analyzed in the gut and salivary glands of *R. microplus* after knockdown of Relish and infection with *A. marginale*. Interestingly, only the microplusin transcript levels were downregulated in dsRelish ticks, implicating this AMP as an effector of the IMD signaling pathway, which may act against *A. marginale* (49). However, although microplusin appears to be under IMD pathway regulation, possible coregulation by the JAK/STAT pathway cannot be discarded (49).

The other branch that constitutes the IMD pathway is JNK signaling (**Figure 2B**). In *Drosophila*, JNK has been shown to be involved in a wide range of biological processes, including cellular immune and stress responses, but it seems to not be required to induce AMP gene expression (59). Although activation of both the JNK and Relish branches of the IMD pathway occurs *via* TAK1 in *Drosophila* (59), additional studies are warranted to determine the activation of JNK pathways in ticks (48, 53, 58).

JAK/STAT Pathway: Just a Support Molecular Circuit?

In *Drosophila*, the JAK/STAT signaling pathway only plays an indirect role in controlling bacterial and fungal infection. Therefore, this pathway is considered a support circuit to the Toll and IMD pathways; however, it is especially sensitive to viral infections (60). Beyond its effects on the immune response, the JAK/STAT signaling pathway also regulates multiple biological processes, including repair and renewal of the gut epithelial layer (61), a function that was also reported to occur in ticks (62).

Although still poorly understood, the tick JAK/STAT pathway **(Figure 2C)** was reported to be functional, playing an important role in the control of pathogens (53, 62, 63). However, it is not clear how ticks activate the JAK/STAT signaling pathway, as the unpaired (Upd) encoding gene, a cytokine-like signaling molecule ligand of the transmembrane receptor Domeless, is missing. In *I. scapularis*, knockdown of the transcription factor STAT and JAK yielded evidence that this pathway is key to the control of *A. phagocytophilum* infection (53). The results also showed that the 5.3-kDa AMP is an effector regulated by the JAK/STAT pathway, which is essential to restrict *A. phagocytophilum* proliferation in tick salivary glands and hemolymph but not in the gut, indicating that additional effectors under JAK/STAT pathway regulation are required in this organ (53). Interestingly, it was reported that *I. scapularis* employs a sophisticated immune strategy that uses a vertebrate host-derived cytokine to stimulate its own JAK/STAT immune pathway (63). During feeding, the interferon-gamma (INFγ) acquired within the infected bloodmeal activates STAT by a yet unknown receptor and, through mediation of a Rho-like GTPase, leads to the synthesis of the AMP domesticated amidase effector 2 (Dae2), limiting the level of *B. burgdorferi*. Other evidence that indicates that the JAK/STAT pathway is associated with the regulation of AMPs was reported by Capelli-Peixoto and collaborators in adult *R. microplus* (49). The authors observed the downregulation of the AMPs ixodidin and lysozyme in the salivary glands and defensin in the gut and salivary glands of STAT-deficient ticks.

Effectors from signaling pathways, such as JAK/STAT, can act as either positive or negative regulators of infection. As presented above, Dae2 (63) and the 5.3-kDa AMP (53) are negative regulators, as they control pathogen proliferation. In contrast, peritrophin-1, another effector from the tick JAK/STAT pathway, was reported to increase *B. burgdorferi* survival in the gut of *I. scapularis* nymphs (62). Knockdown of STAT had a direct impact on the gut epithelium, affecting its mitotic activity as well as decreasing peritrophin-1 expression, which consequently disrupted the structural integrity of the peritrophic matrix (62). Therefore, peritrophin-1, which is a component of the peritrophic matrix, favors *B. burgdorferi* establishment (62). Interestingly, peritrophin-1 exhibits the opposite effect on *A. phagocytophilum*, another pathogen naturally transmitted by *I. scapularis* (64). Infection with *A. phagocytophilum* upregulates a tick antifreeze glycoprotein, which, in turn, alters bacterial biofilm formation and, consequently, disturbs the natural gut microbiota. This microbiota alteration affects the integrity of the peritrophic matrix, favoring pathogen colonization (64). Knockdown of peritrophin-1 and, therefore, the reduction in the thickness of the peritrophic matrix increases the *A. phagocytophilum* load in the tick gut (64).

RNAi as a Tick Innate Immunity Component

RNAi is a biological process that plays an important role in the defense of arthropods against viruses and transposable elements. Four main RNAi-related pathways have been described based on the origin of the activating small RNAs. The origin of three of these small RNAs is endogenous [microRNA (miRNA), small interfering RNA (endo-siRNA), and piwi-interacting RNA (piRNA)], while the origin of the fourth is exogenous (siRNA) (65). The exogenous siRNA pathway is especially important and has been proposed to be the main antiviral response in *Drosophila* and mosquitoes (66). In general, after infection, long viral dsRNA is recognized and cleaved by Dicer-2 (Dcr-2) into 21 nucleotide (nt) siRNAs, known as viRNAs (65, 66). These viRNAs are then transferred to Argonaute-2 (Ago2), which couples to other members of the RNA-induced silencing complex (RISC). Only one strand of the viRNA remains coupled to RISC and guides the degradation of complementary viral RNA (65, 66). miRNAs use a similar mechanism, although involving Dcr-1 and Ago-1 (67).

The genome of *I. scapularis* exhibits significant gene expansion in RNAi elements, including five *Ago* homologous genes: *Ago-78*, homologous to insect *Ago-1*, and *Ago-96*, *-68*, *-16*, and*-30*, homologous to insect *Ago-2* (68). Additionally, two *Dcr* genes, *Dcr-89* and *-90*, were clustered with *Drosophila Dcr-2* and *-1*, respectively. Similar gene expansion was identified in *Hyalomma asiaticum* RNAi components (viz., two copies of *Dcr-2* and five copies of *Ago-2*) (69). Infection of *I. scapularis* IDE8 cells with Langat virus (LGTV) showed that Ago-16 and Ago-30 neutralized both LGTV and its replicon, as well as Dcr-90, despite the clustering of the last element with insect Dcr-1, which is involved in miRNA processing but not in siRNA (68). Shortly thereafter, knockdown of Ago-30 and Dcr-90 confirmed their antiviral role upon LGTV infection in *I. scapularis* IDE8 and *I. ricinus* IRE/CTVM19 cell lines (70).

Interestingly, viral or endogenous siRNAs were shown to be mostly 22 nt in length depending on the tick (68), in contrast with *Drosophila* and mosquito viRNAs and endo-siRNAs, which contain 21 nt (66). Moreover, these viRNAs mapped at the highest frequency around the 5' and 3' UTRs of the viral genome and antigenome (68). The 3' UTRs of LGTV and TBEV express subgenomic flavivirus RNAs (sfRNAs), which are a counterdefense against the tick RNAi system, assuring vectorial competence (68). Of note, sfRNAs are expressed by almost all Flaviviridae members as an evolved balance between arthropods and viruses (67).

Grubaugh and collaborators (71) validated the *in vitro* data previously obtained by Schnettler et al. (68), showing that most viRNAs are, indeed, 22 nt in length and originate from the UTR of the viral genome and antigenome of *I. scapularis* in its life stages (larvae, nymphs, and adults) naturally infected with Powassan virus (POWV) (71). Moreover, the viral genetic diversity in ticks is lower than that in mice, suggesting that ticks exert stronger viral control than their vertebrate hosts. Therefore, POWV evolution seems to depend on RNAi-mediated diversification and selective constraints (71).

Regarding endogenous miRNAs, recent studies have shown that pathogens, such as viruses (72) and bacteria (73), modulate tick miRNA profiles, with a potential role in controlling pathogen replication within the vector (72, 73). On the other hand, the piRNA response to infection is still unknown in ticks. Nonetheless, the piRNA response has been implicated in the response of mosquitoes to viral infections (74, 75). Moreover, Hess and colleagues (76) suggested that the mosquito piRNA response precedes the RNAi-Dcr-2-dependent (siRNA) response during viral infection. In contrast with siRNAs, piRNA activation seems to be mediated by single-stranded RNAs that are Dcr1- and Dcr2-independent and possibly mediated by the endonuclease activity of Piwi proteins, resulting in 24–30 nt small RNAs, as found in *Drosophila*. In addition to antiviral activity, piRNAs seem to have important roles in controlling the activity of transposable elements in the genome and in the development of reproductive tissues (65). Considering the knowledge of the role played by RNAi in the defense of insects against infections, the tick RNAi system represents a wide and still unexplored field awaiting investigation.

Independent Immune Pathways or Dynamic and Indispensable Crosstalk?

Although the term crosstalk is commonly applied to the arthropod immunity literature, its definition remains conflicting, and in many cases, the mechanism by which it occurs remains unknown. Here, we consider crosstalk to occur when (i) the same effector is regulated by more than one immune signaling pathway (50, 56, 77) and (ii) the components of a specific immune signaling pathway modulate the components of other pathways (49, 51, 52, 78–80).

The regulation of AMP expression by Toll and IMD pathways was initially established in *Drosophila*, as well documented in the historical review by Imler (24). Originally, it was accepted that AMPs were regulated by a specific immune pathway; however, subsequent studies carried out by different research groups showed that this regulation was more complex than initially known, and crosstalk among immune pathways could occur, as described in the examples below. Although AMPs are mostly regulated by either Toll or IMD pathways in *Drosophila*, it has been reported that some AMP-encoding genes can be activated synergistically by both immune pathways (50) (**Figure 3A**). It was shown that the NF-κB transcription factors Dorsal, DIF, and Relish can dimerize as homo- or heterodimers with varying degrees of efficiency. The DIF-Relish heterodimer mediates the crosstalk between the Toll and IMD pathways, resulting in the activation of effectors from both pathways and, consequently, targeting a broader spectrum of infectious microorganisms (50).

Another example of a certain effector being regulated by more than one immune pathway occurs in the hemipteran stinkbug *Plautia stali* (56). As shown by Nishide and collaborators, knockdown of IMD, as well as Toll pathway components, modulates effectors of both pathways. Interruption of both pathways at the same time had a more conspicuous effect on AMP production, strengthening crosstalk (56). The authors proposed an intriguing hypothesis that the redundancy between these two immune signaling pathways may have predisposed them to and facilitated the loss of some IMD-related genes in *P. stali*.

The crosstalk between RNAi and immune signaling pathways has been shown in recent publications (51, 52, 78, 79). In *Culex* mosquitoes, Dcr-2, a central component of the siRNA pathway, recognizes West-Nile virus (WNV) dsRNA and activates a signaling cascade to stimulate Relish *via* tumor necrosis factor (TNF) receptor-associated factor (TRAF) to increase Vago expression (**Figure 3B**) (51, 52). Following this transcriptional upregulation, Vago is secreted from infected cells and acts as a vertebrate cytokine functional homolog, binding to a still unknown cellular receptor in surrounding cells and triggering the JAK/STAT pathway. Activation of the JAK/STAT pathway ultimately results in an appropriate antiviral response in uninfected cells, such as upregulation of *vir-1* and other antiviral genes. These studies thereby revealed a paracrine signaling response mediated by a complex network of crosstalk, opening up several intriguing lines of investigation for future studies on arthropod immunity. Other studies have shown crosstalk between RNAi and the Toll pathway in *Ae aegypti* Aag2 cells (78) and *Drosophila* (79). In the first study, the miRNA aae-miR-375 upregulated Cactus, inhibiting the activation of the NF-κB transcription factor and reducing AMP synthesis, consequently enhancing dengue virus (DENV) infection (78). In *Drosophila*, on the other hand, four distinct members of the miR-310 family directly regulate drosomycin expression, a Toll-derived AMP (79). In addition to the connection between RNAi and signaling pathways, the redundancy of distinct miRNAs cotargeting the same transcript highlights the tight regulation imposed by miRNAs on the innate response.

It was also shown that the transcription factors activator protein 1 (AP-1; from the JNK pathway) and STAT neutralize Relish-mediated activation during the innate immune response in *Drosophila*, which is necessary for a proper and balanced immune response. The mechanism for controlling Relish-mediated transcriptional activation is through the formation of a complex composed of AP-1 and STAT with the dorsal switch protein (Dsp1), which recruits a histone deacetylase to prevent Relish transcription (80).

In ticks, to the best of our knowledge, there is only one study reporting putative crosstalk among the immune signaling pathways, which was reported by Capelli-Peixoto and collaborators (49). The authors showed that knockdown of the transcription factors Dorsal, Relish, or STAT downregulates

Relish expression (**Figure 3C**), with a consequent increase in the *A. marginale* load in *R. microplus* salivary glands. In contrast, Dorsal-deficient ticks presented no effects on Relish expression in the gut, where, intriguingly, ticks exhibited only modest silencing of Dorsal itself. Relish levels were also diminished in STAT-deficient guts. Only treatment with dsRelish resulted in specific silencing of its target gene in both the gut and salivary glands (**Figure 3C**). Nonetheless, the *A. marginale* burden was higher in the gut of ticks from all groups (dsDorsal, dsRelish, and dsSTAT) than in the control (49). As similarities among *Dorsal, Relish*, and *STAT* gene sequences were insignificant, the authors hypothesized that crosstalk of the immune pathways in ticks might occur to enhance the immune response. However, an off-target effect cannot be completely disregarded. Although the regulation of AMPs by the IMD and JAK/STAT pathways has been established, as already described above, it is still necessary to silence AMP-encoding genes to assign their role in *A. marginale* control. Therefore, the tick immune system, as shown in some insects, is also integrated, versatile, and possibly capable of making a network of connections among innate signaling pathways, giving rise to effective antimicrobial responses.

ANTIMICROBIAL PEPTIDES: MAY THE "SOURCE" BE WITH YOU!

AMPs are important effectors of the immune systems of both invertebrates and vertebrates, having a broad spectrum of activity against microorganisms (81). In ticks, the main sites of AMP expression are hemocytes, fat body, gut, ovaries, and salivary glands, where they can be modulated in response to either blood feeding or microbial challenge (82). Several reviews of tick AMPs addressing their characterization, as well as their interaction with microorganisms, have been published in the last decade (11, 33, 83, 84).

Interestingly, ticks use host hemoglobin, one of the most abundant proteins within the blood meal, as a source for the production of antimicrobial-derived fragments (85–88). Hemoglobin-derived AMPs, referred to as hemocidins (89), are produced by the proteolytic activity of aspartic and cysteine (catepsin-L like) proteinases from the tick gut (90). Structural studies with the synthetic amidated hemocidin Hb33-61a of *R. microplus* showed that its α-helical C-terminus is responsible for the permeabilization of the microbial membrane (91). However, it is still unknown whether hemocidins act intracellularly or if they are released to the tick gut lumen, where they can fight against microorganisms.

In addition to hemocidins, ticks also produce endogenous (ribosomally synthesized) AMPs (11, 83). Among the several tick AMPs identified to date, microplusins (also known as hebraeins) are among the most well characterized. Microplusin is a cysteine- and histidine-rich AMP that was first isolated from the hemolymph of adult *R. microplus* (92) and *Amblyomma hebraeum* (93). Microplusin was also identified in the ovaries and eggs of *R. microplus* (94), suggesting that in addition to protecting adults, it may also play a role in the protection of embryos before and after oviposition. Microplusin exhibits an α-helical globular domain and chelates metal ions (95). The bacteriostatic activity of microplusin against the Gram-positive bacterium *M. luteus* was reversed by the addition of copper II but not iron II. Indeed, microplusin interferes with the respiration (a copper-dependent process) of both *M. luteus* (95) and the fungus *Cryptococcus neoformans* (96). Microplusin was also reported to affect melanization and capsule formation, which are important virulence factors of *C. neoformans* (96). Interestingly, knockdown of microplusin increased the load of *R. rickettsii* in *Amblyomma aureolatum* (97). On the other hand, this AMP had no effect on either rickettsial transmission or tick fitness. Defensins compose another class of AMPs that have been described in several tick species, displaying activity against different types of microorganisms [for review, see (11, 83)]. For example, defensin-2 of *Dermacentor variabilis* was shown to protect against another bacterium of the genus *Rickettsia*, *R. montanensis*, as its neutralization with antidefensin-2 IgG increased the rickettisal load in the tick gut (98). Defensin-2 causes permeabilization of the bacterial membrane with consequent leakage of cytoplasmic proteins (98).

Dae2 is an AMP of *I. scapularis* that was acquired by horizontal bacterial gene transfer and has become an important effector to control *B. burgdorferi* infection (99), although it does not exhibit direct action on this pathogen (63). Indeed, it was recently shown that Dae2 is physically unable to overcome the outer membrane structure of the outer membrane of Gram-negative bacteria; thus, it does not present lytic activity against *B. burgdorferi*, suggesting the need for other factors, such as membrane-permeabilizing agents (100). As Dae2 is delivered to the vertebrate host bite site *via* saliva and exhibits strong activity against bacteria usually encountered in the host skin, this AMP may protect ticks from the acquisition and proliferation of host skin microbes (100).

Serine proteinase inhibitors have also been reported to play a role in the arthropod immune system. For instance, serine proteinase inhibitors mediate both coagulation and melanization processes of hemolymph and the production of AMPs (101). In addition, serine proteinases may also exert antimicrobial activity, possibly inhibiting proteinases that microorganisms use to colonize host tissues and evade the immune system (102). The first report of a tick serine proteinase inhibitor with antimicrobial properties was the ixodidin of *R. microplus* (103), which presents the key features of trypsin inhibitor-like domain proteins (104). Interestingly, one Kunitz inhibitor was reported to control *R. montanensis* infection in the gut of *D. variabilis* (105). In contrast to defensin, *D. variabilis* Kunitz-type inhibitors present a bacteriostatic effect on *R. montanensis* (106). Therefore, serine proteinase inhibitors are also used by ticks as powerful antimicrobial molecules.

Despite the diverse nature of molecules used by ticks as antimicrobials, little information on their synthesis regulation is available, as discussed above. Therefore, additional studies on the regulation of tick AMPs by immune signaling pathways are required to better understand their role in the control of distinct pathogens.

REDOX METABOLISM AS AN IMPORTANT PLAYER IN THE INFECTION CONTROL ORCHESTRA

In addition to AMPs, triggering of the production of reactive oxygen species (ROS) and reactive nitrogen species (RNS) in response to infection has been described in several arthropods, such as *Drosophila* (107) and mosquitoes (108). ROS have an essential role in infection-related physiological as well as pathophysiological processes, such as signaling, regulation of tissue injury and inflammation, cell survival, proliferation, differentiation, and apoptosis (109, 110).

In ticks, there is still little available information on ROS metabolism and their impact on pathogen control. Nonetheless, it is recognized that hemocytes produce ROS under stimulation. Gram-positive bacteria, zymosan, and phorbol 12-myristate 13-acetate elicit the production of hydrogen peroxide (H_2O_2) and superoxide (O_2^-) by hemocytes of *R. microplus* (111). In contrast, stimulation with lipopolysaccharide (LPS), the major component of the Gram-negative bacterial outer membrane, failed to induce ROS generation, indicating that different mechanisms or roles for ROS upon infection with either Gram-positive or Gram-negative bacteria may exist (111). Further studies with *R. microplus* showed that cytochrome c oxidase subunit III (COXIII), an enzyme of mitochondrial electron transport complex IV involved in mitochondrial ATP and ROS generation, is important for the transmission of *A. marginale* to calves (112). It is possible that COXIII knockdown imbalances tick redox metabolism, affecting its ability to transmit this pathogen (112). The peroxiredoxin Salp25D from *I. scapularis* had no effect on the transmission of *B. burgdorferi* but instead played a role in spirochete acquisition by the tick (113). RNAi-mediated silencing of Salp25D affects bacterial acquisition by ticks fed on *B. burgdorferi*-infected mice. The same effect was obtained when ticks were fed on Salp25-immunized mice (113). It is possible that Salp25 may detoxify ROS at the tick feeding site and gut, thus affording a survival advantage to *B. burgdorferi*.

In the mosquito *An. gambiae*, an extracellular matrix crosslinked by dityrosine covalent bonds catalyzed by dual oxidase (DUOX) and heme peroxidase is located in the gut ectoperitrophic space (between the epithelial cell layer and the peritrophic matrix). This extracellular matrix acts as an additional physical barrier to decrease gut permeability to bacterial PAMPs, impairing immune response activation by the resident microbiota (114). Importantly, the dityrosine network also provides a favorable environment for *Plasmodium* development, as it prevents the activation of nitric oxidase synthase (iNOS), a nitric oxide-generator enzyme (114). iNOS is responsible for parasite nitration, a key step in the action of the antiplasmodium complement-like molecule TEP1. Later, it was shown that the heme peroxidase 2/NADPH oxidase 5 system plays a central role in epithelium nitration, therefore potentiating the antiparasitic effect of nitric oxide (115). Similar to *An. gambiae* (114), an extracellular matrix was described in the tick *I. scapularis*, which acts as a shield that favors *B. burgdorferi* survival and indirectly prevents the induction of borreliacidal agents in the tick gut (116).

Intriguingly, *A. marginale* upregulated the genes encoding antioxidant enzymes, including superoxide dismutase, catalase, glutathione peroxidase, glutathione S-transferase, thioredoxin, thioredoxin reductase, and peroxiredoxin, whereas genes encoding ROS-generating enzymes, such as DUOX and endoplasmic reticulum oxidase, were downregulated in *R. microplus*-derived BME26 cells (117). Conversely, *R. rickettsii* and heat-killed *S. cerevisiae, E. cloacae* or *M. luteus* triggered the opposite gene expression pattern (117). Furthermore, simultaneous RNAi knockdown of catalase, thioredoxin, and glutathione peroxidase, three representative members of the tick antioxidant enzymatic system, as well as the oxidation resistance 1 (OXR1), which regulates the expression of ROS detoxification enzymes, decreased *A. marginale* infection (117). Therefore, while BME26 cells respond to infection, producing an oxidant environment, *A. marginale* seems to subvert this response to create an antioxidant environment, which is required for its survival (117). It is possible that *A. marginale* manipulates *R. microplus* redox metabolism (and production of immune signaling pathway effectors, as aforementioned) to favor its proliferation. Additional studies are required to elucidate the mechanisms that this bacterium uses to subvert tick immune responses.

CELL-MEDIATED IMMUNITY IN TICKS

Hemocytes, which are sessile or circulating cells from arthropod hemolymph, are responsible for several immune responses. The nomenclature of hemocytes varies considerably depending on the arthropod species and/or the approaches of the study (118). Earlier morphological, ultrastructural, and physiological studies of the hemocyte repertoire in different tick species consistently reported the presence of three basic types of hemocytes, namely, phagocytic plasmatocytes and granulocytes and nonphagocytic granulocytes (119–121). These cells apparently differentiate from rarely occurring prohemocytes (120, 122). More recent studies have described additional types of tick hemocytes, namely, adipohemocytes in *Rhipicephalus sanguineus* (123) and spherulocytes and oenocytoids in *R. microplus* (122). The most important immune responses of arthropod hemocytes are phagocytosis, encapsulation, nodulation (which involves melanization by the PPO cascade), coagulation, and production of immune-related molecules.

The role of tick hemocytes in the phagocytosis of a variety of microbes, including bacteria, yeast, spirochetes, and foreign particles, has been investigated by several studies [for example, see (111, 124–127)]. By contrast, very little is known about the encapsulation and nodulation mechanisms. Indeed, there is only one report on encapsulation (128) and one on nodulation (129), both in *D. variabilis*. After the inoculation of ticks with *Escherichia coli*, hemocytes did not form circular layers but aggregated around the bacteria, which is a characteristic feature of nodule formation (129). As the encapsulation study was performed using an implant of Epon–Araldite under the tick cuticle, it is still unknown whether it also occurs against microorganisms (128).

In invertebrates such as insects and crustaceans, hemocytes produce components of the melanization response, which involves an enzymatic cascade referred to as the PPO activating system, ultimately resulting in the production of melanin (130, 131). This process can be locally activated by cuticle injury or systemically triggered by microbial invasion of the hemocoel. Interestingly, in the cotton bollworm *Helicoverpa armigera*, infection with the baculovirus HearNPV decreased the levels of the majority of PPO cascade components, while serpin-9 and serpin-5 (which were also shown to regulate the proteases cSP4 and cSP6, respectively) were increased (132). In addition, *in vitro* assays showed that hemolymph melanization can kill baculovirus, an effect abolished by the specific PO inhibitor phenylthiourea. Together, the results suggest that baculovirus inhibits the melanization response to ensure its survival in *H. armigera* (132). There is no evidence of the existence of the PPO cascade in ticks based on available genomic and transcriptomic data. In line with this, no PPO activity has been reported to be present in the hemolymph of the hard ticks *Amblyomma americanum, D. variabilis*, and *I. scapularis* (133). In contrast, two studies reported PPO-like activity using L-DOPA as a substrate in the hard tick *R. sanguineus* (134) and in the soft tick *Ornithodoros moubata* (135). However, the enzymes responsible for such activity have not yet been identified, and enzymatic assays did not employ phenylthiourea as a control.

Coagulation is another important immune response of arthropods. The final product of coagulation is a protein clot, which is essential to avoid the loss of hemolymph in cases of an injury and the spread of an invader microorganism throughout the hemocoel (136). In horseshoe crabs, the clotting process involves a serine-protease cascade that leads to the activation of the clotting enzyme that converts the coagulogen into the insoluble clot (137), while in crayfish, the process depends on direct transglutaminase (TG)-mediated cross-linking of a specific plasma protein homologous to vitellogenins (19, 136). TG is also involved in the final step of coagulation in horseshoe crabs, cross-linking coagulin with hemocyte surface proteins named proxins (138). Interestingly, factors of the coagulation cascade interact with hemocyanin, causing it to present PO activity in the horseshoe crab *Tachypleus tridentatus*, demonstrating crosstalk between melanization and coagulation cascades (139). In *Drosophila*, coagulation and PO activity were also described to be tightly associated (140). Wound sealing in flies involves two steps: in the first step, TG-mediated crosslinking of hemolymph proteins occurs, and in the second step, PO-dependent crosslinking takes place, hardening the clot and producing melanin. In ticks, putative coagulation was uniquely reported for *D. variabilis*, where a fibrous matrix was observed around an inert implant (128). TGs and proclotting enzyme precursors have been detected in tick genomes (33). Moreover, an injury-responsive multidomain serine protease homologous to *Limulus* Factor C has been characterized in *I. ricinus* (141). Therefore, additional studies based on appropriate *in vitro* assays are needed to ultimately resolve the question of the existence of hemolymph clotting in ticks.

Tick hemocytes (83), as well as the hemocytes of other arthropods, such as mosquitoes (142), also produce a series of immune-related molecules. Intriguingly, the hemocytome of *I. ricinus* showed that only 1.48% of the 15,716 coding sequences (CDSs) identified were related to immune factors (143). Of the identified CDSs, 327 were five times more highly expressed in hemocytes than in salivary glands and the gut, among which 11 encode immune factors, including AMPs and proteins involved in pathogen recognition. As presented in this section, hemocytes are versatile components of the arthropod immune system that play diverse and key roles. The principal insect tissue that produces the majority of soluble immune molecules in hemolymph is the fat body (44). The role of tick fat body in the tick immune system requires further investigation.

THE PRIMORDIAL COMPLEMENT SYSTEM OF TICKS

One important branch of both cellular and humoral innate immunity in vertebrate and invertebrate metazoan organisms is carried out by the complement system. In higher vertebrates, the complement system is composed of approximately thirty components arranged in classical, lectin, and alternative pathways, which recognize foreign cells (microbes), specifically tag them *via* opsonization, and ultimately, eliminate them *via* phagocytosis or cell lysis (144). The common denominator of all three pathways is the proteolytic activation of the central C3 complement component. The occurrence of this molecule can be traced back in most ancient invertebrates, such as horseshoe crabs (subphylum Chelicerata, class Merostomata), implying that an ancestor of the complement system existed on Earth for more than 500 mil. years (145, 146). For ticks, which are also chelicerates, advanced knowledge of the primitive complement system of horseshoe crabs gathered during the past two decades presents the best matching comparative model (137, 145, 147).

Microbial pattern recognition by the vertebrate lectin pathway is mediated by multimeric mannose-binding lectins (MBLs) or ficolins. The horseshoe crab counterparts of mammalian ficolins are lectins named tachylectin-5 or carcinolectin-5 (148–150). These lectins share a fibrinogen-related protein (FRED) with ficolins but lack the N-terminal collagen-like domain responsible for forming complexes with MBL-associated serine proteases (MASPs) (151), which are absent in arthropods (146). The lectin Dorin M, purified from the plasma of the soft tick *O. moubata* (152), was shown to be a clear ortholog of the horseshoe crab tachylectins-5 (153), and similarly to ficolins and tachylectins, it forms high molecular weight multimers in the native state (152). The search for homologous lectins in *I. ricinus* (154) and in the genome of *I. scapularis* (155) revealed the existence of two phylogenetically distinct families, further referred to as ixoderin A and ixoderin B (**Figure 4**). Ixoderin A is mainly present in plasma and is responsible for the hemagglutination of mouse

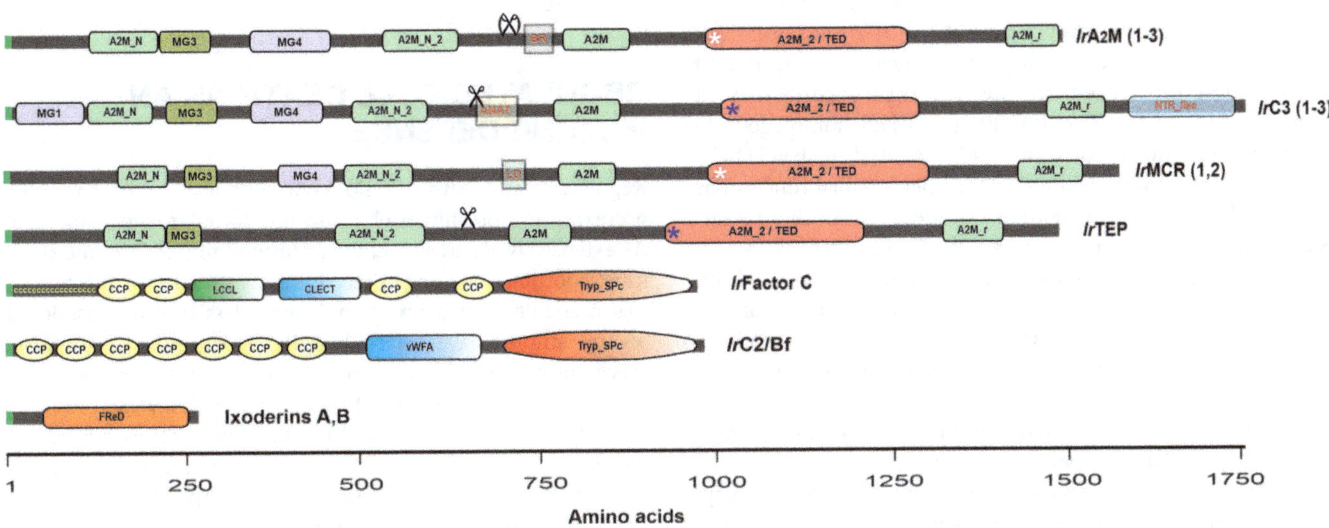

FIGURE 4 | Schematic representation of tick complement-related molecules (TEPs, convertases, lectins). Invertebrate TEPs are divided into four groups: panprotease inhibitors of the α_2-macroglobulin type (α_2M); C3-like complement components (C3); macroglobulin complement-related (MCR); and insect-type TEPs (iTEPs). IrA2M(1–3) represents *I. ricinus* α_2M: IrA2M-1, 2 and 3; IrC3(1-3) represents *I. ricinus* C3: IrC3-1, IrC3-2, and IrC3-3; *Ir*MCR (1,2) represents *I. ricinus* MCR: IrMcr-1 and IrMCR-*2;* and IrTEP represents *I. ricinus* iTEP. Other components of the *I. ricinus* primitive complement system are two putative convertases: IrFactor C, which shows the domain organization of the *I. ricinus* injury-responsive convertase related to *Limulus* Factor C (141), and IrC2/Bf, which shows the domain organization of the *I. ricinus* convertase related to the complement components C2 and/or Bf (156). Ixoderins A and B show the monomer structure of *Ixodes* sp. lectins related to ficolins (155). Domain abbreviations and nomenclature according to the NCBI conserved domain database (https://www.ncbi.nlm.nih.gov/Structure/cdd/wrpsb.cgi) and symbols used in the figure: MG1, 3, 4 – macroglobulin domains 1, 3, 4; A2M_N – MG2 domain of α_2-macroglobulins; A2M_N_2 – α_2-macroglobulin family N-terminal region; Scissors – indicate the posttranslational cleavage site (not present in IrA2M-3); BR – bait region of α_2-macroglobulins (variable by alternative splicing); ANAT – anaphylatoxin homologous domain (signature domain of C3-complement components); LD – low density lipoprotein class A domain (signature domain of MCRs); A2M_2/TED – thioester containing domain; Blue asterisks – thioester bond present; White asterisks – thioester bond absent in IrA2M-2 and IrMCR-1; A2M_r – α_2-macroglobulin receptor domain; NTR_like – the signature C-terminal domain of C3,C4, and C5 complement components; cccccccc – the cysteine-rich N-terminal region of *Limulus* Factor C; CCP – complement control protein module (aka short consensus repeats SCRs or SUSHI repeats); LCCL – LCCL domain; CLECT – C-lectin domain; Tryp_Spc – Trypsin-like serine protease; vWFA – Von Willebrand factor A domain; FReD – Fibrinogen-related domain.

erythrocytes (155). On the other hand, the salivary gland transcriptomes of *I. ricinus* (157, 158) indicate that ixoderin B represents a highly variable multigene family that is preferentially expressed in the salivary glands and secreted into saliva. The function of these FREPs in tick saliva is still obscure, but we can hypothesize that they may play a role in the recognition of a specific tick host.

The central effector molecules of vertebrate and invertebrate complement systems are proteins belonging to the thioester-containing protein (TEP) family, formerly referred to as proteins of the α_2-macroglobulin superfamily (144, 159, 160). The TEP designation is given due to the presence of a highly reactive β-cysteinyl-γ-glutamyl thioester (TE) bond within a thioester domain. Invertebrate TEPs are divided into four major phylogenetically distinct groups: (i) panprotease inhibitors of the α_2-macroglobulin type (α_2M), (ii) C3-like complement components (C3), (iii) insect-type TEPs (iTEPs), and (iv) macroglobulin complement-related proteins (MCRs) (124, 146, 161). Genome-wide screening of the *I. scapularis* genome (124) and the recently available horseshoe crab genomes (162, 163), together with transcriptome data from a variety of arthropods, reveal that all these major groups of TEPs are present in chelicerates, but C3-like molecules are absent in crustaceans and hexapods, while α_2Ms were lost in the evolution of some insect lineages, such as *Drosophila* and mosquitoes (146).

Orthologs of nine TEPs present in the *I. scapularis* genome (124) were identified in closely related *I. ricinus* (125), and their full CDSs were recently deposited in GenBank: IrA2M-1 (MT779788); IrA2M-2 (MT779789); IrA2M-3 (MT779790); IrTep (MT779791); IrC3-1 (MT779792); IrC3-2 (MT779793); IrC3-3 (MT779793); IrMcr-1 (MT779795); and IrMcr-2 (MT779796). The domain structure of tick TEP representatives is shown in **Figure 4**. The hallmark domain of α_2Ms is the presence of the bait region (BR), which is cleaved by the target protease. Several bait region alternative splicing variants were reported in the α_2M region of the soft tick *O. moubata* (164) as well as in IrA2M-1 of *I. ricinus* (165). IrTEP has a domain architecture quite similar to that of IrA2Ms; however, this molecule is phylogenetically more closely related to insect TEPs (124). Tick C3-like molecules (IrC3-1, IrC3-2, IrC3-3) possess two signature domains, namely, the anaphylatoxin domain and C-terminal NTR complement_C345C domain. The MCRs can be clearly identified based on the presence of the short low-density lipoprotein receptor domain (LD), which occurs in the central part of the molecule (**Figure 4**). Tick TEPs are specifically expressed in tick fat body (IrA2M-1, IrA2M-3,

IrC3-1, IrC3-2, IrC3-3), tick hemocytes (IrA2M-2, IrA2M-3), salivary glands (IrC3-2, IrMcr-1), and ovaries (IrTEP) (125).

Other characterized components of the *I. ricinus* primitive complement system are two putative convertases: (i) IrC2/Bf (156), which is related to the vertebrate complement components C2 and/or FactorB (Bf) (144) and homologous to convertases from horseshoe crabs (145, 166), and (ii) IrFC (141), homologous to *Limulus* Factor C, which plays a dual function as the factor that triggers the clotting cascade upon sensing Gram-negative bacterial endotoxins and as an LPS-sensitive convertase of the horseshoe crab C3 complement component (147, 167). Both IrC2/Bf and IrFC are multidomain convertases that share the N-terminal trypsin-like domain and numerous CCP modules (complement control protein, aka sushi domains) (**Figure 4**). While IrC2/Bf is mainly expressed in the tick fat body and its expression is responsive to injection of the yeast *Candida albicans* and a variety of *Borrelia* species (156), IrFC is produced by tick hemocytes, and its expression is responsive to any injury, including injection of sterile phosphate-buffered saline, implicating its role in hemolymph clotting and wound healing (141).

RNAi-based functional studies of *I. ricinus* complement components successively deciphered their nonredundant roles in the phagocytosis of different microbes by tick hemocytes (124, 125, 141, 155, 156, 165). Phagocytosis of Gram-negative bacteria represented by the tick pathogen *Chryseobacterium indologenes* (168) depends mainly on the convertase IrFC, which seems to be linked to the IrC3-3 component. Interestingly, phagocytosis of this bacterium is also clearly mediated by α_2Ms IrAM2-1 and IrAM2-2 by a yet unknown mechanism that likely involves the interaction of these macromolecular protease inhibitors with the potent metalloprotease secreted by the bacterium (168).

A distinct phagocytic pathway dependent on the convertase IrC2/Bf is responsible for the phagocytosis of the yeast *C. albicans* and spirochete *Borrelia*. Phagocytosis of *C. albicans* is further facilitated by IrC3-1 and IrMcr-2, consistent with the reported role of its related molecule MCR (DmTep6) in the phagocytosis of this yeast by *Drosophila* S2 cells (161). Similar to other Gram-negative bacteria, phagocytosis of *Borrelia* is also mediated by IrC3-3. Ixoderins A and B were found to be involved in the phagocytosis of all the tested microbes, except *Borrelia*. Although *Borrelia afzelii* (the principal Lyme disease-causative agent in Europe) is actively phagocytosed by tick hemocytes; neither RNAi-mediated silencing of any tick complement-related molecules nor the total elimination of phagocytosis by preinjection of latex beads have shown any effect on the transmission of these spirochetes to the host (126). These results indirectly support the recent finding that the transmission of *B. afzelii* from infected *I. ricinus* nymphs to naive mice avoids the tick hemocoel and salivary glands and occurs by a direct gut-to-mouthpart route (169). However, it is possible that the tick complement plays a role in the transmission of other tick-borne pathogens, such as intracellular bacteria, including *Anaplasma* spp. and *Rickettsia* spp., or protozoan parasites, including *Babesia* spp. These objectives await an intensive research focus in the future.

REGULATED CELL DEATH AS AN IMMUNE DEFENSE

Regulated cell death (RCD) is widely distributed in nature, occurring in both unicellular and multicellular organisms (170). As extensively stated above, the arthropod innate immune system must coordinate pathogen recognition with effector mechanisms to successfully control infection. Nonetheless, over the past decade, several studies have established RCD processes as important mechanisms for the regulation of the immune response as well as the control of infections (171–173). Autophagy, apoptosis, and necrosis are the main types of RCD that have been described to be related to insect immunity in the last few years (173). In this section, we focus on autophagy and apoptosis and their interconnections with immune signaling pathways.

Autophagy is a highly conserved process in which endogenous material (misfolded proteins and aggregates, damaged organelles, and other macromolecules) or exogenous material (such as invading pathogens) are selectively recognized and sequestered within autophagosomes (double-membrane vesicles) that subsequently fuse with lysosomes, leading to cargo degradation (174). Autophagy is executed by a series of evolutionarily conserved autophagy-related (ATG) proteins that have orthologs in eukaryotic organisms ranging from yeasts to humans (174). Studies on *Drosophila* have provided excellent insights into the importance of autophagy during microbial infection (175). For instance, infection with the intracellular bacterium *Listeria monocytogenes* induces autophagy in both hemocytes and a hemocyte-derived *Drosophila* cell line (176). Interestingly, the IMD pathway receptor PGRP-LE is involved in bacterial recognition for autophagy activation. In addition, RNAi-mediated silencing of the autophagy genes *atg5* and *atg1* increases the bacterial load within cells, showing that this pathway is important to control infection. Autophagy is also important to control infection by vesicular stomatitis virus (VSV) in *Drosophila* (177, 178). In this process, the viral glycoprotein VSV-G is recognized by Toll-7, activating autophagy *via* a still unknown pathway that is independent of the canonical Toll, IMD, and JAK/STAT pathways (178). The role played by autophagy in the protection of mosquitoes against viruses is somewhat controversial, with reports suggesting both pro- and antiviral effects (179). In ticks, the expression of *atg* genes was upregulated under starvation in *Haemaphysalis longicornis* (180, 181), *I. scapularis* (182), *R. microplus*, and *A. sculptum* (183), correlating with the classical role of autophagy in stress. However, studies correlating tick autophagy with immune responses still need to be performed.

Apoptosis is another highly conserved RCD that is essential for removing damaged and infected cells to maintain homeostasis. There are two major apoptotic signaling pathways: extrinsic, also called death receptor pathway, and intrinsic, in which mitochondria play a central role (**Figure 5**). Both of these

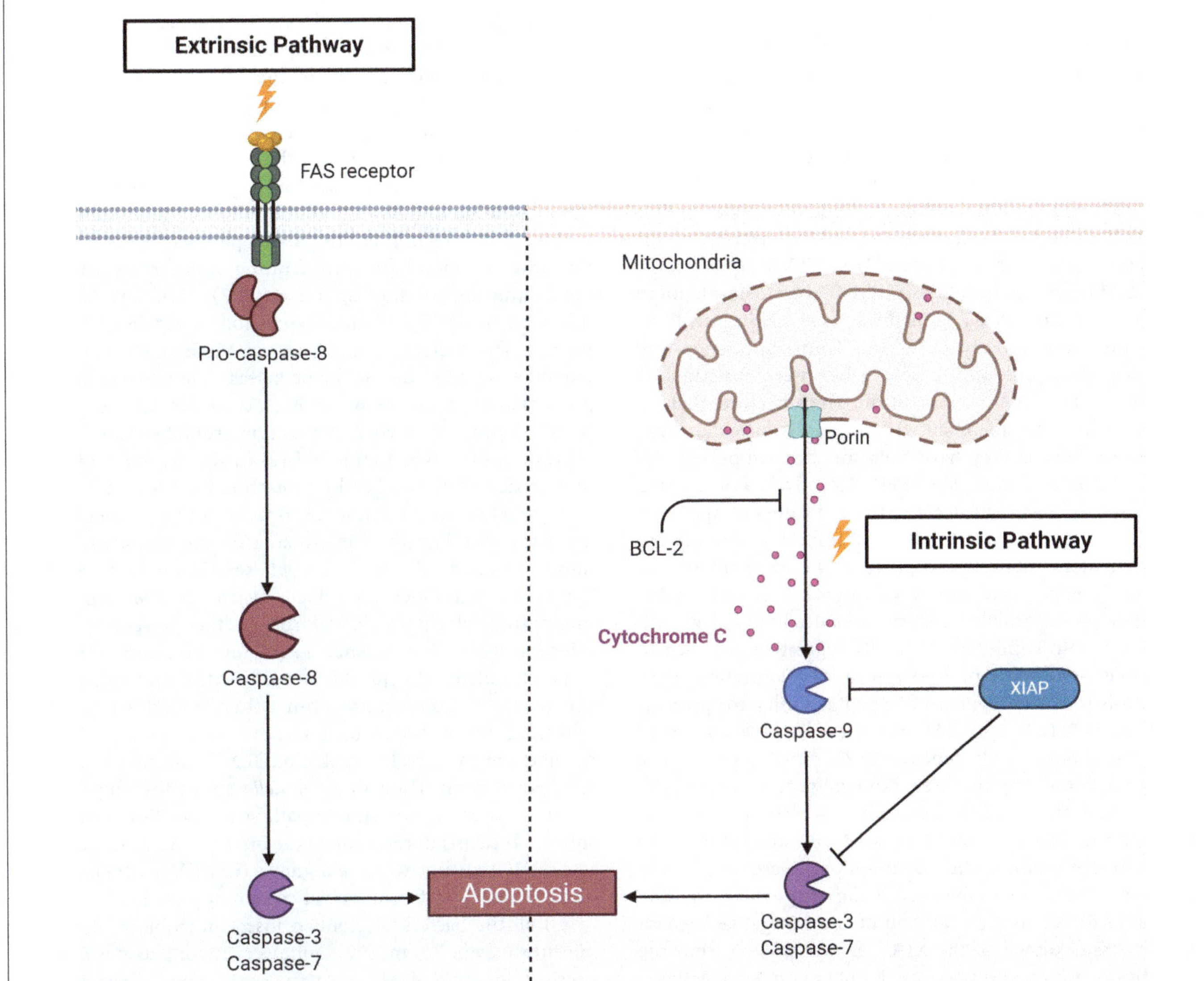

FIGURE 5 | Components of apoptosis activation pathways identified in ticks. Apoptosis is triggered by two main pathways. The extrinsic pathway is activated by recognition of external stimuli by transmembrane death receptors, such as fatty acid synthase (FAS), leading to the activation of caspase-8. The intrinsic pathway, also known as the mitochondrial pathway, is activated by internal stimuli. Subsequently, mitochondrial channels composed, for example, of porins, allow the release of mitochondrial components, such as cytochrome c, to the cytosol, activating the initiator caspase-9. B-cell lymphoma protein 2 (Bcl-2) can inhibit cytochrome c release from mitochondria. Both pathways culminate in the activation of effector or executioner caspases, such as caspases -3 and -7, resulting in chromatin condensation, DNA fragmentation, degradation of nuclear and cytoskeletal proteins and protein cross-linking, which ultimately cause cell death.

pathways culminate in the activation of executer caspases that are key for eliminating apoptotic cells (184). Apoptosis is activated in *Drosophila* by infection with *Drosophila* C virus (DCV), and infected cells are phagocytized by hemocytes in a phosphatidylserine-mediated process (185). Apoptosis can also control viral infection in mosquitoes (186, 187). Interestingly, the expression of proapoptotic genes was significantly higher in the refractory strain Cali-MIB of *Ae. aegypti* than in the susceptible strain Cali-S upon experimental infection with DENV-2, suggesting that apoptosis is involved in the distinct susceptibility of mosquitoes to infection (186). Apoptosis is also involved in the control of the proliferation of WNV in the midgut of a refractory strain of the mosquito *Culex pipiens pipiens* (187). Studies on the apoptotic response upon pathogen infection in ticks are also scarcer than those in insects. Infection of the *I. ricinus* cell line IRE/CTVM20 with the bacterium *A. phagocytophilum* and the flaviviruses TBEV and LIV upregulated the expression of apoptosis-associated components, such as cytochrome c and fatty-acid synthase (FAS) (54, 188).

To guarantee their replication and survival within the host cell, many pathogens, including viruses, bacteria and protozoa, subvert apoptosis induced by infection (189). For instance, infection with Zika virus (ZIKV) inhibits apoptosis in *Ae. aegypti* through the action of sfRNAs (190). Until very recently, the unique example of a pathogen that inhibits apoptosis in tick cells was *A. phagocytophilum* (188, 191, 192). This bacterium inhibits the intrinsic apoptosis pathway in *I. scapularis* salivary glands and ISE6 cells by porin (voltage-dependent anion-selective channel) downregulation, resulting in the inhibition of cytochrome c release. Nonetheless, while the intrinsic pathway is inhibited, the extrinsic pathway seems to be activated through the inhibition of FAS by an unknown mechanism as a possible attempt to limit bacterial infection (192, 193). Conversely, in the *I. scapularis* gut and *I. ricinus* IRE/CTVM20 cells, *A. phagocytophilum* supposedly inhibits apoptosis through upregulation of the JAK/STAT pathway (191). However, these conclusions were mostly based on transcriptomics and proteomics data, and only a few genes were functionally characterized by RNAi. In addition, the effectors that *A. phagocytophilum* uses to inhibit tick apoptosis have not been elucidated to date, as they have been for the manipulation of apoptosis in human neutrophils (194). Recently, it was reported that *R. rickettsii* downregulates negative regulators of apoptosis in the initial phase of BME26 cell infection, which are upregulated later. Infection also prevents the fragmentation of DNA and decreases the activity of caspase-3 as well as the exposure of phosphatidylserine. Remarkably, bacterial growth is higher in apoptosis-inhibited tick cells, suggesting that such an inhibitory effect is important to guarantee cell colonization (195).

Apoptosis is closely regulated by apoptosis inhibitor proteins (IAPs) (**Figure 5**) (196, 197). IAPs present at least two conserved motifs: baculoviral IAP repeat (BIR) motifs, which are represented from one to three tandem repeats in the N-terminus, and the C-terminal really interesting new gene (RING) motif; this last motif presents E3-ubiquitin ligase activity. In *Drosophila*, the E3-ubiquitin ligase activity of DIAP-2 has been described as being important for the activation of Relish after recognition of Gram-negative bacteria (198–201). Knockdown of the XIAP of *I. scapularis* from the IMD pathway, which also possesses E3-ubiquitin ligase activity, increased colonization by *A. phagocytophilum*, showing that E3 is important for the control of infection (202) (see the above section "The unconventional IMD pathway"). However, it is still unknown whether XIAP plays a role in tick apoptosis.

Additional studies are warranted to better understand the role played by tick apoptosis pathway components in infection control and their interconnections with immune signaling pathways as well as the mechanisms that pathogens use to subvert the death of tick cells, thereby guaranteeing their survival and proliferation.

THE ROLE OF TICK MICROBIOTA IN VECTOR COMPETENCE

Ticks, as well as most multicellular eukaryotes, possess associated bacteria, viruses, fungi and archaea, mainly in mucosal organs, composing their microbiota (203). In the last decade, several studies have focused on the bacterial composition of different genera of ticks and have explored the interaction of TBPs with nonpathogenic tick endosymbionts to elucidate the impact of microbiota on their vector competence (62, 64, 204–206). The tick immune responses to microbiota, despite its importance for a more comprehensive understanding of tick biology, is a field that requires attention since little is known in comparison with other arthropods. Therefore, in this section, we summarize the *Ae. aegypti* immune responses to the gut microbiota and relate this knowledge to ticks.

In adult mosquitoes, the IMD pathway is activated in response to microbiota proliferation induced by the blood meal, limiting Sindbis infection (207). ROS production is mediated by DUOX, whose expression is regulated by a gut membrane-associated protein named Mesh (208). However, a reduction in ROS due to heme release upon blood digestion protects the gut microbiota (209). To counteract the action of Relish-dependent AMPs, the gut microbiota stimulates the expression of C-type lectins (CLTs) in *Ae. aegypti*, which bind to bacterial cell walls, thereby protecting the bacteria (210).

In addition to the immune response to microbiota, there is interest in the impact of microbiota on the vector capacity of mosquitoes and ticks. In *Ae. aegypti*, several studies have shown that larval microbiota can influence vector competence in adult mosquitoes, playing a critical role in their response to viral infections (211). For instance, *E. coli* infection during the larval stage stimulates the production of AMPs and nitric oxide, protecting the mosquito from other infections (212). In addition, when Enterobacteriaceae bacteria are the only members of the larval microbiota, DENV infection in adults is reduced in comparison to *Salmonella* sp. as the only member (213). Conversely, exposure to pathogenic *Bacillus thuringiensis* subsp. *israelensis* in resistant larvae increases adult susceptibility to DENV [but not to Chikungunya (CHIKV)] (214), possibly due to changes in the microbial community (215).

Of all the bacteria present in insect microbiota, *Wolbachia pipientis* may be the most ubiquitous symbiont, as it is naturally present in 40% of all terrestrial arthropod species (216). Intracellular and maternally transmitted *Wolbachia* can cause pathogen interference (PI; the ability to reduce the chance of pathogen infection and decrease pathogen load) and cytoplasmic incompatibility (CI; when infected males mate with uninfected females, the hatch of eggs is heavily reduced), manipulating host reproduction and working as a genetic driver (the ability to spread through a population in a non-Mendelian way) (217). In *Ae. aegypti*, *Wolbachia* strongly reduces CHIKV, DENV and ZIKV infection and vector competence *via* the PI phenotype (217–220). For this reason, there is an ongoing program, the World Mosquito Program, to infect mosquito eggs with *Wolbachia* (from *Drosophila* – *w*Mel) in the laboratory and release them in dengue-endemic areas, such as the city of Rio de Janeiro in Brazil (221, 222).

Despite being the most common bacteria in the microbiota of insects, *Wolbachia* has been reported only in a few species of ticks (205, 223, 224). In fact, the adult tick microbiota is mostly composed of *Coxiella*, *Rickettsia*, *Francisella*, *Spiroplasma*,

Midichloria and *Rickettsiella* (203, 205). Most of these bacteria are intracellular and noncultivable in the laboratory, which hampers the manipulation of tick microbiota. Some studies on the larval microbiota of *I. scapularis* (62, 64, 204) showed a wide variety of bacterial genera, including cultivable extracellular bacteria. A deep bioinformatics analysis of the raw data of these studies suggested a taxonomic core composed of 61 bacterial taxa for *I. scapularis* larvae (225). However, this high number of bacterial genera in the larval microbiota of *I. scapularis* has been questioned, and the possibility of contamination potentially due to the low biomass of tick samples has been raised (226, 227). Interestingly, some tick species, such as *R. microplus* and *I. ricinus*, present a poor and unstable microbiota in the gut (228). On the other hand, these two species harbor a more abundant and stable microbiota in their ovaries that is composed mostly of *Midichloria* spp. in *I. ricinus* (228) and *Coxiella* spp. in *R. microplus* (229). The authors hypothesized that the reduced microbiota in the tick gut might be due to the action of immune factors, such as AMPs and ROS (228).

As described for mosquitoes, the tick microbiota can exert an effect on vector capacity; bacterial infection can modify the microbiota of its host. In *I. scapularis*, perturbation of the normal gut microbiota decreased the expression of STAT, which, in turn, reduced the expression of peritrophin-1. Since the integrity of the peritrophic matrix is essential to *B. burgdorferi* infection, as previously discussed, alteration of the microbiota reduces borrelial colonization (62). In addition, infection with *B. burgdorferi* promotes the expression of the *I. scapularis* gene *pixr*, which encodes a gut secreted protein with functions in tick biology, such as larval molting and inhibition of biofilm formation (preferentially by Gram-positive bacteria), facilitating the colonization of *B. burgdorferi* in ticks (204). These studies suggest a mutual influence or interconnection between the gut microbiota and *B. burgdorferi* in *I. scapularis*. Conversely, *A. phagocytophilum* infection in this same tick species promotes the expression of an antifreeze protein, which perturbs the gut microbiota and reduces the integrity of the peritrophic matrix (64). In contrast to *B. burgdorferi* (62), an extracellular bacterium that benefits from a preserved peritrophic matrix, *A. phagocytophilum*, which is an obligate intracellular bacterium, reduces the thickness of the peritrophic matrix to colonize the tick gut (64). In the tick *Dermacentor andersoni*, a microbiota alteration was induced by feeding on calves treated with oxytetracycline. Although this treatment did not change the microbiota composition, the proportion of its components was altered, negatively impacting the acquisition of *A. marginale* and *Francisella novicida* (230). Importantly, perturbation of the *D. andersoni* microbiota exerted a negative impact on the reproductive fitness of the tick, thereby identifying the microbiota as an important target for the development of control strategies (231).

A recent study compared the microbiota of two *R. rickettsii* tick vectors in Brazil, *Amblyomma sculptum* and *A. aureolatum*, which present significant differences regarding their susceptibility to infection (232). Interestingly, *A. aureolatum* is highly susceptible to *R. rickettsii* infection and harbors a robust intestinal microbiota, mainly composed of the *Francisella* genus. *A. sculptum*, on the other hand, is less susceptible to *R. rickettsii* infection and harbors a reduced intestinal microbiota (206). Additionally, *R. rickettsii* causes a slight reduction in the microbiota load without changing its composition. It has been reported that the transcriptional gut response of these two ticks to *R. rickettsii* infection is also distinct: while the majority of genes of *A. sculptum*, including immune factors, were upregulated by infection, *A. aureolatum* genes were mostly downregulated (233). Together, these data suggest that the *A. aureolatum* gut microbiota somehow desensitizes the immune system and promotes *R. rickettsii* infection. Interestingly, the presence of *Francisella* endosymbionts positively impacted the establishment of *F. novicida* in *D. andersoni*, and the authors hypothesized that these endosymbionts may suppress the tick immune system, favoring *F. novicida* acquisition (230). Additional studies are needed to confirm this hypothesis and to identify the mechanisms by which microbiota delineate tick susceptibility to infection.

Studies focused on the immune response to tick microbiota are necessary to elucidate this important feature, which is involved in many aspects of tick biology, including its vector capacity, representing a question of public health interest. These responses may involve only one immune signaling pathway or crosstalk of the different pathways, as is suggested to occur in *R. microplus* in response to *A. marginale* infection (49). In addition, we can raise a possible role of DUOX in the control of tick microbiota since this enzyme is present and functional in *I. scapularis* (116).

CONCLUSIONS

To date, studies on the interactions between ticks and TBPs have shown that both the IMD and JAK/STAT pathways are key for the control of bacterial infections (*B. burgdorferi*, *A. marginale* and *A. phagocytophilum*), while the Toll and RNAi pathways might be involved in tick defense against viral infections. Studies on the identification of tick immune system-specific effectors are warranted to describe the mechanisms involved in these signaling pathways. In addition, this review has provided several lines of evidence of interconnections between immune signaling pathways, as well as links among several elements from the innate immunity of arthropods, such as the RNAi system, redox metabolism and microbiota. This review also highlights the importance of bearing in mind a widely integrated, versatile, and complex immune system as a response to infection in ticks, far beyond a canonical and linear pathway.

As mentioned above, most of our knowledge on arthropod immunity comes from *Drosophila* as well as other arthropod studies. Nevertheless, the search for a direct correlation between immune signaling and effector specificity in ticks may result in the absence of new and important mechanisms of the tick immune system. For instance, recent works have suggested that ticks express different types of effectors from immune signaling pathway activation, such as peritrophins, which are key structural components of the gut peritrophic matrix. Moreover, it is extremely important to keep in mind that *Drosophila* is not a vector model and, as such, some aspects of the pathogen-vector interaction cannot be fully modeled. Of relevance, the studies on the innate responses of *Drosophila* follow infections by an intrathoracic injection with large loads of artificial pathogens, greatly contrasting those from ticks, which experience natural pathogens, doses, and routes of infection.

Phagocytosis, AMPs, complement-like molecules and ROS production are also considered important factors for protecting ticks from infection. The microbiota can interfere with tick colonization by pathogens as well. Therefore, it is important to identify the microorganisms that compose the microbiota of different organs of ticks and to determine their influence on the tick immune system as well as on tick vector competence. Interestingly, in some insects, the immune system can be primed by nonpathogenic microorganisms, protecting the animal from subsequent infection with a pathogenic microbe (234). Nonetheless, there is only one report on tick immune system priming to date (48). The authors showed that immune priming with POPG and PODAG protects *I. scapularis* against infection by *A. phagocytophilum* and *D. andersoni* against infection by *A. marginale*. In addition, it was shown that the lipid immune-priming effect is abolished only by the silencing of IMD pathway components but not of the Toll or JAK/STAT pathways, excluding an off-target effect (48). Therefore, the tick immune system and its relationship with microorganisms is a wide and unexplored field to be pursued.

In summary, every aspect concerning the tick immune system and its relation with microorganisms - endosymbionts or pathogens - remains far from completely understood. Despite the vast advances made in recent decades, which have helped us to build parts of this puzzle, working with ticks is still a bright and open field full of possibilities. We expect more groups to work with ticks due to their importance to public health and await the discovery of new knowledge in the next few years. In this way, we will all be able to assemble this extraordinary and complex puzzle.

AUTHOR CONTRIBUTIONS

All authors searched the literature and wrote the manuscript. SD and AF conceived the work and the final edition. GS, DP, EE, LM, and PK elaborated the figures. All authors contributed to the article and approved the submitted version.

FUNDING

This work was supported by funds from the São Paulo Research Foundation (FAPESP 2013/26450-2) and the National Council for Scientific and Technological Development (CNPq) - the National Institutes of Science and Technology Program in Molecular Entomology (INCTEM 573959/2008-0). AF (309733/2018-9) and SD (304382/2017-5) received CNPq research productivity scholarships. GS and DP received a postdoctoral scholarship from FAPESP (2019/07122-0 and 2018/00652-1, respectively) and EE from the Coordination for the Improvement of Higher Education Personnel (CAPES 88887.321638/2019-00). VU and PK were supported by the Czech Science Foundation (20-05736S).

ACKNOWLEDGMENTS

The authors are grateful to Dr. Ondrej Hajdusek, Institute of Parasitology, BC CAS, for the critical reading of the manuscript and valuable discussions. **Figures 1–3**, and **5** were created with Biorender.com.

REFERENCES

Dantas-Torres F, Fernandes Martins T, Munoz-Leal S, Onofrio VC, Barros-Battesti DM. Ticks (Ixodida: Argasidae, Ixodidae) of Brazil: Updated species checklist and taxonomic keys. *Ticks Tick Borne Dis* (2019) 10:101252. doi: 10.1016/j.ttbdis.2019.06.012

Dantas-Torres F. Species Concepts: What about ticks? *Trends Parasitol* (2018) 34:1017–26. doi: 10.1016/j.pt.2018.09.009

Koch HG, Sauer JR. Quantity of blood ingested by four species of hard ticks (Acari:Ixodidae) fed on domestic dogs. *Ann Entomol Soc Am* (1984) 77:142–6. doi: 10.1093/aesa/77.2.142

Grisi L, Leite RC, Martins JR, Barros AT, Andreotti R, Cancado PH, et al. Reassessment of the potential economic impact of cattle parasites in Brazil. *Rev Bras Parasitol Vet* (2014) 23:150–6. doi: 10.1590/S1984- 29612014042

Bowman AS, Sauer JR. Tick salivary glands: function, physiology and future. *Parasitology* (2004) 129(Suppl):S67–81. doi: 10.1017/s0031182004006468

Kazimirova M, Stibraniova I. Tick salivary compounds: their role in modulation of host defences and pathogen transmission. *Front Cell Infect Microbiol* (2013) 3:43. doi: 10.3389/fcimb.2013.00043

Kotal J, Langhansova H, Lieskovska J, Andersen JF, Francischetti IM, Chavakis T, et al. Modulation of host immunity by tick saliva. *J Proteomics* (2015) 128:58–68. doi: 10.1016/j.jprot.2015.07.005

Simo L, Kazimirova M, Richardson J, Bonnet SI. The essential role of tick salivary glands and saliva in tick feeding and pathogen transmission. *Front Cell Infect Microbiol* (2017) 7:281. doi: 10.3389/fcimb.2017.00281

Dantas-Torres F, Chomel BB, Otranto D. Ticks and tick-borne diseases: a one health perspective. *Trends Parasitol* (2012) 28:437–46. doi: 10.1016/j.pt.2012.07.003

Stanek G, Strle F. Lyme borreliosis-from tick bite to diagnosis and treatment. *FEMS Microbiol Rev* (2018) 42:233–58. doi: 10.1093/femsre/fux047

Hajdusek O, Sima R, Ayllon N, Jalovecka M, Perner J, de la Fuente J, et al. Interaction of the tick immune system with transmitted pathogens. *Front Cell Infect Microbiol* (2013) 3:26. doi: 10.3389/fcimb.2013.00026

Brey PT. The contribution of the Pasteur scholl of insect immunity. In: PT Brey and D Hultmark, editors. *Molecular Mechanisms of Immune Responses in Insects*. London: Chapman & Hall (1998). p. 1–39.

Steiner H, Hultmark D, Engstrom A, Bennich H, Boman HG. Sequence and specificity of two antibacterial proteins involved in insect immunity. *Nature* (1981) 292:246–8. doi: 10.1038/292246a0

Selsted ME, Brown DM, DeLange RJ, Lehrer RI. Primary structures of MCP- 1 and MCP-2, natural peptide antibiotics of rabbit lung macrophages. *J Biol Chem* (1983) 258:14485–9.

Selsted ME, Harwig SS, Ganz T, Schilling JW, Lehrer RI. Primary structures of three human neutrophil defensins. *J Clin Invest* (1985) 76:1436–9. doi: 10.1172/JCI112121

Boman HG, Hultmark D. Cell-free immunity in insects. *Annu Rev Microbiol* (1987) 41:103–26. doi: 10.1146/annurev.mi.41.100187.000535
Ashida M. The prophenoloxidase cascade in insect immunity. *Res Immunol* (1990) 141:908–10. doi: 10.1016/0923-2494(90)90191-z
Johansson MW, Soderhall K. Cellular immunity in crustaceans and the proPO system. *Parasitol Today* (1989) 5:171–6. doi: 10.1016/0169-4758(89) 90139-7
Kopacek P, Hall M, Soderhall K. Characterization of a clotting protein, isolated from plasma of the freshwater crayfish *Pacifastacus leniusculus*. *Eur J Biochem* (1993) 213:591–7. doi: 10.1111/j.1432-1033.1993.tb17798.x
Iwanaga S, Miyata T, Tokunaga F, Muta T. Molecular mechanism of hemolymph clotting system in *Limulus*. *Thromb Res* (1992) 68:1–32. doi: 10.1016/0049-3848(92)90124-s
Hoffmann JA, Kafatos FC, Janeway CA, Ezekowitz RA. Phylogenetic perspectives in innate immunity. *Science* (1999) 284:1313–8. doi: 10.1126/science.284.5418.1313
Hultmark D. *Drosophila* immunity: paths and patterns. *Curr Opin Immunol* (2003) 15:12–9. doi: 10.1016/s0952-7915(02)00005-5
Lemaitre B, Nicolas E, Michaut L, Reichhart JM, Hoffmann JA. The dorsoventral regulatory gene cassette spätzle/Toll/cactus controls the potent antifungal response in *Drosophila* adults. *Cell* (1996) 86:973–83. doi: 10.1016/s0092-8674(00)80172-5
Imler JL. Overview of *Drosophila* immunity: a historical perspective. *Dev Comp Immunol* (2014) 42:3–15. doi: 10.1016/j.dci.2013.08.018
Engstrom Y, Kadalayil L, Sun SC, Samakovlis C, Hultmark D, Faye I. kappa B-like motifs regulate the induction of immune genes in *Drosophila*. *J Mol Biol* (1993) 232:327–33. doi: 10.1006/jmbi.1993.1392
Belvin MP, Anderson KV. A conserved signaling pathway: the *Drosophila* Toll-Dorsal pathway. *Annu Rev Cell Dev Biol* (1996) 12:393–416. doi: 10.1146/annurev.cellbio.12.1.393
Michel K, Kafatos FC. Mosquito immunity against *Plasmodium*. *Insect Biochem Mol Biol* (2005) 35:677–89. doi: 10.1016/j.ibmb.2005.02.009
Garcia GR, Maruyama SR, Malardo T, Zangirolamo AF, Gardinassi LG. The biology of hematophagous arthropods addressed by molecular high-throughput approaches. *Austin J Trop Med Hyg* (2015) 1:1004–10.
Christophides GK, Zdobnov E, Barillas-Mury C, Birney E, Blandin S, Blass C, et al. Immunity-related genes and gene families in *Anopheles gambiae*. *Science* (2002) 298:159–65. doi: 10.1126/science.1077136
Palmer WJ, Jiggins FM. Comparative genomics reveals the origins and diversity of arthropod immune systems. *Mol Biol Evol* (2015) 32:2111–29. doi: 10.1093/molbev/msv093
Rosa RD, Capelli-Peixoto J, Mesquita RD, Kalil SP, Pohl PC, Braz GR, et al. Exploring the immune signalling pathway-related genes of the cattle tick *Rhipicephalus microplus*: From molecular characterization to transcriptional profile upon microbial challenge. *Dev Comp Immunol* (2016) 59:1–14. doi: 10.1016/j.dci.2015.12.018
Zumaya-Estrada FA, Martinez-Barnetche J, Lavore A, Rivera-Pomar R, Rodriguez MH. Comparative genomics analysis of triatomines reveals common first line and inducible immunity-related genes and the absence of Imd canonical components among hemimetabolous arthropods. *Parasit Vectors* (2018) 11:48. doi: 10.1186/s13071-017-2561-2
Smith AA, Pal U. Immunity-related genes in *Ixodes scapularis*-perspectives from genome information. *Front Cell Infect Microbiol* (2014) 4:116. doi: 10.3389/fcimb.2014.00116
Barnard AC, Nijhof AM, Fick W, Stutzer C, Maritz-Olivier C. RNAi in arthropods: insight into the machinery and applications for understanding the pathogen-vector interface. *Genes (Basel)* (2012) 3:702–41. doi: 10.3390/genes3040702
Sun D, Guo Z, Liu Y, Zhang Y. Progress and prospects of CRISPR/Cas systems in insects and other arthropods. *Front Physiol* (2017) 8:608. doi: 10.3389/fphys.2017.00608
Geraci NS, Spencer Johnston J, Paul Robinson J, Wikel SK, Hill CA. Variation in genome size of argasid and ixodid ticks. *Insect Biochem Mol Biol* (2007) 37:399–408. doi: 10.1016/j.ibmb.2006.12.007
Barrero RA, Guerrero FD, Black M, McCooke J, Chapman B, Schilkey F, et al. Gene-enriched draft genome of the cattle tick *Rhipicephalus microplus*: assembly by the hybrid Pacific Biosciences/Illumina approach enabled analysis of the highly repetitive genome. *Int J Parasitol* (2017) 47:569–83. doi: 10.1016/j.ijpara.2017.03.007
Gulia-Nuss M, Nuss AB, Meyer JM, Sonenshine DE, Roe RM, Waterhouse RM, et al. Genomic insights into the *Ixodes scapularis* tick vector of Lyme disease. *Nat Commun* (2016) 7:10507. doi: 10.1038/ncomms10507
Jia N, Wang J, Shi W, Du L, Sun Y, Zhan W, et al. Large-scale comparative analyses of tick genomes elucidate their genetic diversity and vector capacities. *Cell* (2020) 182:1328–40.e13. doi: 10.1016/j.cell.2020.07.023
Romano D, Stefanini C, Canale A, Benelli G. Artificial blood feeders for mosquito and ticks-where from, where to? *Acta Trop* (2018) 183:43–56. doi: 10.1016/j.actatropica.2018.04.009
Bell-Sakyi L, Darby A, Baylis M, Makepeace BL. The tick cell biobank: a global resource for in vitro research on ticks, other arthropods and the pathogens they transmit. *Ticks Tick Borne Dis* (2018) 9:1364–71. doi: 10.1016/j.ttbdis.2018.05.015
de la Fuente J, Estrada-Pena A, Venzal JM, Kocan KM, Sonenshine DE. Overview: ticks as vectors of pathogens that cause disease in humans and animals. *Front Biosci* (2008) 13:6938–46. doi: 10.2741/3200
Verhulst NO, Boulanger N JS. Impact of skin microbiome on attractiveness to arthropod vectors and pathogen transmission. In: N Boulanger, editor. *Skin and Arthropod Vectors*. Academic Press (Cambridge, Massachusetts, EUA) (2018). p. 55–81. doi: 10.1016/B978-0-12-811436-0.00003-4
Lemaitre B, Hoffmann J. The host defense of *Drosophila melanogaster*. *Annu Rev Immunol* (2007) 25:697–743. doi: 10.1146/annurev.immunol.25.022106.141615
Kitsou C, Pal U. *Ixodes* immune responses against Lyme disease pathogens. *Front Cell Infect Microbiol* (2018) 8:176. doi: 10.3389/fcimb.2018.00176
Lindsay SA, Wasserman SA. Conventional and non-conventional *Drosophila* Toll signaling. *Dev Comp Immunol* (2014) 42:16–24. doi: 10.1016/j.dci.2013.04.011
Oliva Chavez AS, Shaw DK, Munderloh UG, Pedra JH. Tick humoral responses: marching to the beat of a different drummer. *Front Microbiol* (2017) 8:223. doi: 10.3389/fmicb.2017.00223
Shaw DK, Wang X, Brown LJ, Chavez AS, Reif KE, Smith AA, et al. Infection-derived lipids elicit an immune deficiency circuit in arthropods. *Nat Commun* (2017) 8:14401. doi: 10.1038/ncomms14401
Capelli-Peixoto J, Carvalho DD, Johnson WC, Scoles GA, Fogaca AC, Daffre S, et al. The transcription factor Relish controls *Anaplasma marginale* infection in the bovine tick *Rhipicephalus microplus*. *Dev Comp Immunol* (2017) 74:32–9. doi: 10.1016/j.dci.2017.04.005
Tanji T, Yun EY, Ip YT. Heterodimers of NF-kappaB transcription factors DIF and Relish regulate antimicrobial peptide genes in *Drosophila*. *Proc Natl Acad Sci USA* (2010) 107:14715–20. doi: 10.1073/pnas.1009473107
Paradkar PN, Duchemin JB, Voysey R, Walker PJ. Dicer-2-dependent activation of *Culex* Vago occurs via the TRAF-Rel2 signaling pathway. *PloS Negl Trop Dis* (2014) 8:e2823. doi: 10.1371/journal.pntd.0002823
Paradkar PN, Trinidad L, Voysey R, Duchemin JB, Walker PJ. Secreted Vago restricts West Nile virus infection in *Culex* mosquito cells by activating the Jak-STAT pathway. *Proc Natl Acad Sci USA* (2012) 109:18915–20. doi: 10.1073/pnas.1205231109
Liu L, Dai J, Zhao YO, Narasimhan S, Yang Y, Zhang L, et al. *Ixodes scapularis* JAK-STAT pathway regulates tick antimicrobial peptides, thereby controlling the agent of human granulocytic anaplasmosis. *J Infect Dis* (2012) 206:1233–41. doi: 10.1093/infdis/jis484
Mansfield KL, Cook C, Ellis RJ, Bell-Sakyi L, Johnson N, Alberdi P, et al. Tick-borne pathogens induce differential expression of genes promoting cell survival and host resistance in *Ixodes ricinus* cells. *Parasit Vectors* (2017) 10:81. doi: 10.1186/s13071-017-2011-1
Kleino A, Silverman N. The *Drosophila* IMD pathway in the activation of the humoral immune response. *Dev Comp Immunol* (2014) 42:25–35. doi: 10.1016/j.dci.2013.05.014
Nishide Y, Kageyama D, Yokoi K, Jouraku A, Tanaka H, Futahashi R, et al. Functional crosstalk across IMD and Toll pathways: insight into the evolution of incomplete immune cascades. *Proc Biol Sci* (2019) 286:20182207. doi: 10.1098/rspb.2018.2207
Salcedo-Porras N, Guarneri A, Oliveira PL, Lowenberger C. *Rhodnius prolixus*: identification of missing components of the IMD immune signaling

pathway and functional characterization of its role in eliminating bacteria. *PloS One* (2019) 14:e0214794. doi: 10.1371/journal.pone.0214794

McClure Carroll EE, Wang X, Shaw DK, O'Neal AJ, Oliva Chavez AS, Brown LJ, et al. p47 licenses activation of the immune deficiency pathway in the tick *Ixodes scapularis*. *Proc Natl Acad Sci USA* (2019) 116:205–10. doi: 10.1073/pnas.1808905116

Silverman N, Zhou R, Erlich RL, Hunter M, Bernstein E, Schneider D, et al. Immune activation of NF-kappaB and JNK requires *Drosophila* TAK1. *J Biol Chem* (2003) 278:48928–34. doi: 10.1074/jbc.M304802200

Dostert C, Jouanguy E, Irving P, Troxler L, Galiana-Arnoux D, Hetru C, et al. The Jak-STAT signaling pathway is required but not sufficient for the antiviral response of *Drosophila*. *Nat Immunol* (2005) 6:946–53. doi: 10.1038/ni1237

Osman D, Buchon N, Chakrabarti S, Huang YT, Su WC, Poidevin M, et al. Autocrine and paracrine unpaired signaling regulate intestinal stem cell maintenance and division. *J Cell Sci* (2012) 125:5944–9. doi: 10.1242/jcs.113100

Narasimhan S, Rajeevan N, Liu L, Zhao YO, Heisig J, Pan J, et al. Gut microbiota of the tick vector *Ixodes scapularis* modulate colonization of the Lyme disease spirochete. *Cell Host Microbe* (2014) 15:58–71. doi: 10.1016/j.chom.2013.12.001

Smith AA, Navasa N, Yang X, Wilder CN, Buyuktanir O, Marques A, et al. Cross-species interferon signaling boosts microbicidal activity within the tick vector. *Cell Host Microbe* (2016) 20:91–8. doi: 10.1016/ j.chom.2016.06.001

Abraham NM, Liu L, Jutras BL, Yadav AK, Narasimhan S, Gopalakrishnan V, et al. Pathogen-mediated manipulation of arthropod microbiota to promote infection. *Proc Natl Acad Sci USA* (2017) 114:E781–E90. doi: 10.1073/pnas.1613422114

Karlikow M, Goic B, Saleh MC. RNAi and antiviral defense in *Drosophila*: setting up a systemic immune response. *Dev Comp Immunol* (2014) 42:85–92. doi: 10.1016/j.dci.2013.05.004

Blair CD. Mosquito RNAi is the major innate immune pathway controlling arbovirus infection and transmission. *Future Microbiol* (2011) 6:265–77. doi: 10.2217/fmb.11.11

Asgari S. Role of microRNAs in arbovirus/vector interactions. *Viruses* (2014) 6:3514–34. doi: 10.3390/v6093514

Schnettler E, Tykalova H, Watson M, Sharma M, Sterken MG, Obbard DJ, et al. Induction and suppression of tick cell antiviral RNAi responses by tick-borne flaviviruses. *Nucleic Acids Res* (2014) 42:9436–46. doi: 10.1093/nar/gku657

Yuan C, Wu J, Peng Y, Li Y, Shen S, Deng F, et al. Transcriptome analysis of the innate immune system of Hyalomma asiaticum. *J Invertebr Pathol* (2020) 177:107481. doi: 10.1016/j.jip.2020.107481

Weisheit S, Villar M, Tykalova H, Popara M, Loecherbach J, Watson M, et al. *Ixodes scapularis* and *Ixodes ricinus* tick cell lines respond to infection with tick-borne encephalitis virus: transcriptomic and proteomic analysis. *Parasit Vectors* (2015) 8:599. doi: 10.1186/s13071-015-1210-x

Grubaugh ND, Ruckert C, Armstrong PM, Bransfield A, Anderson JF, Ebel GD, et al. Transmission bottlenecks and RNAi collectively influence tick- borne flavivirus evolution. *Virus Evol* (2016) 2:vew033. doi: 10.1093/ve/ vew033

Hermance ME, Widen SG, Wood TG, Thangamani S. *Ixodes scapularis* salivary gland microRNAs are differentially expressed during Powassan virus transmission. *Sci Rep* (2019) 9:13110. doi: 10.1038/s41598-019- 49572-5

Artigas-Jeronimo S, Alberdi P, Villar Rayo M, Cabezas-Cruz A, Prados PJE, Mateos-Hernandez L, et al. *Anaplasma phagocytophilum* modifies tick cell microRNA expression and upregulates isc-mir-79 to facilitate infection by targeting the roundabout protein 2 pathway. *Sci Rep* (2019) 9:9073. doi: 10.1038/s41598-019-45658-2

Morazzani EM, Wiley MR, Murreddu MG, Adelman ZN, Myles KM. Production of virus-derived ping-pong-dependent piRNA-like small RNAs in the mosquito soma. *PloS Pathog* (2012) 8:e1002470. doi: 10.1371/ journal.ppat.1002470

Vodovar N, Bronkhorst AW, van Cleef KW, Miesen P, Blanc H, van Rij RP, et al. Arbovirus-derived piRNAs exhibit a ping-pong signature in mosquito cells. *PloS One* (2012) 7:e30861. doi: 10.1371/journal.pone.0030861

Hess AM, Prasad AN, Ptitsyn A, Ebel GD, Olson KE, Barbacioru C, et al. Small RNA profiling of Dengue virus-mosquito interactions implicates the PIWI RNA pathway in anti-viral defense. *BMC Microbiol* (2011) 11:45. doi: 10.1186/1471-2180-11-45

Tanji T, Hu X, Weber AN, Ip YT. Toll and IMD pathways synergistically activate an innate immune response in *Drosophila melanogaster*. *Mol Cell Biol* (2007) 27:4578–88. doi: 10.1128/MCB.01814-06

Hussain M, Walker T, O'Neill SL, Asgari S. Blood meal induced microRNA regulates development and immune associated genes in the Dengue mosquito vector, *Aedes aegypti*. *Insect Biochem Mol Biol* (2013) 43:146–52. doi: 10.1016/j.ibmb.2012.11.005

Li Y, Li S, Li R, Xu J, Jin P, Chen L, et al. Genome-wide miRNA screening reveals miR-310 family members negatively regulate the immune response in *Drosophila melanogaster* via co-targeting drosomycin. *Dev Comp Immunol* (2017) 68:34–45. doi: 10.1016/j.dci.2016.11.014

Kim LK, Choi UY, Cho HS, Lee JS, Lee WB, Kim J, et al. Down-regulation of NF-kappaB target genes by the AP-1 and STAT complex during the innate immune response in *Drosophila*. *PloS Biol* (2007) 5:e238. doi: 10.1371/journal.pbio.0050238

Bulet P, Stocklin R, Menin L. Anti-microbial peptides: from invertebrates to vertebrates. *Immunol Rev* (2004) 198:169–84. doi: 10.1111/j.0105-2896.2004.0124.x

Sonenshine DE, Hynes WL. Molecular characterization and related aspects of the innate immune response in ticks. *Front Biosci* (2008) 13:7046–63. doi: 10.2741/3209

Kopacek P, Hajdusek O, Buresova V, Daffre S. Tick innate immunity. *Adv Exp Med Biol* (2010) 708:137–62. doi: 10.1007/978-1-4419-8059-5_8

Sonenshine DE, Macaluso KR. Microbial invasion vs. tick immune regulation. *Front Cell Infect Microbiol* (2017) 7:390. doi: 10.3389/ fcimb.2017.00390

Fogaca AC, da Silva PI Jr, Miranda MT, Bianchi AG, Miranda A, Ribolla PE, et al. Antimicrobial activity of a bovine hemoglobin fragment in the tick *Boophilus microplus*. *J Biol Chem* (1999) 274:25330–4. doi: 10.1074/jbc.274.36.25330

Nakajima Y, Ogihara K, Taylor D, Yamakawa M. Antibacterial hemoglobin fragments from the midgut of the soft tick, *Ornithodoros moubata* (Acari: Argasidae). *J Med Entomol* (2003) 40:78–81. doi: 10.1603/0022-2585-40.1.78

Sonenshine DE, Hynes WL, Ceraul SM, Mitchell R, Benzine T. Host blood proteins and peptides in the midgut of the tick *Dermacentor variabilis* contribute to bacterial control. *Exp Appl Acarol* (2005) 36:207–23. doi: 10.1007/s10493-005-2564-0

Belmonte R, Cruz CE, Pires JR, Daffre S. Purification and characterization of Hb 98-114: a novel hemoglobin-derived antimicrobial peptide from the midgut of *Rhipicephalus (Boophilus) microplus*. *Peptides* (2012) 37:120–7. doi: 10.1016/j.peptides.2012.05.017

Dubin A, Mak P, Dubin G, Rzychon M, Stec-Niemczyk J, Wladyka B, et al. New generation of peptide antibiotics. *Acta Biochim Pol* (2005) 52:633–8.

Cruz CE, Fogaca AC, Nakayasu ES, Angeli CB, Belmonte R, Almeida IC, et al. Characterization of proteinases from the midgut of *Rhipicephalus (Boophilus) microplus* involved in the generation of antimicrobial peptides. *Parasit Vectors* (2010) 3:63. doi: 10.1186/1756-3305-3-63

Machado A, Sforca ML, Miranda A, Daffre S, Pertinhez TA, Spisni A, et al. Truncation of amidated fragment 33-61 of bovine alpha-hemoglobin: effects on the structure and anticandidal activity. *Biopolymers* (2007) 88:413–26. doi: 10.1002/bip.20688

Fogaca AC, Lorenzini DM, Kaku LM, Esteves E, Bulet P, Daffre S. Cysteine-rich antimicrobial peptides of the cattle tick *Boophilus microplus*: isolation, structural characterization and tissue expression profile. *Dev Comp Immunol* (2004) 28:191–200. doi: 10.1016/j.dci.2003.08.001

Lai R, Takeuchi H, Lomas LO, Jonczy J, Rigden DJ, Rees HH, et al. A new type of antimicrobial protein with multiple histidines from the hard tick, *Amblyomma hebraeum*. *FASEB J* (2004) 18:1447–9. doi: 10.1096/fj.03-1154fje

Esteves E, Fogaca AC, Maldonado R, Silva FD, Manso PP, Pelajo-Machado M, et al. Antimicrobial activity in the tick *Rhipicephalus (Boophilus) microplus* eggs: Cellular localization and temporal expression of microplusin during oogenesis and embryogenesis. *Dev Comp Immunol* (2009) 33:913–9. doi: 10.1016/j.dci.2009.02.009

Silva FD, Rezende CA, Rossi DC, Esteves E, Dyszy FH, Schreier S, et al. Structure and mode of action of microplusin, a copper II-chelating antimicrobial peptide from the cattle tick *Rhipicephalus (Boophilus) microplus*. *J Biol Chem* (2009) 284:34735–46. doi: 10.1074/jbc.M109.016410

Silva FD, Rossi DC, Martinez LR, Frases S, Fonseca FL, Campos CB, et al. Effects of microplusin, a copper-chelating antimicrobial peptide, against *Cryptococcus neoformans*. *FEMS Microbiol Lett* (2011) 324:64–72. doi: 10.1111/j.1574-6968.2011.02386.x

Martins LA, Malossi CD, Galletti M, Ribeiro JM, Fujita A, Esteves E, et al. The transcriptome of the salivary glands of *Amblyomma aureolatum* reveals the antimicrobial peptide microplusin as an important factor for the tick protection against *Rickettsia rickettsii* infection. *Front Physiol* (2019) 10:529. doi: 10.3389/fphys.2019.00529

Pelc RS, McClure JC, Sears KT, Chung A, Rahman MS, Ceraul SM. Defending the fort: a role for defensin-2 in limiting *Rickettsia montanensis* infection of *Dermacentor variabilis*. *Insect Mol Biol* (2014) 23:457–65. doi: 10.1111/imb.12094

Chou S, Daugherty MD, Peterson SB, Biboy J, Yang Y, Jutras BL, et al. Transferred interbacterial antagonism genes augment eukaryotic innate immune function. *Nature* (2015) 518:98–101. doi: 10.1038/nature13965

Hayes BM, Radkov AD, Yarza F, Flores S, Kim J, Zhao Z, et al. Ticks resist skin commensals with immune factor of bacterial origin. *Cell* (2020) 183:1562–71.e12. doi: 10.1016/j.cell.2020.10.042

Gulley MM, Zhang X, Michel K. The roles of serpins in mosquito immunology and physiology. *J Insect Physiol* (2013) 59:138–47. doi: 10.1016/j.jinsphys.2012.08.015

Armstrong PB. The contribution of proteinase inhibitors to immune defense. *Trends Immunol* (2001) 22:47–52. doi: 10.1016/s1471-4906(00)01803-2

Fogaca AC, Almeida IC, Eberlin MN, Tanaka AS, Bulet P, Daffre S. Ixodidin, a novel antimicrobial peptide from the hemocytes of the cattle tick *Boophilus microplus* with inhibitory activity against serine proteinases. *Peptides* (2006) 27:667–74. doi: 10.1016/j.peptides.2005.07.013

Bania J, Stachowiak D, Polanowski A. Primary structure and properties of the cathepsin G/chymotrypsin inhibitor from the larval hemolymph of *Apis mellifera*. *Eur J Biochem* (1999) 262:680–7. doi: 10.1046/j.1432-1327.1999.00406.x

Ceraul SM, Chung A, Sears KT, Popov VL, Beier-Sexton M, Rahman MS, et al. A Kunitz protease inhibitor from *Dermacentor variabilis*, a vector for spotted fever group rickettsiae, limits *Rickettsia montanensis* invasion. *Infect Immun* (2011) 79:321–9. doi: 10.1128/IAI.00362-10

Ceraul SM, Dreher-Lesnick SM, Mulenga A, Rahman MS, Azad AF. Functional characterization and novel rickettsiostatic effects of a Kunitz- type serine protease inhibitor from the tick *Dermacentor variabilis*. *Infect Immun* (2008) 76:5429–35. doi: 10.1128/IAI.00866-08

Ha EM, Oh CT, Bae YS, Lee WJ. A direct role for dual oxidase in *Drosophila* gut immunity. *Science* (2005) 310:847–50. doi: 10.1126/science.1117311

Molina-Cruz A, DeJong RJ, Charles B, Gupta L, Kumar S, Jaramillo- Gutierrez G, et al. Reactive oxygen species modulate *Anopheles gambiae* immunity against bacteria and *Plasmodium*. *J Biol Chem* (2008) 283:3217– 23. doi: 10.1074/jbc.M705873200

Fang FC. Antimicrobial reactive oxygen and nitrogen species: concepts and controversies. *Nat Rev Microbiol* (2004) 2:820–32. doi: 10.1038/nrmicro1004

Jones DP. Redefining oxidative stress. *Antioxid Redox Signal* (2006) 8:1865– 79. doi: 10.1089/ars.2006.8.1865

Pereira LS, Oliveira PL, Barja-Fidalgo C, Daffre S. Production of reactive oxygen species by hemocytes from the cattle tick *Boophilus microplus*. *Exp Parasitol* (2001) 99:66–72. doi: 10.1006/expr.2001.4657

Bifano TD, Ueti MW, Esteves E, Reif KE, Braz GR, Scoles GA, et al. Knockdown of the *Rhipicephalus microplus* cytochrome c oxidase subunit III gene is associated with a failure of *Anaplasma marginale* transmission. *PloS One* (2014) 9:e98614. doi: 10.1371/journal.pone.0098614

Narasimhan S, Sukumaran B, Bozdogan U, Thomas V, Liang X, DePonte K, et al. A tick antioxidant facilitates the Lyme disease agent's successful migration from the mammalian host to the arthropod vector. *Cell Host Microbe* (2007) 2:7–18. doi: 10.1016/j.chom.2007.06.001

Kumar S, Molina-Cruz A, Gupta L, Rodrigues J, Barillas-Mury C. A peroxidase/dual oxidase system modulates midgut epithelial immunity in *Anopheles gambiae*. *Science* (2010) 327:1644–8. doi: 10.1126/science.1184008

Oliveira Gde A, Lieberman J, Barillas-Mury C. Epithelial nitration by a peroxidase/NOX5 system mediates mosquito antiplasmodial immunity. *Science* (2012) 335:856–9. doi: 10.1126/science.1209678

Yang X, Smith AA, Williams MS, Pal U. A dityrosine network mediated by dual oxidase and peroxidase influences the persistence of Lyme disease pathogens within the vector. *J Biol Chem* (2014) 289:12813–22. doi: 10.1074/jbc.M113.538272

Kalil SP, Rosa RDD, Capelli-Peixoto J, Pohl PC, Oliveira PL, Fogaca AC, et al. Immune-related redox metabolism of embryonic cells of the tick *Rhipicephalus microplus* (BME26) in response to infection with *Anaplasma marginale*. *Parasit Vectors* (2017) 10:613. doi: 10.1186/s13071-017-2575-9

Hillyer JF, Christensen BM. Characterization of hemocytes from the Yellow Fever mosquito, *Aedes aegypti*. *Histochem Cell Biol* (2002) 117:431–40. doi: 10.1007/s00418-002-0408-0

Kuhn KH, Haug T. Ultrastructural, cytochemical, and immunocytochemical characterization of haemocytes of the hard tick *Ixodes ricinus* (Acari; Chelicerata). *Cell Tissue Res* (1994) 277:493–504. doi: 10.1007/BF00300222

Borovickova B, Hypsa V. Ontogeny of tick hemocytes: a comparative analysis of *Ixodes ricinus* and *Ornithodoros moubata*. *Exp Appl Acarol* (2005) 35:317–33. doi: 10.1007/s10493-004-2209-8

Inoue N, Hanada K, Tsuji N, Igarashi I, Nagasawa H, Mikami T, et al. Characterization of phagocytic hemocytes in *Ornithodoros moubata* (Acari: Ixodidae). *J Med Entomol* (2001) 38:514–9. doi: 10.1603/0022-2585-38.4.514

Fiorotti J, Menna-Barreto RFS, Golo PS, Coutinho-Rodrigues CJB,

Bitencourt ROB, Spadacci-Morena DD, et al. Ultrastructural and cytotoxic effects of *Metarhizium robertsii* infection on *Rhipicephalus microplus* hemocytes. *Front Physiol* (2019) 10:654. doi: 10.3389/fphys.2019.00654

Feitosa AP, Alves LC, Chaves MM, Veras DL, Silva EM, Alianca AS, et al. Hemocytes of *Rhipicephalus sanguineus* (Acari: Ixodidae): characterization, population abundance, and ultrastructural changes following challenge with *Leishmania infantum*. *J Med Entomol* (2015) 52:1193–202. doi: 10.1093/jme/tjv125

Buresova V, Hajdusek O, Franta Z, Loosova G, Grunclova L, Levashina EA, et al. Functional genomics of tick thioester-containing proteins reveal the ancient origin of the complement system. *J Innate Immun* (2011) 3:623–30. doi: 10.1159/000328851

Urbanova V, Sima R, Sauman I, Hajdusek O, Kopacek P. Thioester- containing proteins of the tick *Ixodes ricinus*: gene expression, response to microbial challenge and their role in phagocytosis of the yeast *Candida albicans*. *Dev Comp Immunol* (2015) 48:55–64. doi: 10.1016/ j.dci.2014.09.004

Urbanova V, Hajdusek O, Honig Mondekova H, Sima R, Kopacek P. Tick thioester-containing proteins and phagocytosis do not affect transmission of *Borrelia afzelii* from the competent vector *Ixodes ricinus*. *Front Cell Infect Microbiol* (2017) 7:73. doi: 10.3389/fcimb.2017.00073

Dunham-Ems SM, Caimano MJ, Pal U, Wolgemuth CW, Eggers CH, Balic A, et al. Live imaging reveals a biphasic mode of dissemination of *Borrelia burgdorferi* within ticks. *J Clin Invest* (2009) 119:3652–65. doi: 10.1172/JCI39401

Eggenberger LR, Lamoreaux WJ, Coons LB. Hemocytic encapsulation of implants in the tick *Dermacentor variabilis*. *Exp Appl Acarol* (1990) 9:279–87. doi: 10.1007/BF01193434

Ceraul SM, Sonenshine DE, Hynes WL. Resistance of the tick *Dermacentor variabilis* (Acari: Ixodidae) following challenge with the bacterium *Escherichia coli* (Enterobacteriales: Enterobacteriaceae). *J Med Entomol* (2002) 39:376–83. doi: 10.1603/0022-2585-39.2.376

Cerenius L, Soderhall K. The prophenoloxidase-activating system in invertebrates. *Immunol Rev* (2004) 198:116–26. doi: 10.1111/j.0105-2896.2004.00116.x

Nakhleh J, El Moussawi L, Osta MA. The melanization response in insect immunity. *Adv Insect Physiol* (2017) 52:83–109. doi: 10.1016/bs.aiip.2016.11.002

Yuan C, Xing L, Wang M, Wang X, Yin M, Wang Q, et al. Inhibition of melanization by serpin-5 and serpin-9 promotes baculovirus infection in cotton bollworm *Helicoverpa armigera*. *PloS Pathog* (2017) 13:e1006645. doi: 10.1371/journal.ppat.1006645

Zhioua E, Browning M, Johnson PW, Ginsberg HS, LeBrun RA. Pathogenicity of the entomopathogenic fungus *Metarhizium anisopliae*

(Deuteromycetes) to *Ixodes scapularis* (Acari: Ixodidae). *J Parasitol* (1997) 83:815–8.

Feitosa APS, Chaves MM, Veras DL, de Deus DMV, Portela NCJ, Araujo AR, et al. Assessing the cellular and humoral immune response in *Rhipicephalus sanguineus* sensu lato (Acari: Ixodidae) infected with *Leishmania infantum* (Nicolle, 1908). *Ticks Tick Borne Dis* (2018) 9:1421–30. doi: 10.1016/j.ttbdis.2018.06.007

Kadota K, Satoh E, Ochiai M, Inoue N, Tsuji N, Igarashi I, et al. Existence of phenol oxidase in the argasid tick *Ornithodoros moubata*. *Parasitol Res* (2002) 88:781–4. doi: 10.1007/s00436-002-0664-x

Jiravanichpaisal P, Lee BL, Soderhall K. Cell-mediated immunity in arthropods: hematopoiesis, coagulation, melanization and opsonization. *Immunobiology* (2006) 211:213–36. doi: 10.1016/j.imbio.2005.10.015

Iwanaga S, Lee BL. Recent advances in the innate immunity of invertebrate animals. *J Biochem Mol Biol* (2005) 38:128–50. doi: 10.5483/bmbrep.2005.38.2.128

Osaki T, Okino N, Tokunaga F, Iwanaga S, Kawabata S. Proline-rich cell surface antigens of horseshoe crab hemocytes are substrates for protein cross-linking with a clotting protein coagulin. *J Biol Chem* (2002) 277:40084- 90. doi: 10.1074/jbc.M206773200

Nagai T, Kawabata S. A link between blood coagulation and prophenol oxidase activation in arthropod host defense. *J Biol Chem* (2000) 275:29264- 7. doi: 10.1074/jbc.M002556200

Theopold U, Krautz R, Dushay MS. The *Drosophila* clotting system and its messages for mammals. *Dev Comp Immunol* (2014) 42:42–6. doi: 10.1016/j.dci.2013.03.014

Urbanova V, Hartmann D, Grunclova L, Sima R, Flemming T, Hajdusek O, et al. IrFC - An *Ixodes ricinus* injury-responsive molecule related to *Limulus* Factor C. *Dev Comp Immunol* (2014) 46:439–47. doi: 10.1016/j.dci.2014.05.016

Hillyer JF, Strand MR. Mosquito hemocyte-mediated immune responses. *Curr Opin Insect Sci* (2014) 3:14–21. doi: 10.1016/j.cois.2014.07.002

Kotsyfakis M, Kopacek P, Franta Z, Pedra JH, Ribeiro JM. Deep sequencing analysis of the *Ixodes ricinus* haemocytome. *PloS Negl Trop Dis* (2015) 9: e0003754. doi: 10.1371/journal.pntd.0003754

Ricklin D, Hajishengallis G, Yang K, Lambris JD. Complement: a key system for immune surveillance and homeostasis. *Nat Immunol* (2010) 11:785–97. doi: 10.1038/ni.1923

Zhu Y, Thangamani S, Ho B, Ding JL. The ancient origin of the complement system. *EMBO J* (2005) 24:382–94. doi: 10.1038/sj.emboj.7600533

Sekiguchi R, Nonaka M. Evolution of the complement system in protostomes revealed by de novo transcriptome analysis of six species of Arthropoda. *Dev Comp Immunol* (2015) 50:58–67. doi: 10.1016/j.dci.2014.12.008

Kawabata S. Immunocompetent molecules and their response network in horseshoe crabs. *Adv Exp Med Biol* (2010) 708:122–36. doi: 10.1007/978-1- 4419-8059-5_7

Gokudan S, Muta T, Tsuda R, Koori K, Kawahara T, Seki N, et al. Horseshoe crab acetyl group-recognizing lectins involved in innate immunity are structurally related to fibrinogen. *Proc Natl Acad Sci USA* (1999) 96:10086–91. doi: 10.1073/pnas.96.18.10086

Kawabata S, Tsuda R. Molecular basis of non-self recognition by the horseshoe crab tachylectins. *Biochim Biophys Acta* (2002) 1572:414–21. doi: 10.1016/s0304-4165(02)00322-7

Zhu Y, Ng PM, Wang L, Ho B, Ding JL. Diversity in lectins enables immune recognition and differentiation of wide spectrum of pathogens. *Int Immunol* (2006) 18:1671–80. doi: 10.1093/intimm/dxl101

Matsushita M. Ficolins: complement-activating lectins involved in innate immunity. *J Innate Immun* (2010) 2:24–32. doi: 10.1159/000228160

Kovar V, Kopacek P, Grubhoffer L. Isolation and characterization of Dorin M, a lectin from plasma of the soft tick *Ornithodoros moubata*. *Insect Biochem Mol Biol* (2000) 30:195–205. doi: 10.1016/s0965-1748(99)00107-1

Rego RO, Kovar V, Kopacek P, Weise C, Man P, Sauman I, et al. The tick plasma lectin, Dorin M, is a fibrinogen-related molecule. *Insect Biochem Mol Biol* (2006) 36:291–9. doi: 10.1016/j.ibmb.2006.01.008

Rego RO, Hajdusek O, Kovar V, Kopacek P, Grubhoffer L, Hypsa V. Molecular cloning and comparative analysis of fibrinogen-related proteins from the soft tick *Ornithodoros moubata* and the hard tick *Ixodes ricinus*. *Insect Biochem Mol Biol* (2005) 35:991–1004. doi: 10.1016/j.ibmb. 2005.04.001

Honig Mondekova H, Sima R, Urbanova V, Kovar V, Rego ROM, Grubhoffer L, et al. Characterization of *Ixodes ricinus* fibrinogen-related proteins (ixoderins) discloses their function in the tick innate immunity. *Front Cell Infect Microbiol* (2017) 7:509. doi: 10.3389/fcimb.2017.00509

Urbanova V, Hajdusek O, Sima R, Franta Z, Honig-Mondekova H, Grunclova L, et al. IrC2/Bf - A yeast and *Borrelia* responsive component of the complement system from the hard tick *Ixodes ricinus*. *Dev Comp Immunol* (2018) 79:86–94. doi: 10.1016/j.dci.2017.10.012

Schwarz A, von Reumont BM, Erhart J, Chagas AC, Ribeiro JM, Kotsyfakis M. De novo *Ixodes ricinus* salivary gland transcriptome analysis using two next-generation sequencing methodologies. *FASEB J* (2013) 27:4745–56. doi: 10.1096/fj.13-232140

Perner J, Kropackova S, Kopacek P, Ribeiro JMC. Sialome diversity of ticks revealed by RNAseq of single tick salivary glands. *PloS Negl Trop Dis* (2018) 12:e0006410. doi: 10.1371/journal.pntd.0006410

Blandin SA, Marois E, Levashina EA. Antimalarial responses in *Anopheles gambiae*: from a complement-like protein to a complement- like pathway. *Cell Host Microbe* (2008) 3:364–74. doi: 10.1016/j.chom. 2008.05.007

Shokal U, Eleftherianos I. Evolution and function of thioester-containing proteins and the complement system in the innate immune response. *Front Immunol* (2017) 8:759. doi: 10.3389/fimmu.2017.00759

Stroschein-Stevenson SL, Foley E, O'Farrell PH, Johnson AD. Identification of *Drosophila* gene products required for phagocytosis of *Candida albicans*. *PloS Biol* (2006) 4:e4. doi: 10.1371/journal.pbio.0040004

Simpson SD, Ramsdell JS, Watson Iii WH, Chabot CC. The draft genome and transcriptome of the atlantic horseshoe crab, *Limulus polyphemus*. *Int J Genomics* (2017) 2017:7636513. doi: 10.1155/2017/7636513

Zhou Y, Liang Y, Yan Q, Zhang L, Chen D, Ruan L, et al. The draft genome of horseshoe crab *Tachypleus tridentatus* reveals its evolutionary scenario and well-developed innate immunity. *BMC Genomics* (2020) 21:137. doi: 10.1186/s12864-020-6488-1

Saravanan T, Weise C, Sojka D, Kopacek P. Molecular cloning, structure and bait region splice variants of alpha2-macroglobulin from the soft tick *Ornithodoros moubata*. *Insect Biochem Mol Biol* (2003) 33:841–51. doi: 10.1016/s0965-1748(03)00083-3

Buresova V, Hajdusek O, Franta Z, Sojka D, Kopacek P. IrAM-An alpha2-macroglobulin from the hard tick *Ixodes ricinus*: characterization and function in phagocytosis of a potential pathogen *Chryseobacterium indologenes*. *Dev Comp Immunol* (2009) 33:489–98. doi: 10.1016/j.dci.2008.09.011

Tagawa K, Yoshihara T, Shibata T, Kitazaki K, Endo Y, Fujita T, et al. Microbe-specific C3b deposition in the horseshoe crab complement system in a C2/factor B-dependent or -independent manner. *PloS One* (2012) 7: e36783. doi: 10.1371/journal.pone.0036783

Le Saux A, Ng PM, Koh JJ, Low DH, Leong GE, Ho B, et al. The macromolecular assembly of pathogen-recognition receptors is impelled by serine proteases, via their complement control protein modules. *J Mol Biol* (2008) 377:902–13. doi: 10.1016/j.jmb.2008.01.045

Buresova V, Franta Z, Kopacek P. A comparison of *Chryseobacterium indologenes* pathogenicity to the soft tick *Ornithodoros moubata* and hard tick *Ixodes ricinus*. *J Invertebr Pathol* (2006) 93:96–104. doi: 10.1016/ j.jip.2006.05.006

Pospisilova T, Urbanova V, Hes O, Kopacek P, Hajdusek O, Sima R. Tracking of *Borrelia afzelii* transmission from infected *Ixodes ricinus* nymphs to mice. *Infect Immun* (2019) 87:e00896–18. doi: 10.1128/IAI.00896-18

Galluzzi L, Vitale I, Aaronson SA, Abrams JM, Adam D, Agostinis P, et al. Molecular mechanisms of cell death: recommendations of the Nomenclature Committee on Cell Death 2018. *Cell Death Differ* (2018) 25:486–541. doi: 10.1038/s41418-017-0012-4

Ashida H, Mimuro H, Ogawa M, Kobayashi T, Sanada T, Kim M, et al. Cell death and infection: a double-edged sword for host and pathogen survival. *J Cell Biol* (2011) 195:931–42. doi: 10.1083/jcb.201108081

Steinert S, Levashina EA. Intracellular immune responses of dipteran insects. *Immunol Rev* (2011) 240:129–40. doi: 10.1111/j.1600-065X.2010.00985.x

Cooper DM, Mitchell-Foster K. Death for survival: what do we know about innate immunity and cell death in insects? *Invertebr Surv J* (2011) 8:162–72. doi: 10.1111/j.1600-065X.2011.01040.x

Kuo CJ, Hansen M, Troemel E. Autophagy and innate immunity: insights from invertebrate model organisms. *Autophagy* (2018) 14:233–42. doi: 10.1080/15548627.2017.1389824

Moy RH, Cherry S. Antimicrobial autophagy: a conserved innate immune response in *Drosophila. J Innate Immun* (2013) 5:444–55. doi: 10.1159/000350326

Yano T, Mita S, Ohmori H, Oshima Y, Fujimoto Y, Ueda R, et al. Autophagic control of *Listeria* through intracellular innate immune recognition in *Drosophila. Nat Immunol* (2008) 9:908–16. doi: 10.1038/ni.1634

Shelly S, Lukinova N, Bambina S, Berman A, Cherry S. Autophagy is an essential component of *Drosophila* immunity against vesicular stomatitis virus. *Immunity* (2009) 30:588–98. doi: 10.1016/j.immuni.2009.02.009

Nakamoto M, Moy RH, Xu J, Bambina S, Yasunaga A, Shelly SS, et al. Virus recognition by Toll-7 activates antiviral autophagy in *Drosophila. Immunity* (2012) 36:658–67. doi: 10.1016/j.immuni.2012.03.003

Echavarria-Consuegra L, Smit JM, Reggiori F. Role of autophagy during the replication and pathogenesis of common mosquito-borne flavi- and alphaviruses. *Open Biol* (2019) 9:190009. doi: 10.1098/rsob.190009

Umemiya R, Matsuo T, Hatta T, Sakakibara S, Boldbaatar D, Fujisaki K. Autophagy-related genes from a tick, *Haemaphysalis longicornis. Autophagy* (2008) 4:79–81. doi: 10.4161/auto.5143

Kawano S, Umemiya-Shirafuji R, Boldbaatar D, Matsuoka K, Tanaka T, Fujisaki K. Cloning and characterization of the autophagy-related gene 6 from the hard tick, *Haemaphysalis longicornis. Parasitol Res* (2011) 109:1341–9. doi: 10.1007/s00436-011-2429-x

Wang XR, Kurtti TJ, Oliver JD, Munderloh UG. The identification of tick autophagy-related genes in *Ixodes scapularis* responding to amino acid starvation. *Ticks Tick Borne Dis* (2020) 11:101402. doi: 10.1016/j.ttbdis.2020.101402

Moura-Martiniano NO, Machado-Ferreira E, Gazeta GS, Soares CAG. Relative transcription of autophagy-related genes in *Amblyomma sculptum* and *Rhipicephalus microplus* ticks. *Exp Appl Acarol* (2017) 73:401–28. doi: 10.1007/s10493-017-0193-z

Elmore S. Apoptosis: a review of programmed cell death. *Toxicol Pathol* (2007) 35:495–516. doi: 10.1080/01926230701320337

Nainu F, Tanaka Y, Shiratsuchi A, Nakanishi Y. Protection of insects against viral infection by apoptosis-dependent phagocytosis. *J Immunol* (2015) 195:5696–706. doi: 10.4049/jimmunol.1500613

Ocampo CB, Caicedo PA, Jaramillo G, Ursic Bedoya R, Baron O, Serrato IM, et al. Differential expression of apoptosis related genes in selected strains of *Aedes aegypti* with different susceptibilities to Dengue virus. *PloS One* (2013) 8:e61187. doi: 10.1371/journal.pone.0061187

Vaidyanathan R, Scott TW. Apoptosis in mosquito midgut epithelia associated with *West Nile* virus infection. *Apoptosis* (2006) 11:1643–51. doi: 10.1007/s10495-006-8783-y

Alberdi P, Mansfield KL, Manzano-Roman R, Cook C, Ayllon N, Villar M, et al. Tissue-specific signatures in the transcriptional response to *Anaplasma phagocytophilum* Infection of *Ixodes scapularis* and *Ixodes ricinus* tick cell lines. *Front Cell Infect Microbiol* (2016) 6:20. doi: 10. 3389/fcimb.2016.00020

Lamkanfi M, Dixit VM. Manipulation of host cell death pathways during microbial infections. *Cell Host Microbe* (2010) 8:44–54. doi: 10.1016/j.chom.2010.06.007

Slonchak A, Hugo LE, Freney ME, Hall-Mendelin S, Amarilla AA, Torres FJ, et al. Zika virus noncoding RNA suppresses apoptosis and is required for virus transmission by mosquitoes. *Nat Commun* (2020) 11:2205. doi: 10.1038/s41467-020-16086-y

Alberdi P, Ayllon N, Cabezas-Cruz A, Bell-Sakyi L, Zweygarth E, Stuen S, et al. Infection of *Ixodes* spp. tick cells with different *Anaplasma phagocytophilum* isolates induces the inhibition of apoptotic cell death. *Ticks Tick Borne Dis* (2015) 6:758–67. doi: 10.1016/j.ttbdis.2015.07.001

Ayllon N, Villar M, Busby AT, Kocan KM, Blouin EF, Bonzon-Kulichenko E, et al. *Anaplasma phagocytophilum* inhibits apoptosis and promotes cytoskeleton rearrangement for infection of tick cells. *Infect Immun* (2013) 81:2415–25. doi: 10.1128/IAI.00194-13

Ayllon N, Villar M, Galindo RC, Kocan KM, Sima R, Lopez JA, et al. Systems biology of tissue-specific response to *Anaplasma phagocytophilum* reveals differentiated apoptosis in the tick vector *Ixodes scapularis. PloS Genet* (2015) 11:e1005120. doi: 10.1371/journal.pgen.1005120

Rikihisa Y. *Anaplasma phagocytophilum* and *Ehrlichia chaffeensis*: subversive manipulators of host cells. *Nat Rev Microbiol* (2010) 8:328–39. doi: 10.1038/nrmicro2318

Martins LA, Palmisano G, Cortez M, Kawahara R, de Freitas Balanco JM, Fujita A, et al. The intracellular bacterium *Rickettsia rickettsii* exerts an inhibitory effect on the apoptosis of tick cells. *Parasit Vectors* (2020) 13:603. doi: 10.1186/s13071-020-04477-5

Berthelet J, Dubrez L. Regulation of apoptosis by inhibitors of apoptosis (IAPs). *Cells* (2013) 2:163–87. doi: 10.3390/cells2010163

Orme M, Meier P. Inhibitor of apoptosis proteins in *Drosophila*: gatekeepers of death. *Apoptosis* (2009) 14:950–60. doi: 10.1007/s10495-009-0358-2

Gesellchen V, Kuttenkeuler D, Steckel M, Pelte N, Boutros M. An RNA interference screen identifies inhibitor of apoptosis protein 2 as a regulator of innate immune signalling in *Drosophila. EMBO Rep* (2005) 6:979–84. doi: 10.1038/sj.embor.7400530

Huh JR, Foe I, Muro I, Chen CH, Seol JH, Yoo SJ, et al. The *Drosophila* inhibitor of apoptosis (IAP) DIAP2 is dispensable for cell survival, required for the innate immune response to gram-negative bacterial infection, and can be negatively regulated by the reaper/hid/grim family of IAP-binding apoptosis inducers. *J Biol Chem* (2007) 282:2056–68. doi: 10.1074/ jbc.M608051200

Kleino A, Valanne S, Ulvila J, Kallio J, Myllymaki H, Enwald H, et al. Inhibitor of apoptosis 2 and TAK1-binding protein are components of the *Drosophila* Imd pathway. *EMBO J* (2005) 24:3423–34. doi: 10.1038/ sj.emboj.7600807

Leulier F, Lhocine N, Lemaitre B, Meier P. The *Drosophila* inhibitor of apoptosis protein DIAP2 functions in innate immunity and is essential to resist gram-negative bacterial infection. *Mol Cell Biol* (2006) 26:7821–31. doi: 10.1128/MCB.00548-06

Severo MS, Choy A, Stephens KD, Sakhon OS, Chen G, Chung DW, et al. The E3 ubiquitin ligase XIAP restricts *Anaplasma phagocytophilum* colonization of *Ixodes scapularis* ticks. *J Infect Dis* (2013) 11:1830–40. doi: 10.1093/infdis/jit380

Bonnet SI, Binetruy F, Hernandez-Jarguin AM, Duron O. The tick microbiome: why non-pathogenic microorganisms matter in tick biology and pathogen transmission. *Front Cell Infect Microbiol* (2017) 7:236. doi: 10.3389/fcimb.2017.00236

Narasimhan S, Schuijt TJ, Abraham NM, Rajeevan N, Coumou J, Graham M, et al. Modulation of the tick gut milieu by a secreted tick protein favors *Borrelia burgdorferi* colonization. *Nat Commun* (2017) 8:184. doi: 10.1038/s41467-017-00208-0

Duron O, Binetruy F, Noel V, Cremaschi J, McCoy KD, Arnathau C, et al. Evolutionary changes in symbiont community structure in ticks. *Mol Ecol* (2017) 26:2905–21. doi: 10.1111/mec.14094

Pavanelo DB, Schroder NCH, Pin Viso ND, Martins LA, Malossi CD, Galletti M, et al. Comparative analysis of the midgut microbiota of two natural tick vectors of *Rickettsia rickettsii. Dev Comp Immunol* (2020) 106:103606. doi: 10.1016/j.dci.2019.103606

Barletta A, Nascimento-Silva M, Talyuli O, Oliveira J, Pereira L, Oliveira P, et al. Microbiota activates IMD pathway and limits Sindbis infection in *Aedes aegypti. Parasit Vectors* (2017) 10:103. doi: 10.1186/s13071-017-2040-9

Xiao X, Yang L, Pang X, Zhang R, Zhu Y, Wang P, et al. A Mesh-Duox pathway regulates homeostasis in the insect gut. *Nat Microbiol* (2017) 2:17020. doi: 10.1038/nmicrobiol.2017.20

Oliveira JH, Goncalves RL, Lara FA, Dias FA, Gandara AC, Menna-Barreto RF, et al. Blood meal-derived heme decreases ROS levels in the midgut of *Aedes aegypti and* allows proliferation of intestinal microbiota. *PloS Pathog* (2011) 7:e1001320. doi: 10.1371/journal.ppat.1001320

Pang X, Xiao X, Liu Y, Zhang R, Liu J, Liu Q, et al. Mosquito C-type lectins maintain gut microbiome homeostasis. *Nat Microbiol* (2016) 1:16023. doi: 10.1038/nmicrobiol.2016.23

Caragata E, Tikhe C, Dimopoulos G. Curious entanglements: interactions between mosquitoes, their microbiota, and arboviruses. *Curr Opin Virol* (2019) 37:26–36. doi: 10.1016/j.coviro.2019.05.005

Moreno-García M, Vargas V, Ramırez-Bello I, Hernández-Martınez G, 231. Clayton KA, Gall CA, Mason KL, Scoles GA, Brayton KA. The Lanz-Mendoza H. Bacterial exposure at the larval stage induced sexual immune dimorphism and priming in adult *Aedes aegypti* mosquitoes. *PloS One* (2015) 10:e0133240. doi: 10.1371/journal.pone.0133240

Dickson L, Jiolle D, Minard G, Moltini-Conclois I, Volant S, Ghozlane A, et al. Carryover effects of larval exposure to different environmental bacteria drive adult trait variation in a mosquito vector. *Sci Adv* (2017) 3:e1700585. doi: 10.1126/sciadv.1700585

Moltini-Conclois I, Stalinski R, Tetreau G, Després L, Lambrechts L. Larval exposure to the bacterial insecticide Bti enhances Dengue virus susceptibility of adult *Aedes aegypti* mosquitoes. *Insects* (2018) 9:193. doi: 10.3390/ insects9040193

Tetreau G, Grizard S, Patil C, Tran F, Tran Van V, Stalinski R, et al. Bacterial microbiota of *Aedes aegypti* mosquito larvae is altered by intoxication with *Bacillus thuringiensis israelensis*. *Parasit Vectors* (2018) 11:121. doi: 10.1186/ s13071-018-2741-8

Zug R, Hammerstein P. Still a host of hosts for *Wolbachia*: analysis of recent data suggests that 40% of terrestrial arthropod species are infected. *PloS One* (2012) 7:e38544. doi: 10.1371/journal.pone.0038544

Caragata E, Dutra H, Moreira L. Exploiting intimate relationships: controlling mosquito-transmitted disease with *Wolbachia*. *Trends Parasitol* (2016) 32:207–18. doi: 10.1016/j.pt.2015.10.011

Bian G, Xu Y, Lu P, Xie Y, Xi Z. The endosymbiotic bacterium *Wolbachia* induces resistance to Dengue virus in *Aedes aegypti*. *PloS Pathog* (2010) 6: e1000833. doi: 10.1371/journal.ppat.1000833

Hoffmann A, Montgomery B, Popovici J, Iturbe-Ormaetxe I, Johnson P, Muzzi F, et al. Successful establishment of *Wolbachia* in *Aedes* populations to suppress Dengue transmission. *Nature* (2011) 476:454–7. doi: 10.1038/ nature10356

Walker T, Johnson PH, Moreira LA, Iturbe-Ormaetxe I, Frentiu FD, McMeniman CJ, et al. The *w*Mel *Wolbachia* strain blocks Dengue and invades caged *Aedes aegypti* populations. *Nature* (2011) 476:450–3. doi: 10.1038/nature10355

Dutra H, Dos Santos L, Caragata E, Silva J, Villela D, Maciel-de-Freitas R, et al. From lab to field: the influence of urban landscapes on the invasive potential of *Wolbachia* in Brazilian *Aedes aegypti* mosquitoes. *PloS Negl Trop Dis* (2015) 9:e0003689. doi: 10.1371/journal.pntd.0003689

Caragata E, Rocha M, Pereira T, Mansur S, Dutra H, Moreira L. Pathogen blocking in *Wolbachia*-infected *Aedes aegypti* is not affected by Zika and Dengue virus co-infection. *PloS Negl Trop Dis* (2019) 13:e0007443. doi: 10.1371/journal.pntd.0007443

Andreotti R, Perez de Leon AA, Dowd SE, Guerrero FD, Bendele KG, Scoles GA. Assessment of bacterial diversity in the cattle tick *Rhipicephalus (Boophilus) microplus* through tag-encoded pyrosequencing. *BMC Microbiol* (2011) 11:6. doi: 10.1186/1471-2180-11-6

Cerutti F, Modesto P, Rizzo F, Cravero A, Jurman I, Costa S, et al. The microbiota of hematophagous ectoparasites collected from migratory birds. *PloS One* (2018) 13:e0202270. doi: 10.1371/journal.pone.0202270

Estrada-Peña A, Cabezas-Cruz A, Obregón D. Resistance of tick gut microbiome to anti-tick vaccines, pathogen infection and antimicrobial peptides. *Pathogens* (2020) 9:309. doi: 10.3390/pathogens9040309

Ross BD, Hayes B, Radey MC, Lee X, Josek T, Bjork J, et al. *Ixodes scapularis* does not harbor a stable midgut microbiome. *ISME J* (2018) 12:2596–607. doi: 10.1038/s41396-018-0161-6

Kurokawa C, Lynn GE, Pedra JHF, Pal U, Narasimhan S, Fikrig E. Interactions between *Borrelia burgdorferi* and ticks. *Nat Rev Microbiol* (2020) 18:1–14. doi: 10.1038/s41579-020-0400-5

Guizzo MG, Neupane S, Kucera M, Perner J, Frantova H, da Silva Vaz I, et al. Poor unstable midgut microbiome of hard ticks contrasts with abundant and stable monospecific microbiome in ovaries. *Front Cell Infect Microbiol* (2020) 10:211. doi: 10.3389/fcimb.2020.00211

Guizzo MG, Parizi LF, Nunes RD, Schama R, Albano RM, Tirloni L, et al. A *Coxiella* mutualist symbiont is essential to the development of *Rhipicephalus microplus*. *Sci Rep* (2017) 7:17554. doi: 10.1038/s41598-017-17309-x

Gall CA, Reif KE, Scoles GA, Mason KL, Mousel M, Noh SM, et al. The bacterial microbiome of *Dermacentor andersoni* ticks influences pathogen susceptibility. *ISME J* (2016) 10:1846 55. doi: 10.1038/ismej.2015.266

characterization and manipulation of the bacterial microbiome of the Rocky Mountain wood tick, *Dermacentor andersoni*. *Parasit Vectors* (2015) 8:632. doi: 10.1186/s13071-015-1245-z

Labruna MB, Ogrzewalska M, Martins TF, Pinter A, Horta MC. Comparative susceptibility of larval stages of *Amblyomma aureolatum*, *Amblyomma cajennense*, and *Rhipicephalus sanguineus* to infection by *Rickettsia rickettsii*. *J Med Entomol* (2008) 45:1156–9. doi: 10.1603/0022-2585(2008) 45[1156:csolso]2.0.co;2

Martins LA, Galletti M, Ribeiro JM, Fujita A, Costa FB, Labruna MB, et al. The distinct transcriptional response of the midgut of *Amblyomma sculptum* and *Amblyomma aureolatum* ticks to *Rickettsia rickettsii* correlates to their differences in susceptibility to infection. *Front Cell Infect Microbiol* (2017) 7:129. doi: 10.3389/fcimb.2017.00129

Cooper D, Eleftherianos I. Memory and specificity in the insect immune system: current perspectives and future challenges. *Front Immunol* (2017) 8:539. doi: 10.3389/fimmu.2017.00539

6

Tick Cell Lines in Research on Tick Control

*Ahmed Al-Rofaai and Lesley Bell-Sakyi**

Department of Infection Biology, Institute of Infection and Global Health, University of Liverpool, Liverpool, United Kingdom

***Correspondence:**
Lesley Bell-Sakyi
L.Bell-Sakyi@liverpool.ac.uk

Ticks and the diseases they transmit are of huge veterinary, medical and economic importance worldwide. Control of ticks attacking livestock and companion animals is achieved primarily by application of chemical or plant-based acaricides. However, ticks can rapidly develop resistance to any new product brought onto the market, necessitating an ongoing search for novel active compounds and alternative approaches to tick control. Many aspects of tick and tick-borne pathogen research have been facilitated by the application of continuous cell lines derived from some of the most economically important tick species. These include cell lines derived from acaricide-susceptible and resistant ticks, cell sub-lines with *in vitro*-generated acaricide resistance, and genetically modified tick cells. Although not a replacement for the whole organism, tick cell lines enable studies at the cellular and molecular level and provide a more accessible, more ethical and less expensive *in vitro* alternative to *in vivo* tick feeding experiments. Here we review the role played by tick cell lines in studies on acaricide resistance, mode-of-action of acaricides, identification of potential novel control targets through better understanding of tick metabolism, and anti-tick vaccine development, that may lead to new approaches to control ticks and tick-borne diseases.

Keywords: *Rhipicephalus microplus*, *Ixodes* spp., control, tick cell line, acaricide, resistance, metabolism, anti-tick vaccine

INTRODUCTION

Ticks are obligate, haematophagous ectoparasites. Like mosquitoes, they cause problems to their hosts both from skin irritation and damage during blood feeding and by transmitting numerous pathogens including viruses, bacteria and protozoa. Consequently, ticks and tick-borne pathogens (TBPs) are of huge veterinary, medical and economic importance due to their negative impact on the health of humans and domestic animals (de la Fuente et al., 2008). Therefore, many control strategies have been devised to eliminate or avoid ticks and reduce the spread of TBPs, such as personal protection, landscape management, chemicals, vaccination, and biological control (Stafford et al., 2017). Amongst these, chemical control using a variety of acaricidal compounds is still the main strategy for controlling ticks affecting livestock and companion animals. However, many tick species develop resistance to these chemicals, which has led to attempts to find natural alternatives by studying the effects of some natural products on ticks and TBPs (Rodriguez-Vivas et al., 2018). Globally, the most economically important species, the invasive Asian cattle tick

Rhipicephalus (*Boophilus*) *microplus*, is also the most notorious for rapid development of resistance to every new acaricidal product brought onto the market (Jonsson and Hope, 2007; Abbas et al., 2014). Acaricide-resistant *R. microplus* are widespread throughout tropical and sub-tropical Asia, Latin America and Australia (Abbas et al., 2014), and are rapidly spreading in Southern, Central and West Africa (Nyangiwe et al., 2018; Silatsa et al., 2019).

Tick cell lines have an invaluable role to play in many aspects of tick and TBP research including tick biology, host-vector-pathogen relationships, genetic manipulation, genomics and proteomics (Bell-Sakyi et al., 2007). In addition, tick cell lines play a major role as essential tools in *in vitro* studies to examine and assess the impact of chemical molecules and vaccines against ticks and TBPs, as well as to investigate the mechanisms of resistance and tick metabolism which can lead to the development of novel approaches to control ticks and TBPs (Bell-Sakyi et al., 2018). While >60 continuous cell lines have now been established from 16 ixodid and three argasid tick species (Bell-Sakyi et al., 2018), studies on tick and pathogen control have predominantly centered around cell lines derived from, not surprisingly, *R. microplus*. A smaller number of studies have used cell lines derived from other tropical *Rhipicephalus* species of veterinary importance, from *Ixodes ricinus*, a European tick that feeds on a wide range of domestic and wild animal hosts as well as attacking humans, and from the medically important North American species *Ixodes scapularis* (**Table 1**).

This Mini Review focuses on the role of tick cell lines in studies on control of ticks and the few studies dealing with approaches to combined control of ticks and TBPs. While tick cell lines have been used in many studies contributing to aspects of pathogen control *per se*, these are beyond the scope of our review. Here we review selected studies to highlight how tick cell lines can contribute to tick control research, bearing in mind that results gained *in vitro* should be validated *in vivo*.

TICK CELL LINES IN STUDIES ON ACARICIDE RESISTANCE

Tick cell lines have been investigated for their potential as cheap and ethical tools to study acaricide resistance. Some studies focused on establishing drug-resistant cell lines which provide a useful tool to study and understand the mechanisms of resistance, an important step toward improving detection and prevention of tick resistance against acaricides. Tick cell lines are also a useful resource for identifying genes responsible for acaricide resistance and some published studies have focused on this aspect.

Generation and Application of Acaricide-Resistant Tick Cell Lines

Cossio-Bayugar et al. (2002b) generated three organophosphate-resistant *R. microplus* cell sub-lines by exposing the *R. microplus* BmVIII-SCC cell line (Holman, 1981), originally derived from embryos of acaricide-susceptible ticks, to gradually increasing concentrations of the organophosphate compound coumaphos (**Table 2**). They then assessed the levels of esterase, an enzyme that, when present at high levels, is responsible for causing resistance by modifying the organophosphate target site to be less sensitive. After exposure to coumaphos, there were higher levels of esterase in the resistant sub-lines compared to the original susceptible cell line. These findings, which were in line with previous *in vivo* studies (Miranda et al., 1995; Rosario-Cruz et al., 1997), validated the use of tick cell lines to study development of resistance in ticks, which could thereafter help to determine a suitable approach to formulating acaricides that would be less likely to induce resistance.

This group then used the coumaphos-resistant *R. microplus* cell sub-lines to evaluate the mechanisms that may contribute to acaricide resistance by further characterizing them compared to susceptible control cells (Cossio-Bayugar et al., 2002a). In addition to higher esterase levels, they found that the resistant cells exhibited higher levels of intracellular calcium and glutathione, decreased glutathione S-transferase activity, and reduced plasma and mitochondrial membrane potentials. Their results were consistent with the *in vivo* observations of increased esterase activity in organophosphate-resistant ticks, as well as resistance mechanisms found in other cell systems. One of the coumaphos-resistant *R. microplus* cell sub-lines played an important role in a further study (Cossio-Bayugar et al., 2005) that identified amino acid substitutions in the protein encoded by the phospholipid hydroperoxide glutathione peroxidase (PHGPx) gene in susceptible and resistant *R. microplus*, highlighting the possibility of its relationship with acaricide resistance in these tick populations.

A study conducted by Pohl et al. (2014) also focused on understanding the mechanisms of acaricide resistance in *R. microplus*. In this study, the authors established an ivermectin-resistant sub-line (BME26-IVM) of the *R. microplus* embryo-derived cell line BME26 (Kurtti et al., 1988; Esteves et al., 2008) by exposing susceptible cells to increasing concentrations of ivermectin (**Table 2**) over 46 weeks. Using the BME26-IVM sub-line, the contribution of the ATP-binding cassette (ABC) transporter mechanism was investigated by evaluating mRNA expression using quantitative RT-PCR. This study demonstrated increased levels of ABC transporter gene transcripts in the ivermectin-resistant cells compared to the original susceptible BME26 cells.

Effect of Acaricide Treatment of "Susceptible" Tick Cell Lines on Expression of Genes Associated With Resistance

Taking a different approach and using a cell line expected to be susceptible to ivermectin, Mangia et al. (2016) evaluated the expression of selected members of the ABC transporter subfamily B genes encoding P-glycoproteins (PgPs) in the *I. ricinus* embryo-derived cell line IRE/CTVM19 following treatment with ivermectin. The authors showed that ABC pump expression was not significantly modulated by ivermectin treatment, and expression of one of the subfamily genes was not detected. Interestingly, this study revealed that the IRE/CTVM19 cell line was able to tolerate a much higher concentration of ivermectin

TABLE 1 | Tick cell lines used in studies on tick control reviewed in this article.

Tick species	Distribution	Economic importance	Cell line	Geographic origin of parent ticks	Original references
Rhipicephalus microplus	Worldwide tropical and sub-tropical	Serious ectoparasitic pest of cattle; transmits anaplasmosis and babesiosis; high propensity to develop acaricide resistance	BmVIII-SCC	Mexico	Holman, 1981
			BME26	Mexico	Kurtti et al., 1988
			BME/CTVM2	Costa Rica	Bell-Sakyi, 2004
			BME/CTVM5	Colombia	Bell-Sakyi et al., 2007
			BME/CTVM6	Colombia	Bell-Sakyi, 2004
			BME/CTVM23	Mozambique	Alberdi et al., 2012
			BME/CTVM30	Mozambique	Alberdi et al., 2012
Rhipicephalus appendiculatus	East, Central and Southern Africa	Transmits East Coast fever of cattle and Nairobi sheep disease	RAN/CTVM3	Kenya	Bekker et al., 2002
			RA243	East Africa	Varma et al., 1975
Rhipicephalus evertsi	Sub-Saharan Africa	Transmits equine babesiosis, bovine anaplasmosis and causes tick toxicosis in ruminants	REN/CTVM32	South Africa	Bell-Sakyi et al., 2015
Rhipicephalus sanguineus	Worldwide tropical, sub-tropical and temperate	Transmits canine babesiosis, ehrlichioses and human rickettsioses	RSE/PILS35	France	Koh-Tan et al., 2016
			RML-RSE	United States	Yunker et al., 1981; Bell-Sakyi et al., 2015
Ixodes ricinus	Europe	Transmits borreliosis, neoehrlichiosis, anaplasmosis, babesiosis, tick-borne encephalitis, louping ill	IRE/CTVM19	United Kingdom	Bell-Sakyi et al., 2007
			IRE/CTVM20	United Kingdom	Bell-Sakyi et al., 2007
Ixodes scapularis	North America	Transmits Lyme borreliosis, human anaplasmosis and babesiosis, Powassan encephalitis	IDE8	United States	Munderloh et al., 1994
			ISE6	United States	Kurtti et al., 1996

TABLE 2 | Acaricides and pesticides used with tick cell lines in studies on tick control reviewed in this article.

Name	Chemical class	Route of application to animals	Mode of action
Amitraz	Amidines	Spot-on, spraying and dipping	Has an antagonistic effect on octopaminergic G protein-coupled receptors of the nerve cells causing paralysis and hyperexcitation in ticks
Coumaphos	Organophosphate compounds	Spraying and dipping	Acts on the nervous system as an inhibitor of transmission of nervous signals causing paralysis in the parasite
Fipronil	Phenylpyrazole compounds	Pour-on, spot-on and spraying	Inhibitor of GABA (gamma-aminobutyric acid), a key neurotransmitter in the central nervous system.
Ivermectin	Avermectins (macrocyclic lactones)	Pour-on, orally and by injection	Acts as inhibitor of GABA causing neuromuscular blockage, also opens chloride ion channels in membranes of the nervous system and further depresses neuronal function.
Paraquat	Dipyridylium (viologen)	Not applied to animals	A highly toxic herbicide known to induce oxidative stress in cells because of its ability to induce generation of superoxide ions
Permethrin	Synthetic pyrethroids	Pour-on, spot-on, spraying and dipping	Acts on the membrane of nerve cells blocking the closure of the ion gates of the sodium channel during re-polarization, and thereby disrupts transmission of nervous impulses.

(30 μg/ml) than the *R. microplus*-derived line BME26 that did not survive after exposure to 12.5 μg/ml ivermectin (Pohl et al., 2014). This could have been due to biological differences between the two tick species from which the cell lines were derived, differences in the phenotypic composition of the cell lines and/or in the culture conditions used. This should be considered when conducting such *in vitro* experiments using tick cell lines.

In a further study, Mangia et al. (2018) treated IRE/CTVM19 cultures with different concentrations of the acaricides permethrin, amitraz and fipronil (**Table 2**). They assessed cell viability, morphology, metabolic activity and expression of ABC genes at day 10 post-treatment. In general, the results showed that fipronil had the greatest significant negative effects on cell viability and metabolic activity, followed by permethrin, while amitraz only caused a significant decrease in these parameters at the highest concentration tested. The negative effects of fipronil and permethrin were confirmed by their effects on ABC gene expression with upregulation of ABCB6, ABCB8, and ABCB10, while amitraz had little or no effect on expression of any of the ABC genes tested.

Exploiting Tick Cell Lines Derived From Susceptible and Resistant Ticks to Identify Genes Involved in Acaricide Resistance

For some of the currently available *R. microplus* cell lines, the acaricide resistance status of the parent ticks from which the cultures were derived is known. As already mentioned, the parent BmVIII-SCC and BME26 cells used by, respectively, Cossio-Bayugar et al. (2002b) and Pohl et al. (2014) to derive acaricide-resistant sub-lines *in vitro* were originally susceptible to the compounds used, implying that the parent ticks of both lines, originally from Mexico, were also acaricide-susceptible. Two additional *R. microplus* cell lines, BME/CTVM2 (Bell-Sakyi, 2004) and BME/CTVM4 (Bell-Sakyi et al., 2007), were derived from known acaricide-susceptible ticks from Costa Rica, while two other cell lines, BME/CTVM5 (Bell-Sakyi et al., 2007) and BME/CTVM6 (Bell-Sakyi, 2004) were derived from Colombian ticks known to be resistant to organophosphates, organochlorines and amitraz (Koh-Tan et al., 2016). While these cells whose natural resistance status derives from their parent ticks offer a potentially very interesting complement to the *in vitro*-derived resistant *R. microplus* cell lines of Cossio-Bayugar et al. (2002b) and Pohl et al. (2014), to date they have only been exploited in a single study. Koh-Tan et al. (2016) investigated the expression of the β-adrenergic octopamine receptor (βAOR) gene, associated with amitraz resistance, and the ATP-binding cassette B10 (ABCB10) gene, associated with macrocyclic lactone resistance, in tick cell lines derived from *R. microplus*, including BmVIII-SCC, BME/CTVM2, BME/CTVM5 and BME/CTVM6, *Rhipicephalus appendiculatus*, *Rhipicephalus sanguineus*, and *Rhipicephalus evertsi* (**Table 1**). Expression of the βAOR gene was detected in all the *Rhipicephalus* spp. cell lines, but in BME/CTVM6, derived from amitraz-resistant ticks, a novel larger amplicon was detected. This was found to encode a 12-amino acid insertion identified as a duplication of the immediately upstream sequence; the insertion was also present in genomic DNA from BME/CTVM5 cells, similarly derived from amitraz-resistant ticks, but transcription of the novel amplicon was not detectable. Expression of the ABC10 gene was approximately seven-fold higher in BME/CTVM6 cells compared to all other cell lines examined including BME/CTVM5. These findings suggest that BME/CTVM6 cells in particular could be a useful model system for studying resistance to multiple acaricide groups in *R. microplus*; further experiments are needed to determine whether additional genes are mutated in this cell line.

TICK CELL LINES ELUCIDATE NOVEL ASPECTS OF TICK CELL METABOLISM TO IDENTIFY POTENTIAL CONTROL TARGETS

Tick cell lines have also played a valuable role in the study of tick cell metabolism which can help in developing novel control methods. De Abreu et al. (2013) investigated the role of protein kinase B (AKT) and glycogen synthase kinase 3 (GSK3) in glycogen metabolism and cell viability using the *R. microplus* cell line BME26, and the results revealed an antagonistic role for AKT and GSK3. A reduction in AKT caused a decrease in glycogen content, cell viability and altered cell membrane permeability, whereas the inhibition of GSK3 promoted an increase in glycogen content.

To better understand energy metabolism during embryonic development in ticks, Da Silva et al. (2015) used the BME26 cell line to evaluate several genes involved in gluconeogenesis, glycolysis and glycogen metabolism, the major pathways for carbohydrate catabolism and anabolism. Their results showed that several genes displayed mutual regulation in response to glucose treatment, and the transcription of gluconeogenic genes in tick cells is controlled by GSK3.

The BME26 cell line also played an essential and effective role in the first report on characterization of a cell cycle protein in arachnids, and the reversal of its functions with an inhibitor (Gomes et al., 2013). The BME26 cell line was used in an *in vitro* inhibition assay to determine the inhibitory effects of roscovitine, a purine derivative, on tick cyclin-dependent kinases (CDKs), which are essential for cell cycle progression, and the results suggested that CDKs may present an alternative strategy for designing a novel acaricide that targets both oogenesis and embryogenesis processes.

The *I. scapularis* embryo-derived tick cell line ISE6 (Kurtti et al., 1996) is the one of the most widely used tick cell lines due to its susceptibility to a wide range of TBPs (Oliver et al., 2015). ISE6 cells were used by Cabezas-Cruz et al. (2017) to study possible control of infection with the obligate intracellular bacterium *Anaplasma phagocytophilum*, causative agent of disease in humans, ruminants, horses and dogs, by increasing the synthesis of phosphoenolpyruvate from tyrosine. Ferritins (FER) are iron-storage proteins that act to store excess iron available in the cellular iron pool by the binding and oxidation of the ferrous ion ($Fe2+$) and the formation of ferric ion ($Fe3+$) in the FER core cavity (Galay et al., 2015). Hernandez et al. (2018) were able to induce intracellular ferritin (FER1) protein expression by exposing ISE6 cells to various concentrations of ferrous sulfate. They showed that silencing of FER1 expression by RNA interference led to a decrease in ISE6 cell proliferation and an increase in mortality, concluding that ISE6 cells could be a good tool to further understanding of the mechanism of FER1 action. Thereafter, Hernandez et al. (2019) characterized the activity of an iron-inducible tick promoter derived from the tick *Haemaphysalis longicornis*, previously identified by Kusakisako et al. (2018b), in ISE6 cells, which could be a valuable tool in the development of a gene-manipulation system to control ticks and TBPs. Kusakisako et al. (2018a) established methods to visualize H_2O_2 in ISE6 cells using an intracellular H_2O_2 probe and observed that paraquat, known to induce oxidative stress in mammalian cells (**Table 2**), was also effective in this respect in ISE6 tick cells. Iron derived from host blood may react with oxygen in the tick's body and lead to high levels of H_2O_2, causing oxidative stress such as DNA strand breaks, lipid peroxidation and degradation of other molecules (Kusakisako et al., 2018a; Hernandez et al., 2019).

GENETIC MANIPULATION OF TICK CELL LINES

The development of new strategies for control of ticks could be greatly enhanced by exploring genetic manipulation of ticks and tick cell lines. Demonstrating proof of concept, Kurtti et al. (2006) first reported stable transfection of the *I. scapularis* cell line ISE6 with a gene encoding a fluorescent protein using the Sleeping Beauty transposon system. In a different approach, Cossio-Bayugar and Miranda-Miranda (2007) reported retroviral transfection of primary *R. microplus* cell cultures with green fluorescent protein; fluorescence was detectable for up to 2 weeks following retroviral transfection. Using yet another approach, Machado-Ferreira et al. (2015) achieved the expression of transgenes in *R. microplus* ticks and the cell line BME/CTVM2 using *Agrobacterium tumefaciens* T-DNA constructs; evidence of transcription and protein synthesis were detectable for 2–3 weeks by fluorescence microscopy, western blot analyses and RT-PCR. These studies demonstrate that genetic manipulation approaches used with other animal cell systems can equally be applied to tick cell lines, and raise the possibility of modifying ticks to render them incapable of developing acaricide resistance.

TICK CELL LINES CONTRIBUTE TO ANTI-TICK VACCINE DEVELOPMENT

Vaccination with recombinant tick antigens represents a promising tick control strategy. Vaccines containing recombinant tick antigens demonstrated advantages including reduction in acaricide application, cost-effectiveness and reducing the prevalence of tick-borne diseases through reducing exposure of cattle to infected ticks. However, the efficacies of these vaccines vary considerably between tick species and geographic location (de la Fuente et al., 2007). Tick cell lines have played a central role in identifying tick protective antigens to produce a variety of vaccines that contribute to the prevention and control of tick infestations and TBP infections. For example, three embryo-derived tick cell lines, *R. microplus* BME/CTVM2 and *I. scapularis* IDE8 (Munderloh et al., 1994) and ISE6, were used in a study conducted by Antunes et al. (2014) to identify tick proteins involved in tick-pathogen interactions. The aim was to identify candidate protective antigens that could be used as vaccines for the control of cattle infestations with *R. microplus* ticks and infection with the TBPs *Anaplasma marginale* and *Babesia bigemina* transmitted by *R. microplus*. As an important part of the experiment, antibodies produced against the *R. microplus* protein subolesin were tested using immunofluorescence and showed positive reactions in the three cell lines, but no effect was observed on pathogen DNA levels. In contrast, using the *I. scapularis* cell line ISE6 and the *I. ricinus* cell line IRE/CTVM20 (Bell-Sakyi et al., 2007), Contreras et al. (2017) determined that two candidate tick-protective antigens – *I. scapularis* lipocalin (ISCW005600) and lectin pathway inhibitor (AAY66632), and their *I. ricinus* homologs – constitute candidate protective antigens for the control of tick infestations as well as *A. phagocytophilum* infection. They showed that anti ISCW005600 and AAY66632 IgG significantly increased the percentage of apoptotic tick cells and decreased pathogen infection, which could help in the development of effective anti-tick and anti-pathogen vaccines.

CONCLUSION

Ticks and TBPs have huge negative impacts on global livestock and public health and national economies. Scientific research has focused on creating and developing a variety of strategies to prevent and control ticks and TBPs. Tick cell lines represent essential tools in this area of research: *in vitro*-generated acaricide-resistant cell lines, cell lines derived from acaricide-resistant and susceptible ticks, genetically modified cell lines and cell lines supporting growth of intracellular TBPs all have a role to play. Experimental parameters can be easily controlled, effects at the cellular and molecular level can be determined, and cell lines reduce, while not ultimately replacing, the need for expensive *in vivo* studies involving maintenance of tick colonies and feeding on laboratory animals. As the numbers of cell lines derived from economically important tick species increase, so do the opportunities for exploiting them in a wide range of studies. For example, the potential for developing high-throughput preliminary screens of novel, potentially acaricidal compounds using cell lines from multiple tick species remains unexplored; such screens could greatly increase the number of active compounds identified for further testing at relatively low cost, and could be applied both to compound libraries held by pharmaceutical companies and to natural plant products. It is anticipated that gene editing of tick cell lines by technologies such as CRISPR will add another facet to the control portfolio. The Tick Cell Biobank (Bell-Sakyi et al., 2018), which houses all the cell lines mentioned in this review as well as cell lines derived from many other species of veterinary and medical concern, will continue to underpin research on tick and TBP control.

AUTHOR CONTRIBUTIONS

AA-R drafted the manuscript, LB-S edited the draft and both authors produced and agreed the final version.

FUNDING

AA-R is supported by the Council for At-Risk Academics (CARA) and the University of Liverpool. LB-S is supported by the United Kingdom Biotechnology and Biological Sciences Research Council grant number BB/P024270/1.

ACKNOWLEDGMENTS

We would like to thank staff of the Council for At-Risk Academics (CARA) and Dr. Benjamin Makepeace for their instrumental roles in bringing AA-R to the University of Liverpool.

REFERENCES

Abbas, R. Z., Zaman, M. A., Colwell, D. D., Gilleard, J., and Iqbal, Z. (2014). Acaricide resistance in cattle ticks and approaches to its management: the state of play. *Vet. Parasitol.* 203, 6–20. doi: 10.1016/j.vetpar.2014.03.006

Alberdi, M. P., Dalby, M. J., Rodriguez-Andres, J., Fazakerley, J. K., Kohl, A., and Bell-Sakyi, L. (2012). Detection and identification of putative bacterial endosymbionts and endogenous viruses in tick cell lines. *Ticks Tick Borne Dis.* 3, 137–146. doi: 10.1016/j.ttbdis.2012.05.002

Antunes, S., Merino, O., Mosqueda, J., Moreno-Cid, J. A., Bell-Sakyi, L., Fragkoudis, R., et al. (2014). Tick capillary feeding for the study of proteins involved in tick-pathogen interactions as potential antigens for the control of tick infestation and pathogen infection. *Parasit. Vectors* 7:42. doi: 10.1186/1756-3305-7-42

Bekker, C. P. J., Bell-Sakyi, L., Paxton, E. A., Martinez, D., Bensaid, A., and Jongejan, F. (2002). Transcriptional analysis of the major antigenic protein 1 multigene family of *Cowdria ruminantium*. *Gene* 285, 193–201. doi: 10.1016/s0378-1119(02)00408-0

Bell-Sakyi, L. (2004). *Ehrlichia ruminantium* grows in cell lines from four ixodid tick genera. *J. Comp. Pathol.* 130, 285–293. doi: 10.1016/j.jcpa.2003.12.002

Bell-Sakyi, L., Darby, A., Baylis, M., and Makepeace, B. L. (2018). The tick cell biobank: a global resource for *in vitro* research on ticks, other arthropods and the pathogens they transmit. *Ticks Tick Borne Dis.* 9, 1364–1371. doi: 10.1016/j.ttbdis.2018.05.015

Bell-Sakyi, L., Palomar, A., Bradford, E. L., and Shkap, V. (2015). Propagation of the Israeli vaccine strain of *Anaplasma centrale* in tick cell lines. *Vet. Microbiol.* 179, 270–276. doi: 10.1016/j.vetmic.2015.07.008

Bell-Sakyi, L., Zweygarth, E., Blouin, E. F., Gould, E. A., and Jongejan, F. (2007). Tick cell lines: tools for tick and tick-borne disease research. *Trends Parasitol.* 23, 450–457. doi: 10.1016/j.pt.2007.07.009

Cabezas-Cruz, A., Espinosa, P. J., Obregon, D. A., Alberdi, P., and de la Fuente, J. (2017). *Ixodes scapularis* tick cells control *Anaplasma phagocytophilum* infection by increasing the synthesis of phosphoenolpyruvate from tyrosine. *Front. Cell. Infect. Microbiol.* 7:375. doi: 10.3389/fcimb.2017.00375

Contreras, M., Alberdi, P., Fernandez de Mera, I. G., Krull, C., Nijhof, A., Villar, M., et al. (2017). Vaccinomics approach to the identification of candidate protective antigens for the control of tick vector infestations and *Anaplasma phagocytophilum* infection. *Front. Cell. Infect. Microbiol.* 7:360. doi: 10.3389/fcimb.2017.00360

Cossio-Bayugar, R., Barhoumi, R., Burghardt, R. C., Wagner, G. G., and Holman, P. J. (2002a). Basal cellular alterations of esterase, glutathione, glutathione S-transferase, intracellular calcium, and membrane potentials in coumaphos-resistant *Boophilus microplus* (Acari: Ixodidae) cell lines. *Pesticide Biochem. Physiol.* 72, 1–9. doi: 10.1006/pest.2001.2578

Cossio-Bayugar, R., Miranda, E., and Holman, P. J. (2005). Molecular cloning of a phospholipid-hydroperoxide glutathione peroxidase gene from the tick *Boophilus microplus* (Acari: Ixodidae). *Insect Biochem. Molec. Biol.* 35, 1378–1387. doi: 10.1016/j.ibmb.2005.08.008

Cossio-Bayugar, R., and Miranda-Miranda, E. (2007). Heterologus gene expression in a cattle tick *Rhipicephalus microplus* embryonic cell culture. *J. Anim. Vet. Adv.* 6, 1214–1218.

Cossio-Bayugar, R., Wagner, G. G., and Holman, P. J. (2002b). *In vitro* generation of organophosphate resistant *Boophilus microplus* (Acari: Ixodidae) cell lines. *J. Med. Entomol.* 39, 278–284. doi: 10.1603/0022-2585-39.2.278

Da Silva, R. M., Noce, B. D., Waltero, C. F., Costa, E. P., de Abreu, L. A., Githaka, N. W., et al. (2015). Non-classical gluconeogenesis-dependent glucose metabolism in *Rhipicephalus microplus* embryonic cell line BME26. *Int. J. Mol. Sci.* 16, 1821–1839. doi: 10.3390/ijms16011821

De Abreu, L. A., Calixto, C., Waltero, C. F., Della Noce, B. P., Githaka, N. W., Seixas, A., et al. (2013). The conserved role of the AKT/GSK3 axis in cell survival and glycogen metabolism in *Rhipicephalus Boophilus microplus* embryo tick cell line BME26. *Biochim. Biophys. Acta* 1830, 2574–2582. doi: 10.1016/j.bbagen.2012.12.016

de la Fuente, J., Almazán, C., Canales, M., Pérez de la Lastra, J. M., Kocan, K. M., and Willadsen, P. (2007). A ten-year review of commercial vaccine performance for control of tick infestations on cattle. *Anim. Health Res. Rev.* 8, 23–28. doi: 10.1017/s1466252307001193

de la Fuente, J., Estrada-Pena, A., Venzal, J. M., Kocan, K. M., and Sonenshine, D. E. (2008). Overview: ticks as vectors of pathogens that cause disease in humans and animals. *Front. Biosci.* 13:6938–6946. doi: 10.2741/3200

Esteves, E., Lara, F. A., Lorenzini, D. M., Costa, G. H. N., Fukuzawa, A. H., Pressinotti, L. N., et al. (2008). Cellular and molecular characterization of an embryonic cell line (BME26) from the tick *Rhipicephalus (Boophilus) microplus*. *Insect Biochem. Mol. Biol.* 38, 568–580. doi: 10.1016/j.ibmb.2008.01.006

Galay, R. L., Umemiya-Shirafuji, R., Mochizuki, M., Fujisaki, K., and Tanaka, T. (2015). Iron metabolism in hard ticks (Acari: Ixodidae): the antidote to their toxic diet. *Parasitol. Int.* 64, 182–189. doi: 10.1016/j.parint.2014.12.005

Gomes, H., Romeiro, N. C., Braz, G. R. C., de Oliveira, E. A. G., Rodrigues, C., da Fonseca, R. N., et al. (2013). Identification and structural-functional analysis of cyclin-dependent kinases of the cattle tick *Rhipicephalus (Boophilus) microplus*. *PLoS One* 8:e76128. doi: 10.1371/journal.pone.0076128

Hernandez, E. P., Kusakisako, K., Hatta, T., and Tanaka, T. (2019). Characterization of an iron-inducible *Haemaphysalis longicornis* tick-derived promoter in an *Ixodes scapularis*-derived tick cell line (ISE6). *Parasit. Vectors* 12:321. doi: 10.1186/s13071-019-3574-9

Hernandez, E. P., Kusakisako, K., Talactac, M. R., Galay, R. L., Yoshii, K., and Tanaka, T. (2018). Induction of intracellular ferritin expression in embryo-derived *Ixodes scapularis* cell line (ISE6). *Sci. Rep.* 8:16566. doi: 10.1038/s41598-018-34860-3

Holman, P. J. (1981). Partial characterization of a unique female diploid cell strain from the tick *Boophilus microplus* (Acari: Ixodidae). *J. Med. Entomol.* 18, 84–88. doi: 10.1093/jmedent/18.1.84

Jonsson, N. N., and Hope, M. (2007). Progress in the epidemiology and diagnosis of amitraz resistance in the cattle tick *Boophilus microplus*. *Vet. Parasitol.* 146, 193–198. doi: 10.1016/j.vetpar.2007.03.006

Koh-Tan, H. H. C., Strachan, E., Cooper, K., Bell-Sakyi, L., and Jonsson, N. N. (2016). Identification of a novel β-adrenergic octopamine receptor-like gene (βAOR-like) and increased ATP-binding cassette B10 (ABCB10) expression in a *Rhipicephalus microplus* cell line derived from acaricide-resistant ticks. *Parasit. Vectors* 9:425.

Kurtti, T. J., Felsheim, R. F., Mattila, J. T., Baldridge, G. D., Burkhardt, N. Y., and Munderloh, U. G. (2006). Stable transformation of a tick (*Ixodes scapularis*) cell line with the *Sleeping Beauty* transposon system. *Soc. Vitro Biol. J.* 42:32.

Kurtti, T. J., Munderloh, U. G., and Ahlstrand, G. G. (1988). Tick tissue and cell culture in vector research. *Adv. Dis. Vector Res.* 5, 87–109.

Kurtti, T. J., Munderloh, U. G., Andreadis, T. G., Magnarelli, L. A., and Mather, T. N. (1996). Tick cell culture isolation of an intracellular prokaryote from the tick *Ixodes scapularis*. *J. Invert. Pathol.* 67, 318–321. doi: 10.1006/jipa.1996.0050

Kusakisako, K., Hernandez, E. P., Talactac, M. R., Yoshii, K., Umemiya-Shirafuji, R., Fujisaki, K., et al. (2018a). Peroxiredoxins are important for the regulation of hydrogen peroxide concentrations in ticks and tick cell line. *Ticks Tick Borne Dis.* 9, 872–881. doi: 10.1016/j.ttbdis.2018.03.016

Kusakisako, K., Ido, A., Masatan, T., Morokuma, H., Hernandez, E. P., Talactac, M. R., et al. (2018b). Transcriptional activities of two newly identified *Haemaphysalis longicornis* tick-derived promoter regions in the *Ixodes scapularis* tick cell line (ISE6). *Insect Mol. Biol.* 27, 590–602. doi: 10.1111/imb.12497

Machado-Ferreira, E., Balsemão-Pires, E., Dietrich, G., Hojgaard, A., Vizzoni, V. F., Scoles, G., et al. (2015). Transgene expression in tick cells using *Agrobacterium tumefaciens*. *Exp. Appl. Acarol.* 67, 269–287. doi: 10.1007/s10493-015-9949-5

Mangia, C., Vismarra, A., Genchi, M., Epis, S., Bandi, C., Grandi, G., et al. (2018). Exposure to amitraz, fipronil and permethrin affects cell viability and ABC transporter gene expression in an *Ixodes ricinus* cell line. *Parasit. Vectors* 11:437. doi: 10.1186/s13071-018-3020-4

Mangia, C., Vismarra, A., Kramer, L., Bell-Sakyi, L., Porretta, D., Otranto, M., et al. (2016). Evaluation of the *in vitro* expression of ATP binding-cassette (ABC) proteins in an *Ixodes ricinus* cell line exposed to ivermectin. *Parasit. Vectors* 9:215. doi: 10.1186/s13071-016-1497-2

Miranda, E., Cossio-Bayugar, R., Tellez-Alanis, M. R., Garcia-Vazquez, Z., Rosario-Cruz, R., and Ortiz-Estrada, M. (1995). An enzymatic marker for ixodicide resistance detection in the cattle tick *Boophilus microplus*. *Adv. Agric. Res.* 4, 1–8.

Munderloh, U. G., Liu, Y., Wang, M., Chen, C., and Kurtti, T. J. (1994). Establishment, maintenance and description of cell lines from the tick *Ixodes scapularis*. *J. Parasitol.* 80, 533–543.

Nyangiwe, N., Yawa, M., and Muchenje, V. (2018). Driving forces for changes in geographic range of cattle ticks (Acari: Ixodidae) in Africa: a review. *South Afr. J. Anim. Sci.* 48, 829–841.

Oliver, J. D., Chavez, A. S., Felsheim, R. F., Kurtti, T. J., and Munderloh, U. G. (2015). An *Ixodes scapularis* cell line with a predominantly neuron-like phenotype. *Exp. Appl. Acarol.* 66, 427–442. doi: 10.1007/s10493-015-9908-1

Pohl, P. C., Carvalho, D. D., Daffre, S., da Silva Vaz, I., and Masuda, A. (2014). *In vitro* establishment of ivermectin-resistant *Rhipicephalus microplus* cell line and the contribution of ABC transporters on the resistance mechanism. *Vet. Parasitol.* 204, 316–322. doi: 10.1016/j.vetpar.2014.05.042

Rodriguez-Vivas, R. I., Jonsson, N. N., and Bhushan, C. (2018). Strategies for the control of *Rhipicephalus microplus* ticks in a world of conventional acaricide and macrocyclic lactone resistance. *Parasitol. Res.* 117, 3–29. doi: 10.1007/s00436-017-5677-5676

Rosario-Cruz, R., Miranda-Miranda, E., Garcia-Vazquez, Z., and Ortiz-Estrada, M. (1997). Detection of esterase activity in susceptible and organophosphate resistant strains of the cattle tick *Boophilus microplus*. *Bull. Entomol. Res.* 87, 197–202. doi: 10.1017/s0007485300027358

Silatsa, B. A., Simo, G., Githaka, N., Mwaura, S., Kamga, R. M., Oumarou, F., et al. (2019). A comprehensive survey of the prevalence and spatial distribution of ticks infesting cattle in different agro-ecological zones of Cameroon. *Parasit. Vectors* 12:489. doi: 10.1186/s13071-019-3738-7

Stafford, K. C., Williams, S. C., and Molaei, G. (2017). Integrated pest management in controlling ticks and tick-associated diseases. *J. Integr. Pest Manag.* 8:28. doi: 10.1093/jipm/pmx018

Varma, M. G. R., Pudney, M., and Leake, C. J. (1975). The establishment of three cell lines from the tick *Rhipicephalus appendiculatus* (Acari: Ixodidae) and their infection with some arboviruses. *J. Med. Entomol.* 11, 698–706. doi: 10.1093/jmedent/11.6.698

Yunker, C. E., Cory, J., and Meibos, H. (1981). Continuous cell lines from embryonic tissues of ticks (Acari: Ixodidae). *In Vitro* 17, 139–142. doi: 10.1007/bf02618071

7

Functional Evolution of Subolesin/Akirin

Sara Artigas-Jerónimo[1†], Margarita Villar[1†], Alejandro Cabezas-Cruz[2], James J. Valdés[3,4,5], Agustín Estrada-Peña[6], Pilar Alberdi[1] and José de la Fuente[1,7]*

[1] SaBio, Instituto de Investigación en Recursos Cinegéticos (IREC), CSIC, Universidad de Castilla-La Mancha (UCLM), Junta de Comunidades de Castilla – La Mancha (JCCM), Ciudad Real, Spain, [2] UMR BIPAR, INRA, ANSES, Ecole Nationale Vétérinaire d'Alfort, Université Paris-Est, Paris, France, [3] Faculty of Science, University of South Bohemia, České Budějovice, Czechia, [4] Institute of Parasitology, Biology Centre, Czech Academy of Sciences, České Budějovice, Czechia, [5] Department of Virology, Veterinary Research Institute, Brno, Czechia, [6] Facultad de Veterinaria, Universidad de Zaragoza, Zaragoza, Spain, [7] Department of Veterinary Pathobiology, Center for Veterinary Health Sciences, Oklahoma State University, Stillwater, OK, United States

***Correspondence:**
José de la Fuente
jose_delafuente@yahoo.com

†These authors have contributed equally to this work

The Subolesin/Akirin constitutes a good model for the study of functional evolution because these proteins have been conserved throughout the metazoan and play a role in the regulation of different biological processes. Here, we investigated the evolutionary history of Subolesin/Akirin with recent results on their structure, protein-protein interactions and function in different species to provide insights into the functional evolution of these regulatory proteins, and their potential as vaccine antigens for the control of ectoparasite infestations and pathogen infection. The results suggest that Subolesin/Akirin evolved conserving not only its sequence and structure, but also its function and role in cell interactome and regulome in response to pathogen infection and other biological processes. This functional conservation provides a platform for further characterization of the function of these regulatory proteins, and how their evolution can meet species-specific demands. Furthermore, the conserved functional evolution of Subolesin/Akirin correlates with the protective capacity shown by these proteins in vaccine formulations for the control of different arthropod and pathogen species. These results encourage further research to characterize the structure and function of these proteins, and to develop new vaccine formulations by combining Subolesin/Akirin with interacting proteins for the control of multiple ectoparasite infestations and pathogen infection.

Keywords: immune response, vaccine, interactome, regulome, phylogeny, tick, *Anaplasma phagocytophilum*

INTRODUCTION

Akirin, from the Japanese "akiraka ni suru" meaning "making things clear," was first identified by Goto et al. (2008) as a key component of the immune deficiency (IMD) and Tumor necrosis factor (TNF)/Toll-like receptor (TLR)-nuclear factor-kappa B (NF-kB) (TNF/TLR) signaling pathways in *Drosophila melanogaster* and *Mus musculus*, respectively. However, previous reports identified *akirin* as a gene involved in developmental processes in flies (Peña-Rangel et al., 2002; DasGupta et al., 2005). Subolesin, from the Latin "suboles" meaning "progeny," was first reported in 2003 with its discovery as the candidate protective antigen 4D8 by expression library immunization in *Ixodes scapularis* (Almazán et al., 2003).

Gene orthology is a key concept in functional evolution (Koonin, 2005). Orthologs genes, defined as derived from a single ancestral gene that diverged during speciation, usually perform equivalent or identical functions, while paralogs that originated after gene duplication are considered to have more divergent functions (Koonin, 2005; Adipietro et al., 2012). Studies at genome level have identified many orthologs genes between divergent species, but the functional equivalency of the proteins encoded by these genes has not been fully characterized (Koonin, 2005).

Subolesin/Akirin are encoded by orthologs evolutionarily conserved throughout the metazoan that play a role in the regulation of different biological processes including immune response (de la Fuente et al., 2006a; Beutler and Moresco, 2008; Goto et al., 2008; Galindo et al., 2009; Macqueen, 2009; Macqueen and Johnston, 2009; Wan and Lenardo, 2010). Two *akirin* paralogs encoding Akirin1 and Akirin2 have been identified in vertebrates, but the functional homolog for invertebrate Subolesin/Akirin appears to be Akirin2 ortholog (Beutler and Moresco, 2008; Goto et al., 2008; Galindo et al., 2009; Macqueen and Johnston, 2009).

Understanding the function of the cell interactome (protein-protein physical and functional interactions) and regulome (transcription factors-target genes interactions) in response to infection is critical toward a better understanding of host-pathogen interactions and the identification of potential targets for new interventions for the prevention and control of tick infestations and tick-borne diseases (Rioualen et al., 2017; de la Fuente, 2018). Subolesin/Akirin are involved in both cell interactome and regulome, and constitute a good model for the study of the functional evolution of these processes in response to infection. In this review, we integrated the evolutionary history of Subolesin/Akirin with recent results on their structure and function in different species to provide insights into the functional evolution of these regulatory proteins, and their potential as vaccine antigens for the control of ectoparasite infestations and pathogen infection.

EVOLUTION OF SUBOLESIN/AKIRIN

The phylogenetic analysis of *subolesin/akirin* coding sequences using an updated sequence database (**Figure 1A** and **Supplementary Figure S1**) expanded the information on the evolution of these genes, and supported the results reported previously by Macqueen and Johnston (2009) that *akirin1* and *akirin2* are vertebrate-specific paralogs that form a separate clade from invertebrate *subolesin/akirin*. In some vertebrate species, Akirins constitute a family of paralog proteins that probably originated as a result of whole-genome duplications (Macqueen and Johnston, 2009; Macqueen et al., 2010a,b; Liu et al., 2015). After *akirin* duplication, *akirin1* evolved faster than *akirin2*, the ortholog of tick *subolesin* (**Figure 1A**; Macqueen and Johnston, 2009). Furthermore, the loss of some *akirin* paralogs may have also occurred after genome duplications (Macqueen et al., 2010b; Liu et al., 2015). For example, the *subolesin/akirin* gene family consists of a single member in invertebrates (*subolesin/akirin*), birds and reptiles (*subolesin/akirin2*), two members in amphibians and mammals (*akirin1* and *akirin2*), two to three members in teleosts, and more than three members in Salmonidae (Macqueen et al., 2010a,b; Liu et al., 2015).

The phylogenetic analysis of *subolesin* gene sequences was performed in 42 species belonging to 6 and 1 genera of hard (family Ixodidae) and soft (family Argasidae) ticks, respectively. The analysis corroborated previous results showing a reductive evolution in protein length (de la Fuente et al., 2006a; **Figure 1B**). The Subolesin amino acid (aa) sequence evolved from 173 to 184 aa in *Ornithodoros*, *Ixodes* and *Haemaphysalis* spp. to 161 aa in *Rhipicephalus* spp. (**Figure 1B**). It is generally accepted that evolution proceeds toward greater complexity at both the organismal and genomic levels. However, numerous examples of reductive evolution of parasites and symbionts have been described to challenge this notion (Wolf and Koonin, 2013). Wolf and Koonin (2013) proposed that quantitatively, the evolution of genomes appears to be dominated by reduction and simplification, punctuated by episodes of complexification. The reductive evolution process has been particularly documented in genomes that replicate within the domain of a host genome (Andersson and Kurland, 1998; Driscoll et al., 2017), but it has also been proposed to be involved in the origin of bacteria from eukaryotes (Staley, 2017). In arthropods, reductive evolution has been implicated in the evolutionary origin of other proteins such as type IV classical cadherins (Sasaki et al., 2017).

The protein length is subjected to systematic variation that relates to the cellular context in which it functions (Wang et al., 2011). For growth rate-optimized cells, the reduction in protein length constitutes an advantage by increasing their mass-normalized kinetic efficiencies (Ehrenberg and Kurland, 1984; Kurland et al., 2007; Wang et al., 2011). Consequently, shorter proteins that retain maximum functional rates are expected to support faster cell growth rates than longer proteins with similar kinetic characteristics. Wang et al. (2011) proposed the use of the terms "domain" and "linker" to refer to protein folded domains and nondomain regions, respectively. Proteins with nondomain sequences are proteins intrinsically unstructured or natively unfolded that lack a stable tertiary structure but have a dynamic range of conformations (Orengo and Thornton, 2005). These proteins appear to be more abundant in eukaryotes when compared to prokaryotes and are usually involved in binding and molecular recognition (Brown et al., 2011). Subolesin/Akirin were characterized as a linker with three predicted disordered nondomain regions that resulted in unstructured proteins (Prudencio et al., 2010; see also below). These results agreed with the findings of Wang et al. (2011) that the evolutionary reductive constraints on protein lengths are preferentially expressed in linker sequences.

It is difficult to establish a comprehensive record of ticks developmental rates because most of the experiments in previously published papers have been done at different regimes of temperature, relative humidity and photoperiod, all factors affecting the time in which ticks complete each developmental stage. However, data compiled by Hoogstraal (1956), Morel (2003) and Horak et al. (2018) under similar

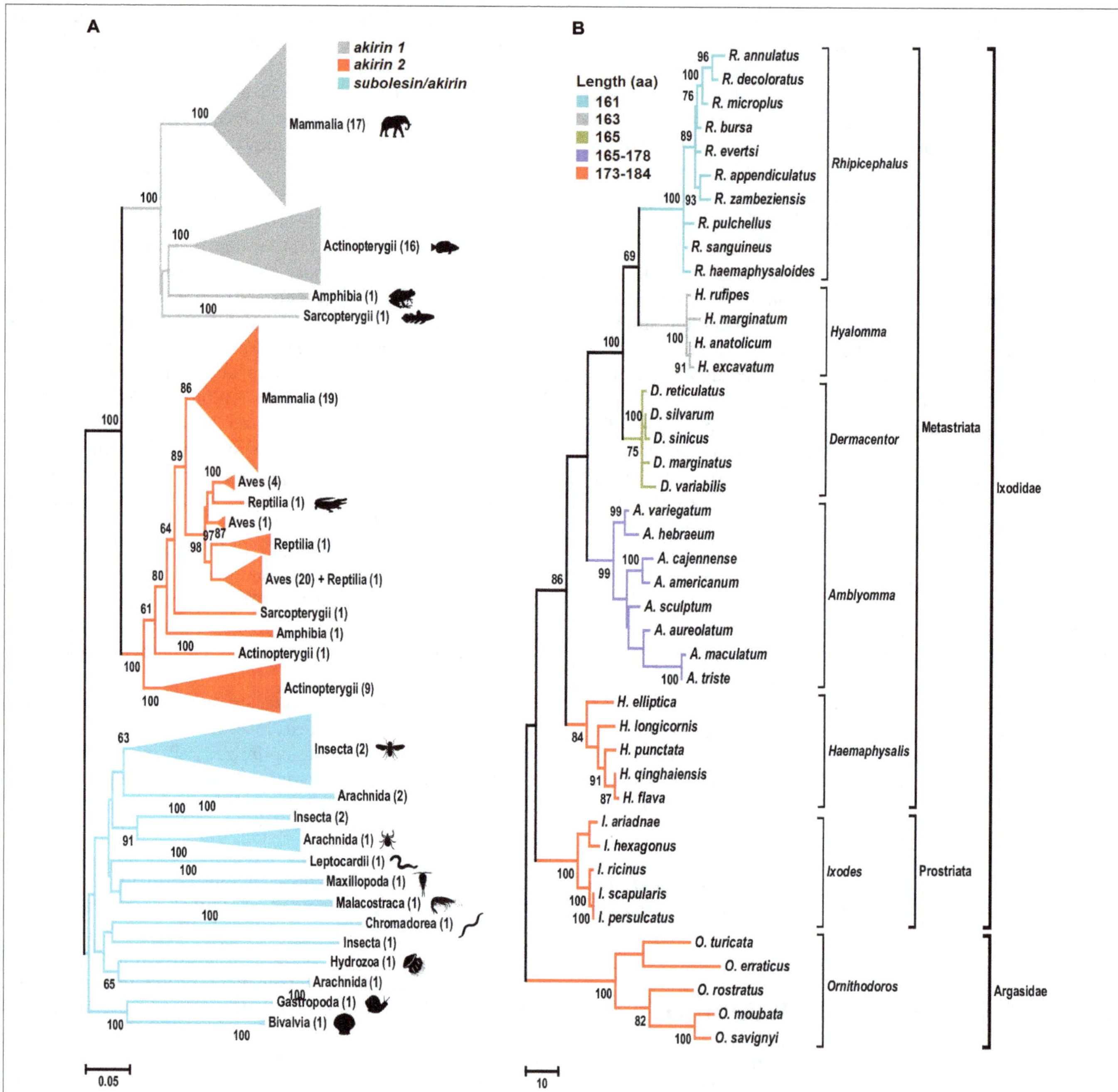

FIGURE 1 | Phylogenetic analysis of *akirin* and *subolesin* nucleotide sequences. **(A)** A Neighbor Joining (NJ) phylogenetic tree was constructed with 361 nucleotide sequences belonging to 152 families, 73 orders and 15 classes (Mammalia, Actinopterygii, Amphibia, Sarcopterygii, Aves, Reptilia, Arachnida, Malacostraca, Insecta, Leptocardii, Maxillopoda, Chromadorea, Hydrozoa, Gastropoda and Bivalvia) of animals. All branches were collapsed at the class level and the number of orders per cluster is shown inside brackets. GenBank accession numbers and species names are provided in **Supplementary Figure S1**. Sequences were aligned using MAFFT configured for the maximum accuracy (Katoh and Standley, 2013). The final alignment contained 303 gap-free sites. All ambiguous positions were removed for each sequence pair. The best-fit model of the sequence evolution was selected based on Corrected Akaike Information Criterion (cAIC) and Bayesian Information Criterion (BIC) implemented in Molecular Evolutionary Genetics Analysis (MEGA) version 7. The Kimura 2-parameter model, which showed the lowest values of cAIC and BIC, was chosen for tree reconstruction. The evolutionary history was inferred using the NJ method implemented in MEGA 7 (Kumar et al., 2016). The percentage of replicate trees in which the associated taxa clustered together in the bootstrap test (500 replicates) is shown next to the branches (Felsenstein, 1985). **(B)** Phylogenetic tree of tick *subolesin* sequences. A Maximum Parsimony (MP) phylogenetic tree was constructed with 42 nucleotide sequences belonging to 6 and 1 genera of hard (family Ixodidae) and soft (family Argasidae) ticks, respectively. Because the evolution of *subolesin* in ticks has been less studied when compared to akirins, MP was used to generate a robust hypothesis on the evolution of this molecule in ticks. Sequences were aligned using MAFFT configured for the maximum accuracy (Katoh and Standley, 2013). Then, using the MAFFT alignment as template, a condon aligment was build (HIV database; www.hiv.lanl.gov accessed on 29-12-2017). The final alignment contained 576 total sites of which 329 were gap-free. The evolutionary history was inferred using the MP method

(Continued)

FIGURE 1 | Continued
implemented in Molecular Evolutionary Genetics Analysis (MEGA) version 7 (Kumar et al., 2016). The percentage of replicate trees in which the associated taxa clustered together in the bootstrap test (500 replicates) is shown next to the branches (Felsenstein, 1985). The MP tree was obtained using the Subtree-Pruning-Regrafting (SPR) algorithm with search level 1 in which the initial trees were obtained by the random addition of sequences (10 replicates). Sequences were collected from Genbank and transcriptome projects and accession numbers are as follow: *Ixodes scapularis* (AY652654), *I. persulcatus* (KM888876), *I. ricinus* (JX193817), *I. ariadnae* (KM455971), *I. hexagonus* (JX193818), *Rhipicephalus evertsi* (JX193846), *R. appendiculatus* (DQ159967), *R. microplus* (EU301808), *R. sanguineus* (JX193845), *R. haemaphysaloides* (KP677498), *R. annulatus* (JX193844), *R. decoloratus* (JX193843), *R. zambeziensis* (GFPF01005851), *R. bursa* (GFZJ01017781), *R. pulchellus* (GACK01006228), *Dermacentor silvarum* (JX856138), *D. sinicus* (KM115649), *D. marginatus* (KU973622), *D. variabilis* (AY652657), *D. reticulatus* (JX193847), *Amblyomma variegatum* (JX193824), *A. hebraeum* (EU262598), *A. cajennense* (JX193823), *A. americanum* (JX193819), *A. maculatum* (JX193825), *A. aureolatum* (GFAC01005925), *A. triste* (GBBM01002796), *A. sculptum* (GFAA01000261), *Hyalomma anatolicum* (KT981976), *H. rufipes* (JX193849, *H. marginatum* (DQ159971), *H. excavatum* (GEFH01000904), *Haemaphysalis longicornis* (EU289292), *Hae. elliptica* (JX193850), *Hae. qinghaiensis* (EU326281, *Hae. flava* (KJ829652), *Hae. punctata* (DQ159972), *Ornithodoros moubata* (JX193852), *O. savignyi* (JX193851), *O. turicata* (GDIE01114362), *O. erraticus* (HM622148) and *O. rostratus* (GCJJ01005500).

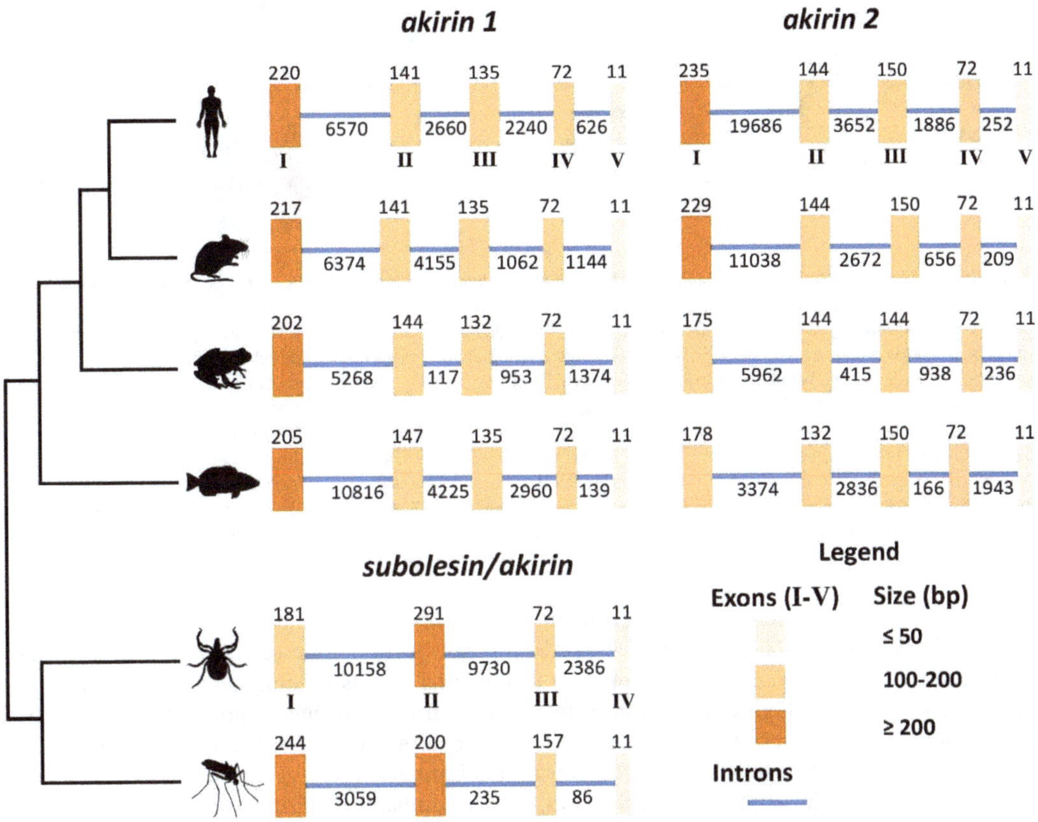

FIGURE 2 | Genomic organization of *subolesin/akirin* orthologs across selected eukaryotic species. The genomic organization of the coding regions of tick (*I. scapularis*), human (*Homo sapiens*), mouse (*M. musculus*), frog (*Xenopus laevis*), fish (*Danio rerio*) and mosquito (*Anopheles gambiae*) *subolesin/akirin* is shown. The genomic organization of human, mouse, frog and fish *akirins* was previously reported (Liu et al., 2015). The genomic organization of tick and mosquito *subolesin/akirin* was collected from VectorBase (https://www.vectorbase.org; Giraldo-Calderón et al., 2015). Latin numerals correspond to the size of exons/introns in base pairs.

conditions established that in the range of 24–28°C, ticks of the genera *Hyalomma* and *Rhipicephalus* complete their life cycle in about 33% less time than ticks of the genera *Ixodes* or *Amblyomma*. The *Hyalomma* and *Rhipicephalus* spp. are considered the two most recent genera of ticks, while *Ixodes* spp. and *Amblyomma* are among the most ancient splits of tick lineages (Mans et al., 2016; **Figure 1B**). Therefore, it is possible that the reductive evolution of Subolesin is associated with faster developmental rates in *Rhipicephalus* and *Hyalomma* spp. when compared to more ancient tick species even if they are sympatric. The faster developmental rate in recently evolved tick species may be associated with increasing cell growth rates that have been associated with reductive evolution (Wang et al., 2011). However, the complete association between existing data about developmental rates and evolutionary features of ticks requires further research.

At the genome level, *subolesin/akirin* exon-intron architecture shows a clear evolutionary pattern (**Figure 2**). As shown for *subolesin/akirin* coding sequences (**Figure 1A**), the vertebrate-specific paralogs form a separate clade from invertebrate genes

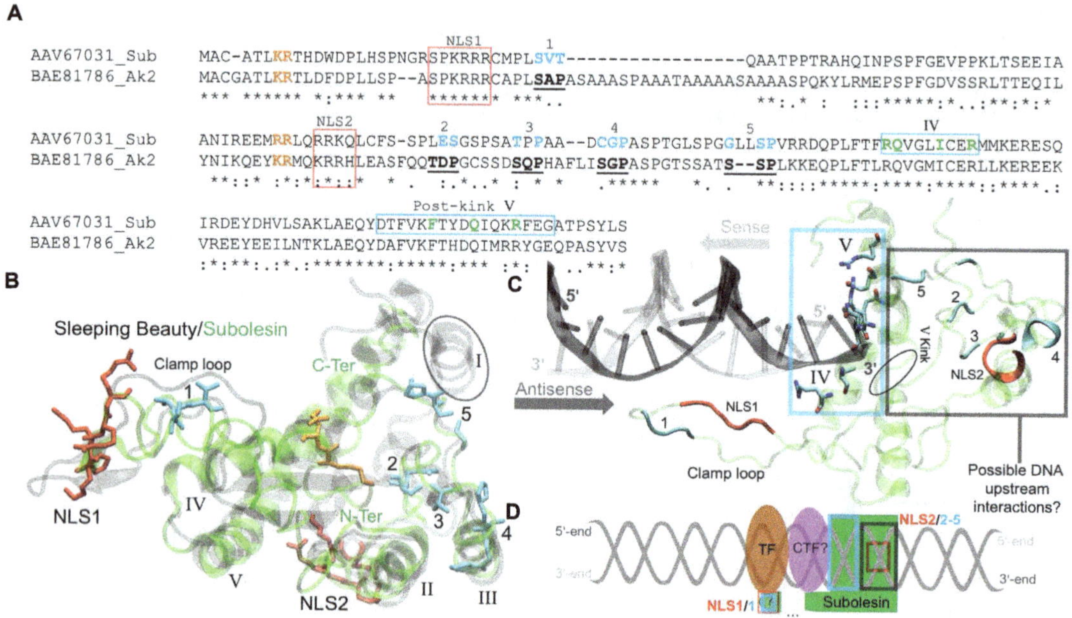

FIGURE 3 | The *I. scapularis* Subolesin structure and its interactions with DNA and transcription factors. **(A)** The pairwise sequence alignment of the *I. scapularis* Subolesin (Sub) and the rat Arkinin2 (Ak2), accession numbers indicated, was generated using the MAFFT alignment program at default settings (Katoh et al., 2017). The NLS 1 and 2 domains (red box), binding sites 1-5 (bold-underlined in Ak2 and cyan for Sub), and the novel DNA binding sites (green and enclosed in a cyan box) are shown. The residues color-coded orange are extensions of the NLS domains. **(B)** The superposed tertiary structures of Sleeping Beauty (transparent black) and Subolesin (transparent green) are represented with the clamp loop labeled and the five α-helices of Sleeping Beauty (PDB: 5CR4) annotated in roman numerals. The tertiary residue positions of the labeled Subolesin NLS domains and binding sites are, respectively, color-coded as in the pairwise alignment. The Subolesin termini positions are color-labeled (green). **(C)** The Subolesin-DNA complex, modeled from the Mos1-DNA (PDB: 3HOS) show the residues of the novel DNA-binding site on α-helices IV-V, enclosed by a cyan box that were predicted by I-TASSER (Zhang, 2008). The DNA prime ends are color-labeled for the respective directions (indicated by arrows) of the sense (gray) and antisense (dark gray) strands. The residue positions of the Subolesin clamp loop, NLS domains and binding sites are color-coded as in previous panels A and B. **(D)** The schematic representation of the upstream DNA (gray helix) interactions with Subolesin NLS2, binding sites 2-5, and the potential clamp loop interaction (via NLS1 and binding site 1) with an unknown co-transcription factor (CTF?) and unknown (?) transcription factor (TF).

(**Figure 2**). The *subolesin*/*akirin* genes evolved from 4 exons in invertebrates to 5 exons in vertebrates. The exon sizes showed a pattern of larger to shorter for vertebrate *akirin1* exons I to V and mosquito *akirin* exons I to IV (**Figure 2**). However, for tick *subolesin* and vertebrate *akirin2* genes, the size of exons II and III, respectively, were larger or similar than that of preceding exon (**Figure 2**). Furthermore, while the length of 11 nucleotides (nt) in the last exon was conserved across evolution, the length of the penultimate exon evolved from 157 nt in mosquitoes to 72 nt in ticks and vertebrates (**Figure 2**). However, the length of the exon-intron sequence increased from 3,992 nt in mosquitoes to 22,829 nt in ticks and then decreased to 8,862 nt in fish to increase back again to 26,088 nt in humans (**Figure 2**). These results do not correlate with genome sizes of these organisms (Gregory, 2005), and may originated from still unknown evolutionary events.

SUBOLESIN/AKIRIN STRUCTURE AND ITS INTERACTIONS WITH DNA AND TRANSCRIPTION FACTORS

Akirins are involved in cellular processes that are regulated by specific domains and binding sites. The rat Akirin2 (or 14-3-3β Interactant 1) described by Komiya et al. (2008) is 48% identical to the *I. scapularis* Subolesin and was previously used to identify the conserved Akirin nuclear localization signal (NLS) domains and its binding sites (Macqueen and Johnston, 2009). The pairwise sequence alignment shows that both NLS domains of the rat Akirin2 are conserved in Subolesin, but with variations in a few binding sites (**Figure 3A**). Subolesin binding sites 1 and 4 are similar to Akirin2 with Subolesin binding sites 2 and 3 each possessing a single substitution. The Subolesin binding site 5, however, has a double Leu insertion when compared to Akirin2 (**Figure 3A**). Currently there are no resolved Subolesin/Akirin structures and standard sequence-based bioinformatics methods lack parameters for locating structural homologs in the Protein Databank (PDB). Therefore, several logical steps were taken to correctly model the *I. scapularis* Subolesin. The Subolesin sequence (**Figure 3A**) was initially submitted to I-TASSER (Zhang, 2008), a protein multiple threading algorithm that is considered a top competitor in the Critical Assessment of Structure Prediction[1]. The I-TASSER algorithm resulted in five distinct Subolesin models that were then individually submitted to the DALI server (Holm and Laakso, 2016) for identifying PDB structural homologs of similar length with minimalα-carbon backbone deviations between the two global structures. Since

[1]http://predictioncenter.org

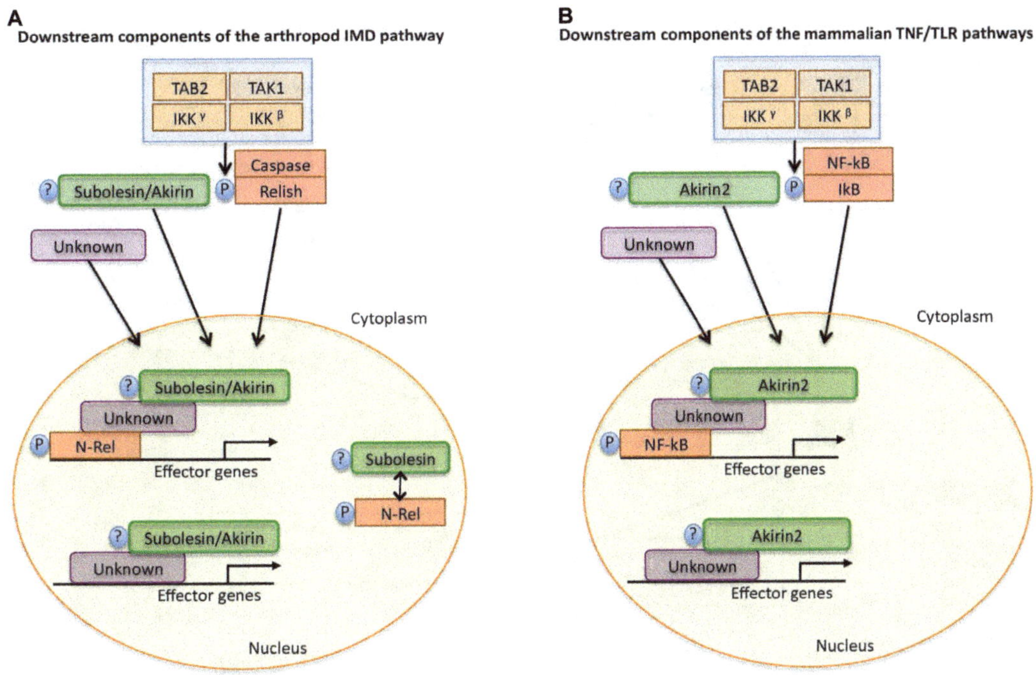

FIGURE 4 | Model for Subolesin/Akirin function in immune response pathways. A simplified annotation of the downstream components of the arthropod IMD and mammalian TNF/TLR pathways (Goto et al., 2008; Beutler and Moresco, 2008; de la Fuente et al., 2008; Naranjo et al., 2013; Shaw et al., 2017). **(A)** After activation of the arthropod IMD pathway, the TGF-β (TAK1), Tak1-binding protein 2 (TAB2) and the I-KB kinase (IKK) complex are recruited, which leads to phosphorylation of the NF-κB transcription factor, Relish. After phosphorylation, the N-terminal domain of Relish (N-Rel) is cleaved by Caspase-8 homolog Dredd or a similar Caspase and is translocated to the nucleus. Subolesin/Akirin may be post-translationally modified and translocated to the nucleus. In the nucleus, N-Rel interacts with Subolesin/Akirin through unknown proteins to drive the production of anti-microbial peptides and other effector genes. In ticks, N-Rel and Subolesin may be reciprocally regulated. **(B)** In mammals, the activation of the TNF/TLR signaling pathways also results in the recruitment of the TAB2-TAK1 and IKK complexes, which results in the phosphorylation of the inhibitory regulator of NF-kB, IkB, resulting in the NF-kB translocation to the nucleus. As in arthropods, Akirin2 may be post-translationally modified and translocated to the nucleus. Once in the nucleus, NF-kB interacts with Akirin2 through unknown proteins for the activation of gene expression. In both arthropods and mammals, Subolesin/Akirin are involved in the regulation of genes that are Relish/NF-kB independent.

Subolesin/Akirin are effectors of the IMD/TNF/TLR Relish/NF-kB signaling pathways (Goto et al., 2008; Naranjo et al., 2013), a match with homologous structures that potentially participate within these pathways was also a criterion in selecting an appropriate Subolesin model. This logical approach resulted in a Subolesin model homologous in structure, with only 7% residue conservation, to the genetically engineered catalytic domain of the transposase Sleeping Beauty (Ivics et al., 1997; Zanesi et al., 2013; **Figure 3B**).

As part of the *Tc1/mariner* transposon superfamily, the Sleeping Beauty transposase has been engineered for genetic screening studies, leading to the discovery of several genes activated by Sleeping Beauty transposon insertions that participate in the NF-kB signaling pathway (Zanesi et al., 2013). The Sleeping Beauty transposase sequence is composed of an N-terminus paired-like domain with a leucine zipper (~90 residues long) and the C-terminus folds as the catalytic domain (Ivics et al., 1997). The catalytic domain of Sleeping Beauty was resolved with a DNA transposon end and modeled with a target DNA revealing the mechanism of hyperactive Sleeping Beauty mutation screening studies while discovering novel variants for future screenings (Voigt et al., 2016). The Sleeping Beauty crystal structure details that its catalytic domain has a global homology to Ribonuclease H (RNase H) (Voigt et al., 2016). The RNase H-like protein fold forms a catalytic triad (Asp-Asp-Glu) that coordinates metal ions involved in excision and insertions of DNA (Voigt et al., 2016). By resolving the Sleeping Beauty catalytic domain, Voigt et al. (2016) also discovered that the Gly-rich box (located on the clamp loop) is involved in protein-protein interactions, specifically with partnering monomers in the DNA complex. The conserved positions of the catalytic triad and the Gly-rich box, however, are not present in Subolesin/Akirin sequences.

Prior to acting in the *Tc1/mariner* transposon system, Sleeping Beauty must enter the nucleus. Passage to the nucleus is controlled by NLS domains that have a strong affinity to karyopherin/importin receptors, proteins responsible for transporting NLS-tagged "cargo" in and out of the nucleus via nuclear pores (Leung et al., 2003). The N-terminus of the Sleeping Beauty catalytic domain contains a NLS domain that is quite long (17 residues) and is actually a bipartite NLS (Ivics et al., 1997). A monopartite NLS domain has the formulation Lys-Lys/Arg-[X]-Lys-Lys/Arg, where [X] is any other (~2) amino acids. A bipartite NLS domain has a linker sequence, where [X] is ~10 residues long (Makkerh et al., 1996). Mutations of

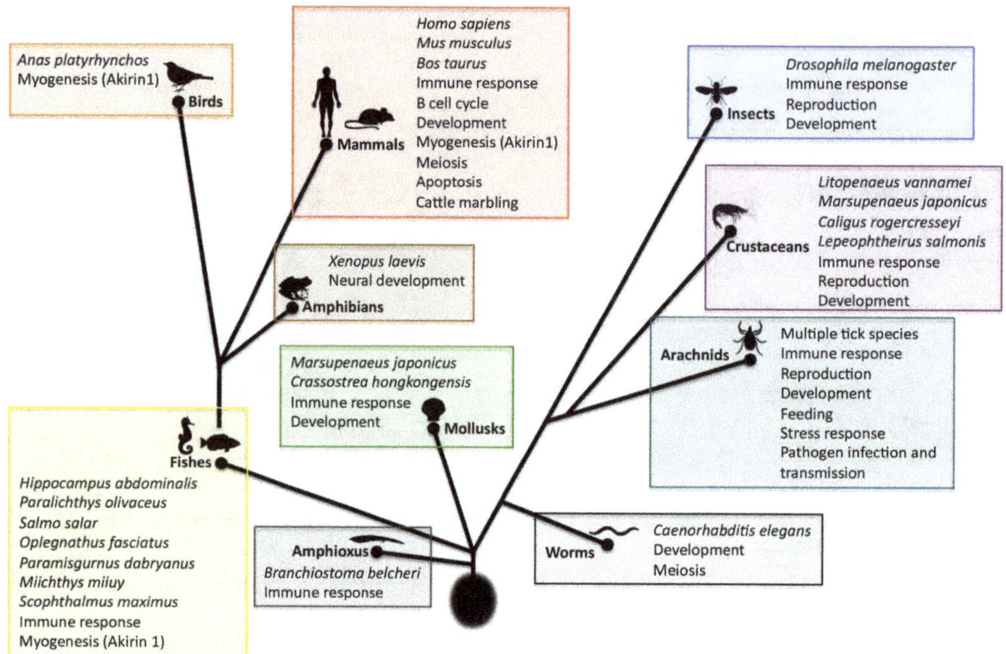

FIGURE 5 | Scheme of the evolution and function of Subolesin/Akirin | Functional annotations were done based on published results for Subolesin/Akirin2. References are in the text of the paper. Myogenesis, attributed exclusively to Akirin1, was included and labeled as such. For each taxa, species in which studies were conducted are shown.

these upstream NLS residues prior to the linker sequence [X] has shown to reduce protein entry into the nucleus (Dingwall et al., 1988), and inhibit NLS binding to karyopherin/importin receptors (Leung et al., 2003). These upstream, positively charged residue pairs are in the aligned sequences of **Figure 3A** (orange-labeled residues), indicating that Subolesin/Akirin2 NLS1 is bipartite. The two positively charged residues highlighted near NLS2 (**Figure 3A**) indicate that the NLS2 of Subolesin/Akirin is actually a longer monopartite domain. The modeled Subolesin structure has its NLS1 positioned on the clamp loop, which differs from Sleeping Beauty that is coordinated at the N-terminus α-helix (I) (**Figure 3B**). The Subolesin NLS2 domain, not present in the catalytic domain of Sleeping Beauty, is located on an α-helix (II) outside the central core of the protein. The absence of the catalytic triad of Sleeping Beauty (Voigt et al., 2016) and metal binding sites in Subolesin/Akirin support that these proteins do not act as a transposase. Additionally, the Subolesin/Akirin binding sites have long been recognized by mutation studies (Komiya et al., 2008), and Subolesin/Akirin RNA interference (RNAi) experiments have shown to disrupt the Relish signaling pathway (Goto et al., 2008; Naranjo et al., 2013). However, as discussed bellow, the Subolesin/Akirin interactome has not been fully characterized, and whether Subolesin/Akirin binding partners are only proteins or also include nucleic acids.

The superposed structures of Subolesin and Sleeping Beauty depict a global homology with a low α-carbon backbone deviation of 0.3 nm (**Figure 3B**). There are, however, missing and disordered secondary structures. The Sleeping Beauty catalytic domain has five β-sheets surrounded by five α-helices. As previously mentioned, the N-terminus α-helix I of Sleeping Beauty that contains its NLS domain is missing in the Subolesin model (encircled in **Figure 3B**), thereby shifting the Subolesin NLS1 domain to the clamp loop. Moreover, the β-sheets of Subolesin are highly disordered. Future experiments should resolve the stacking and conformations of the disordered Subolesin β-sheets by X-ray crystallography. Nevertheless, the remaining four α-helices (II-V) are structurally conserved, and the Subolesin/Akirin binding sites 2-5 are positioned on or approximating α-helix III (**Figure 3B**). As in the primary sequence (**Figure 3A**), the Subolesin/Akirin binding site 1 is structurally distant from the other sites, located on the N-terminus clamp loop near the position of NLS1 (**Figure 3B**). As a transposase, the clamp loop of the resolved Sleeping Beauty catalytic domain is not in its DNA-bound conformation. Therefore, Voigt et al. (2016) modeled the clamp loop after the DNA-bound transposase, Mos1, from *Drosophila mauritiana* (Richardson et al., 2009). The Mos1 also has poor sequence identity to Subolesin (<5%), but are structurally homologous with α-carbon backbone deviation of 0.34 nm. This led to a subsequent I-TASSER simulation using the template Mos1 as conducted by Voigt et al. (2016). The resulting model has Subolesin bound to a DNA duplex with an adequate clamp loop conformation that extends downstream the duplex (**Figure 3C**).

The Subolesin-DNA complex show several residues on α-helices IV and V that approximate the DNA 5′-end of the sense strand and the 3′-end of the antisense strand (**Figure 3C**).

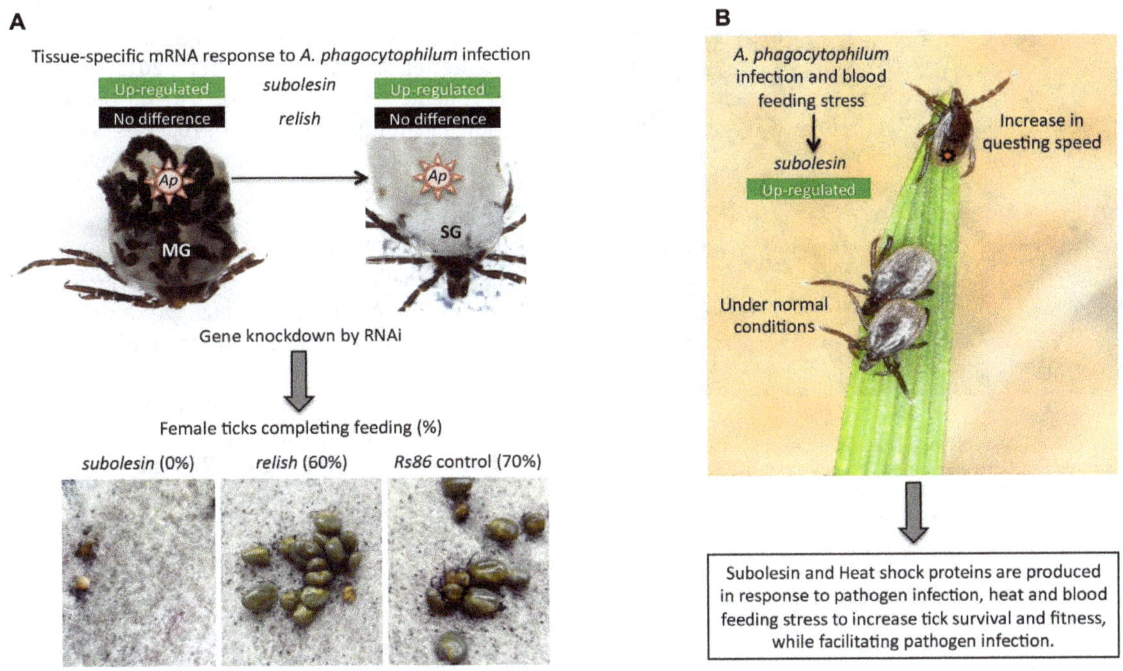

FIGURE 6 | Examples of the role of tick Subolesin in different biological processes | **(A)** Role of tick Subolesin in *A. phagocytophilum* infection and blood feeding. The transcriptomics analysis in different *I. scapularis* tick tissues showed that *subolesin* (ISCW023283) but not *relish* (ISCW018935) mRNA levels significantly increased in response to *A. phagocytophilum* (*Ap*) infection in both midgut (MG) and salivary glands (SG). In addition, the *subolesin* gene knockdown phenotype in ticks injected with dsRNA resulted in a significant reduction in the number of female ticks completing feeding, oviposition and fertility. Results were reported by Ayllón et al. (2015). Photo of dissected *I. scapularis* partially fed adult female ticks courtesy of K. M. Kocan (Oklahoma State University, United States). **(B)** Role of tick Subolesin in *A. phagocytophilum* infection, blood feeding and questing speed. The response to *A. phagocytophilum* and stress increases *subolesin* levels, which together with heat shock proteins improve tick questing speed and survival. Results were reported by Busby et al. (2012). Photo of questing *Ixodes ricinus* courtesy of L. Grubhoffer & J. Erhard (Biology Center of the AS CR, Institute of Parasitology, Czechia).

Four of the seven residues positioned on α-helix IV mainly interact with the phosphate backbone of the antisense strand. The remaining three residues that interact with both strands are after the pivotal kink of α-helix V (encircled in **Figure 3C**). The alignment in **Figure 3A** highlights these novel DNA-binding residues and indicates the α-helix on which they are positioned. The binding sites 2–5 and NLS2 are distal to the DNA interacting site, while the clamp loop containing NLS1 and binding site one is downstream the DNA duplex. Given the structural coordination of Subolesin bound to DNA (**Figure 3C**), binding sites 2–5 and NLS2 may interact with nucleotides upstream the DNA or with additional co-transcription factors (CTF) (**Figure 3D**). The transcription factors (TF) Relish/NF-kB form DNA-protein complexes with CTFs, and Subolesin is hypothesized to act as a CTF of Relish via an intermediate CTF (**Figure 3D** and described in the next section). Furthermore, the extended DNA downstream position of the Subolesin clamp loop with binding site one will hypothetically coordinate the CTF and possibly the TF (**Figure 3D**). If Subolesin is a CTF, how will it conform while the mRNA is being transcribed? Positively charged residues, specifically Lys, recognize RNA strands via electrostatic interactions (Law et al., 2006). Given conformational flexibility of the Subolesin clamp loop and the fact that it does not contain the Sleeping Beauty Gly-rich box, the proximity of positively charged Subolesin NLS1 domain residues downstream the DNA duplex may guide transcribing mRNAs for post-transcriptional processing.

FUNCTION OF SUBOLESIN/AKIRIN

The innate immune response acts as the first line of defense against pathogen infection in all metazoans, and constitutes the only immune response in invertebrates (Medzhitov et al., 1997; Shaw et al., 2017). It has been shown that invertebrate Subolesin/Akirin and vertebrate Akirin2 act in concert with Relish/NF-kB to induce the expression of a subset of downstream pathway elements in the IMD and TNF/TLR signaling pathways involved in the immune response to pathogen infection. This function of Subolesin/Akirin has been documented in ticks (de la Fuente et al., 2008, 2017a; Naranjo et al., 2013; Gulia-Nuss et al., 2016; Shaw et al., 2017), fruit fly (Beutler and Moresco, 2008; Goto et al., 2008; Wan and Lenardo, 2010; Bonnay et al., 2014), human (Goto et al., 2008), salmon (Macqueen et al., 2010b), shrimp (Hou et al., 2013), Japanese flounder (Yang et al., 2013), amphioxus (Yan et al., 2013), rock bream (Kasthuri et al., 2013), Chinese loach (Xue et al., 2014), Hong Kong oyster (Qu et al., 2014), turbot (Yang et al., 2011), sea louse (Valenzuela-Muñoz and Gallardo-Escárate, 2014), mouse

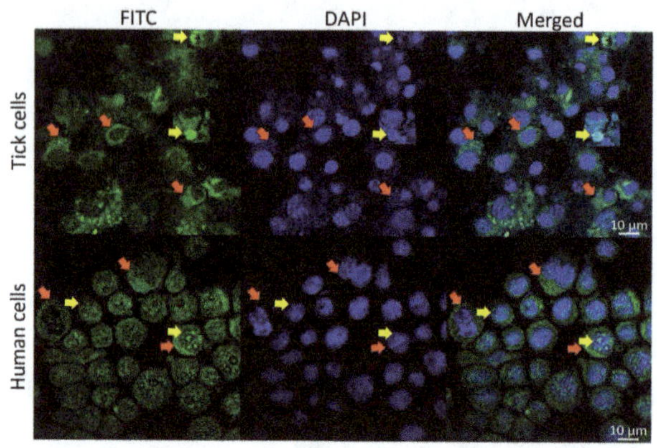

FIGURE 7 | Subcellular localization of Subolesin/Akirin2. Representative images of immunofluorescence analysis of *I. scapularis* ISE6 and human HL60 cells incubated with anti-Subolesin and anti-Akirin2 antibodies, respectively. The cells were fixed with 4% paraformaldehyde in PBS for 15 min, permeabilized with 0.5% Triton X-100 in PBS for 5 min and blocked with blocking buffer (3% BSA in PBS) for 1 h. Then, the cells were incubated overnight at 4°C with anti-Subolesin (Antunes et al., 2014) or anti-Akirin2 (Abcam, Cambridge, United Kingdom) antibodies (1/50 dilution in 3% BSA in PBS). After 3 washes with PBS, the slides were incubated with fluorescein isothiocyanate (FITC) conjugated anti-rabbit secondary antibodies (Sigma-Aldrich, St. Louis, MO, United States; green) at 1/160 dilution in 3% BSA in PBS for 1 h at room temperature. Cells were counterstained with ProLong Antifade containing 4′,6-diamidino-2-phenylindole (DAPI) (Molecular Probes, Eugene, OR, United States; blue), and imaged with a Zeiss LSM800 confocal microscope using a 63× oil immersion lens (Carl Zeiss, Oberkochen, Germany). Yellow arrows show examples of protein localization in the nucleus while red arrows illustrate protein localization in the cytoplasm.

(Beutler and Moresco, 2008; Goto et al., 2008; Wan and Lenardo, 2010; Tartey et al., 2015), croaker (Liu et al., 2015); shrimp (Liu Y. et al., 2016; Liu et al., 2016), and seahorse (Pavithiran et al., 2018; **Figures 4, 5**).

Subolesin/Akirin are also involved in the Relish/NF-kB independent gene regulation (**Figure 4**), thus playing a role in various biological processes in addition to the immune response (**Figure 5**). These processes include animal reproduction and development, causing lethal embryonic or reduced growth phenotypes in knockout mice, fruit fly, ticks, and nematodes (Maeda et al., 2001; de la Fuente et al., 2006a; Goto et al., 2008; Carpio et al., 2013; Qu et al., 2014), metazoan myogenesis (Marshall et al., 2008; Salerno et al., 2009; Macqueen et al., 2010a; Mobley et al., 2014; Sun et al., 2016), *Xenopus* neural development (Liu et al., 2017), meiosis/carcinogenesis (Komiya et al., 2008; Macqueen et al., 2010b; Clemons et al., 2013), tick stress response, feeding, growth and reproduction (Almazán et al., 2003, 2005; de la Fuente et al., 2006a, 2008; Smith et al., 2009; Busby et al., 2012; Rahman et al., 2018), pathogen infection and transmission in ticks (de la Fuente et al., 2006b, 2016, 2017a; Zivkovic et al., 2010a,b; Busby et al., 2012; Hajdušek et al., 2013) and turbot (Yang et al., 2011), human glioblastoma cell apoptosis (Krossa et al., 2015), cattle marbling (Sasaki et al., 2009; Watanabe et al., 2011; Kim et al., 2013), and mouse mitogen-induced B cell cycle progression and humoral immune responses (Tartey et al., 2015). For example, as previously reported in *I. scapularis* and other tick species (de la Fuente and Kocan, 2006; de la Fuente et al., 2006a,b, 2011, 2013; Merino et al., 2013a; de la Fuente and Contreras, 2015), Subolesin appears to function in multiple biological processes such as tick response to infection, feeding, reproduction, development and stress response (**Figure 6**).

Akirin1 and Akirin2 have also different functions in vertebrates, which is illustrated by the role of Akirin1 in myogenesis while Akirin2 promotes meiosis/carcinogenesis (Macqueen and Johnston, 2009; Macqueen et al., 2010a,b; **Figure 4**). These different functions may be related to the Akirin subcellular localization. While Akirin1 is found in the nucleus, Subolesin/Akirin2 is located in both cytoplasm and nucleus (de la Fuente et al., 2011; Antunes et al., 2014; Krossa et al., 2015; Pavithiran et al., 2018; **Figure 7**). The subcellular localization of Subolesin/Akirin2 is probably related to its structure, which as discussed above contains NLS domains that are involved in protein transport in and out of the nucleus via nuclear pores (Leung et al., 2003).

In summary and based on current information, Subolesin/Akirin evolved with similar functions in both invertebrates and vertebrates (**Figure 5**). The annotation of some biological processes described in certain taxa only may be due to the presence of species-specific functions or more likely a consequence of the still incomplete characterization of Subolesin/Akirin function in the different species.

SUBOLESIN/AKIRIN ROLE IN CELL INTERACTOME AND REGULOME

Subolesin/Akirin are proteins without catalytic or DNA-binding capacity. How Subolesin/Akirin regulate gene expression is unknown but likely involve interactions with proteins with DNA-binding or chromatin-remodeling capacity (de la Fuente et al., 2008; Beutler and Moresco, 2008; Nowak and Baylies, 2012; Nowak et al., 2012; Naranjo et al., 2013). In this way, Subolesin/Akirin link the activities of transcription factors with those of chromatin remodeling complexes to influence gene expression in a context-dependent manner (Nowak and Baylies, 2012; Nowak et al., 2012). For example, Subolesin/Akirin and Akirin2 as key components of the innate immune response can directly or indirectly interact with other regulatory proteins such as "14-3-3" proteins, DNA methyltransferase-associated protein 1 (DMAP1) and the basic helix–loop–helix transcription factor (Twist) to up- or down-regulate transcription (Gonzalez and Baylies, 2005; Goto et al., 2008, 2014; Komiya et al., 2008; de la Fuente et al., 2008; Beutler and Moresco, 2008; Nowak et al., 2012; Naranjo et al., 2013; Tartey et al., 2014; Gulia-Nuss et al., 2016; Shaw et al., 2017).

The Subolesin/Akirin role in the cell interactome and regulome in response to different stimuli has not been characterized. Recently, we proposed a method based on the graph theory for the analysis of human and tick cell

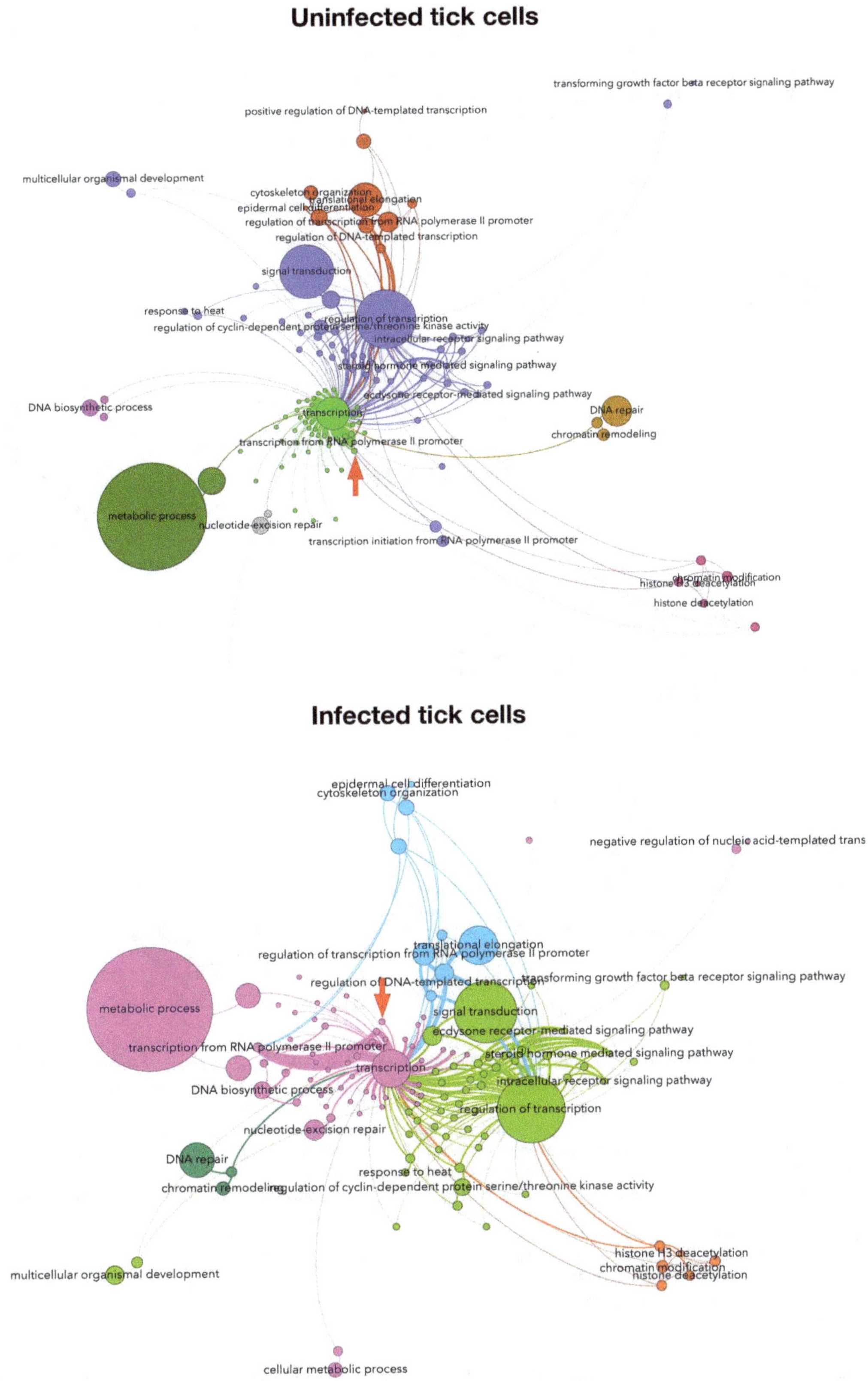

FIGURE 8 | Subolesin regulome in tick cells. The network of proteins and processes associated to transcription in tick cells uninfected and infected with *Anaplasma phagocytophilum*. The nodes (circles) are either proteins or processes (labeled). The size of each circle is proportional to its centrality index. The networks show

(Continued)

FIGURE 8 | Continued
clusters of interacting proteins and processes in colors. The width of each link is proportional to the strength of the interaction. The networks show the topology of the tick interactome and regulome. The networks were built with the annotated proteins represented in either uninfected or infected cells, and a directed network was built for each protein linked to the processes in which it is involved. The weight of each link is proportional to the number of reads of the protein. This weighted degree of each link was used to calculate the centrality indexes, mainly the Betweenness Centrality, which is represented in the panels. Only the proteins annotated as involved in processes associated with transcription (i.e., linked by one or more protein(s) simultaneously annotated as transcripiton or other cellular process). The topology of the networks was obtained with the Lovaine algorithm. In both networks, the topological position of Subolesin is marked with a red arrow. Methods were described in Estrada-Peña et al. (2018).

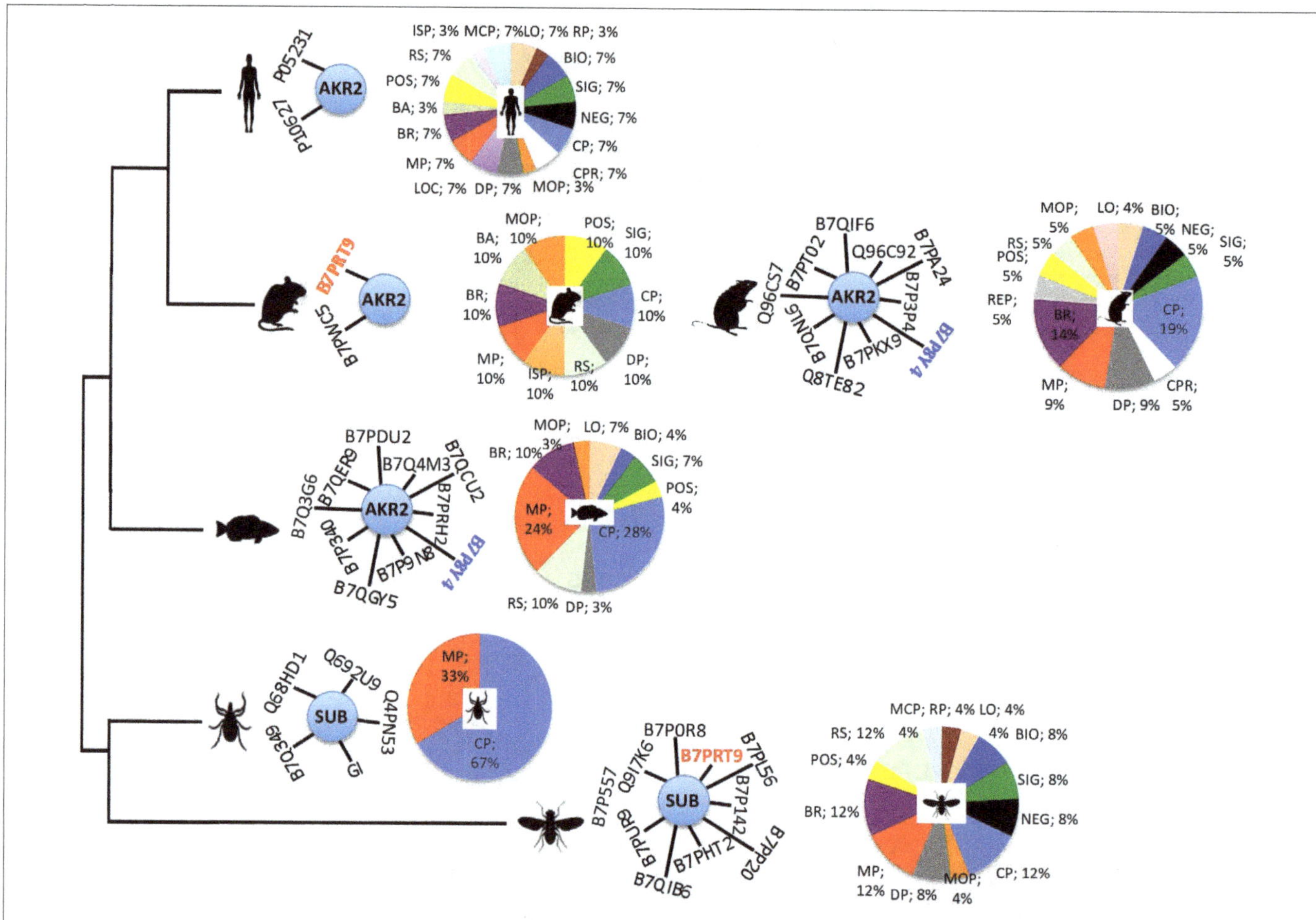

FIGURE 9 | Characterization of the Subolesin/Akirin2 interactome. The information on Subolesin/Akirin-protein physical and functional interactions was compiled from the String protein-protein interactions database v.10.5 (https://string-db.org). The central node of the networks represent Subolesin/Akirin2 while the edges correspond to the predicted functional associations. Only predictions with medium (or better) confidence (> 0.4) limited to the top 10 interactions with protein-protein interaction (PPI) enrichment p-value ≤ 0.5 were considered. To compare the different species, protein annotations were standardize by identity to *I. scapularis/I. ricinus-D. melanogaster-H. sapiens* order of priority (see **Supplementary Dataset S1** for complete annotations). For illustration purposes, the species included in the analysis correspond to *D. melanogaster*, *I. scapularis*, *Danio rerio*, *Mus musculus*, *Rattus norvegicus*, and *H. sapiens*. Identical proteins in two different species are highlighted in red and blue letters. The functional annotation of the Subolesin/Akirin2 interacting proteins according to the biological processes (level 2) in which they are involved was done using Blast2GO (www.blast2go.com), and represented in pies with different colors for each process and the percentage of proteins on each process. Abbreviations: LO, localization (sepia); RP, rhythmic process (sangria); BIO, biogenesis (blue); SIG, signaling (green); NEG, negative regulation of biological process (black); CP, cellular process (azure); CPR, cell proliferation (white); MCP, multi-organism process (sky); DP, developmental process (gray); LOC, locomotion (violet); MP, metabolic process (red); BR, biological regulation (byzantine); BA, biological adhesion (moss); POS, positive regulation of biological process (yellow); RS, response to stimulus (tea); ISP, immune system process (gold); MOP, multicellular organismal process (orange); REP, reproductive process (smoke). Color code was established according to color thesaurus (https://graf1x.com/list-of-colors-with-color-names/).

proteome in response to *A. phagocytophilum* infection (Estrada-Peña et al., 2018). This approach resulted in a network of interacting proteins and cell processes clustered in biological pathways, and ranked with indexes representing the topology of the proteome influenced by features of the interactome and regulome. The results evidenced differences in the response to *A. phagocytophilum* infection between human and tick cells, and supported that human neutrophils but not tick cells

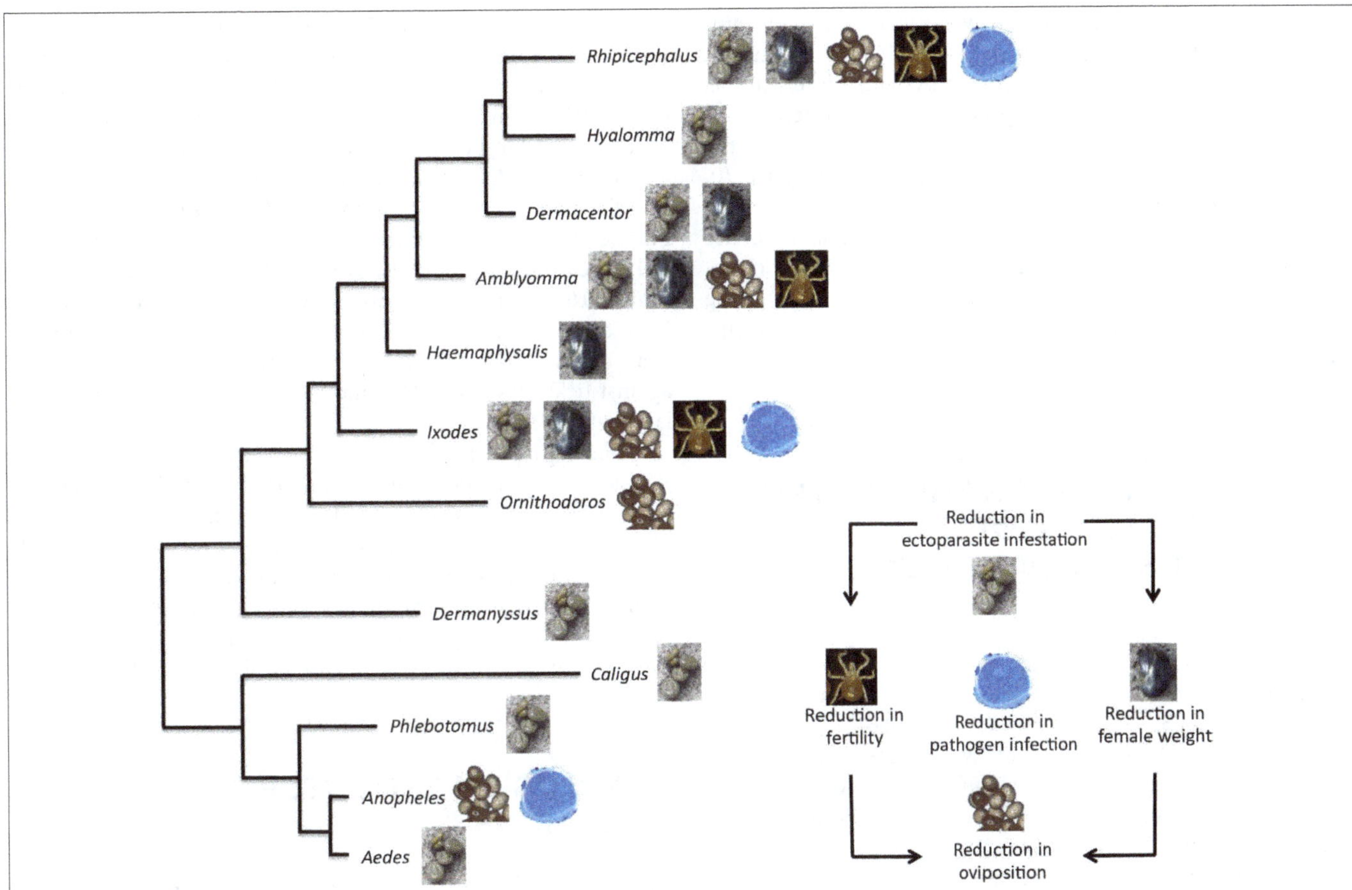

FIGURE 10 | Protective capacity of Subolesin/Akirin in vaccines for the control of arthropod ectoparasite infestations and pathogen infection. The effect of Subolesin/Akirin vaccination is shown on evolutionarily diverse arthropod genera. The effect of the vaccine was recorded on different phases of ectoparasite life cycle in the form of reduction in ectoparasite infestation (number of ectoparasites completing feeding), weight (weight of engorged female ectoparasites), oviposition (number of eggs per female), and fertility (number of larvae per female) in ectoparasites fed on vaccinated hosts when compared to controls. The reduction in pathogen infection was recorded as differences in pathogen levels between ectoparasites fed on vaccinated and control hosts.

limit pathogen infection through differential representation of ras-related proteins (Estrada-Peña et al., 2018). Herein, this method was applied to predict the position of Subolesin in the regulome of tick cells and in response to *A. phagocytophilum* infection (**Figure 8**). The results showed that Subolesin is deeply involved in the core of transcription processes but also in other secondary processes such as transcription from RNA polymerase II promoter, DNA repair, and chromatin remodeling (**Figure 8**). Furthermore, other processes that change in infected cells when compared to uninfected cells (i.e., signal transduction, regulation of transcription, and response to heat) are deeply linked to the central transcription process. The putative Subolesin role in these processes varied between infected and uninfected cells (the width of the lines is proportional to the importance of the link between proteins and processes; **Figure 8**). For example, it appears that particularly in infected cells other proteins but Subolesin have a more prominent role in the strong protein link with transcription and transcription from RNA polymerase II promoter processes (**Figure 8**). These results predict the role that Subolesin plays in the regulation of different biological processes, and its differential role in response to *A. phagocytophilum* infection in tick cells. However, the lack of a more prominent role for Subolesin may respond to the fact that this protein does not bind directly to DNA but interacts with other proteins to exert its regulatory function.

In an attempt to provide information on the Subolesin/Akirin interactome, the information on Subolesin/Akirin-protein physical and functional interactions was compiled from the String protein-protein interactions database[2] (**Figure 9** and **Supplementary Dataset S1**). Based on the analysis of protein-protein interactions, the results did not allow establishing an evolutionary signature of the Subolesin/Akirin2 interactome (**Figure 9**), probably due to the limited information available. Nevertheless, similar Subolesin/Akirin2 interacting proteins were described in fly and mouse (B7PRT9, Brahma/SWI2-related protein BRG-1) and in fish and rat (B7P8Y4, Arginyl-tRNA synthetase)

[2]https://string-db.org

suggesting possible evolutionarily conserved protein-protein interactions (**Figure 9**). To further gain insight into the evolution of the Subolesin/Akirin2 interactome, instead of looking only at protein-protein interactions, the interacting proteins were annotated according to the biological processes in which they are involved (**Figure 9**). The results of this analysis showed that the biological processes affected by the Subolesin/Akirin interactome are evolutionarily conserved, with metabolic process (MP), cellular process (CP) and biological regulation (BR) being among the most represented processes in all organisms (**Figure 9**).

PROTECTIVE CAPACITY OF SUBOLESIN/AKIRIN FOR THE CONTROL OF ECTOPARASITE VECTOR INFESTATIONS AND PATHOGEN INFECTION

Subolesin was discovered and characterized as a tick protective antigen for the control of *I. scapularis* infestations (Almazán et al., 2003, 2005; Sonenshine et al., 2006). Since then, Subolesin/Akirin showed a protective capacity in vaccines for the control of infestations by different arthropod species and pathogen infection and transmission (reviewed by de la Fuente et al., 2006a, 2011, 2013; de la Fuente and Kocan, 2006, 2014; Merino et al., 2013a,b; de la Fuente and Contreras, 2015). The putative mechanism for Subolesin vaccine protection was described by de la Fuente et al. (2011). They showed that by still unknown mechanisms anti-Subolesin antibodies could enter into tick cells where they can interact with cytosolic Subolesin to prevent its translocation to the nucleus and therefore the possibility to exert it regulatory functions.

The development of vaccines for the control of multiple arthropod ectoparasites constitutes a priority for targeting the various species infesting the same host (de la Fuente et al., 2011; Contreras and de la Fuente, 2016b). In this context, Subolesin/Akirin appears as a promising vaccine protective antigen due to its conservation in sequence and function through evolution (**Figures 1**, **5**, **9**). In fact, recent results support the potential of Subolesin/Akirin as a vaccine protective antigen for the control of multiple ectoparasite vector species and transmitted pathogens (**Figure 10**). The arthropod ectoparasite species in which Subolesin/Akirin have shown protective capacity by affecting different phases of their life cycles include the genera *Aedes, Anopheles, Phlebotomus, Caligus, Dermanyssus, Ornithodoros, Ixodes, Haemaphysalis, Amblyomma, Dermacentor, Hyalomma* and *Rhipicephalus* (Almazán et al., 2003, 2005, 2010, 2012; de la Fuente et al., 2006a, 2010, 2011, 2013; Canales et al., 2009; Harrington et al., 2009; Zivkovic et al., 2010a; Moreno-Cid et al., 2011, 2013; Carpio et al., 2011; Bensaci et al., 2012; Merino et al., 2011a,b, 2013b; Carreón et al., 2012; Manzano-Román et al., 2012, 2015; de la Fuente and Kocan, 2014; da Costa et al., 2014; Shakya et al., 2014; Torina et al., 2014; Contreras et al., 2015; de la Fuente and Contreras, 2015; Lu et al., 2016; Olds et al., 2016; Contreras and de la Fuente, 2016a; Kumar et al., 2017; Villar et al., 2017; **Figure 10**). The reduction in pathogen infection has been shown for tick-borne pathogens, *Anaplasma marginale, A. phagocytophilum, Borrelia burgdorferi* s.s. and *Babesia bovis*, and the mosquito-borne pathogen, *Plasmodium berghei* (de la Fuente et al., 2011; Merino et al., 2011b, 2013a; Bensaci et al., 2012; de la Fuente and Kocan, 2014; da Costa et al., 2014; **Figure 10**). Furthermore, protective epitopes were mapped in Subolesin/Akirin (Prudencio et al., 2010) and chimeric antigens were designed showing protective capacity in vaccinated hosts against tick infestations (Merino et al., 2013b; Contreras and de la Fuente, 2016a).

Considering the protective capacity shown by Subolesin/Akirin on different vector and pathogen species, future research directions will include the characterization of its protective capacity in other arthropod ectoparasite species, and the combination with other vector-derived and pathogen-derived antigens to increase vaccine efficacy for the control of both vector infestations and pathogen infection (Schetters et al., 2016; de la Fuente et al., 2017b; de la Fuente, 2018).

CONCLUSION AND FUTURE DIRECTIONS

Significant advances have been made recently toward understanding the evolution and function of Subolesin/Akirin. Our results suggest that Subolesin/Akirin evolved conserving not only its sequence and structure, but also its function and role in cell interactome and regulome in response to pathogen infection and other biological processes. However, major challenges remain in fully characterizing the interactome and function of these proteins, their role in the cell regulome in response to different stimuli, and how their evolution can meet species-specific demands. Furthermore, the structure of Subolesin/Akirin and interacting molecules should be resolved by X-ray crystallography to better understand their function. Finally, the conserved functional evolution of Subolesin/Akirin correlates with the protective capacity shown by these proteins in vaccine formulations for the control of different arthropod and pathogen species, and encourage further research to develop new vaccine formulations by combining Subolesin/Akirin with interacting proteins for the control of multiple ectoparasite infestations and pathogen infection.

AUTHOR CONTRIBUTIONS

JdlF conceived the paper. SA-J, MV, AC-C, JV, and AE-P performed the data analyses. PA and SA-J performed the microscopy studies. JF, SA-J, JV, and AC-C wrote the manuscript. All authors approved and contributed to the final version of the manuscript.

FUNDING

This work was financially supported by the Ministerio de Economía, Industria y Competitividad (Spain) grant BFU2016-79892-P. MV was funded by the Universidad de Castilla La Mancha, Spain. JV was supported by Project FIT (Pharmacology, Immunotherapy, nanoToxicology), funded by the European Regional Development Fund. The publication fee was partially supported by the CSIC Open Access Publication Support Initiative through its Unit of Information Resources for Research (URICI).

ACKNOWLEDGMENTS

We acknowledge a grant for the development of a research organization RVO: RO0516 from the Veterinary Research Institute, Brno, Czechia.

SUPPLEMENTARY MATERIAL

FIGURE S1 | Phylogenetic tree of akirin and subolesin nucleotide sequences. The figure displays a Neighbor Joining (NJ) phylogenetic tree of 361 nucleotide sequences belonging to 152 families, 73 orders and 15 classes. GenBank accession numbers and species names are shown. Tree reconstruction method was as described in **Figure 1**.

DATASET S1 | Annotation of the Subolesin/Akirin interactome. The information on Subolesin/Akirin-protein interactions was compiled from the literature and String protein-protein interactions database v.10.5 (https://string-db.org). Only predictions with medium (or better) confidence (0.4) limited to the top 10 interactions with protein-protein interaction (PPI) enrichment p-value ≤ 0.5 were considered. To compare the different species, protein annotations were standardize by identity to *I. scapularis/I. ricinus-D. melanogaster-H. sapiens* order of priority.

REFERENCES

Adipietro, K. A., Mainland, J. D., and Matsunami, H. (2012). Functional evolution of mammalian odorant receptors. *PLoS Genet.* 8:e1002821. doi: 10.1371/journal.pgen.1002821

Almazán, C., Blas-Machado, U., Kocan, K. M., Yoshioka, J. H., Blouin, E. F., Mangold, A. J., et al. (2005). Characterization of three *Ixodes scapularis* cDNAs protective against tick infestations. *Vaccine* 23, 4403–4416. doi: 10.1016/j.vaccine.2005.04.012

Almazán, C., Kocan, K. M., Bergman, D. K., Garcia-Garcia, J. C., Blouin, E. F., and de la Fuente, J. (2003). Identification of protective antigens for the control of *Ixodes scapularis* infestations using cDNA expression library immunization. *Vaccine* 21, 1492–1501. doi: 10.1016/S0264-410X(02)00683-7

Almazán, C., Lagunes, R., Villar, M., Canales, M., Rosario-Cruz, R., Jongejan, F., et al. (2010). Identification and characterization of *Rhipicephalus (Boophilus) microplus* candidate protective antigens for the control of cattle tick infestations. *Parasitol. Res.* 106, 471–479. doi: 10.1007/s00436-009-1689-1

Almazán, C., Moreno-Cantú, O., Moreno-Cid, J. A., Galindo, R. C., Canales, M., Villar, M., et al. (2012). Control of tick infestations in cattle vaccinated with bacterial membranes containing surface-exposed tick protective antigens. *Vaccine* 30, 265–272. doi: 10.1016/j.vaccine.2011.10.102

Andersson, S. G., and Kurland, C. G. (1998). Reductive evolution of resident genomes. *Trends Microbiol.* 6, 263–268. doi: 10.1016/S0966-842X(98)01312-2

Antunes, S., Merino, O., Mosqueda, J., Moreno-Cid, J. A., Bell-Sakyi, L., Fragkoudis, R., et al. (2014). Tick capillary feeding for the study of proteins involved in tick-pathogen interactions as potential antigens for the control of tick infestation and pathogen infection. *Parasit. Vectors* 7:42. doi: 10.1186/1756-3305-7-42

Ayllón, N., Villar, M., Galindo, R. C., Kocan, K. M., Šíma, R., López, J. A., et al. (2015). Systems biology of tissue-specific response to *Anaplasma phagocytophilum* reveals differentiated apoptosis in the tick vector *Ixodes scapularis*. *PLoS Genet.* 11:e1005120. doi: 10.1371/journal.pgen.1005120

Bensaci, M., Bhattacharya, D., Clark, R., and Hu, L. T. (2012). Oral vaccination with *Vaccinia virus* expressing the tick antigen subolesin inhibits tick feeding and transmission of *Borrelia burgdorferi*. *Vaccine* 30, 6040–6046. doi: 10.1016/j.vaccine.2012.07.053

Beutler, B., and Moresco, E. M. (2008). Akirins versus infection. *Nat. Immunol.* 9, 7–9. doi: 10.1038/ni0108-7

Bonnay, F., Nguyen, X. H., Cohen-Berros, E., Troxler, L., Batsche, E., Camonis, J., et al. (2014). Akirin specifies NF-κB selectivity of *Drosophila* innate immune response via chromatin remodeling. *EMBO J.* 33, 2349–2362. doi: 10.15252/embj.201488456

Brown, C. J., Johnson, A. K., Dunker, A. K., and Daughdrill, G. W. (2011). Evolution and disorder. *Curr. Opin. Struct. Biol.* 21, 441–446. doi: 10.1016/j.sbi.2011.02.005

Busby, A. T., Ayllón, N., Kocan, K. M., Blouin, E. F., de la Fuente, G., Galindo, R. C., et al. (2012). Expression of heat-shock proteins and subolesin affects stress responses, *Anaplasma phagocytophilum* infection and questing behavior in the tick, *Ixodes scapularis*. *Med. Vet. Entomol.* 26, 92–102. doi: 10.1111/j.1365-2915.2011.00973.x

Canales, M., Naranjo, V., Almazán, C., Molina, R., Tsuruta, S. A., Szabó, M. P. J., et al. (2009). Conservation and immunogenicity of the mosquito ortholog of the tick protective antigen, subolesin. *Parasitol. Res.* 105, 97–111. doi: 10.1007/s00436-009-1368-2

Carpio, Y., Basabe, L., Acosta, J., Rodríguez, A., Mendoza, A., Lisperger, A., et al. (2011). Novel gene isolated from *Caligus rogercresseyi*: a promising target for vaccine development against sea lice. *Vaccine* 29, 2810–2820. doi: 10.1016/j.vaccine.2011.01.109

Carpio, Y., García, C., Pons, T., Haussmann, D., Rodríguez-Ramos, T., Basabe, L., et al. (2013). Akirins in sea lice: first steps toward a deeper understanding. *Exp. Parasitol.* 135, 188–199. doi: 10.1016/j.exppara.2013.06.018

Carreón, D., Pérez de la Lastra, J. M., Almazán, C., Canales, M., Ruiz-Fons, F., Boadella, M., et al. (2012). Vaccination with BM86, subolesin and akirin protective antigens for the control of tick infestations in white tailed deer and red deer. *Vaccine* 30, 273–279. doi: 10.1016/j.vaccine.2011.10.099

Clemons, A. M., Brockway, H. M., Yin, Y., Kasinathan, B., Butterfield, Y. S., Jones, S. J., et al. (2013). Akirin is required for diakinesis bivalent structure and synaptonemal complex disassembly at meiotic prophase I. *Mol. Biol. Cell.* 24, 1053–1067. doi: 10.1091/mbc.E12-11-0841

Contreras, M., and de la Fuente, J. (2016a). Control of *Ixodes ricinus* and *Dermacentor reticulatus* tick infestations in rabbits vaccinated with the Q38 Subolesin/Akirin chimera. *Vaccine* 34, 3010–3013. doi: 10.1016/j.vaccine.2016.04.092

Contreras, M., and de la Fuente, J. (2016b). Vaccinomics approach to the development of vaccines for the control of multiple ectoparasite infestations. *Nova Acta Leopold.* 411, 185–200. doi: 10.1186/1471-2164-12-105

Contreras, M., Moreno-Cid, J. A., Domingos, A., Canales, M., Díez-Delgado, I., Pérez de la Lastra, J. M., et al. (2015). Bacterial membranes enhance the immunogenicity and protective capacity of the surface exposed tick Subolesin-*Anaplasma marginale* MSP1a chimeric antigen. *Ticks Tick Borne Dis.* 6, 820–828. doi: 10.1016/j.ttbdis.2015.07.010

da Costa, M., Pinheiro-Silva, R., Antunes, S., Moreno-Cid, J. A., Villar, M., de la Fuente, J., et al. (2014). Mosquito Akirin as a potential antigen for malaria control. *Malar. J.* 13:470. doi: 10.1186/1475-2875-13-470

DasGupta, R., Kaykas, A., Moon, R. T., and Perrimon, N. (2005). Functional genomic analysis of the Wnt-wingless signaling pathway. *Science* 308, 826–833. doi: 10.1126/science.1109374

de la Fuente, J. (2018). Controlling ticks and tick-borne diseases...looking forward. *Ticks Tick Borne Dis.* 9, 1354–1357. doi: 10.1016/j.ttbdis.2018.04.001

de la Fuente, J., Almazaìn, C., Blas-Machado, U., Naranjo, V., Mangold, A. J., Blouin, E. F., et al. (2006a). The tick protective antigen, 4D8, is a conserved protein involved in modulation of tick blood ingestion and reproduction. *Vaccine* 24, 4082–4095.

de la Fuente, J., Almazán, C., Blouin, E. F., Naranjo, V., and Kocan, K. M. (2006b). Reduction of tick infections with *Anaplasma marginale* and *A. phagocytophilum* by targeting the tick protective antigen subolesin. *Parasitol. Res.* 100, 85–91.

de la Fuente, J., Antunes, S., Bonnet, S., Cabezas-Cruz, A., Domingos, A., Estrada-Peña, A., et al. (2017a). Tick-pathogen interactions and vector competence: identification of molecular drivers for tick-borne diseases. *Front. Cell. Infect. Microbiol.* 7:114. doi: 10.3389/fcimb.2017.00114

de la Fuente, J., Contreras, M., Estrada-Peña, A., and Cabezas-Cruz, A. (2017b). Targeting a global health problem: vaccine design and challenges for the control of tick-borne diseases. *Vaccine* 35, 5089–5094. doi: 10.1016/j.vaccine.2017.07.097

de la Fuente, J., and Contreras, M. (2015). Tick vaccines: current status and future directions. *Expert Rev. Vaccines* 14, 1367–1376. doi: 10.1586/14760584.2015.1076339

de la Fuente, J., and Kocan, K. M. (2006). Strategies for development of vaccines for control of ixodid tick species. *Parasite Immunol.* 28, 275–283. doi: 10.1111/j.1365-3024.2006.00828.x

de la Fuente, J., and Kocan, K. M. (2014). "Development of vaccines for control of tick infestations and interruption of pathogen transmission," in *Biology of Ticks*, 2nd Edn, eds D. E. Sonenshine and R. M. Roe (New York, NY: Oxford University Press), 333–352.

de la Fuente, J., Manzano-Roman, R., Naranjo, V., Kocan, K. M., Zivkovic, Z., Blouin, E. F., et al. (2010). Identification of protective antigens by RNA interference for control of the lone star tick, *Amblyomma americanum*. *Vaccine* 28, 1786–1795. doi: 10.1016/j.vaccine.2009.12.007

de la Fuente, J., Maritz-Olivier, C., Naranjo, V., Ayoubi, P., Nijhof, A. M., Almazán, C., et al. (2008). Evidence of the role of tick subolesin in gene expression. *BMC Genomics* 9:372. doi: 10.1186/1471-2164-9-372

de la Fuente, J., Moreno-Cid, J. A., Canales, M., Villar, M., Pérez de la Lastra, J. M., Kocan, K. M., et al. (2011). Targeting arthropod subolesin/akirin for the development of a universal vaccine for control of vector infestations and pathogen transmission. *Vet. Parasitol.* 181, 17–22. doi: 10.1016/j.vetpar.2011.04.018

de la Fuente, J., Moreno-Cid, J. A., Galindo, R. C., Almazán, C., Kocan, K. M., Merino, O., et al. (2013). Subolesin/Akirin vaccines for the control of arthropod vectors and vector-borne pathogens. *Transbound. Emerg. Dis.* 60(Suppl. 2), 172–178. doi: 10.1111/tbed.12146

de la Fuente, J., Villar, M., Cabezas-Cruz, A., Estrada-Peña, A., Ayllón, N., and Alberdi, P. (2016). Tick-host-pathogen interactions: conflict and cooperation. *PLoS Pathog.* 12:e1005488. doi: 10.1371/journal.ppat.1005488

Dingwall, C., Robbins, J., Dilworth, S. M., Roberts, B., and Richardson, W. D. (1988). The nucleoplasmin nuclear location sequence is larger and more complex than that of SV-40 large T antigen. *J. Cell Biol.* 107, 841–849. doi: 10.1083/jcb.107.3.841

Driscoll, T. P., Verhoeve, V. I., Guillotte, M. L., Lehman, S. S., Rennoll, S. A., Beier-Sexton, M., et al. (2017). Wholly *Rickettsia*! Reconstructed metabolic profile of the quintessential bacterial parasite of eukaryotic cells. *mBio* 8:e859-17. doi: 10.1128/mBio.00859-17

Ehrenberg, M., and Kurland, C. G. (1984). Costs of accuracy determined by a maximal growth rate constraint. *Q. Rev. Biophys.* 17, 45–82. doi: 10.1017/S0033583500005254

Estrada-Peña, A., Villar, M., Artigas-Jerónimo, S., López, V., Alberdi, P., Cabezas-Cruz, A., et al. (2018). Use of graph theory to characterize human and arthropod vector cell protein response to infection. *Front. Cell. Infect. Microbiol.* 8:265. doi: 10.3389/fcimb.2018.00265

Felsenstein, J. (1985). Confidence limits on phylogenies: an approach using the bootstrap. *Evolution* 39, 783–791. doi: 10.1111/j.1558-5646.1985.tb00420.x

Galindo, R. C., Doncel-Pérez, E., Zivkovic, Z., Naranjo, V., Gortazar, C., Mangold, A. J., et al. (2009). Tick subolesin is an ortholog of the akirins described in insects and vertebrates. *Dev. Comp. Immunol.* 33, 612–617. doi: 10.1016/j.dci.2008.11.002

Giraldo-Calderón, G. I., Emrich, S. J., MacCallum, R. M., Maslen, G., Dialynas, E., Topalis, P., et al. (2015). VectorBase: an updated bioinformatics resource for invertebrate vectors and other organisms related with human diseases. *Nucleic Acids Res.* 43, D707–D713. doi: 10.1093/nar/gku1117

Gonzalez, K., and Baylies, M. (2005). "bhringi: A novel Twist co-regulator", in *Proceedings of the Program and Abstracts 46th Annual Drosophila Research Conference*, San Diego, CA, 46:320B.

Goto, A., Fukuyama, H., Imler, J. L., and Hoffmann, J. A. (2014). The chromatin regulator DMAP1 modulates activity of the nuclear factor B (NF-B) transcription factor Relish in the *Drosophila* innate immune response. *J. Biol. Chem.* 289, 20470–20476. doi: 10.1074/jbc.C114.553719

Goto, A., Matsushita, K., Gesellchen, V., El Chamy, L., Kuttenkeuler, D., Takeuchi, O., et al. (2008). Akirins are highly conserved nuclear proteins required for NF-kappaB-dependent gene expression in Drosophila and mice. *Nat. Immunol.* 9, 97–104. doi: 10.1038/ni1543

Gregory, T. R. (2005). *Animal Genome Size Database.* Avilable at: http://www.genomesize.com

Gulia-Nuss, M., Nuss, A. B., Meyer, J. M., Sonenshine, D. E., Roe, R. M., Waterhouse, R. M., et al. (2016). Genomic insights into the *Ixodes scapularis* tick vector of Lyme disease. *Nat. Commun.* 7:10507. doi: 10.1038/ncomms10507

Hajdušek, O., Šíma, R., Ayllón, N., Jalovecká, M., Perner, J., de la Fuente, J., et al. (2013). Interaction of the tick immune system with transmitted pathogens. *Front. Cell. Infect. Microbiol.* 3:26. doi: 10.3389/fcimb.2013.00026

Harrington, D., Canales, M., de la Fuente, J., de Luna, C., Robinson, K., Guy, J., et al. (2009). Immunisation with recombinant proteins subolesin and Bm86 for the control of *Dermanyssus gallinae* in poultry. *Vaccine* 27, 4056–4063. doi: 10.1016/j.vaccine.2009.04.014

Holm, L., and Laakso, L. M. (2016). Dali server update. *Nucleic Acids Res.* 44, W351–W355. doi: 10.1093/nar/gkw357

Hoogstraal, H. (1956). *African Ixodoidea. I. Ticks of the Sudan (with Special Reference to Equatoria Province and with Preliminary Reviews of the Genera Boophilus, Margaropus and Hyalomma).* Washington, DC: Department of the Navy, 1101.

Horak, I. G., Heyne, H., Williams, R., Gallivan, G. J., Spickett, A. M., Bezuidenhout, J. D., et al. (2018). *The Ixodid Ticks (Acari: Ixodidae) of Southern Africa.* Hamburg: Springer, 675. doi: 10.1007/978-3-319-70642-9

Hou, F., Wang, X., Qian, Z., Liu, Q., Liu, Y., He, S., et al. (2013). Identification and functional studies of Akirin, a potential positive nuclear factor of NF-κB signaling pathways in the Pacific white shrimp, *Litopenaeus vannamei*. *Dev. Comp. Immunol.* 41, 703–714. doi: 10.1016/j.dci.2013.08.005

Ivics, Z., Hackett, P. B., Plasterk, R. H., and Izsvak, Z. (1997). Molecular reconstruction of Sleeping Beauty, a Tc1-like transposon from fish, and its transposition in human cells. *Cell* 91, 501–510. doi: 10.1016/S0092-8674(00)80436-5

Kasthuri, S. R., Umasuthan, N., Whang, I., Wan, Q., Lim, B. S., Jung, H. B., et al. (2013). Akirin2 homologues from rock bream, *Oplegnathus fasciatus*: genomic and molecular characterization and transcriptional expression analysis. *Fish Shellfish Immunol.* 35, 740–747. doi: 10.1016/j.fsi.2013.06.006

Katoh, K., Rozewicki, J., and Yamada, K. D. (2017). MAFFT online service: multiple sequence alignment, interactive sequence choice and visualization. *Brief. Bioinform.* doi: 10.1093/bib/bbx108 [Epub ahead of print].

Katoh, K., and Standley, D. M. (2013). MAFFT multiple sequence alignment software version 7: improvements in performance and usability. *Mol. Biol. Evol.* 30, 772–780. doi: 10.1093/molbev/mst010

Kim, H., Lee, S. K., Hong, M. W., Park, S. R., Lee, Y. S., Kim, J. W., et al. (2013). Association of a single nucleotide polymorphism in the akirin 2 gene with economically important traits in Korean native cattle. *Anim. Genet.* 44, 750–753. doi: 10.1111/age.12055

Komiya, Y., Kurabe, N., Katagiri, K., Ogawa, M., Sugiyama, A., Kawasaki, Y., et al. (2008). A novel binding factor of 14-3-3beta functions as a transcriptional repressor and promotes anchorage-independent growth, tumorigenicity, and metastasis. *J. Biol. Chem.* 283, 18753–18764. doi: 10.1074/jbc.M802530200

Koonin, E. V. (2005). Orthologs, paralogs, and evolutionary genomics. *Annu. Rev. Genet.* 39, 309–338. doi: 10.1371/journal.pgen.1002821

Krossa, S., Schmitt, A. D., Hattermann, K., Fritsch, J., Scheidig, A. J., Mehdorn, H. M., et al. (2015). Down regulation of Akirin-2 increases chemosensitivity in human glioblastomas more efficiently than Twist-1. *Oncotarget* 6, 21029–21045. doi: 10.18632/oncotarget.3763

Kumar, B., Manjunathachar, H. V., Nagar, G., Ravikumar, G., de la Fuente, J., Saravanan, B. C., et al. (2017). Functional characterization of candidate antigens of *Hyalomma anatolicum* and evaluation of its cross-protective efficacy against *Rhipicephalus microplus*. *Vaccine* 35, 5682–5692. doi: 10.1016/j.vaccine.2017.08.049

Kumar, S., Stecher, G., and Tamura, K. (2016). MEGA7: molecular evolutionary genetics analysis version 7.0 for bigger datasets. *Mol. Biol. Evol.* 33, 1870–1874. doi: 10.1093/molbev/msw054

Kurland, C. G., Canbäck, B., and Berg, O. G. (2007). The origins of modern proteomes. *Biochimie* 89, 1454–1463. doi: 10.1016/j.biochi.2007.09.004

Law, M. J., Linde, M. E., Chambers, E. J., Oubridge, C., Katsamba, P. S., Nilsson, L., et al. (2006). The role of positively charged amino acids and electrostatic interactions in the complex of U1A protein and U1 hairpin II RNA. *Nucleic Acids Res.* 34, 275–285. doi: 10.1093/nar/gkj436

Leung, S. W., Harreman, M. T., Hodel, M. R., Hodel, A. E., and Corbett, A. H. (2003). Dissection of the karyopherin alpha nuclear localization signal (NLS)-binding groove: functional requirements for NLS binding. *J. Biol. Chem.* 278, 41947–41953. doi: 10.1074/jbc.M307162200

Liu, N., Wang, X. W., Sun, J. J., Wang, L., Zhang, H. W., Zhao, X. F., et al. (2016). Akirin interacts with Bap60 and 14-3-3 proteins to regulate the expression of antimicrobial peptides in the kuruma shrimp (*Marsupenaeus japonicus*). *Dev. Comp. Immunol.* 55, 80–89. doi: 10.1016/j.dci.2015.10.015

Liu, T., Gao, Y., and Xu, T. (2015). Evolution of akirin family in gene and genome levels and coexpressed patterns among family members and rel gene in croaker. *Dev. Comp. Immunol.* 52, 17–25. doi: 10.1016/j.dci.2015.04.010

Liu, X., Xia, Y., Tang, J., Ma, L., Li, C., Ma, P., et al. (2017). Dual roles of Akirin2 protein during *Xenopus* neural development. *J. Biol. Chem.* 292, 5676–5684. doi: 10.1074/jbc.M117.777110

Liu, Y., Song, L., Sun, Y., Liu, T., Hou, F., and Liu, X. (2016). Comparison of immune response in Pacific white shrimp, *Litopenaeus vannamei*, after knock down of Toll and IMD gene *in vivo*. *Dev. Comp. Immunol.* 60, 41–52. doi: 10.1016/j.dci.2016.02.004

Lu, P., Zhou, Y., Yu, Y., Cao, J., Zhang, H., Gong, H., et al. (2016). RNA interference and the vaccine effect of a subolesin homolog from the tick *Rhipicephalus haemaphysaloides*. *Exp. Appl. Acarol.* 68, 113–126. doi: 10.1007/s10493-015-9987-z

Macqueen, D. (2009). Commentary on Galindo et Al. [Dev. Comp. Immunol. 33(4) (2009) 612-617]. *Dev. Comp. Immunol.* 33, 877; authorrely 878–879. doi: 10.1016/j.dci.2009.02.011

Macqueen, D. J., and Johnston, I. A. (2009). Evolution of the multifaceted eukaryotic akirin gene family. *BMC Evol. Biol.* 9:34. doi: 10.1186/1471-2148-9-34

Macqueen, D. J., Bower, N. I., and Johnston, I. A. (2010a). Positioning the expanded akirin gene family of Atlantic salmon within the transcriptional networks of myogenesis. *Biochem. Biophys. Res. Commun.* 200, 599–605. doi: 10.1016/j.bbrc.2010.08.110

Macqueen, D. J., Kristjánsson, B. K., and Johnston, I. A. (2010b). Salmonid genomes have a remarkably expanded akirin family, coexpressed with genes from conserved pathways governing skeletal muscle growth and catabolism. *Physiol. Genomics* 42, 134–148. doi: 10.1152/physiolgenomics.00045.2010

Maeda, I., Kohara, Y., Yamamoto, M., and Sugimoto, A. (2001). Large-scale analysis of gene function in *Caenorhabditis elegans* by high-throughput RNAi. *Curr. Biol.* 11, 171–176. doi: 10.1016/S0960-9822(01)00052-5

Makkerh, J. P., Dingwall, C., and Laskey, R. A. (1996). Comparative mutagenesis of nuclear localization signals reveals the importance of neutral and acidic amino acids. *Curr. Biol.* 6, 1025–1027. doi: 10.1016/S0960-9822(02)00648-6

Mans, B. J., De Castro, M. H., Pienaar, R., De Klerk, D., Gaven, P., Genu, S., et al. (2016). Ancestral reconstruction of tick lineages. *Ticks Tick Borne Dis.* 7, 509–535. doi: 10.1016/j.ttbdis.2016.02.002

Manzano-Román, R., Díaz-Martín, V., Oleaga, A., and Pérez-Sánchez, R. (2015). Identification of protective linear B-cell epitopes on the subolesin/akirin orthologues of *Ornithodoros* spp. soft ticks. *Vaccine* 33, 1046–1055. doi: 10.1016/j.vaccine.2015.01.015

Manzano-Román, R., Díaz-Martín, V., Oleaga, A., Siles-Lucas, M., and Pérez-Sánchez, R. (2012). Subolesin/akirin orthologs from *Ornithodoros* spp. soft ticks: cloning, RNAi gene silencing and protective effect of the recombinant proteins. *Vet. Parasitol.* 185, 248–259. doi: 10.1016/j.vetpar.2011.10.032

Marshall, A., Salerno, M. S., Thomas, M., Davies, T., Berry, C., Dyer, K., et al. (2008). Mighty is a novel promyogenic factor in skeletal myogenesis. *Exp. Cell Res.* 314, 1013–1029. doi: 10.1016/j.yexcr.2008.01.004

Medzhitov, R., and Janeway, C. A. Jr. (1997). Innate immunity: impact on the adaptive immune response. *Curr. Opin. Immunol.* 9, 4–9. doi: 10.1016/S0952-7915(97)80152-5

Merino, O., Alberdi, P., Pérez de la Lastra, J. M., and de la Fuente, J. (2013a). Tick vaccines and the control of tick-borne pathogens. *Front. Cell. Infect. Microbiol.* 3:30. doi: 10.3389/fcimb.2013.00030

Merino, O., Antunes, S., Mosqueda, J., Moreno-Cid, J. A., Pérez de la Lastra, J. M., Rosario-Cruz, R., et al. (2013b). Vaccination with proteins involved in tick-pathogen interactions reduces vector infestations and pathogen infection. *Vaccine* 31, 5889–5896. doi: 10.1016/j.vaccine.2013.09.037

Merino, O., Almazán, C., Canales, M., Villar, M., Moreno-Cid, J. A., Estrada-Peña, A., et al. (2011a). Control of *Rhipicephalus (Boophilus) microplus* infestations by the combination of subolesin vaccination and tick autocidal control after subolesin gene knockdown in ticks fed on cattle. *Vaccine* 29, 2248–2254. doi: 10.1016/j.vaccine.2011.01.050

Merino, O., Almazán, C., Canales, M., Villar, M., Moreno-Cid, J. A., Galindo, R. C., et al. (2011b). Targeting the tick protective antigen subolesin reduces vector infestations and pathogen infection by *Anaplasma marginale* and *Babesia bigemina*. *Vaccine* 29, 8575–8579. doi: 10.1016/j.vaccine.2011.09.023

Mobley, C. B., Fox, C. D., Ferguson, B. S., Amin, R. H., Dalbo, V. J., Baier, S., et al. (2014). L-leucine, beta-hydroxy-beta-methylbutyric acid (HMB) and creatine monohydrate prevent myostatin-induced Akirin-1/Mighty mRNA down-regulation and myotube atrophy. *J. Int. Soc. Sports Nutr.* 11:38. doi: 10.1186/1550-2783-11-38

Morel, P. C. (2003). *Les Tiques d'Afrique et du Bassin Meìditerraneìen (1965–1995).* Can Tho: CIRAD-EMVT, 1342.

Moreno-Cid, J. A., Jiménez, M., Cornelie, S., Molina, R., Alarcón, P., Lacroix, M.-N., et al. (2011). Characterization of *Aedes albopictus* akirin for the control of mosquito and sand fly infestations. *Vaccine* 29, 77–82. doi: 10.1016/j.vaccine.2010.10.011

Moreno-Cid, J. A., Pérez de la Lastra, J. M., Villar, M., Jiménez, M., Pinal, R., Estrada-Peña, A., et al. (2013). Control of multiple arthropod vector infestations with subolesin/akirin vaccines. *Vaccine* 31, 1187–1196. doi: 10.1016/j.vaccine.2012.12.073

Naranjo, N., Ayllón, N., Pérez de la Lastra, J. M., Galindo, R. C., Kocan, K. M., Blouin, E. F., et al. (2013). Reciprocal regulation of NF-kB (Relish) and Subolesin in the tick vector, *Ixodes scapularis*. *PLoS One* 8:e65915. doi: 10.1371/journal.pone.0065915

Nowak, S. J., Aihara, H., Gonzalez, K., Nibu, Y., and Baylies, M. K. (2012). Akirin links twist-regulated transcription with the Brahma chromatin remodeling complex during embryogenesis. *PLoS Genet.* 8:e1002547. doi: 10.1371/journal.pgen.1002547

Nowak, S. J., and Baylies, M. K. (2012). Akirin: a context-dependent link between transcription and chromatin remodeling. *Bioarchitecture* 2, 209–213. doi: 10.4161/bioa.22907

Olds, C. L., Mwaura, S., Odongo, D. O., Scoles, G. A., Bishop, R., and Daubenberger, C. (2016). Induction of humoral immune response to multiple recombinant *Rhipicephalus appendiculatus* antigens and their effect on tick feeding success and pathogen transmission. *Parasit. Vectors* 9:484. doi: 10.1186/s13071-016-1774-0

Orengo, C. A., and Thornton, J. M. (2005). Protein families and their evolution-a structural perspective. *Annu. Rev. Biochem.* 74, 867–900. doi: 10.1146/annurev.biochem.74.082803.133029

Pavithiran, A., Bathige, S. D. N. K., Kugapreethan, R., Priyathilaka, T. T., Yang, H., Kim, M. J., et al. (2018). A comparative study of three akirin genes from big belly seahorse *Hippocampus abdominalis*: molecular, transcriptional and functional characterization. *Fish Shellfish Immunol.* 74, 584–592. doi: 10.1016/j.fsi.2018.01.025

Peña-Rangel, M. T., Rodriguez, I., and Riesgo-Escovar, J. R. (2002). A misexpression study examining dorsal thorax formation in *Drosophila melanogaster*. *Genetics* 160, 1035–1050.

Prudencio, C. R., Pérez de la Lastra, J. M., Canales, M., Villar, M., and de la Fuente, J. (2010). Mapping protective epitopes in the tick and mosquito subolesin ortholog proteins. *Vaccine* 28, 5398–5406. doi: 10.1016/j.vaccine.2010.06.021

Qu, F., Xiang, Z., Zhang, Y., Li, J., Zhang, Y., and Yu, Z. (2014). The identification of the first molluscan Akirin2 with immune defense function in the Hong Kong oyster *Crassostrea hongkongensis*. *Fish Shellfish Immunol.* 41, 455–465. doi: 10.1016/j.fsi.2014.09.029

Rahman, M. K., Saiful Islam, M., and You, M. (2018). Impact of subolesin and cystatin knockdown by RNA interference in adult female *Haemaphysalis longicornis* (Acari: Ixodidae) on blood engorgement and reproduction. *Insects* 9:E39. doi: 10.3390/insects9020039

Richardson, J. M., Colloms, S. D., Finnegan, D. J., and Walkinshaw, M. D. (2009). Molecular architecture of the Mos1 paired-end complex: the structural basis of DNA transposition in a eukaryote. *Cell* 138, 1096–1108. doi: 10.1016/j.cell.2009.07.012

Rioualen, C., Da Costa, Q., Chetrit, B., Charafe-Jauffret, E., Ginestier, C., and Bidaut, G. (2017). HTS-Net: an integrated regulome-interactome approach for establishing network regulation models in high-throughput screenings. *PLoS One* 12:e0185400. doi: 10.1371/journal.pone.0185400

Salerno, M. S., Dyer, K., Bracegirdle, J., Platt, L., Thomas, M., Siriett, V., et al. (2009). Akirin1 (Mighty), a novel promyogenic factor regulates muscle regeneration and cell chemotaxis. *Exp. Cell Res.* 315, 2012–2021. doi: 10.1016/j.yexcr.2009.04.014

Sasaki, M., Akiyama-Oda, Y., and Oda, H. (2017). Evolutionary origin of type IV classical cadherins in arthropods. *BMC Evol. Biol.* 17:142. doi: 10.1186/s12862-017-0991-2

Sasaki, S., Yamada, T., Sukegawa, S., Miyake, T., Fujita, T., Morita, M., et al. (2009). Association of a single nucleotide polymorphism in akirin 2 gene with marbling in Japanese Black beef cattle. *BMC Res. Notes* 2:131. doi: 10.1186/1756-0500-2-131

Schetters, T., Bishop, R., Crampton, M., Kopáčk, P., Lew-Tabor, A., Maritz-Olivier, C., et al. (2016). Cattle tick vaccine researchers join forces in CATVAC. *Parasit. Vectors* 9:105. doi: 10.1186/s13071-016-1386-8

Shakya, M., Kumar, B., Nagar, G., de la Fuente, J., and Ghosh, S. (2014). Subolesin: a candidate vaccine antigen for the control of cattle tick infestations in Indian situation. *Vaccine* 32, 3488–3494. doi: 10.1016/j.vaccine.2014.04.053

Shaw, D. K., Wang, X., Brown, L. J., Oliva Chávez, A. S., Reif, K. E., Smith, A. A., et al. (2017). Infection-derived lipids elicit an immune deficiency circuit in arthropods. *Nat. Commun.* 8:14401. doi: 10.1038/ncomms14401

Smith, A., Guo, X., de la Fuente, J., Naranjo, N., Kocan, K. M., and Kaufman, W. R. (2009). The impact of RNA interference of the subolesin and voraxin genes in male *Amblyomma hebraeum* (Acari: Ixodidae) on female engorgement and oviposition. *Exp. Appl. Acarol.* 47, 71–86. doi: 10.1007/s10493-008-9195-1

Sonenshine, D. E., Kocan, K. M., and de la Fuente, J. (2006). Tick control: further thoughts on a research agenda. *Trends Parasitol.* 22, 550–551. doi: 10.1016/j.pt.2006.09.003

Staley, J. T. (2017). Domain Cell Theory supports the independent evolution of the Eukarya, Bacteria and Archaea and the Nuclear Compartment Commonality hypothesis. *Open Biol.* 7:170041. doi: 10.1098/rsob.170041

Sun, W., Huang, H., Ma, S., Gan, X., Zhu, M., Liu, H., et al. (2016). Akirin2 could promote the proliferation but not the differentiation of duck myoblasts via the activation of the mTOR/p70S6K signaling pathway. *Int. J. Biochem. Cell. Biol.* 79, 298–307. doi: 10.1016/j.biocel.2016.08.032

Tartey, S., Matsushita, K., Imamura, T., Wakabayashi, A., Ori, D., Mino, T., et al. (2015). Essential function for the nuclear protein Akirin2 in B cell activation and humoral immune responses. *J. Immunol.* 195, 519–527. doi: 10.4049/jimmunol.1500373

Tartey, S., Matsushita, K., Vandenbon, A., Ori, D., Imamura, T., Mino, T., et al. (2014). Akirin2 is critical for inducing inflammatory genes by bridging IκB-ζ and the SWI/SNF complex. *EMBO J.* 33, 2332–2348. doi: 10.15252/embj.201488447

Torina, A., Moreno-Cid, J. A., Blanda, V., Fernández de Mera, I. G., Pérez de la Lastra, J. M., Scimeca, S., et al. (2014). Control of tick infestations and pathogen prevalence in cattle and sheep farms vaccinated with the recombinant Subolesin-Major Surface Protein 1a chimeric antigen. *Parasit. Vectors* 7:10. doi: 10.1186/1756-3305-7-10

Valenzuela-Muñoz, V., and Gallardo-Escárate, C. (2014). TLR and IMD signaling pathways from *Caligus rogercresseyi* (Crustacea: Copepoda): *in silico* gene expression and SNPs discovery. *Fish Shellfish Immunol.* 36, 428–434. doi: 10.1016/j.fsi.2013.12.019

Villar, M., Marina, A., and de la Fuente, J. (2017). Applying proteomics to tick vaccine development: where are we? *Expert Rev. Proteomics* 14, 211–221. doi: 10.1080/14789450.2017.1284590

Voigt, F., Wiedemann, L., Zuliani, C., Querques, I., Sebe, A., Mates, L., et al. (2016). Sleeping Beauty transposase structure allows rational design of hyperactive variants for genetic engineering. *Nat. Commun.* 7:11126. doi: 10.1038/ncomms11126

Wan, F., and Lenardo, M. J. (2010). The nuclear signaling of NF-kappaB: current knowledge, new insights, and future perspectives. *Cell Res.* 20, 24–33. doi: 10.1038/cr.2009.137

Wang, M., Kurland, C. G., and Caetano-Anollés, G. (2011). Reductive evolution of proteomes and protein structures. *Proc. Natl. Acad. Sci U.S.A.* 108, 11954–11958. doi: 10.1073/pnas.1017361108

Watanabe, N., Satoh, Y., Fujita, T., Ohta, T., Kose, H., Muramatsu, Y., et al. (2011). Distribution of allele frequencies at TTN g.231054C > T, RPL27A g.3109537C > T and AKIRIN2 c.*188G > A between Japanese Black and four other cattle breeds with differing historical selection for marbling. *BMC Res. Notes* 4:10. doi: 10.1186/1756-0500-4-10

Wolf, Y. I., and Koonin, E. V. (2013). Genome reduction as the dominant mode of evolution. *Bioessays* 35, 829–837. doi: 10.1002/bies.201300037

Xue, X., Wang, L., Chen, Y., Zhang, X., Luo, H., Li, Z., et al. (2014). Identification and molecular characterization of an Akirin2 homolog in Chinese loach (*Paramisgurnus dabryanus*). *Fish Shellfish Immunol.* 36, 435–443. doi: 10.1016/j.fsi.2013.12.021

Yan, J., Dong, X., Kong, Y., Zhang, Y., Jing, R., and Feng, L. (2013). Identification and primary immune characteristics of an amphioxus akirin homolog. *Fish Shellfish Immunol.* 35, 564–571. doi: 10.1016/j.fsi.2013.05.020

Yang, C. G., Wang, X. L., Wang, L., Zhang, B., and Chen, S. L. (2011). A new Akirin1 gene in turbot (*Scophthalmus maximus*): molecular cloning, characterization and expression analysis in response to bacterial and viral immunological challenge. *Fish Shellfish Immunol* 30, 1031–1041. doi: 10.1016/j.fsi.2011.01.028

Yang, C. G., Wang, X. L., Zhang, B., Sun, B., Liu, S. S., and Chen, S. L. (2013). Screening and analysis of PoAkirin1 and two related genes in response to immunological stimulants in the Japanese flounder (*Paralichthys olivaceus*). *BMC Mol. Biol.* 14:10. doi: 10.1186/1471-2199-14-10

Zanesi, N., Balatti, V., Riordan, J., Burch, A., Rizzotto, L., Palamarchuk, A., et al. (2013). A Sleeping Beauty screen reveals NF-kB activation in CLL mouse model. *Blood* 121, 4355–4358. doi: 10.1182/blood-2013-02-486035

Zhang, Y. (2008). I-TASSER server for protein 3D structure prediction. *BMC Bioinformatics* 9:40. doi: 10.1186/1471-2105-9-40

Zivkovic, Z., Esteves, E., Almazán, C., Daffre, S., Nijhof, A. M., Kocan, K. M., et al. (2010a). Differential expression of genes in salivary glands of male *Rhipicephalus (Boophilus) microplus* in response to infection with *Anaplasma marginale*. *BMC Genomics* 11:186. doi: 10.1186/1471-2164-11-186

Zivkovic, Z., Torina, A., Mitra, R., Alongi, A., Scimeca, S., Kocan, K. M., et al. (2010b). Subolesin expression in response to pathogen infection in ticks. *BMC Immunol.* 11:7. doi: 10.1186/1471-2172-11-7

8

Ultrastructural and Cytotoxic Effects of *Metarhizium robertsii* Infection on *Rhipicephalus microplus* Hemocytes

Jéssica Fiorotti*[1], *Rubem Figueiredo Sadok Menna-Barreto*[2], *Patrícia Silva Gôlo*[3], *Caio Junior Balduino Coutinho-Rodrigues*[1], *Ricardo Oliveira Barbosa Bitencourt*[1], *Diva Denelle Spadacci-Morena*[4], *Isabele da Costa Angelo*[5] and *Vânia Rita Elias Pinheiro Bittencourt*[3]

[1] *Programa de Pós-Graduação em Ciências Veterinárias, Instituto de Veterinária, Universidade Federal Rural do Rio de Janeiro, Seropédica, Brazil,* [2] *Laboratório de Biologia Celular, IOC, Fundação Oswaldo Cruz, Rio de Janeiro, Brazil,* [3] *Departamento de Parasitologia Animal, Instituto de Veterinária, Universidade Federal Rural do Rio de Janeiro, Seropédica, Brazil,* [4] *Laboratório de Fisiopatologia, Instituto Butantan, São Paulo, Brazil,* [5] *Departamento de Epidemiologia e Saúde Pública, Instituto de Veterinária, Universidade Federal Rural do Rio de Janeiro, Seropédica, Brazil*

***Correspondence:**
Vânia Rita Elias Pinheiro Bittencourt
vaniabit@ufrrj.br

Metarhizium is an entomopathogenic fungus widely employed in the biological control of arthropods. Hemocytes present in the hemolymph of invertebrates are the cells involved in the immune response of arthropods. Despite this, knowledge about *Rhipicephalus microplus* hemocytes morphological aspects as well as their role in response to the fungal infection is scarce. The present study aimed to analyze the hemocytes of *R. microplus* females after *Metarhizium robertsii* infection, using light and electron microscopy approaches associated with the cytotoxicity evaluation. Five types of hemocytes (prohemocytes, spherulocytes, plasmatocytes, granulocytes, and oenocytoids) were described in the hemolymph of uninfected ticks, while only prohemocytes, granulocytes, and plasmatocytes were observed in fungus-infected tick females. Twenty-four hours after the fungal infection, only granulocytes and plasmatocytes were detected in the transmission electron microscopy analysis. Hemocytes from fungus-infected tick females showed several cytoplasmic vacuoles with different electron densities, and lipid droplets in close contact to low electron density vacuoles, as well as the formation of autophagosomes and subcellular material in different stages of degradation could also be observed. *M. robertsii* propagules were more toxic to tick hemocytes in the highest concentration tested (1.0×10^8 conidia mL^{-1}). Interestingly, the lowest fungus concentration did not affect significantly the cell viability. Microanalysis showed that cells granules from fungus-infected and uninfected ticks had similar composition. This study addressed the first report of fungal cytotoxicity analyzing ultrastructural effects on hemocytes of *R. microplus* infected with entomopathogenic fungi. These results open new perspectives for the comprehension of ticks physiology and pathology, allowing the identification of new targets for the biological control.

Keywords: entomopathogenic fungi, cell death, fungal infection, tick, immunity

INTRODUCTION

Ticks are obligate hematophagous ectoparasites relevant to public and veterinary health (De la Fuente et al., 2008; Kernif et al., 2016). The cattle tick, *Rhipicephalus microplus*, has an enormous negative impact on livestock. The economic impact has increased, particularly in tropical countries and financial losses of USD 3.24 billion per year only in Brazil have been reported (Grisi et al., 2014). The improper use of chemical acaricides is frequently reported and causes the raising of resistant tick populations in addition to the environmental, meat, and milk contamination. Accordingly, alternative control methods using entomopathogenic fungi have been studied to decrease the use of these chemicals (Schank and Vainstein, 2010; Camargo et al., 2012; Perinotto et al., 2017).

Metarhizium anisopliae sensu lato (s.l.) is a complex of species of cosmopolitan entomopathogenic fungi which includes species that can infect specific hosts, as *Metarhizium acridum* with Orthoptera insects, or a wider range of insect groups, such as *Metarhizium robertsii* and *M. anisopliae* sensu stricto (s.s.). These fungi are also considered endophytes and rhizosphere competent (Hu et al., 2014; Vega, 2018). All *R. microplus* life stages have been shown to be sensitive to entomopathogenic fungal infection (Alonso-Díaz et al., 2007; Leemon and Jonsson, 2008), either *in vitro* assays (Perinotto et al., 2017), associated with chemical acaricides (Bahiense et al., 2008; Webster et al., 2015), or *in vivo* tests using available commercial products (Camargo et al., 2016).

Metarhizium infection starts with the fungal propagule attachment on the hosts' surface and active penetration (Madelin et al., 1967). After penetration, the hyphae present in the hemolymph differentiate into blastospores and the host dies due to a set of occurrences such as: physical damage, pathological changes occurring in the hemolymph, histolytic action, blocking of the digestive system, and even production of micotoxins (Bidochka et al., 1997; Alves, 1998; Roberts and St Leger, 2004). Nevertheless, the host can fight against the fungal infection triggering its immune system by starting processes such as phagocytosis, nodule formation, melanization, encapsulation, and secretion of antimicrobial peptides (Kopácek et al., 2010; Hajdušek et al., 2013).

Tick immune system is composed of humoral and cellular defense responses (Schmidt et al., 2001; Lavine and Strand, 2002). In general, the humoral immune response involves several antimicrobial peptides, reactive oxygen species and enzymatic cascades that regulate coagulation and hemolytic melanization processes (Gillespie et al., 1997; Smith and Pal, 2014). The cellular reactions are triggered immediately after the microorganism invasion and directly involve the attack of these microorganisms by hemocytes (Tan et al., 2013). Hemocytes are circulating cells present in the hemolymph that also be found connected to the fatty body, nephrocytes, and salivary glands (Sterba et al., 2011). Innate immune mechanisms have already been reported for several invertebrates (Brayner et al., 2007; Nation, 2016; Iacovone et al., 2018), including ticks (Gillespie et al., 1997; Johns et al., 2001; Feitosa et al., 2015), considering phagocytosis as the most important innate response (Bayne, 1990; Ehlers et al., 1992), that in ticks is mediated mainly by granulocytes and plasmatocytes (Dolp, 1970; Fujisaki et al., 1975; Kuhn and Haug, 1995; Zhioua et al., 1996; Inoue et al., 2001; Borovicková and Hypsa, 2005; Feitosa et al., 2018). Despite this, little has been reported about cellular immune response in *R. microplus* ticks, since most studies are based on the tick humoral responses (Nakajima et al., 2003; Fogaça et al., 2004; Angelo et al., 2014; Chávez et al., 2017).

Hemocytes are extremely relevant for studies about interactions between the host and its pathogens (Jones, 1962; Crossley, 1975; Lackie, 1980; Gupta, 1986; Paskewitz and Christensen, 1996; Chen and Lu, 2018; Iacovone et al., 2018). Arthropods' hemocytes classification and terminology were framed mostly based on insect studies, while this literature is still scarce for ticks (Nevermann et al., 1991; Borovicková and Hypsa, 2005; Araújo et al., 2008; Cunha et al., 2009; Laughton et al., 2011). Additionally, compared to insects, literature about the cell response of ticks challenged with pathogens is poorly explored.

Studies reported that circulating hemocytes of adult mosquitoes infected with pathogens may decrease (Hillyer et al., 2005; Castillo et al., 2006, 2011; Brayner et al., 2007; Bryant and Michael, 2014) and have their morphology altered (Au et al., 2003; Kwon et al., 2014). It is known that the number of circulating hemocytes of *R. microplus* ticks infected with entomopathogenic fungi dropped off in comparison to uninfected females (De Paulo et al., 2018), despite this, to the present date, alterations in the morphology of hemocytes from *R. microplus* ticks infected with pathogens have not been reported yet, as studies were conducted mainly with *R. sanguineus* and *Dermacentor variabilis* ticks (Eggenberger et al., 1990; Ceraul et al., 2002; Feitosa et al., 2015, 2018). Undoubtedly, further approaches to understand the immune system of ticks have to overcome the discussion of hemocyte types, especially when its identification is based just on morphological analyzes, while histochemical differentiation and functional aspects are largely neglected. Accordingly, the aim of this study was to analyze the hemocytes of *R. microplus* females infected or not by *M. robertsii*, using light microscopy, cytotoxicity test, transmission electron microscopy (TEM), and transmission electron microscopy with energy-dispersive X-ray spectrometer (TEM-EDS).

MATERIALS AND METHODS

Fungal Isolate and Tick Obtainment

One fungal isolate, *M. robertsii* ARSEF 2575, was used in the present study. The fungal isolate was obtained from the Agriculture Research Service Collection of Entomopathogenic Fungal Cultures (ARSEF) (USDA-US Plant, Soil and Nutrition Laboratory, Ithaca, NY, United States). Cultures were grown on PDA (potato dextrose agar) at 25°C ± 1°C and ≥80 relative humidity (RH) for 14 days. A conidial suspension was used to infect the ticks.

Rhipicephalus microplus fully engorged ticks were obtained from artificially infested animals [the present experiment was part of a project approved by the Veterinary Institute Ethics Committee of the Federal Rural University of Rio de Janeiro (CEUA UFRRJ no. 037/2014)]. After collection on the stalls floor, fully engorged tick females were immersed in running water followed by 0.05% sodium hypochlorite solution for three min, then dried, identified and weighed for homogeneous division of the groups.

Entomopathogenic Fungi Inoculation Into *R. microplus* Ticks

Fungal suspensions were prepared by suspending *M. robertsii* ARSEF 2575 conidia in 0.1% polyoxyethylene sorbitan monooleate (Tween®80) sterile aqueous solution (v/v). For fungal inoculation, engorged females were divided into seven homogeneously weighed groups with 20 females each (for the bioassay) and three homogeneously weighed groups with 20 females each (for the microscopy analysis). The negative control group did not receive any treatment (tick females under physiological conditions), and treated females were inoculated with 5 μL of ARSEF 2575 fungal suspension or 5 μL 0.1% Tween®80 aqueous solution (v/v) into the foramen located between the dorsal scutum and the capitulum, using an insulin syringe (Johns et al., 1998). All the experiments were performed in triplicate (except the bioassay) and repeated three times.

Bioassay With Engorged Females

Tick females were homogeneously weighed based on the Yule's formula (Sampaio, 2002). Groups were inoculated as mentioned before and divided as follows: A group was treated with 5 μL 0.1% Tween®80 aqueous solution (v/v) and the fungus-infected groups were infected with six different fungal concentrations (1.0×10^3, 10^4, 10^5, 10^6, 10^7 or 10^8 conidia mL^{-1}). Fungal suspensions were adjusted to each concentration using Neubauer's chamber. Fungal concentrations that were used in the present bioassay were the same used in the forward described cell viability test. The highest concentration (1.0×10^8 conidia mL^{-1}) was defined based on the concentration commonly used for topical treatments in ticks. Tick females were maintained at 27 ± 1°C and ≥80% RH in the dark. Tick mortality was recorded 24 and 48 h after the treatments.

Hemolymph Collection

Ticks infected with fungi (each tick infected with 5 μL of 1.0×10^7 conidia mL^{-1}, a sublethal concentration), ticks inoculated with Tween®80 aqueous solution (v/v) and the negative control group (ticks under physiological conditions, a untreated group) had their hemolymph collected according to Angelo et al. (2010) through the ruptured cuticle at the dorsal surface of the tick female using a needle, 24 h after infection. The hemolymph drops were collected with a capillary glass coupled to a flexible rubber. Samples were placed in microtubes containing 30 μL protease inhibitor cocktail (Inhibit®Sigma-Aldrich) and 82 μL saline buffer (1.5 M NaCl, 50 mM EDTA, pH 7.2). Microtubes were kept on ice throughout the collection.

Cell Viability Test

Three hundred engorged tick females were used for the cell viability test. Hemolymph of uninfected females was collected and the hemocytes harvested according to De Paulo et al. (2018). Hemocytes were resuspended in 50 mL sterilized Leibovitz's L-15 culture medium (Gibco®) at double strength, supplemented with 20% fetal bovine serum (FBS), 2 g. L^{-1} glucose, and 100 UI mL^{-1} penicillin, adjusted to pH 7.0–7.2. Cells were then seeded into 96 well plates at 5×10^4 cells mL^{-1} in a final volume of 170 μL culture medium. Cells were allowed to attach to the well surface for 1 h. Hemocytes were then exposed to 10 μL conidial suspensions using six different concentrations (1.0×10^3, 10^4, 10^5, 10^6, 10^7, or 10^8 conidia mL^{-1}) chosen to make it possible to assemble a kinetic curve. 24 h after fungal exposure, 20 μL of resazurin (Sigma-Aldrich) at 0.13 mg mL^{-1} were added in each well, and the plate incubated for 1, 2, 3, and 4 h. Fluorescence was read using a microplate reader Chameleon (Hidex®) at 530 nm excitation and 590 nm emission. Relative hemocyte viability was calculated considered unexposed cells as controls (≈100% viability). Experiments were carried out in triplicate and repeated three times with new engorged females and a new batch of fungus.

Light Microscopy Analysis

Hemolymph Smear

Drops from total hemolymph (plasma and hemocytes) of untreated ticks (negative control group), ticks inoculated with 0.1% Tween®80 and ticks infected with 10^7 conidia mL^{-1} were collected 24 h after infection and placed directly onto glass slides, dried at room temperature for 20–30 min, and fixed in methanol PA (Sigma-Aldrich) for 3 min. Slides were then stained with Giemsa (Sigma-Aldrich) [diluted 1:9 in buffered distilled water Brayner et al. (2005)] for 30 min, rapidly washed with buffered distilled water, and observed by light microscope. Five stained slides were performed per group. One hundred cells per slide were count for differential hemocytes counts. Differential hemocytes counts were expressed based on the amount of each hemocyte type in the total cells counted.

Hemocytes in Historesin

For light microscopy, hemocytes from ticks infected with 10^7 conidia mL^{-1} (collected 24 h after infection) and hemocytes from Tween-inoculated ticks were removed from plasma (De Paulo et al., 2018) and immediately immersed in 4% paraformaldehyde in 0.2 M Millonig buffer (pH 7. 2) for 6 h at room temperature. Samples were then centrifuged at 500 × *g* for 3 min, supernatant was discarded, the hemocytes pellet dehydrated in ascending ethanol series (70–100%), embedded in pure historesin overnight, and finally embedded in historesin plus hardener (Leica) at 4°C for 24 h. Three micrometers thick histological sections were stained with methylene blue for morphological studies. The sections were observed and photographed under a DM LS (Leica) light microscope coupled to a DFC420 camera (Leica) and Leica Application Suite version 3.1.0 imaging software.

Transmission Electron Microscopy

Hemocytes from infected ticks (10^7 conidia mL^{-1}), ticks inoculated with Tween®80 and untreated ticks were collected 24 h after infection, removed from plasma (De Paulo et al., 2018), and fixed in 2% glutaraldehyde for 3 h at 4°C. The samples were then centrifuged at 500 × *g* for 3 min, the supernatant was discarded, the cells' pellet was washed in 0.2 M Millonig buffer for 15 min, centrifuged at 500 × *g* for 3 min, and then post-fixed in 1% OsO_4 at room temperature for 3 h. After that, pellets were washed in Millonig buffer, dehydrated in ascending acetone series (30, 50, 70, 90, and 100%), pre-embedded in Polybed 812 resin-acetone (1:1) overnight at room temperature, and embedded in pure resin at room temperature for 8 h. After resin polymerization (72 h) at 60°C, ultrathin sections were obtained, stained with uranyl acetate and lead citrate. The examination was performed in Jeol 100 CX II and LEO EM 906E transmission electron microscope.

X-Ray Microanalysis of Cells Granules

The chemical composition of *R. microplus* granulocytes' granules was determined by energy-dispersive X-ray spectrometer (TEM-EDS, H7650/Hitachi H-700 FA). Hemocytes from Tween-inoculated ticks and fungus-infected ticks (10^7 conidia mL^{-1}) were prepared as described for transmission electron microscopy and a quantitative characteristic of ions and maps of their distribution were obtained with a Hitachi H-8100 TEM microscope (Hitachi, Tokyo, Japan) equipped with energy-dispersive X-ray spectrometer (EDS, OXFORD INCA x-sight, Abingdon, Oxfordshire, United Kingdom).

Statistical Analysis

Bioassay data were analyzed by one-way ANOVA followed by Newman-Keuls Multiple Comparison Test ($P \leq 0.05$). Cell viability data were analyzed by one-way ANOVA followed by Tukey's test for pair-wise comparisons ($P \leq 0.05$). For analysis of hemocytes populations, multiple *t*-tests were used for pair-wise comparisons ($P \leq 0.05$). All data were analyzed through GraphPad Prism version 5.00 for Windows (GraphPad Software, San Diego, CA, United States).

RESULTS

Bioassay With Engorged Females

Conidia of *M. robertsii* isolate ARSEF 2575 used to infect adult females had 98% germination after incubation for 24 h at 27 ± 1°C and ≥80% RH. Females' mortality percent is shown in **Figure 1**. In general, tick mortality was proportional to conidial concentration, (i.e., the higher the conidial concentration, the higher the tick mortality) (**Figures 1A,B**). Ticks infected with 10^7 conidia mL^{-1} showed 21% ± 2.35 mortality 24 h after infection and 48% ± 2.35 mortality 48 h after infection, while ticks infected with 10^8 conidia mL^{-1} had 31,66% ± 2.0 and 83,3% ± 4.71 mortality 24 and 48 h after infection, respectively.

Cell Viability Test

The kinetic curve shows hemocytes viability 24 h after fungal exposure in different times of incubation with resazurin (**Figure 2**). It was possible to observe that hemocytes viability was similar 3 and 4 h after incubation (**Figure 2**). *M. robertsii* ARSEF 2575 conidia were more toxic to *R. microplus* hemocytes at 10^7 conidia mL^{-1} and 10^8 conidia mL^{-1}, reducing cell viability in 15, 53% ± 1.58 and 36.1% ± 1.48 24 h after the fungal addition, respectively (**Figure 3**). Despite lower fungal concentrations (10^3, 10^4, 10^5, and 10^6 conidia mL^{-1}) can also influence cell viability, drastic reductions started at the higher concentrations (i.e., 10^7 and 10^8).

Light Microscopy Analysis

Prohemocytes, spherulocytes, granulocytes, plasmatocytes, and oenocytoids were observed in both engorged *R. microplus* females under physiological conditions and tween-inoculated ticks after Giemsa staining. The concentration of these hemocytes was the same for both groups (**Figure 4**). On the other hand, when engorged females were infected with *M. robertsii*, spherulocytes and oenocytoids were not observed. In addition, prohemocytes and granulocytes were present in the same amounts in controls and fungus-infected groups, only plasmatocytes amounts were statistically different between uninfected (negative control and tween-inoculated) and infected groups. All cells had the basophilic nucleus and the following characteristics: Prohemocytes (ranging from 8 to 10 μm) as relatively small cells, with large nucleus (**Figures 5A, 6A**). Granulocytes (measuring approximately 12 to 15 μm) as circular cells that were observed in two different forms: with a more central

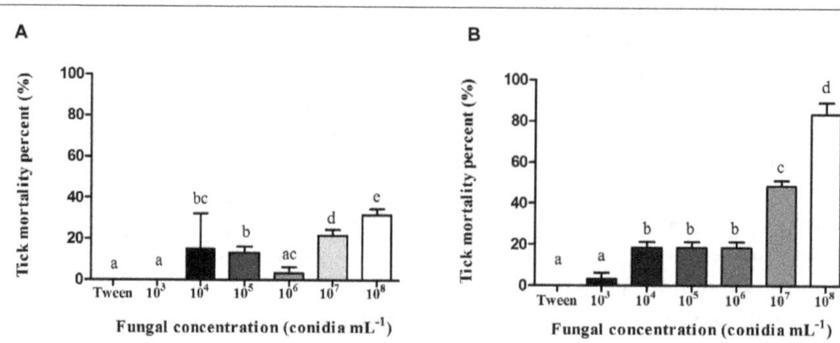

FIGURE 1 | Mean percent (%) mortality and standard deviation of *Rhipicephalus microplus* adult females infected with *Metarhizium robertsii* ARSEF 2575 conidia in different concentrations (1.0 × 10^3, 10^4, 10^5, 10^6, 10^7 and 10^8 conidia mL^{-1}). Each group had 20 tick females. Mortality percent was recorded **(A)** 24 h and **(B)** 48 h after fungal inoculation. Mean values (±) standard deviation followed for the same letter do not differ statistically by ANOVA test ($P \geq 0.05$). The bioassay was conducted three times, on three different days, using new ticks and conidial preparations each day.

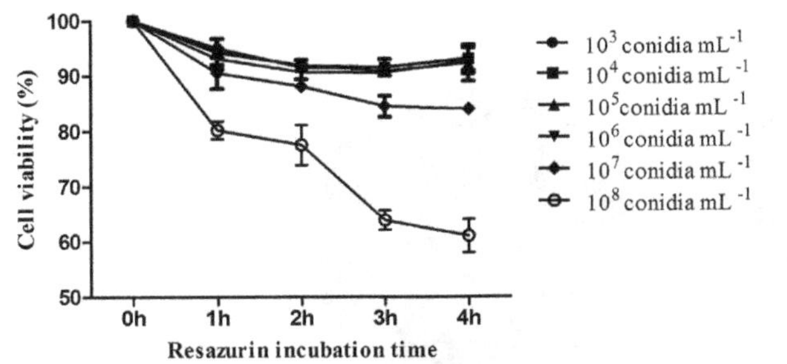

FIGURE 2 | *In vitro* cytotoxic assay of *Metarhizium robertsii* ARSEF 2575 against *Rhipicephalus microplus* hemocytes using a resazurin-based assay (to evaluate cell viability). *R. microplus* hemocytes were exposed to different concentrations (1.0 × 10^3, 10^4, 10^5, 10^6, 10^7, and 10^8 conidia mL^{-1}) of fungal suspensions. Twenty-four hours after exposure, resazurin was used for four different incubation times (1, 2, 3, and 4 h). ANOVA followed by Tukey's test was used. Experiments were repeated with at least three independent biological samples.

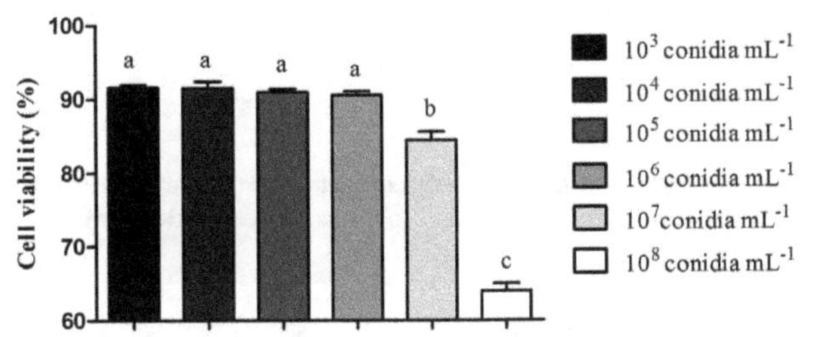

FIGURE 3 | Effect of *Metarhizium robertsii* on the cellular proliferation of *Rhipicephalus microplus* hemocytes at 3 h incubation with resazurin. Mean values (±) standard deviation followed for the same letter do not differ statistically by ANOVA test ($P \geq 0.05$). Experiments were repeated with at least three independent biological samples.

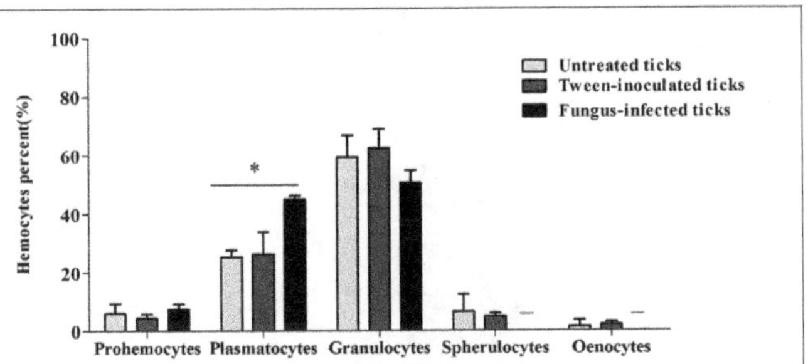

FIGURE 4 | Mean percent and standard deviation of *Rhipicephalus microplus* hemocytes population (prohemocytes, granulocytes, plasmatocytes, spherulocytes and oenocytoids) of untreated tick females (ticks under physiological conditions), tween-inoculated ticks and fungus-infected ticks. *R. microplus* females were infected with *Metarhizium robertsii* ARSEF 2575. Mean values (±) standard deviation followed by * differ statistically by multiple *t*-tests ($P \leq 0.05$). A total of 100 cells were counted in each slide (five slides were analyzed for each group). Experiments were repeated with at least three independent biological samples.

nucleus or eccentric nucleus (**Figures 5B,C, 6B,C**). Spherulocytes (measuring approximately 12 to 15 μm) had oval shape, with spherules in the cytoplasm (**Figures 5D, 6D**). Plasmatocytes (measuring approximately 20 μm) presented a varied shape, with the nucleus displaced of the central region of the cell; some plasmatocytes had pseudopodia (**Figures 5E, 6E**). Oenocytoids were larger-sized (approximately 20 μm) exhibiting the nucleus displaced of the central region of the cells (**Figures 5F, 6F**). Additionally, spherulocytes, plasmatocytes, and oenocytoids exhibited poorly Giemsa-stained areas (**Figures 5D–F, 6D–F**). Granulocytes from fungus-infected ticks showed fewer granules than hemocytes from untreated or tween-inoculated ticks. Prohemocytes were similar in uninfected or fungus-infected females (**Figure 5A, 6A, 7A**). The cells' cytoplasm from infected ticks showed heterogeneity (**Figure 7B**) and also intense vacuolization (**Figure 7C**).

Historesin analysis was used to compare the hemocytes types [i.e., prohemocytes, granulocytes, and plasmatocytes (**Figure 8**)] observed in both fungus-infected and tween-inoculated ticks. After fungal infection, prohemocytes had the same morphology than the prohemocytes from tween-inoculated tick females (**Figures 8A,D**). Despite this, granulocytes apparently lost granules, since cells from infected females had fewer granules than the granulocytes from uninfected ticks (**Figures 8B,E**). Plasmatocytes of fungus-infected females also showed morphological changes, exhibiting vacuoles in their cytoplasm (**Figures 8C,F**).

Transmission Electron Microscopy Analysis

Based on presence or absence of granules, cell shape, presence or absence of pseudopodia, nucleus location, endocytic activity, endoplasmic reticulum and homogeneity of the cytoplasm, *R. microplus* hemocytes were classified as follows: Prohemocytes: small cells with a large and central nucleus, none or few granules, and mitochondria (**Figures 9A, 10A**). Granulocytes: exhibited central or eccentric nuclei, cytoplasmic projections and lots of granules with different electron densities (**Figures 9B,C, 10B,C**). Spherulocytes: large cells with homogeneous electron densities spherules occupying virtually the entire cytoplasm (**Figures 9D, 10D**). Plasmatocytes: variable sized cells with no or few granular inclusions in the cytoplasm and pseudopodia (**Figures 9E,F, 10E,F**). Oenocytoids were not observed in TEM analysis. No differences were observed between untreated and tween-inoculated tick females, except granulocytes from ticks under physiological conditions apparently exhibited more plasma membrane projections (**Figures 9C, 10C**).

Some morphological differences were observed in hemocytes of *R. microplus* ticks after fungal infection. Twenty-four hours after infection, prohemocytes, spherulocytes and oenocytoids could not be observed, only granulocytes and plasmatocytes. Plasmatocytes had intense cytoplasmic vacuolization and double wall fungal conidia in the cytoplasm (**Figures 11A–D**), suggesting phagocytosis of conidia. In addition, these cells displayed autophagosome with material at different stages of degradation, plasma membrane rupture, suggesting a necrosis process, healthy mitochondria, nucleus with normal appearance and an increased endoplasmic reticulum. Granulocytes from fungus-infected ticks had fewer granules than granulocytes of uninfected

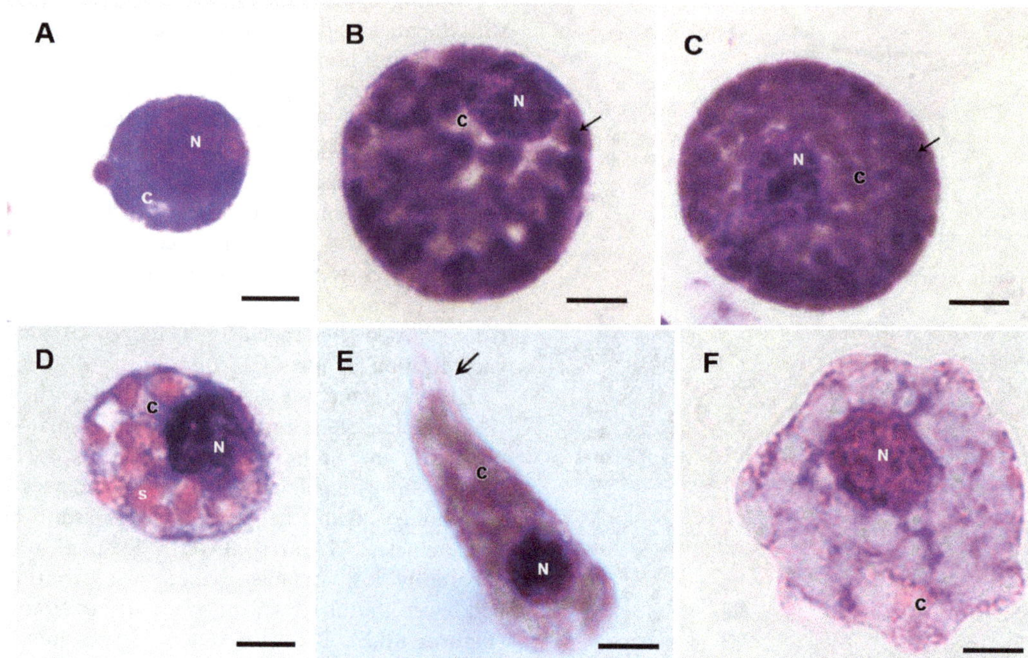

FIGURE 5 | Hemocytes representation found in the hemolymph of *R. microplus* engorged females under physiological conditions (untreated ticks) after Giemsa staining. **(A)** Prohemocyte, **(B,C)** Granulocyte, **(D)** Spherulocyte, **(E)** Plasmatocyte and **(F)** Oenocyte. Nucleus (N), cytoplasm (c), granules (thin black arrow), spherules (s) and pseudopodia (thick black arrow). Bars = 5 μm.

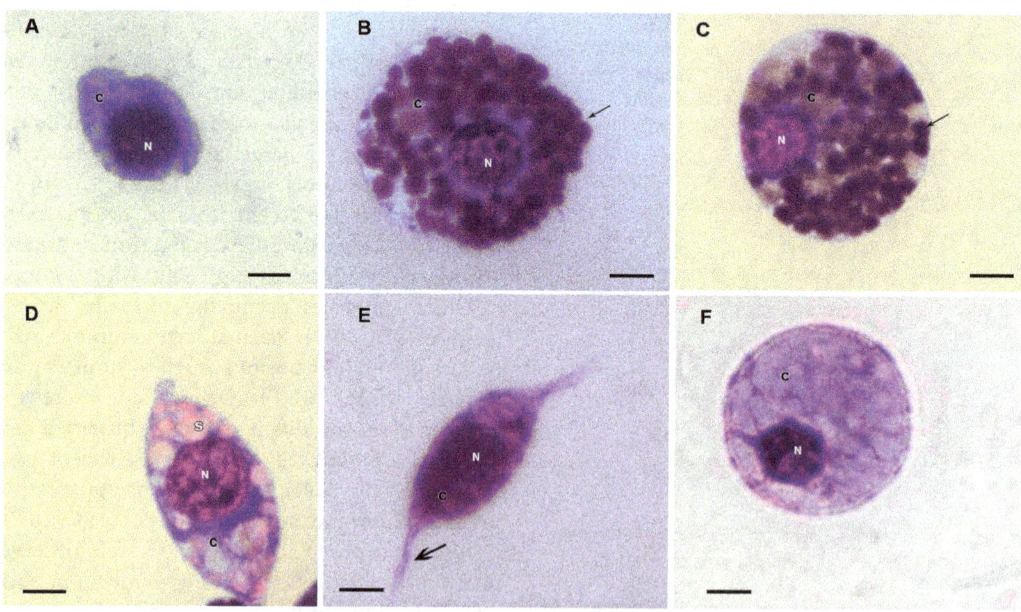

FIGURE 6 | Hemocytes representation found in the hemolymph of *R. microplus* engorged females from tween-inoculated ticks after Giemsa staining. **(A)** Prohemocyte, **(B,C)** Granulocyte, **(D)** Spherulocyte, **(E)** Plasmatocyte and **(F)** Oenocyte. Nucleus (N), cytoplasm (c), granules (thin black arrow), spherules (s) and pseudopodia (thick black arrow). Bars = 5 μm.

ticks, also exhibited autophagosomes with material at different stages of degradation and the presence of multivesicular bodies (**Figures 11E,F**). Hemocytes from fungus-infected tick females had nuclei showing extensive regions of euchromatin, several cytoplasmic vacuoles with different electron densities, subcellular material in degradation stage or already degraded, and the presence of autophagosome or multivesicular bodies, suggesting an autophagy process (**Figure 11**).

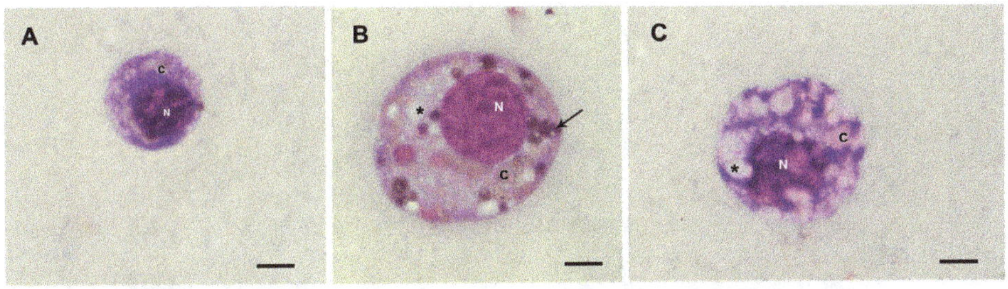

FIGURE 7 | Hemocytes representation found in the hemolymph of *R. microplus* engorged females from fungus-infected ticks after Giemsa staining. **(A)** Prohemocyte, **(B)** Granulocyte and **(C)** Plasmatocyte. Nucleus (N), cytoplasm (c), vacuoles (*) and granules (thin black arrow). Bars = 5 μm.

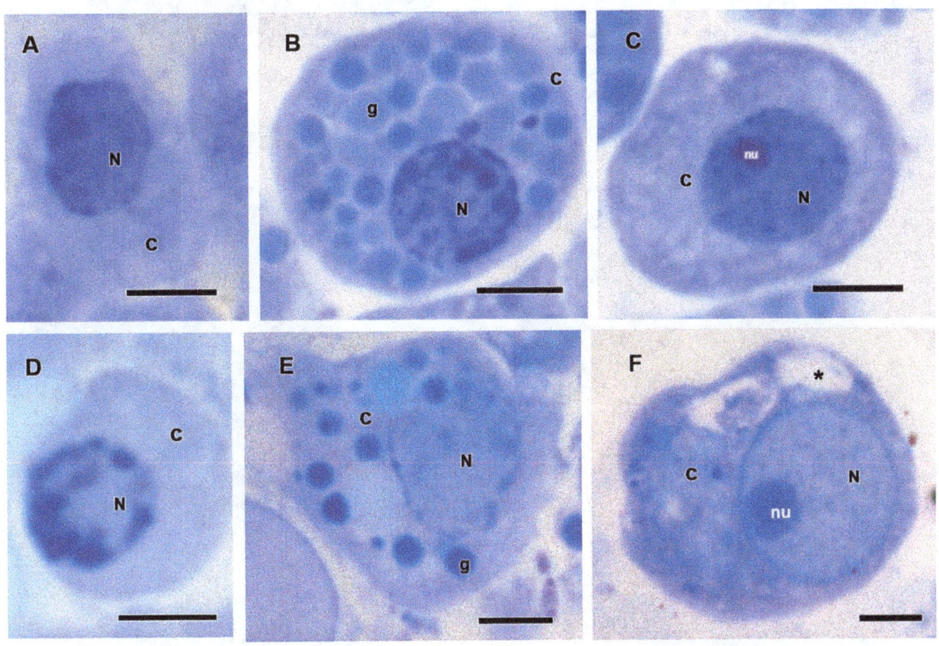

FIGURE 8 | Hemocytes representation found in the hemolymph of *Rhipicephalus microplus* engorged females **(A–C)** inoculated with 0.1% Tween®80 aqueous solution (v/v) or **(D–F)** infected with *Metarhizium robertsii* after methylene blue staining. Prohemocytes **(A)** from tween-inoculated ticks and **(D)** from fungus-infected ticks; granulocytes **(B)** from tween-inoculated ticks and **(E)** from fungus-infected ticks; plasmatocytes from **(C)** tween-inoculated group and **(F)** from fungus-infected ticks. Nucleus (N), cytoplasm (c), nucleolus (nu), granule (g) and vacuoles (*). Bars = 5 μm.

Characterization of Cells Granules by Microanalysis

Microanalysis demonstrated that *M. robertsii* ARSEF 2575 infection did not affect the composition of *R. microplus* granulocytes' electron dense granules (**Figure 12**). Granules of granulocytes from tween-inoculated ticks and fungus-infected ticks were composed only by oxygen and carbon.

DISCUSSION

Some entomopathogenic fungi are known to be highly virulent to ticks, as well as to different species of insects (Roberts and St Leger, 2004; Wang and St Leger, 2006; Leemon and Jonsson, 2008; Samish et al., 2014; Perinotto et al., 2017). Interestingly, entomopathogenic fungi have a variety of mechanisms that can neutralize the host defenses, such as the production of secondary metabolites able to suppress the insect immune system (Dubovskiy et al., 2013). This suppression of immune reactions is one of the main mechanisms governing the outcome of relations between a host and an invader. Furthermore, *Metarhizium* spreads in nutrient-rich hemocoel through immunological evasion and adaptation to osmotic stress (Wang and St Leger, 2006; Huang et al., 2015). Here, *M. robertsii* ARSEF 2575 was virulent to *R. microplus* engorged females after fungal inoculation. Several factors are involved in the virulence of a fungal isolate to arthropods, especially ticks that are much less susceptible than insects (Rot et al., 2013; Erler and Ates, 2015; Mohammadyani et al., 2016; Alves et al., 2017; Fischhoff et al., 2017). Distinct fungal virulence to different populations of the same host (Perinotto et al., 2012), host species, life stage of the host (i.e., some species and stages are more susceptible than

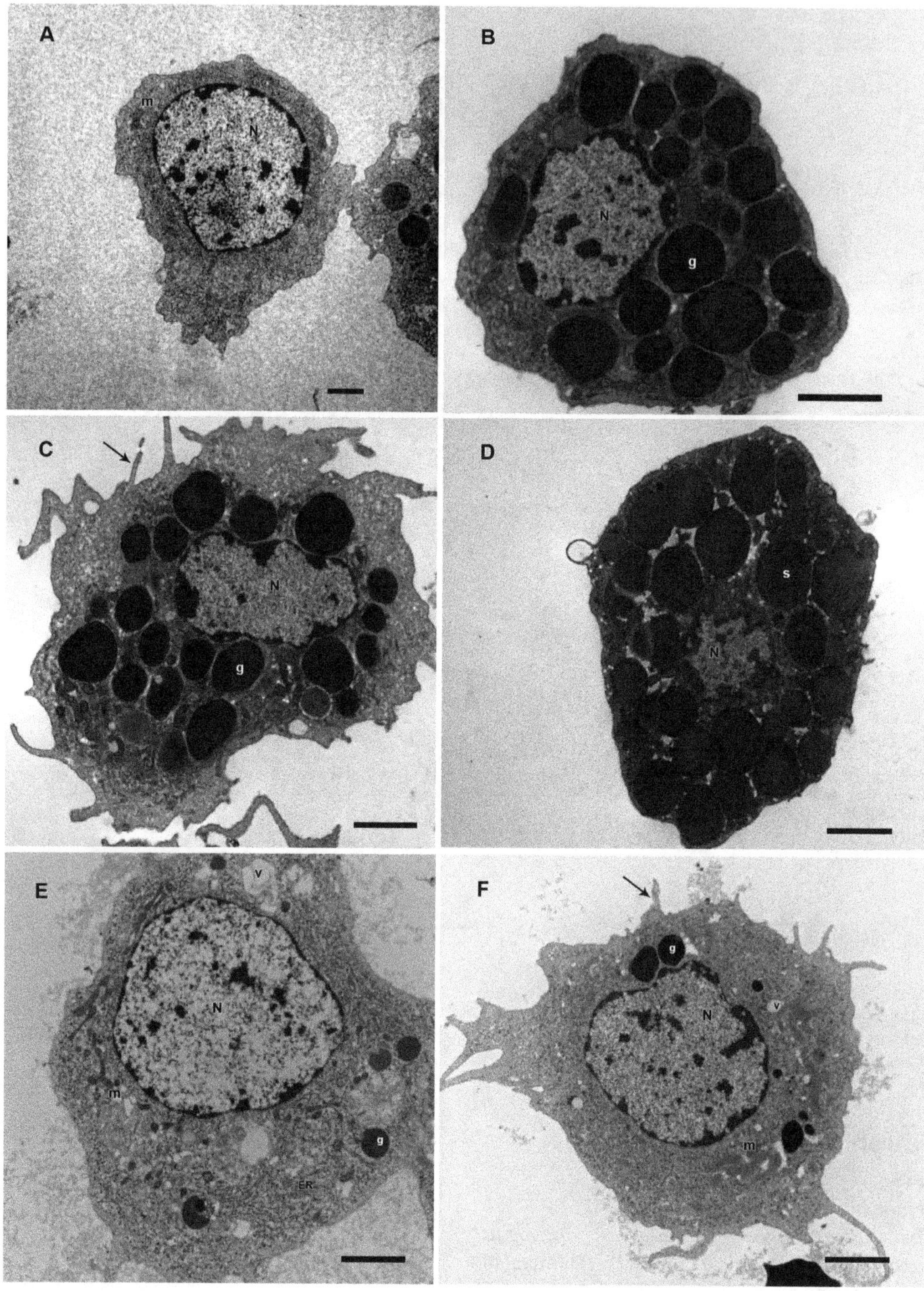

FIGURE 9 | Electromicrographs of *R. microplus* hemocytes in normal physiological conditions (untreated-ticks). **(A)** Prohemocyte with nucleus (N) and mitochondria (m) in its cytoplasm. **(B,C)** Granulocytes with nucleus (N), electron dense granules (g), and plasma membrane projection (black arrow). **(D)** Spherulocyte with nucleus (N) and spherules (s) in the cytoplasm. **(E,F)** Plasmatocytes with nucleus (N), mitochondria (m), endoplasmic reticulum (ER), electron dense granules (g), vacuole (v), and plasma membrane projections (black arrow). Bars = 2 μm.

others), and the quantity of fungal propagules applied to the arthropod pest (Alden et al., 2001; Ment et al., 2012) are some of these factors. Analyzing the results of the present study, the highest fungal concentration (i.e., 1.0×10^8 conidia mL^{-1}, the one more frequently used for tick control) in the longest time of infection (i.e., 48 h) yielded the best tick mortality rate; while the lowest fungal concentrations (i.e., 1.0×10^4, 10^5, and 10^6 conidia mL^{-1}) resulted in similar mortality rates. Despite the longer

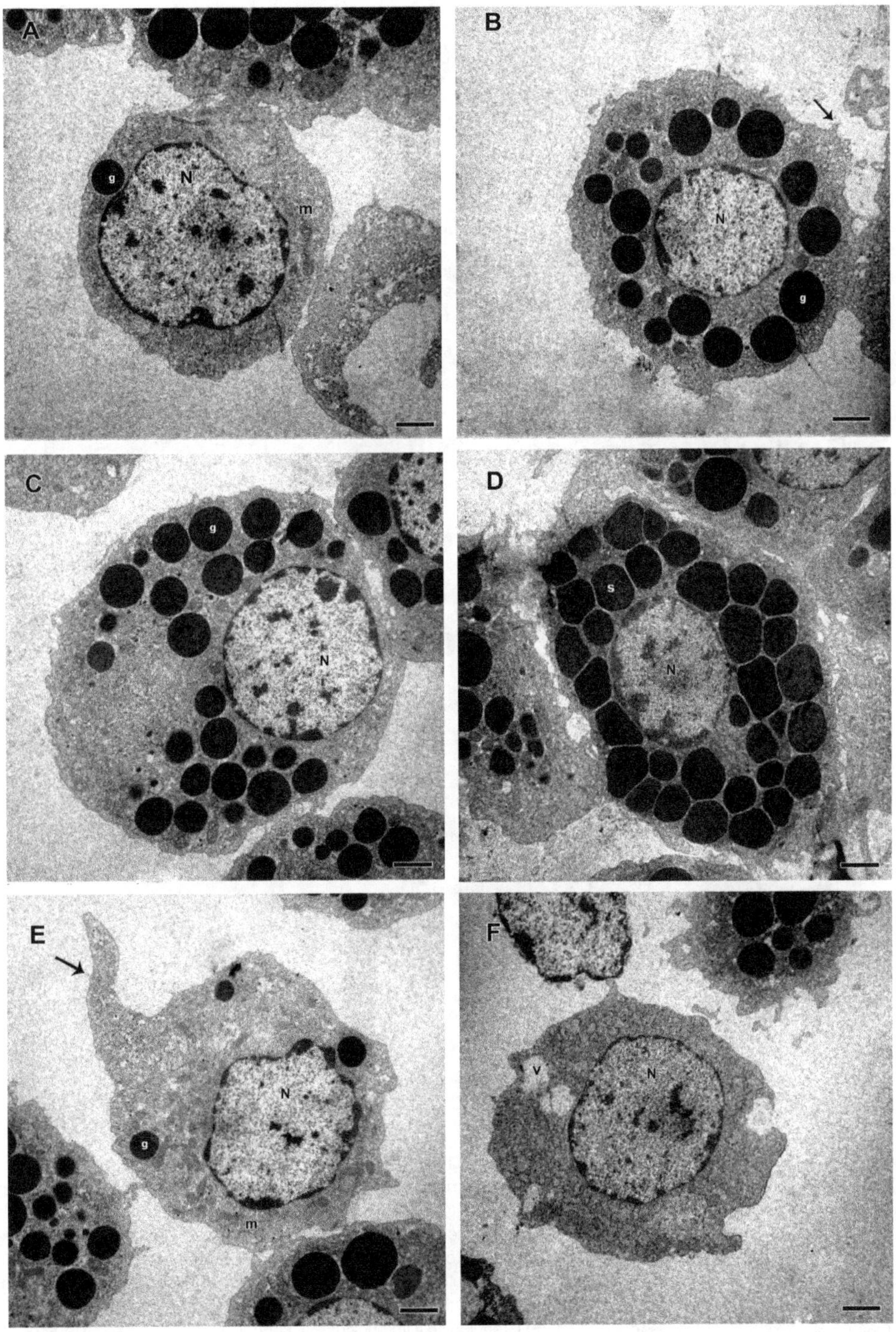

FIGURE 10 | Electromicrographs of hemocytes from *R. microplus* engorged females inoculated with 0.1% Tween®80 aqueous solution (v/v). **(A)** Prohemocyte with nucleus (N), electron dense granule (g) and mitochondria (m) in its cytoplasm. **(B,C)** Granulocytes with nucleus (N), electron dense granules (g), and plasma membrane projection (black arrow). **(D)** Spherulocyte with nucleus (N) and spherules (s) in the cytoplasm. **(E,F)** Plasmatocytes with nucleus (N), mitochondria (m), electron dense granules (g), vacuole (v), and pseudopodia (black arrow). Bars = 2 μm.

time of infection, greater the negative effects for the host. The mortality rates of ticks 48 h after fungal inoculation in the higher doses, prevented the hemolymph collection since hemolymph collected from near-to-death or dead females is not colorless but red, suggesting midgut disruption and fungal colonization of organs such as ovaries (Liu et al., 2009; Ment et al., 2012; Sanchez-Roblero et al., 2012; De Paulo et al., 2018). The same happens with the hemolymph collected 24 h after inoculation with the highest

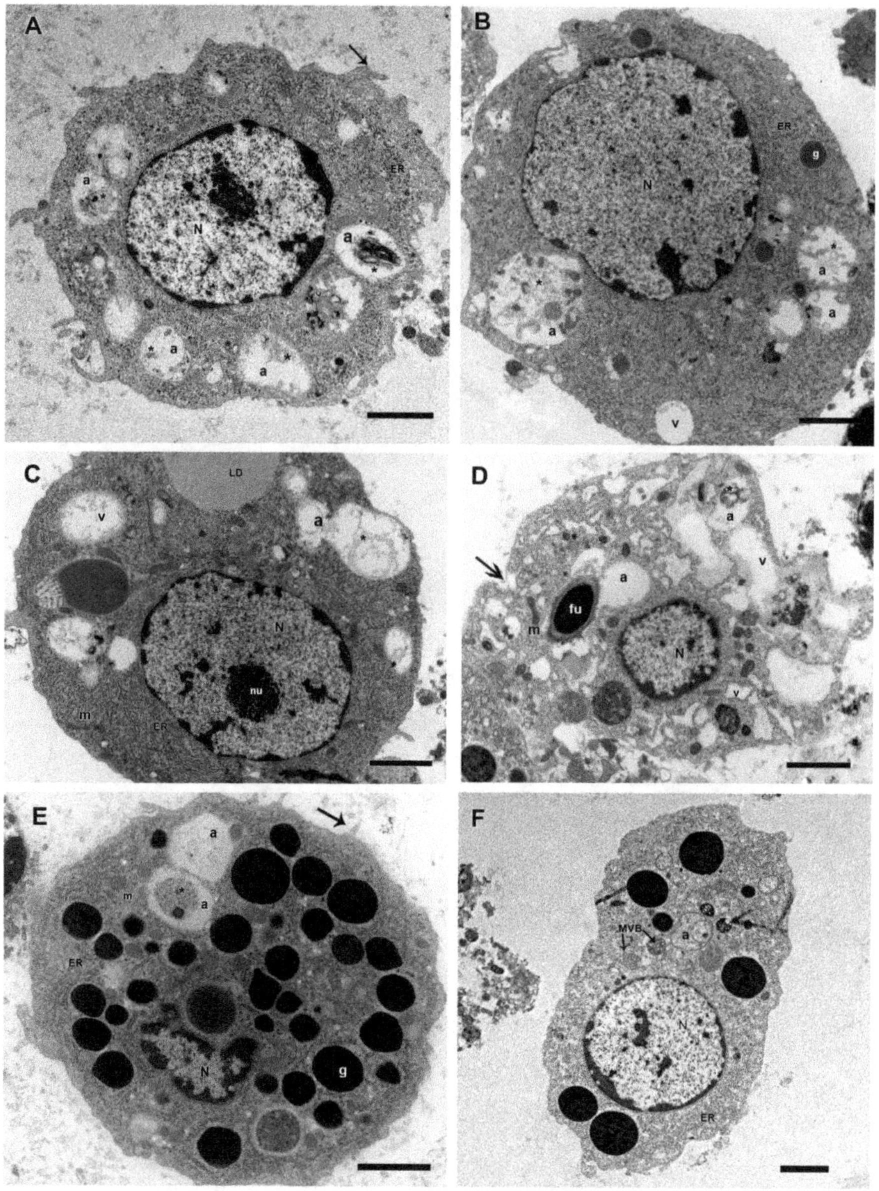

FIGURE 11 | Electromicrographs of *R. microplus* hemocytes from fungus-infected ticks. **(A)** Plasmatocyte with nucleus (N), endoplasmic reticulum (ER), autophagosome (a) with material at different stages of degradation (*) and plasma membrane projection (black arrow). **(B)** Plasmatocyte with nucleus (N), electron dense granules (g), vacuolization (v), endoplasmic reticulum (ER), autophagosome (a) with material at different stages of degradation (*). **(C)** Plasmatocyte with nucleus (N), nucleolus (nu), mitochondria (m), endoplasmic reticulum (ER), presence of lipid droplets (LD) adjacent to low electron density vacuoles (v) and autophagosome (a) with material at different stages of degradation (*). **(D)** Plasmatocyte with nucleus (N), double wall fungal conidia in the cytoplasm (fu), intense vacuolization (v), mitochondria (m), plasma membrane rupture (black arrow) and autophagosome (a) with material at different stages of degradation (*). **(E)** Granulocyte with nucleus (N), electron dense granules (g), mitochondria (m), endoplasmic reticulum (ER), plasma membrane projection (black arrow) and autophagosome (a) with material at different stages of degradation (*). **(F)** Granulocyte with nucleus (N), endoplasmic reticulum (ER), autophagosome (a) and multivesicular bodies (MVB). Bars = 2 μm.

fungal concentration (1.0×10^8 conidia mL^{-1}). Accordingly, the ultrastructural and cytotoxic analyses of hemocytes from fungus-infected ticks were performed with hemolymph collected 24 h after fungal inoculation after inoculation with 1.0×10^7 conidia mL^{-1}.

During the fungal infectious process, the arthropod can fight the pathogen through humoral and cellular immunity; the last one is mediated by hemocytes (Sterba et al., 2011). The present study demonstrated that the entomopathogen *M. robertsii* negatively affected *R. microplus* tick hemocytes, possibly causing cell death. The kinetic curve of the hemocytes viability test 24 h after exposure to *M. robertsii* showed that the highest resazurin activation (i.e., the lowest hemocytes viability) occurred with 3 h of incubation, after this time, activity remained stable. There

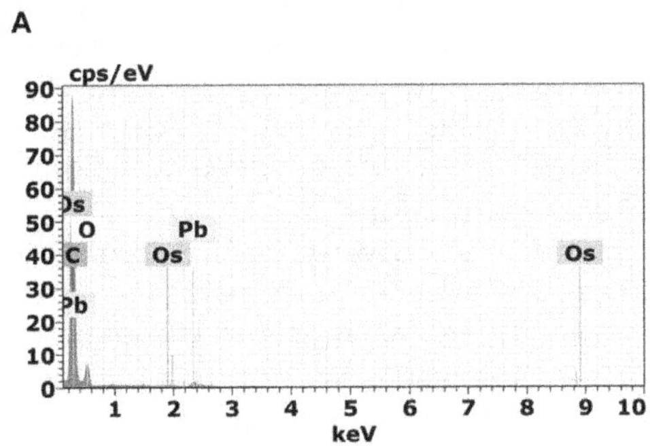

El	AN	Series	unn. C [wt.%]	norm. C [wt.%]	Atom. C [at.%]	Error (1 Sigma) [wt.%]
C	6	K-series	80.56	80.56	88.22	8.94
O	8	K-series	13.90	13.90	11.43	1.90
Os	76	M-series	0.00	0.00	0.00	0.00
Pb	82	M-series	5.54	5.54	0.35	0.24
		Total:	100.00	100.00	100.00	

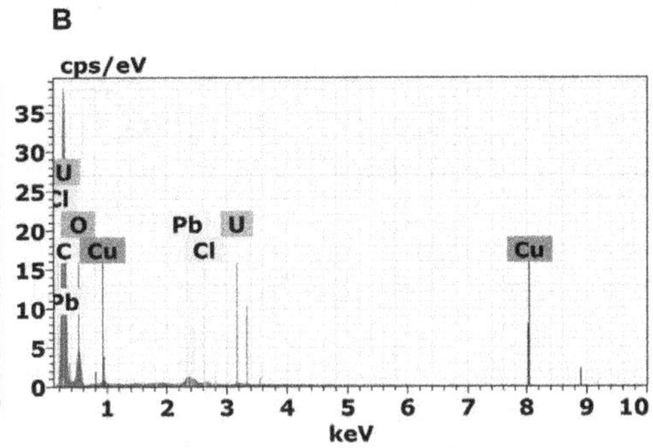

El	AN	Series	unn. C [wt.%]	norm. C [wt.%]	Atom. C [at.%]	Error (1 Sigma) [wt.%]
C	6	K-series	77.50	77.50	86.03	8.70
O	8	K-series	15.99	15.99	13.32	2.18
Cl	17	K-series	0.00	0.00	0.00	0.00
Cu	29	L-series	1.58	1.58	0.33	0.34
Pb	82	M-series	4.93	4.93	0.32	0.23
U	92	M-series	0.00	0.00	0.00	0.00
		Total:	100.00	100.00	100.00	

FIGURE 12 | Emission spectra obtained by Energy Dispersive X-Ray Spectroscopy (X-EDS) in TEM performed on 3 μm sections of **(A)** granulocytes from tween-inoculated ticks and **(B)** granulocytes from fungus-infected ticks. Spectra obtained focusing the incident electron beam on the granulocyte electron-dense granules of which characteristic energies of non-X-ray emission are evident. Multiple X-EDS analyses have been performed in each group; the ones that exhibited a pattern in common with the rest of the acquired spectra are shown. It is also possible to observe the presence of copper (Cu), a component of the TEM supporting grid; osmium (Os), used as fixative; lead (Pb), and uranium (U) that are used as staining.

are no studies involving resazurin and tick hemocytes, or even evaluating entomopathogenic fungal toxicity to these cells. Most studies with arthropod hemocytes are focused on MTT [3-(4,5-dimethylthiazol-2-yl)-2,5-diphenyl tetrazolium bromide] (Jose et al., 2011) and assays performed over heavy metal toxicity (Katsumiti et al., 2014, 2015; Minguez et al., 2014). Analyze the cells' viability is crucial for toxicity tests and MTT is widely used, however, it has lower sensibility and needs a higher incubation time in comparison to resazurin, once MTT measures the mitochondrial dehydrogenate (Mosmann, 1983). In addition, resazurin test is easy to be performed because it does not need culture media removal or organic solvents (Mosmann, 1983; Xu et al., 2015).

Studies about *R. microplus* cellular morphology and ultrastructure are scarce; for this reason, hemocytes identification through light and transmission microscopy was based on other tick species and other arthropods (Carneiro and Daemon, 1997; Borovicková and Hypsa, 2005; Habeeb and El-Hag, 2008; Feitosa et al., 2015, 2018). Silva et al. (2006) studies with light microscopy reported six hemocytes types in *R. microplus* hemolymph described as prohemocytes, granulocytes, plasmatocytes, spherulocytes, adipohemocytes, and oenocytoids. The last two were found to be less abundant. In the present study, only five cell types were observed: prohemocytes, granulocytes with different morphologies, plasmatocytes, spherulocytes, and oenocytoids, also diverging from studies with *R. sanguineus*, where adipohemocytes were also reported (Feitosa et al., 2015). After fungal infection, it was possible to observe that prohemocytes morphology was similar to prohemocytes from uninfected *R. microplus* ticks, unlike granulocytes and plasmatocytes. Granulocytes from fungus-infected ticks apparently lost granules and plasmatocytes of infected females showed cytoplasm vacuolization. The morphological alterations of plasmatocytes suggested the phagocytic activity and also may indicate a process to cell death, already reported by Sharma et al. (2008) and Shaurub et al. (2014). Some cells from untreated or treated ticks exhibited poorly stained areas (**Figures 5–7**), what is suggested to be a result of the differences between intracellular components. Accordingly, further studies are needed to characterize those areas for a better understanding of the organelles present in these cells.

Electron microscopy is very important for hemocytes characterization. Despite this, until the present date, the ultrastructural description of *R. microplus* hemocytes was not available in the literature. Accordingly, the morphological descriptions in the present study were compared with other tick species (Borovicková and Hypsa, 2005; Habeeb and El-Hag, 2008; Feitosa et al., 2015, 2018). Here, prohemocytes had similar morphology to those described by Habeeb and El-Hag (2008) and Feitosa et al. (2015) for other tick species. In the ultrastructure analysis, these cells showed ribosomes and mitochondria, but little endoplasmic reticulum and Golgi. The similar morphological characteristics of this hemocyte reported by this and other studies may be related to its function, since the prohemocyte is considered the precursor of other hemocytes (Lavine and Strand, 2002; Kavanagh and Reeves, 2004). Nevertheless, the origin of the other hemocytes is still unclear (Nation, 2016).

Plasmatocytes were abundant, polymorphic, had either central or eccentric nuclei, vesicles with different sizes, small vacuoles and mitochondria (Sonenshine and Roe, 2014). However, in the present study, cytoplasmic and pseudopodia projections, and an agranular or slightly granular cytoplasm were observed, in contrast to the findings of Feitosa et al. (2015) that described plasmatocytes with only small granulations. This and other studies suggested that this cell type is strongly involved in the immune response, through the removal of apoptotic cells, but mainly due to phagocytosis and encapsulation of pathogens, analogous to the actions of monocytes in vertebrates (Tojo et al., 2000; Lavine and Strand, 2002; Jiang et al., 2009; Honti et al., 2014).

Insect granulocytes are generally elliptic cells showing protease activity with acid phosphatase in the lysosomal compartments (Nation, 2016). For other tick species such as *Ornithodoros moubata* and *Ixodes ricinus*, granulocytes were distinguished in two types, based on the electron density and maturation of their granules (Borovicková and Hypsa, 2005; Sonenshine and Roe, 2014), while for *R. sanguineus* differentiation of granulocytes types was described based on cell maturation (Feitosa et al., 2015). In the present study, these cells had granules with different sizes, different electron densities and also diverse nucleus position in the cytoplasm. Despite this, we did not distinguish these cells in different types, since it was necessary to investigate the granules' composition before staggering additional classifications.

Spherulocytes are less abundant cells in the hemolymph, however, in *R. sanguineus* they appear to be more abundant (Carneiro and Daemon, 1997; Feitosa et al., 2015). In the present study, these cells present spherules in the cytoplasm and less organelles corroborating with other studies with insects (Brayner et al., 2005) and tick (Sonenshine and Hynes, 2008). In insects, this cell type is suggested to be involved with tissue renewal, transport of substances such as hormones and even production of some hemolymph proteins (Negreiro et al., 2004).

Adipohemocytes are cells found in insects and some tick species with varying sized and shape lipid droplets, throughout the entire cytoplasm, some mitochondria, and eccentric nucleus (Cunha et al., 2009). In *Aedes aegypti*, this cell type is considered the second most abundant and may have some granules (Hillyer et al., 2003). In ticks, a study with *R. sanguineus* reported this cellular type was rarely found in the hemolymph (Feitosa et al., 2015). In the present study, this cell type was not observed, endorsing other studies with ticks (Borovicková and Hypsa, 2005; Habeeb and El-Hag, 2008). The absence of these cells in the present study is suggested to reflect its low abundance or absence in *R. microplus* hemolymph, or a misclassification since these cells are microscopically identical fat body cells or can even be mistaken by plasmatocytes with lipid droplets (Gupta, 1985; Hillyer et al., 2003; Nation, 2016).

Oenocytoids are cells the exhibit varied size and shape, without pseudopodia, and usually with an eccentric nucleus (Gupta, 1985). They are non-phagocytic cells but may be involved in the encapsulation process (Eggenberger et al., 1990). At light microscopy these cells show homogeneous cytoplasm or small refractory granulations (Carneiro and Daemon, 1997). Transmission microscopy revels few organelles, but some mitochondria and electron luscent vesicles may be present (Giulianini et al., 2003). In ticks, this hemocyte type is not abundant (Silva et al., 2006; Feitosa et al., 2015). In the present study few oenocytoids were detected and only at light microscopy. It is suggested that the low abundance of these cells is due to its easy disruption associated with calcium mobilization that activates protein kinase C and open calcium channels, inducing increased intracellular osmotic pressure, causing cell disruption (Shrestha et al., 2015).

Hemocytes have several functions, featuring protection against pathogens, production and secretion of peroxidases, encapsulation and phagocytosis (Nation, 2016). The interactions between entomopathogenic fungi and tick hemocytes are not well elucidated, so the morphological characterization of these cells and the changes caused by the infectious process can help to investigate the lower susceptibility that these arthropods have toward entomopathogenic agents.

Granulocytes from fungus-infected ticks showed apparently fewer granules and some cells also exhibited vacuolization. These cells are guided to initiate, mediate and terminate the encapsulation process, forming a monolayer on the foreign agent (Sonenshine and Hynes, 2008). Despite this, in the present study, encapsulation processes of *M. robertsii* conidia by granulocytes were not observed, possibly due to the infection stage here analyzed (24 h after infection), considered advanced.

Plasmatocytes from fungus-infected ticks exhibited cytoplasmic vacuolization and double wall fungal conidia in the cytoplasm, suggesting a process of conidia phagocytosis. Vacuolization in plasmatocytes was also observed in other arthropod species after pathogens challenging (Sharma et al., 2008; Shaurub et al., 2014). In addition, in the present study, cells from tick-infected ticks lost its filopodia, endorsing Ghasemi et al. (2013) reports, and exhibited an increased endoplasmic reticulum. The endoplasmic reticulum is a membranous network which is responsible for protein biosynthesis, for example, and also acts as calcium storage (Berridge et al., 2003). For this reason, endoplasmic reticulum has significant importance in cellular stimuli, nutrient availability or redox status. When one cell has abundance of this organelle, it means this cell is trying to produce and secrete more protein seeking to control adversities in the intracellular media (Zhang and Kaufman, 2008). Nevertheless, further studies are needed to investigate the complete process of phagocytosis or fungal internalization and the resulting autophagy hemocytes.

Non-visualization of other cell types such as prohemocytes, spherulocytes and oenocytoids in the tick hemolymph after fungal infection is suggested to reflect the reduction in the concentration of these cell types considering that these cells do not have specific functions in the cellular immune response, and, for that reason, they are supposed to be more vulnerable to the pathogenic infection (Lavine and Strand, 2002; Cunha et al., 2009). Prohemocytes may also be in a lower concentration because these cells may have differentiated into granulocytes and plasmatocytes (Feitosa et al., 2015). Additionally, secondary metabolites produced by *Metarhizium* can cause hemocytes apoptosis reducing the number of circulating hemocytes in the hemolymph (Wiegand et al., 2000).

The encapsulation of pathogens or foreign bodies is one of the most common defense processes in arthropods succeeding to encompass larger targets such as nematodes (Bronskill, 1962;

Peters and Ehlers, 1997; Mastore et al., 2015). In insects, granulocytes are responsible for this process, in which several layers of the cells surround the pathogen, forming a capsule and inactivating it by the production of free radicals (Nappi and Ottaviani, 2000). In ticks, the process remains evident in plasmatocytes (Kopácek et al., 2000). In the present study, neither encapsulation nor nodulation processes were observed.

The fungal parasitism in arthropod cells has been reported for the fungus *Microsporidium*, which are eukaryotes, obligate parasites of several animal species and was also considered an entomopathogenic fungus (Polar et al., 2008). A large number of pathogens are able to survive in host cells, such as *Histoplasma capsulatum* fungus that can be phagocytosed by human alveolar macrophages and still is capable of multiplying itself within the cell (Newman et al., 2006). Supposedly, intracellular colonization of the fungus support itself, allowing some type of latency with a negative impact for the arthropod host health, although some factors as the nutritional stress can cause a rapid fungal growth, leading to host desiccation and arthropod death Kurtti and Keyhani, 2008).

Exposure of insect hemocytes to pathogens such as viruses, bacteria, protozoa, and other microorganisms can trigger a cell response to the infection (Nation, 2016). Cells populations increase in hemolymph as a feedback to the infection process until the pathogens are eliminated. Nevertheless, when microorganisms are highly pathogenic, cells will be leaning to start autophagy processes. Additionally, the autophagic pathway seems to play an important role during the pathogen-host cell interaction, favoring or hindering the infection. Autophagy refers to the mechanism of degradation of cytoplasmic components through the lysosomal route, selectively or non-selectively. This process occurs physiologically throughout the cell cycle, but it is exacerbated under stress conditions such as nutritional deprivation. Autophagy promotes cell cycle modulation, growth, antigenic presentation, cytokine production, and degradation of intracellular pathogens in certain cell types (Munz, 2009). The imbalance of the autophagic pathway (increase or decrease) can lead to cell death (Kroemer and Levine, 2008). In the present study, an autophagosome was observed in hemocytes from fungus-infected ticks, suggesting an autophagic processes.

Previous studies involving autophagy were limited to its role in non-selective recycling of intracellular material to the lysosome, in response to starvation (Mizushima et al., 2004; Kroemer et al., 2010). Nevertheless, autophagy is now recognized as a process with several specialized functions, including elimination of large endogenous material in a selective way, such as mitophagy and xenophagy. Autophagosomes are identified by multiple assays, including fluorescent dyes and TEM ultrastructural analysis Klionsky et al., 2012). Studies with *Drosophila melanogaster* and *Caenorhabditis elegans* demonstrated the contribution of autophagy to innate immune response, mainly when adaptive immunity is absent (Benjamin et al., 2013; Yin et al., 2016, Zimmermann et al., 2016; Kmiec et al., 2017). In *D. melanogaster* autophagy is promoted by host pattern recognition receptors (PRRs), whereas in *C. elegans*, xenophagy is used to target *Microsporidia* (Bakowski et al., 2014). Recent studies started to unveil the involvement of autophagy with host tolerance rather than resistance to infection caused by extracellular pathogens (Kuo et al., 2018). Nevertheless, more investigation is required to elucidate why ticks are more tolerant to entomopathogenic fungi than insects, focusing especially in autophagy studies, since ticks have short life cycle.

The present study demonstrated the first evaluation of *R. microplus* hemocytes using transmission electron microscopy and elucidated some aspects associated to this tick's cellular immune response to entomopathogenic fungi through cytotoxicity, TEM, and bioassay analysis, seeking to understand this host's higher tolerance to entomopathogenic fungi in comparison to insects. Our study unveiled important observations necessary for the comprehension of tick physiology and tick pathology, supporting the progress of new strategies for the biological control of ticks.

AUTHOR CONTRIBUTIONS

JF, CC-R, PG, IA, RM-B, and VB conceived and designed the study. JF, CC-R, and RB performed the experiments. DS-M helped with histological analyses. DS-M and RM-B helped with transmission electron microscopy analyses. JF and PG analyzed the data and drafted the manuscript. All authors read and approved the final manuscript.

FUNDING

This study was financed in part by the Coordenacão de Aperfeiçoamento de Pessoal de Nível Superior (CAPES) from Brazil, finance code 001, Fundação Carlos Chagas Filho de Amparo à Pesquisa do Estado do Rio de Janeiro (FAPERJ), and Conselho Nacional de Desenvolvimento Científico e Tecnológico (CNPq) from Brazil. VB is a CNPq researcher.

ACKNOWLEDGMENTS

We would like to thank Dr. Flávio J. H. Tommasini Vieira Ramos (Instituto Militar de Engenharia - IME) for helping in EDS analysis.

REFERENCES

Alden, L., Demoling, F., and Baath, E. (2001). Rapid method of determining factors limiting bacterial growth in soil. *Appl. Environ. Microbiol.* 67, 1830–1838. doi: 10.1128/AEM.67.4.1830-1838.2001

Alonso-Díaz, M. A., García, L., Galindo-Velasco, E., Lezama-Gutierrez, R., Angel-Sahagún, C. A., Rodríguez-Vivas, R. I., et al. (2007). Evaluation of *Metarhizium anisopliae* (Hyphomycetes) for the control of *Boophilus microplus* (Acari: Ixodidae) on naturally infested cattle in the Mexican tropics. *Vet. Parasitol.* 147, 336–340. doi: 10.1016/j.vetpar.2007.03.030

Alves, F. M., Bernardo, C. C., Paixão, F. R. S., Barreto, L. P., Luz, C., Humber, R. A., et al. (2017). Heat-stressed *Metarhizium anisopliae*: viability (*in vitro*) and virulence (*in vivo*) assessments against the tick *Rhipicephalus sanguineus*. *Parasitol. Res.* 116, 111–121. doi: 10.1007/s00436-016-5267-z

Alves, S. B. (1998). *Controle Microbiano de Insetos*. Piracicaba: FEALQ.

Angelo, I. C., Fernandes, E. K. K., Bahiense, T. C., Perinotto, W. M. S., Moraes, A. P. R., Terra, A. L. M., et al. (2010). Efficiency of *Lecanicillium lecanii* to control the tick *Rhipicephalus microplus*. *Vet. Parasitol.* 172, 317–322. doi: 10.1016/j.vetpar.2010.04.038

Angelo, I. C., Gôlo, P. S., Perinotto, W. M. S., Camargo, M. G., Coutinho-Rodrigues, C. J. B., Campanhon, I. B., et al. (2014). Detection of serpins involved in cellular immune response of *Rhipicephalus microplus* challenged with fungi. *Biocontrol Sci. Technol.* 24, 351–360. doi: 10.1080/09583157.2013.863269

Araújo, H. C., Cavalcanti, M. G., Santos, S. S., Alves, L. C., and Brayner, F. A. (2008). Hemocytes ultrastructure of *Aedes aegypti* (Diptera: Culicidae). *Micron* 39, 184–189. doi: 10.1016/j.micron.2007.01.003

Au, C., Dean, P., Reynolds, S. E., and Ffrench-Constant, R. H. (2003). Effect of the insect pathogenic bacterium *Photorhabdus* on insect phagocytes. *Cell. Microbiol.* 6, 89–95. doi: 10.1046/j.1462-5822.2003.00345.x

Bahiense, T. C., Fernandes, É. K. K., Angelo, I. C., Perinotto, W. M. S., and Bittencourt, V. R. E. P. (2008). Performance of *Metarhizium anisopliae* and its combination with deltamethrin against a pyrethroid-resistant strain of *Boophilus microplus* in a stall test. *Ann. N. Y. Acad. Sci.* 1149, 242–245. doi: 10.1196/annals.1428.031

Bakowski, M. A., Desjardins, C. A., Smelkinson, M. G., Dunbar, T. L., Lopez-Moyado, I. F., Rifkin, S. A., et al. (2014). Ubiquitin-mediated response to *microsporidia* and virus infection in *C. elegans*. *PLoS Pathog.* 10:e1004200. doi: 10.1371/journal.ppat.1004200

Bayne, C. J. (1990). Phagocytosis and non-self recognition in invertebrates. Phagocytosis appears to be an ancient line of defense. *Bioscience* 40, 723–731. doi: 10.2307/1311504

Benjamin, J. L., Sumpter, R. Jr., Levine, B., and Hooper, L. V. (2013). Intestinal epithelial autophagy is essential for host defense against invasive bacteria. *Cell Host Microbe* 13, 723–734. doi: 10.1016/j.chom.2013.05.004

Berridge, M. J., Bootman, M. D., and Roderick, H. L. (2003). Calcium signalling: dynamics, homeostasis and remodelling. *Nat. Rev. Mol. Cell Biol.* 4, 517–529. doi: 10.1038/nrm1155

Bidochka, M. J., Walsh, S. R. A., Ramos, M. E., St Leger, R. J., Carruthers, R. I., Silver, J. C., et al. (1997). Cloned DNA probes distinguish endemic and exotic *Entomophaga grylli* fungal pathotype infections in grasshopper life stages. *Mol. Ecol.* 6, 303–308. doi: 10.1046/j.1365-294X.1997.00187.x

Borovicková, B., and Hypsa, V. (2005). Ontogeny of tick hemocytes: a comparative analysis of *Ixodes ricinus* and *Ornithodoros moubata*. *Exp. Appl. Acarol.* 35, 317–333. doi: 10.1007/s10493-004-2209-8

Brayner, F. A., Araujo, H. R., Cavalcanti, M. G., Alves, L. C., and Peixoto, C. A. (2005). Ultrastructural characterization of the hemocytes of *Culex quinquefasciatus* (Diptera: Culicidae). *Micron* 36, 359–367. doi: 10.1016/j.micron.2004.11.007

Brayner, F. A., Araujo, H. R., Santos, S. S., Cavalcanti, M. G., Alves, L. C., Souza, J. R., et al. (2007). Haemocyte population and ultrastructural changes during the immune response of the mosquito *Culex quinquefasciatus* to microfilariae of *Wuchereria bancrofti*. *Med. Vet. Entomol.* 21, 112–120. doi: 10.1111/j.1365-2915.2007.00673.x

Bronskill, J. F. (1962). Encapsulation of rhabditoid nematodes in mosquitoes. *Can. J. Zool.* 40, 1269–1275. doi: 10.1139/z62-103

Bryant, W. B., and Michael, K. (2014). Blood feeding induces hemocyte proliferation and activation in the African malaria mosquito, *Anopheles gambiae* Giles. *J. Exp. Biol.* 217, 1238–1245. doi: 10.1242/jeb.094573

Camargo, M. G., Gôlo, P. S., Angelo, I. C., Perinotto, W. M. S., Sa, F. A., Quinelato, S., et al. (2012). Effect of oil-based formulations of acaripathogenic fungi to control *Rhipicephalus microplus* ticks under laboratory conditions. *Vet. Parasitol.* 188, 140–147. doi: 10.1016/j.vetpar.2012.03.012

Camargo, M. G., Nogueira, M. R. S., Marciano, A. F., Perinotto, W. M. S., Coutinho-Rodrigues, C. J. B., Scott, F. B., et al. (2016). *Metarhizium anisopliae* for controlling *Rhipicephalus microplus* ticks under field conditions. *Vet. Parasitol.* 223, 38–42. doi: 10.1016/j.vetpar.2016.04.014

Carneiro, M. E., and Daemon, E. (1997). Caracterização dos tipos celulares presentes na hemolinfa de adultos de *Rhipicephalus sanguineus* (Latreille, 1806) (IXODOIDEA: Ixodidae) em diferentes estados nutricionais. *Rev. Bras. Parasitol. Vet.* 6, 1–9.

Castillo, J., Brown, M. R., and Strand, M. R. (2011). Blood feeding and insulin-like peptide 3 stimulate proliferation of hemocytes in the mosquito *Aedes aegypti*. *PLoS Pathog.* 7:e1002274. doi: 10.1371/journal.ppat.1002274

Castillo, J. C., Robertson, A. E., and Strand, M. R. (2006). Characterization of hemocytes from the mosquitoes *Anopheles gambiae* and *Aedes aegypti*. *Insect. Biochem. Mol. Biol.* 36, 891–903. doi: 10.1016/j.ibmb.2006.08.010

Ceraul, S. M., Sonenshine, D. E., and Hynes, W. L. (2002). Resistance of the tick *Dermacentor variabilis* (Acari: Ixodidae) following challenge with the bacterium *Escherichia coli* (Enterobacteriales: Enterobacteriaceae). *J. Med. Entomol.* 39, 376–383. doi: 10.1603/0022-2585-39.2.376

Chávez, A. S. O., Shaw, D. K., Munderloh, U. G., and Pedra, J. H. (2017). Tick humoral responses: marching to the beat of a different drummer. *Front. Microbiol.* 8:223. doi: 10.3389/fmicb.2017.00223

Chen, K., and Lu, Z. (2018). Immune responses to bacterial and fungal infections in the silkworm, *Bombyx mori*. *Dev. Comp. Immunol.* 83, 3–11. doi: 10.1016/j.dci.2017.12.024

Crossley, A. C. (1975). The cytophysiology of insect blood. *Adv. Insect Physiol.* 11, 117–221. doi: 10.1016/s0065-2806(08)60163-0

Cunha, F. M., Wanderley-Teixeira, V., Teixeira, A. A. C., Albuquerque, A. C., Alves, L. C., and Lima, L. A. (2009). Caracterização dos hemócitos de operários de *Nasutitermes coxipoensis* (Holmgren) (Isoptera: Termitidae) e avaliação hemocitária após parasitismo por *Metarhizium anisopliae*. *Neotrop. Entomol.* 38, 293–297. doi: 10.1590/S1519-566X2009000200021

De la Fuente, J., Estrada-Pena, A., Venzal, J. M., Kocan, K. M., and Sonenshine, D. E. (2008). Overview: ticks as vectors of pathogens that cause disease in humans and animals. *Front. Biosci.* 13, 6938–6946.

De Paulo, J. F., Camargo, M. G., Coutinho-Rodrigues, C. J. B., Marciano, A. F., Freitas, M. C., Da Silva, E. M., et al. (2018). *Rhipicephalus microplus* infected by *Metarhizium*: unveiling hemocyte quantification, GFP-fungi virulence, and ovary infection. *Parasitol. Res.* 117, 1847–1856. doi: 10.1007/s00436-018-5874-y

Dolp, R. M. (1970). Biochemical and physiological studies of certain ticks (Ixodoidea). Qualitative and quantitative studies of hemocytes. *J. Med. Entomol.* 7, 277–288. doi: 10.1093/jmedent/7.3.277

Dubovskiy, I. M., Whitten, M. M. A., Yaroslavtseva, O. N., Greig, C., Kryukov, V. Y., Grizanova, K. V., et al. (2013). Can insects develop resistance to insect pathogenic fungi? *PLoS One* 8:e60248. doi: 10.1371/journal.pone.0060248

Eggenberger, L. R., Lamoreaux, W. J., and Coons, L. B. (1990). Hemocytic encapsulation of implants in the tick *Dermacentor variabilis*. *Exp. Appl. Acarol.* 9, 279–287. doi: 10.1007/BF01193434

Ehlers, S., Mielke, M. E., Blankenstein, T., and Hahn, H. (1992). Kinetic analysis of cytokine gene expression in the livers of naive and immune mice infected with *Listeria monocytogenes*. The immediate early phase in innate resistance and acquired immunity. *J. Immunol.* 149, 3016–3022.

Erler, F., and Ates, A. O. (2015). Potential of two entomopathogenic fungi, *Beauveria bassiana* and *Metarhizium anisopliae* (Coleoptera: Scarabaeidae), as biological control agents against the June beetle. *J. Insect Sci.* 15:44. doi: 10.1093/jisesa/iev029

Feitosa, A. P. S., Alves, L. C., Chaves, M. M., Veras, D. L., Silva, E. M., Alianca, A. S. S., et al. (2015). Hemocytes of *Rhipicephalus sanguineus* (Acari: Ixodidae): characterization, population abundance, and ultrastructural changes following challenge with *Leishmania infantum*. *J. Med. Entomol.* 52, 1193–1202. doi: 10.1093/jme/tjv125

Feitosa, A. P. S., Alves, L. C., Chaves, M. M., Veras, D. L., Vasconcelos de Deus, D. M., Portela Juniora, N. C., et al. (2018). Assessing the cellular and humoral immune response in *Rhipicephalus sanguineus* sensu lato (Acari: Ixodidae)

infected with *Leishmania infantum* (Nicolle, 1908). *Ticks Tick Borne Dis.* 9, 1421–1430. doi: 10.1016/j.ttbdis.2018.06.007

Fischhoff, I. R., Keesing, F., and Ostfeld, R. S. (2017). The tick biocontrol agent *Metarhizium brunneum* (=*M. anisopliae*) (strain F52) does not reduce non-target arthropods. *PLoS One* 12:e0187675. doi: 10.1371/journal.pone.0187675

Fogaça, A. C., Lorenzini, D. M., Kaku, L. M., Esteves, E., Bulet, P., and Daffre, S. (2004). Cysteine-rich antimicrobial peptides of the cattle tick *Boophilus microplus*: isolation, structural characterization and tissue expression profile. *Dev. Comp. Immunol.* 28, 191–200. doi: 10.1016/j.dci.2003.08.001

Fujisaki, K., Kitaoka, S., and Morii, T. (1975). Hemocyte types and their primary cultures in the argasid tick, *Ornithodoros moubata* Murray (Ixodoidea). *Appl. Entomol. Zool.* 10, 30–39. doi: 10.1303/aez.10.30

Ghasemi, V., Moharramipour, S., and Jalali Sendi, J. (2013). Circulating hemocytes of Mediterranean flour moth, *Ephestia kuehniella* Zell. (Lep.:Pyralidae) and their response to thermal stress. *Invertebrate Surviv. J.* 10, 128–140.

Gillespie, J. P., Kanost, M. R., and Trenczek, T. (1997). Biological mediators of insect immunity. *Annl. Rev. Entomol.* 42, 611–643. doi: 10.1146/annurev.ento.42.1.611

Giulianini, P. G., Bertolo, F., Battistella, S., and Amirante, S. A. (2003). Ultrastructure of the hemocytes of *Cetonischema aeruginosa* larvae (Coleoptera, Scarabaeidae): involvement of both granulocytes and oenocytoids in in vivo phagocytosis. *Tissue Cell* 35, 243–251. doi: 10.1016/S0040-8166(03)00037-5

Grisi, L., Leite, R. C., Martins, J. R. S., Barros, A. T. M., Andreotti, R., Cançado, P. D., et al. (2014). Reassessment of the potencial economic impact of cattle parasites in Brazil. *Rev. Bras. Parasitol. Vet.* 23, 150–156. doi: 10.1590/S1984-29612014042

Gupta, A. P. (1985). *Cellular Elements in the Hemolymph: Comprehensive Insect Physiology, Biochemistry and Pharmacology.* Oxford: Pergamon Press, 402–444.

Gupta, A. P. (1986). "Arthropod immunocytes: identification, structure, and analogies to the functions of vertebrate B- and T-lymphocytes," in *Hemocytic and Humoral Immunity in Arthropod*, ed. A. P. Gupta (Hoboken, NJ: John Wiley & Sons), 3–57.

Habeeb, S. M., and El-Hag, H. A. A. (2008). Ultrastructural changes in hemocyte cells of hard tick (*Hyalomma dromedarii*: Ixodidae): a model of *Bacillus thuringiensis* var. *thuringiensis* H14;-endotoxin mode of action. *Am. Eurasian J. Agric. Environ. Sci.* 3, 829–836.

Hajdušek, O., Sima, R., Ayllon, N., Jalovecka, M., Perner, J., de la Fuente, J., et al. (2013). Interaction of the tick immune system with transmitted pathogens. *Front. Cell. Infect. Microbiol.* 3:26. doi: 10.3389/fcimb.2013.00026

Hillyer, J. F., Schmidt, S. L., and Christensen, B. M. (2003). Hemocyte-mediated phagocytosis and melanization in the mosquito *Armigeres subalbatus* following immune challenge by bacteria. *Cell Tissue Res.* 313, 117–127. doi: 10.1007/s00441-003-0744-y

Hillyer, J. F., Schmidt, S. L., Fuchs, J. F., Boyle, J. P., and Christensen, B. M. (2005). Age-associated mortality in immune challenged mosquitoes (*Aedes aegypti*) correlates with a decrease in haemocyte numbers. *Cell. Microbiol.* 7, 39–51. doi: 10.1111/j.1462-5822.2004.00430.x

Honti, V., Csordas, G., Kurucz, E., Markus, R., and Ando, I. (2014). The cell-mediated immunity of *Drosophila melanogaster*: hemocyte lineages, immune compartments, microanatomy and regulation. *Dev. Comp. Immunol.* 42, 47–56. doi: 10.1016/j.dci.2013.06.005

Hu, X., Xiao, G., Zheng, P., Shang, Y., Su, Y., Zhang, X., et al. (2014). Trajectory and genomic determinants of fungal-pathogen speciation and host adaptation. *Proc. Natl. Acad. Sci. U.S.A.* 111, 16796–16801. doi: 10.1073/pnas.1412662111

Huang, W., Shang, Y., Chen, P., Gao, Q., and Wang, C. (2015). MrpacC regulates sporulation, insect cuticle penetration and immune evasion in *Metarhizium robertsii*. *Environ. Microbiol.* 17, 994–1008. doi: 10.1111/1462-2920.12451

Iacovone, A., Ris, N., Poirié, M., and Gatti, J. L. (2018). Time-course analysis of *Drosophila suzukii* interaction with endoparasitoid wasps evidences a delayed encapsulation response compared to *D. melanogaster*. *PLoS One* 13:e0201573. doi: 10.1371/journal.pone.0201573

Inoue, N., Hanada, K., Tsuji, N., Igarashi, I., Nagasawa, H., Mikami, T., et al. (2001). Characterization of phagocytic hemocytes in *Ornithodorosmoubata* (Acari: Ixodidae). *J. Med. Entomol.* 38, 514–519. doi: 10.1603/0022-2585-38.4.514

Jiang, R., Kim, E. H., Gong, J. H., Kwon, H. M., Kim, C. H., Ryu, K. H., et al. (2009). Three pairs of protease-serpin complexes cooperatively regulate the insect innate immune responses. *J. Biol. Chem.* 284, 35652–35658. doi: 10.1074/jbc.M109.071001

Johns, R., Sonenshine, D. E., and Hynes, W. L. (1998). Control of bacterial infections in the hard tick *Dermacentor variabilis* (Acari: Ixodidae): evidence for the existence of antimicrobial proteins in tick hemolymph. *J. Med. Entomol.* 35, 458–464. doi: 10.1093/jmedent/35.4.458

Johns, R., Sonenshine, D. E., and Hynes, W. L. (2001). Identification of a defensin from the hemolymph of the American dog tick, *Dermacentorvariabilis*. *Insect Biochem. Mol. Biol.* 31, 857–865. doi: 10.1016/S0965-1748(01)00031-5

Jones, J. C. (1962). Current concepts concerning insect hemocytes. *Am. Zoo1.* 2, 209–246. doi: 10.1093/icb/2.2.209

Jose, S., Mohandas, A., Philip, R., and Bright Singh, I. S. (2011). Primary haemocyte culture of *Penaeus monodon* as an in vitro model for white spot syndrome virus titration, viral and immune related gene expression and cytotoxicity assays. *J. Invertebr. Pathol.* 105, 312–321. doi: 10.1016/j.jip.2010.08.006

Katsumiti, A., Gilliland, D., Arostegui, I., and Cajaraville, M. P. (2014). Cytotoxicity and cellular mechanisms involved in the toxicity of CdS quantum dots in hemocytes and gill cells of the mussel *Mytilus galloprovincialis*. *Aquat. Toxicol.* 153, 39–52. doi: 10.1016/j.aquatox.2014.02.003

Katsumiti, A., Gilliland, D., Arostegui, I., and Cajaraville, M. P. (2015). Mechanisms of toxicity of Ag nanoparticles in comparison to bulk and ionic Ag on mussel hemocytes and gill cells. *PLoS One* 10:e0129039. doi: 10.1371/journal.pone.0129039

Kavanagh, K., and Reeves, E. P. (2004). Exploiting the potential of insects for in vivo pathogenicity testing of microbial pathogens. *FEMS Microbiol. Rev.* 28, 101–112. doi: 10.1016/j.femsre.2003.09.002

Kernif, T., Leulmi, H., Raoult, D., and Parola, P. (2016). Emerging tick-borne bacterial pathogens. *Microbiol. Spectr.* 4:EI10-0012-2016. doi: 10.1128/microbiolspec.ei10-0012-2016

Klionsky, D. J., Abdalla, F. C., Abeliovich, H., Abraham, R. T., Acevedo-Arozena, A., Adeli, K., et al. (2012). Guidelines for the use and interpretation of assays for monitoring autophagy. *Autophagy* 8, 445–544. doi: 10.4161/auto.19496

Kmiec, Z., Cyman, M., and Slebioda, T. J. (2017). Cells of the innate and adaptive immunity and their interactions in inflammatory bowel disease. *Adv. Med. Sci.* 62, 1–16. doi: 10.1016/j.advms.2016.09.001

Kopácek, P., Hajdusek, O., Buresova, V., and Daffre, S. (2010). "Tick innate immunity," in *Invertebrate Immunity. Advances in Experimental Medicine and Biology*, Vol. 708, ed. K. Söderhäll (Boston, MA: Springer).

Kopácek, P., Weise, C., Saravanan, T., Vitova, K., and Grubhoffer, L. (2000). Characterization of an alpha-macroglobulin-like glycoprotein isolated from the plasma of the soft tick *Ornithodoros moubata*. *Eur. J. Biochem.* 267, 465–475. doi: 10.1046/j.1432-1327.2000.01020.x

Kroemer, G., and Levine, B. (2008). Autophagic cell death: the story of a misnomer. *Nat. Rev. Mol. Cell Biol.* 9, 1004–1010. doi: 10.1038/nrm2529

Kroemer, G., Mariño, G., and Levine, B. (2010). Autophagy and the integrated stress response. *Mol. Cell* 40, 280–293. doi: 10.1016/j.molcel.2010.09.023

Kuhn, K. H., and Haug, T. (1995). Ultrastructural, cytochemical, and immunocytochemical characterization of haemocytes of the hard tick *Ixodes ricinus* (Acari: Chelicerata). *Cell Tissue Res.* 277, 493–504. doi: 10.1007/BF00300222

Kuo, C. J., Hansen, M., and Troemel, E. (2018). Autophagy and innate immunity: insights from invertebrate model organisms. *Autophagy* 14, 233–242. doi: 10.1080/15548627.2017.1389824

Kurtti, T. J., and Keyhani, N. O. (2008). Intracellular infection of tick cell lines by the entomopathogenic fungus *Metarhizium anisopliae*. *Microbiology* 154, 1700–1709. doi: 10.1099/mic.0.2008/016667-0

Kwon, H., Bang, K., and Cho, S. (2014). Characterization of the hemocytes in larvae of *Protaetia brevitarsis seulensis*: involvement of granulocyte-mediated phagocytosis. *PLoS One* 9:e103620. doi: 10.1371/journal.pone.0103620

Lackie, A. M. (1980). Invertebrate immunity. *Parazitology* 80, 393–412.

Laughton, A. M., Boots, M., and Siva-Jothy, M. T. (2011). The ontogeny of immunity in the honey bee, *Apis mellifera* L. following an immune challenge. *J. Insect Physiol.* 57, 1023–1032. doi: 10.1016/j.jinsphys.2011.04.020

Lavine, M. D., and Strand, M. R. (2002). Insect hemocytes and their role in immunity. *Insect Biochem. Mol. Biol.* 32, 1295–1309. doi: 10.1016/S0965-1748(02)00092-9

Leemon, D. M., and Jonsson, N. N. (2008). Laboratory studies on Australian isolates of *Metarhizium anisopliae* as a biopesticide for the cattle tick *Boophilus microplus*. *J. Invertebr. Pathol.* 97, 40–49. doi: 10.1016/j.jip.2007.07.006

Liu, W., Xie, Y., Xue, J., Gao, Y., Zhang, Y., Zhang, X., et al. (2009). Histopathological changes of *Ceroplastes japonicus* infected by *Lecanicillium lecanii*. *J. Invertebr. Pathol.* 101, 96–105. doi: 10.1016/j.jip.2009.03.002

Madelin, M. F., Robinson, R. E., and Williams, R. S. (1967). Appressorium like structures in insect parasitizing deuteromycetes. *J. Invertebr. Pathol.* 9, 404–412. doi: 10.1016/0022-2011(67)90078-X

Mastore, M., Arizza, V., Manachini, B., and Brivio, M. F. (2015). Modulation of immune responses of *Rhynchophorus ferrugineus* (Insecta: Coleoptera) induced by the entomopathogenic nematode *Steinernema carpocapsae* (Nematoda: Rhabditida). *Insect Sci.* 22, 748–760. doi: 10.1111/1744-7917.12141

Ment, D., Churchill, A. C. L., Glazer, I., Rehner, S. A., Rot, A., Donzelli, B. G. G., et al. (2012). Resistant ticks inhibit *Metarhizium* infection prior to haemocoel invasion by reducing fungal viability on the cuticle surface. *Environ. Microbiol.* 14, 1570–1583. doi: 10.1111/j.1462-2920.2012.02747.x

Minguez, L., Halm-Lemeille, M. P., Costil, K., Bureau, R., Lebel, J. M., and Serpentini, A. (2014). Assessment of cytotoxic and immunomodulatory properties of four antidepressants on primary cultures of abalone hemocytes (*Haliotis tuberculata*). *Aquat. Toxicol.* 153, 3–11. doi: 10.1016/j.aquatox.2013.10.020

Mizushima, N., Yamamoto, A., Matsui, M., Yoshimori, T., and Ohsumi, Y. (2004). In vivo analysis of autophagy in response to nutrient starvation using transgenic mice expressing a fluorescent autophagosome marker. *Mol. Biol. Cell* 15, 1101–1111. doi: 10.1091/mbc.e03-09-0704

Mohammadyani, M., Karimi, J., Taheri, P., Sadeghi, H., and Zare, R. (2016). Entomopathogenic fungi as promising biocontrol agents for the rosaceous longhorn beetle, *Osphranteria coerulescens*. *Biocontrol* 6, 579–590. doi: 10.1007/s10526-016-9745-0

Mosmann, T. (1983). Rapid colorimetric assay for cellular growth and survival: application to proliferation and cytotoxicity assays. *J. Immunol. Methods* 65, 55–63. doi: 10.1016/0022-1759(83)90303-4

Munz, C. (2009). Enhancing immunity through autophagy. *Annu. Rev. Immunol.* 27, 423–449. doi: 10.1146/annurev.immunol.021908.132537

Nakajima, Y., Ogihara, K., Taylor, D., and Yamakawa, M. (2003). Antibacterial hemoglobin fragments from the midgut of the soft tick, *Ornithodoros moubata* (Acari: Argasidae). *J. Med. Entomol.* 40, 78–81. doi: 10.1603/0022-2585-40.1.78

Nappi, A. J., and Ottaviani, E. (2000). Cytotoxicity and cytotoxic molecules in invertebrates. *Bioessays* 22, 469–480. doi: 10.1002/(sici)1521-1878(200005)22:5<469::aid-bies9>3.0.co;2-4

Nation, J. L. (2016). *Insect Physiology and Biochemistry*. Gainesville, FL: University of Florida.

Negreiro, M. C. C., Andrade, F. G., and Falleiros, A. M. F. (2004). Sistema imunológico de defesa em insetos: uma abordagem em lagartas da soja, *Anticarsia gemmatalis* Hübner (Lepidoptera: Noctuidae), resistentes ao AgMNPV. *Semin. Ciênc. Agrár.* 25, 293–308. doi: 10.5433/1679-0359

Nevermann, L., Xylander, W. E. R., and Seifert, G. (1991). The hemocytes of the centipede *Lithobius forficatus* (Chilo-poda, Lithobiomorpha). *Zoomorphology* 110, 317–327. doi: 10.1111/j.1744-7410.2012.00264.x

Newman, S. L., Gootee, L., Hilty, J., and Morris, R. E. (2006). Human macrophages do not require phagosome acidification to mediate fungistatic/fungicidal activity against *Histoplasma capsulatum*. *J. Immunol.* 176, 1806–1813. doi: 10.4049/jimmunol.176.3.1806

Paskewitz, S. M., and Christensen, B. M. (1996). "Immune responses of vectors," in *The Biology of Disease vectors*, eds B. J. Beaty and W. C. Marquardt (Niwot, CO: University Press of Colorado), 371–392.

Perinotto, W. M. S., Angelo, I. C., Golo, P. S., Camargo, M. G., Quinelato, S., Sa, F. A., et al. (2017). In vitro pathogenicity of different *Metarhizium anisopliae* s.l. isolates in oil formulations against *Rhipicephalus microplus*. *Biocontrol Sci. Technol.* 27, 338–347. doi: 10.1080/09583157.2017.1289151

Perinotto, W. M. S., Angelo, I. C., Golo, P. S., Quinelato, S. B., Camargo, M. G., Sa, F. A., et al. (2012). Susceptibility of different populations of ticks to entomopathogenic fungi. *Exp. Parasitol.* 130, 257–260. doi: 10.1016/j.exppara.2011.12.003

Peters, A., and Ehlers, R. U. (1997). Encapsulation of the entomopathogenic nematodes *Steinernema feltiae* in *Tipula oleracea*. *J. Invertebr. Pathol.* 69, 218–222. doi: 10.1006/jipa.1996.4648

Polar, P., Moore, D., Kairo, M. T. K., and Ramsubhag, A. (2008). Topically applied myco-acaricides for the control of cattle ticks: overcoming the challenges. *Exp. Appl. Acarol.* 46, 119–148. doi: 10.1007/s10493-008-9170-x

Roberts, D. W., and St Leger, R. J. (2004). *Metarhizium* spp., cosmopolitan insect pathogenic fungi: mycological aspects. Adv. Appl. Microbiol. 54, 1–70. doi: 10.1016/S0065-2164(04)54001-7

Rot, A., Gindin, G., Ment, D., Mishoutchenko, A., Glazer, I., and Samish, M. (2013). On-host control of the brown dog tick *Rhipicephalus sanguineus* Latreille (Acari: Ixodidae) *by Metarhizium brunneum* (Hypocreales: Clavicipitaceae). *Vet. Parasitol.* 193, 229–237. doi: 10.1016/j.vetpar.2012.11.020

Samish, M., Rot, A., Ment, D., Barel, S., Glazer, I., and Gindin, G. (2014). Efficacy of the entomopathogenic fungus *Metarhizium brunneum* in controlling the tick *Rhipicephalus annulatus* under field conditions. *Vet. Parasitol.* 206, 258–266. doi: 10.1016/j.vetpar.2014.10.019

Sampaio, I. B. M. (2002). *Estatística Aplicada à Experimentação Animal*. Belo Horizonte: FEPMVZ.

Sanchez-Roblero, R., Huerta, G., Valle, J., Gomez, J., and Toledo, J. (2012). Effect of *Beauveria bassiana* on the ovarian development and reproductive potential of *Anastrepha ludens* (Diptera: Tephritidae). *Biocontrol Sci. Technol.* 22, 1045–1091. doi: 10.1080/09583157.2012.713090

Schank, A., and Vainstein, M. H. (2010). *Metarhizium anisopliae* s.l. enzymes and toxins. *Toxicon* 56, 1267–1274. doi: 10.1016/j.toxicon.2010.03.008

Schmidt, O., Theopold, U., and Strand, M. R. (2001). Innate immunity and its evasion and suppression by hymenopteran endoparasitoids. *Bioessays* 23, 344–351. doi: 10.1002/bies.1049

Sharma, P. R., Sharma, O. P., and Saxena, B. P. (2008). Effect of sweet flag rhizome oil (*Acorus calamus*) on hemogram and ultrastructure of hemocytes of the tobacco armyworm, *Spodoptera litura* (Lepidoptera: Noctuidae). *Micron* 39, 544–551. doi: 10.1016/j.micron.2007.07.005

Shaurub, E. H., Abdel-Meguide, A., and Abd El-Aziz, N. (2014). Quantificative and ultrastructural changes in the heamocytes of *Spodoptera littoralis* (Boisd.) treated individually or in combination with *Spodoptera littoralis* multicapside nucleopolyhedrovirus (SpliMNPV) and Azadirachtin. *Micron* 65, 62–68. doi: 10.1016/j.micron.2014.04.010

Shrestha, S., Park, J., Ahn, S. J., and Kim, Y. (2015). Pge2 mediates oenocytoid cell lysis via a sodium-potassium-chloride cotransporter. *Arch. Insect Biochem. Physiol.* 89, 218–229. doi: 10.1002/arch.21238

Silva, S. B., Savastano, G., and Bittencourt, V. R. E. P. (2006). Tipos celulares envolvidos na resposta imune de fêmeas de *Boophilus microplus* inoculados com *Metarhizium anisopliae* e *Penicillium* sp. *Rev. Bras. Med. Vet.* 15, 128–131.

Smith, A. A., and Pal, U. (2014). Immunity-related genes in *Ixodes scapularis* – perspectives from genome information. *Microbiology* 4:116. doi: 10.3389/fcimb.2014.00116

Sonenshine, D. E., and Hynes, W. L. (2008). Molecular characterization and related aspects of the innate immune response in ticks. *Front. Biosci.* 13, 7046–7063.

Sonenshine, D. E., and Roe, R. M. (2014). *Biology of Ticks*, 2nd Edn. Oxford: Oxford University Press, 560.

Sterba, J., Dupejova, J., Fiser, M., Vancova, M., and Grubhoffer, L. (2011). Fibrinogen-related proteins in ixodid ticks. *Parasit. Vectors* 4:127. doi: 10.1186/1756-3305-4-127

Tan, J., Xu, M., Zhang, K., Wang, X., Chen, S., Li, T., et al. (2013). Characterization of hemocytes proliferation in larval silkworm *Bombyx mori*. *J. Insect Physiol.* 59, 595–603. doi: 10.1016/j.jinsphys.2013.03.008

Tojo, S., Naganuma, F., Arakawa, K., and Yokoo, S. (2000). Involvement of both granular cells and plasmatocytes in phagocytic reactions in the greater wax moth, *Galleria mellonella*. *J. Insect Physiol.* 46, 1129–1135. doi: 10.1016/s0022-1910(99)00223-1

Vega, F. E. (2018). The use of fungal entomopathogens as endophytes in biological control: a review. *Mycologia* 110, 4–30. doi: 10.1080/00275514.2017.1418578

Wang, C., and St Leger, R. J. (2006). A collagenous protective coat enables *Metarhizium anisopliae* to evade insect immune responses. *Proc. Natl. Acad. Sci. U.S.A.* 103, 6647–6652. doi: 10.1073/pnas.0601951103

Webster, A., Reck, J., Santi, L., Souza, U. A., Dall'Agnol, B., Klafke, G. M., et al. (2015). Integrated control of an acaricide-resistant strain of the cattle tick *Rhipicephalus microplus* by applying *Metarhizium anisopliae* associated with cypermethrin and chlorpyriphos under field conditions. *Vet. Parasitol.* 207, 302–308. doi: 10.1016/j.vetpar.2014.11.021

Wiegand, C., Levin, D., Gillespie, J. P., Willott, E., Kanost, M. R., and Trenczek, T. (2000). Monoclonal antibody M13 identifies a plasmatocyte membrane protein and inhibits encapsulation and spreading reactions of *Manduca sexta* hemocytes. *Arch. Insect Biochem. Physiol.* 45, 95–108. doi: 10.1002/1520-6327(200011)45:3<95::aid-arch1>3.0.co;2-0

Xu, M., McCanna, D. J., and Sivak, J. G. (2015). Use of the viability reagent PrestoBlue in comparison with alamarBlue and MTT to assess the viability of human corneal epithelial cells. *J. Pharmacol. Toxicol. Methods* 71, 1–7. doi: 10.1016/j.vascn.2014.11.003

Yin, Z., Pascual, C., and Klionsky, D. J. (2016). Autophagy: machinery and regulation. *Microb. Cell* 3, 588–596. doi: 10.15698/mic2016.12.546

Zhang, K., and Kaufman, R. J. (2008). From endoplasmic-reticulum stress to the inflammatory response. *Nature* 454, 455–462. doi: 10.1038/nature07203

Zhioua, E., Lebrun, R. A., Johnson, P. W., and Ginsberg, H. S. (1996). Ultrastructure of the haemocytes of *Ixodes scapularis* (Acari: Ixodidae). *Acarologia* 3, 173–179.

Zimmermann, A., Kainz, K., Andryushkova, A., Hofer, S., Madeo, F., and Carmona-Gutierrez, D. (2016). Autophagy: one more Nobel Prize for yeast. *Microb. Cell* 3, 579–581. doi: 10.15698/mic2016.12.544

9

The Tick Microbiome: Why Non-Pathogenic Microorganisms Matter in Tick Biology and Pathogen Transmission

***Sarah I. Bonnet*[1]**, Florian Binetruy*[2]*, Angelica M. Hernández-Jarguín*[3]* and Olivier Duron*[2]**

[1] UMR BIPAR INRA-ENVA-ANSES, Maisons-Alfort, France, [2] Laboratoire MIVEGEC (Maladies Infectieuses et Vecteurs: Écologie, Génétique, Évolution et Contrôle), Centre National de la Recherche Scientifique (UMR5290), IRD (UMR224), Université de Montpellier, Montpellier, France, [3] SaBio Instituto de Investigación en Recursos Cinegéticos CSIC-UCLM-JCCM, Ciudad Real, Spain

***Correspondence:**
Sarah I. Bonnet
sarah.bonnet@vet-alfort.fr

Ticks are among the most important vectors of pathogens affecting humans and other animals worldwide. They do not only carry pathogens however, as a diverse group of commensal and symbiotic microorganisms are also present in ticks. Unlike pathogens, their biology and their effect on ticks remain largely unexplored, and are in fact often neglected. Nonetheless, they can confer multiple detrimental, neutral, or beneficial effects to their tick hosts, and can play various roles in fitness, nutritional adaptation, development, reproduction, defense against environmental stress, and immunity. Non-pathogenic microorganisms may also play a role in driving transmission of tick-borne pathogens (TBP), with many potential implications for both human and animal health. In addition, the genetic proximity of some pathogens to mutualistic symbionts hosted by ticks is evident when studying phylogenies of several bacterial genera. The best examples are found within members of the *Rickettsia*, *Francisella*, and *Coxiella* genera: while in medical and veterinary research these bacteria are traditionally recognized as highly virulent vertebrate pathogens, it is now clear to evolutionary ecologists that many (if not most) *Coxiella*, *Francisella*, and *Rickettsia* bacteria are actually non-pathogenic microorganisms exhibiting alternative lifestyles as mutualistic ticks symbionts. Consequently, ticks represent a compelling yet challenging system in which to study microbiomes and microbial interactions, and to investigate the composition, functional, and ecological implications of bacterial communities. Ultimately, deciphering the relationships between tick microorganisms as well as tick symbiont interactions will garner invaluable information, which may aid in the future development of arthropod pest and vector-borne pathogen transmission control strategies.

Keywords: tick, tick symbionts, tick borne pathogens, microbiome, microbial interactions

INTRODUCTION

Over the last few decades, considerable research efforts have focused on the diversity, distribution, and impact of tick-borne pathogens (TBP). The list of known or potential TBP is constantly evolving, and includes a variety of viruses, bacteria, and parasites afflicting humans and many other animals worldwide (de la Fuente et al., 2008; Heyman et al., 2010; Dantas-Torres et al., 2012; Rizzoli et al., 2014). Less well studied or understood are whole microbial communities hosted by ticks, which attract much less attention, yet are equally important. These communities include TBP, but also non-pathogenic microorganisms such as commensal and mutualistic microbes that are also abundant in ticks (Andreotti et al., 2011; Carpi et al., 2011; Williams-Newkirk et al., 2014; Duron et al., 2015a, 2017). Until recently, these non-pathogenic microorganisms were generally overlooked by scientists working with ticks and TBP. Before 1990, their existence was largely ignored and all bacteria found in ticks were usually considered to be potential TBP without necessarily undergoing rigorous health risk assessment. Toward the end of the 1990s, the advent of simple PCR assays led to a growing understanding that a few intracellular bacteria, such as the *Coxiella*-like endosymbiont and the *Francisella*-like endosymbiont (*Coxiella*-LE and *Francisella*-LE hereafter), are actually non-pathogenic microorganisms hosted by ticks (Niebylski et al., 1997a; Noda et al., 1997). Deeper investigation of microbial biodiversity through high-throughput sequencing and DNA barcoding led to another leap in understanding: non-pathogenic microorganisms from many different clades are present in ticks, and can generally coexist with TBP (Clay et al., 2008; Andreotti et al., 2011; Carpi et al., 2011; Lalzar et al., 2012; Vayssier-Taussat et al., 2013; Qiu et al., 2014; Williams-Newkirk et al., 2014; Narasimhan and Fikrig, 2015; Abraham et al., 2017). In addition, current available data on tick microbiomes suggest that non-pathogenic microorganisms exhibit higher taxonomic diversity than TBP since they encompass most major bacterial and Archaea groups (Andreotti et al., 2011; Carpi et al., 2011; Nakao et al., 2013; Qiu et al., 2014; Williams-Newkirk et al., 2014). Altogether, it is now clear that ticks carry complex microbial communities that are largely dominated by non-pathogenic microorganisms. Most importantly, this implies that both ticks and TBP are commonly engaged in interactions with non-pathogenic microorganisms.

The composition of these microbial communities is highly variable: environmental constraints are key drivers of their structure as shown by differences in bacterial diversity observed between laboratory-reared and wild ticks (Heise et al., 2010; Zolnik et al., 2016). It was further reported that bacterial community structures could vary depending on the examined tick species (Lalzar et al., 2012), the season during which ticks were collected (Lalzar et al., 2012), the examined geographical regions (van Overbeek et al., 2008; Carpi et al., 2011; Williams-Newkirk et al., 2014), the examined tick life stage (Moreno et al., 2006; Clay et al., 2008; Williams-Newkirk et al., 2014; Zolnik et al., 2016), and between different feeding statuses (Heise et al., 2010; Menchaca et al., 2013; Zhang et al., 2014). Furthermore, bacterial community structures may differ depending of the presence of pathogens (Steiner et al., 2008; Abraham et al., 2017). Overall, the quantity of potential variations highlights the lability of microbial communities hosted by ticks, and future studies should focus on understanding how these variations impact tick biology. Below, we will discuss the interesting hypothesis that the inherent flexibility of microbial communities may help ticks adapt to environmental stresses, such as TBP presence.

Microorganisms inhabiting ticks are not only taxonomically diverse, they are also ecologically diverse. This diversity is clearly illustrated by the large panel of lifestyle strategies that microorganisms use to infect and persist within tick populations (**Figure 1**). As vertebrate pathogens, TBP normally spread via infectious (horizontal) transmission through tick bite and blood feeding. A few TBP can also be vertically transmitted in ticks, and thus be maintained throughout each generation as observed for *Babesia* species (Chauvin et al., 2009), *Rickettsia rickettsii* (Burgdorfer et al., 1981), or viruses (Xia et al., 2016). Other tick microorganisms are highly specialized intracellular symbionts depending almost exclusively on maternal (transovarial) transmission to ensure their persistence in tick populations (Niebylski et al., 1997b; Lo et al., 2006; Sassera et al., 2006; Klyachko et al., 2007; Felsheim et al., 2009; Machado-Ferreira et al., 2011; Lalzar et al., 2014; Duron et al., 2015a; Kurtti et al., 2015). Tick microorganism diversity is further augmented due to the fact that environmental microorganisms can also colonize ticks: microbes present on vertebrate skin surfaces may colonize ticks during blood feeding, while those present in the soil or vegetation can colonize ticks on the ground, once they have dropped off their vertebrate hosts (Narasimhan and Fikrig, 2015). Overall, the diverse range of microbial lifestyle strategies creates a complex web of interactions offering excellent opportunities to tackle questions about the impact of whole microbial communities on tick biology and TBP transmission. In spite of this, the direct effects of pathogens and other microbes on tick physiology and activity has received much less attention than their effects on vertebrate hosts. In most cases, the function of tick endosymbionts in relation to their host has not been determined. Many of these endosymbionts have obligate intracellular life cycles or are difficult to cultivate, which may explain the gaps in current knowledge (Tully et al., 1995; Kurtti et al., 1996; Niebylski et al., 1997a; Duron et al., 2015a). However, for some bacteria, tissue-specific localization has been defined, which may aid us to understand bacterial impact on both tick biology and pathogen transmission (Noda et al., 1997; Klyachko et al., 2007; Lalzar et al., 2014; Narasimhan and Fikrig, 2015). Similarly, the use of microarray or RNASeq technologies to analyze induced tick microbiome expression patterns and varying composition following a variety of conditions, may also further elucidate their roles (Rodriguez-Valle et al., 2010). This

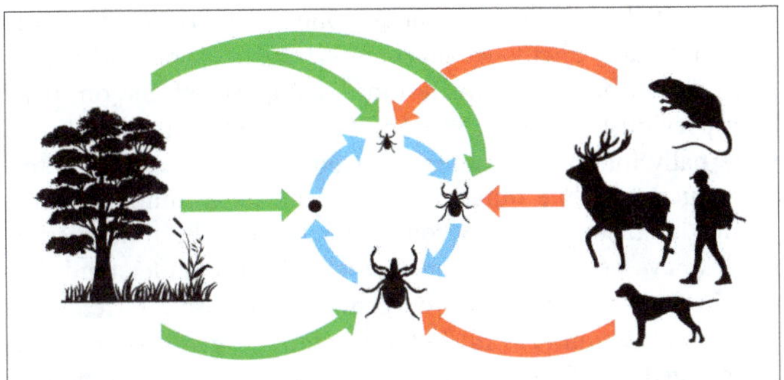

FIGURE 1 | Origin and acquisition of tick microorganisms. Red arrows: vertebrate pathogens acquired from tick bites; blue arrows: maternally inherited tick symbionts acquired via transovarial and transtadial transmission; green arrows: microorganisms acquired from the environment.

knowledge is of both medical and veterinary interest since it may enable the reassessment of tick-associated health risks, but also of ecological and evolutionary importance by highlighting co-evolutionary processes acting between ticks and their microbes. Indeed, some symbionts, but not all (Weller et al., 1998), have a joint evolutionary history of several million years with their tick hosts (Almeida et al., 2012; Duron et al., 2017), suggesting that complex interactions may have evolved in these associations. If biologists aim to fully understand the ecological and evolutionary processes involved in tick biology and the emergence of tick-borne diseases, a thorough examination of non-pathogenic microorganisms is also required.

Maternally-inherited symbionts are well-known to use specific adaptive strategies to spread and persist within arthropod populations, either providing fitness benefits to female hosts or manipulating host reproduction (Moran et al., 2008; Ferrari and Vavre, 2011). Two categories of widespread endosymbionts are usually recognized in arthropods, although intermediates and transition forms are also frequent:

- The first category consists of obligate (primary) mutualistic symbionts required to support normal host development, thus assisting their host in various essential functions. This includes nutritional diet upgrades by providing biosynthetic pathways absent from their hosts (Moran et al., 2008; Wernegreen, 2012). Indeed, most blood-feeding insects such as bed bugs, lice, and tsetse flies harbor obligate symbionts that provide B vitamins and cofactors not readily obtainable in sufficient quantities from a uniquely blood-based diet (Akman et al., 2002; Hosokawa et al., 2010; Boyd et al., 2013; Nikoh et al., 2014).
- The second category consists of facultative (secondary) symbionts not required for host survival. Some are defensive symbionts conferring protection against natural enemies or heat (Oliver et al., 2010; Ferrari and Vavre, 2011), while others are reproductive parasites that manipulate host reproduction through the induction of parthenogenesis, feminization of genetic males, male-killing, and cytoplasmic incompatibility (conditional sterility between infected and uninfected specimens) (Engelstadter and Hurst, 2009; Cordaux et al., 2011).

In this article we review four major biological aspects where our views on tick microbes have undergone substantial change over the last decade. Firstly, we must emphasize that non-pathogenic microorganisms have much more complex effects on ticks than previously thought. Indeed, it is now evident that several maternally-inherited symbionts are required for tick survival and reproduction, while other symbionts can have multiple effects on tick life history traits. Secondly, whilst tick TBP transmission modes have been studied for decades, we now understand that certain non-pathogenic microorganisms may also interfere with TBP transmission. Thirdly, although microorganisms are often categorized as "TBP," "commensals," or "maternally-inherited symbionts," both intermediate and transitional states frequently occur. In this context, it thus appears vital to not overlook the full range of potential effects, as have been recently described in microbiome studies. And finally, bacterial phylogeny demonstrates that several infectious agents have close genetic proximity with mutualistic tick symbionts. This indicates that some bacterial genera (eg. *Rickettsia*, *Francisella*, and *Coxiella*) have the capacity to frequently undergo evolutionary shifts between pathogenic and non-pathogenic forms, a process that may lead to the emergence of novel infectious diseases.

THE EFFECT OF NON-PATHOGENIC MICROORGANISMS ON TICK BIOLOGY

Perhaps the most remarkable observation of recent times is the pivotal role of symbiotic interactions in normal tick biology, including ecological specialization to an exclusive blood diet. Symbionts—i.e., microorganisms engaged in close and long-term interactions with their tick hosts—are exceptionally diverse in ticks: at least 10 distinct genera of maternally-inherited bacteria have been reported in ticks over the last decade (listed in **Table 1** and **Figure 2**) (Duron et al., 2017). Three of these symbionts are only found in ticks: *Coxiella*-LE, which infects at least two thirds of tick species, *Midichloria*, which inhabits the mitochondria of some tick species, and *Francisella*-LE, which has only been reported in a few tick species (**Table 1**). The seven remaining symbiont genera are more- or less-frequently found in other arthropod groups, including several well-studied insects. Five symbionts, *Wolbachia*, *Cardinium*, *Arsenophonus*, *Spiroplasma*, and *Rickettsia*, are commonly identified in some arthropod groups, while two others, *Rickettsiella* and *Lariskella*, have only been reported in a few other arthropod taxa in addition to ticks (**Table 1**).

Coxiella-LE has been reported as essential for tick survival and reproduction in the *Amblyomma americanum* lone star tick (Zhong et al., 2007). As an obligate symbiont, *Coxiella*-LE is, by definition, present in most individuals of a given tick species (Clay et al., 2008; Machado-Ferreira et al., 2011; Lalzar et al., 2012; Duron et al., 2015b, 2017): thus their mutualistic relationship is required for the survival of both organisms. Remarkably, some *Coxiella*-LE may form evolutionarily stable associations with their tick hosts that last for millions of years (Duron et al., 2017). These associations typically exhibit strict co-cladogenesis, resulting in congruent host-symbiont phylogenies as recently observed between members of the *Rhipicephalus* genus and their associated *Coxiella*-LE (Duron et al., 2017). The discovery of *Coxiella*-LE in numerous other tick groups (Jasinskas et al., 2007; Clay et al., 2008; Machado-Ferreira et al., 2011; Almeida et al., 2012; Lalzar et al., 2012; Duron et al., 2014, 2015a, 2017), indicates that it is the most widespread and biologically relevant tick symbiont. An examination of *Coxiella*-LE intra-host localization revealed pronounced tissue tropism in all examined tick species. This symbiont typically infects the ovaries (to ensure maternal transmission) and the distal part of Malpighian tubules, suggesting a possible role in nutrition, osmoregulation, or excretion (Klyachko et al., 2007; Machado-Ferreira et al., 2011; Lalzar et al., 2014). Examination of eggs from several tick species confirmed that *Coxiella*-LE is transmitted to >99% of tick progeny, demonstrating highly efficient maternal transmission (Machado-Ferreira et al., 2011; Lalzar et al., 2014;

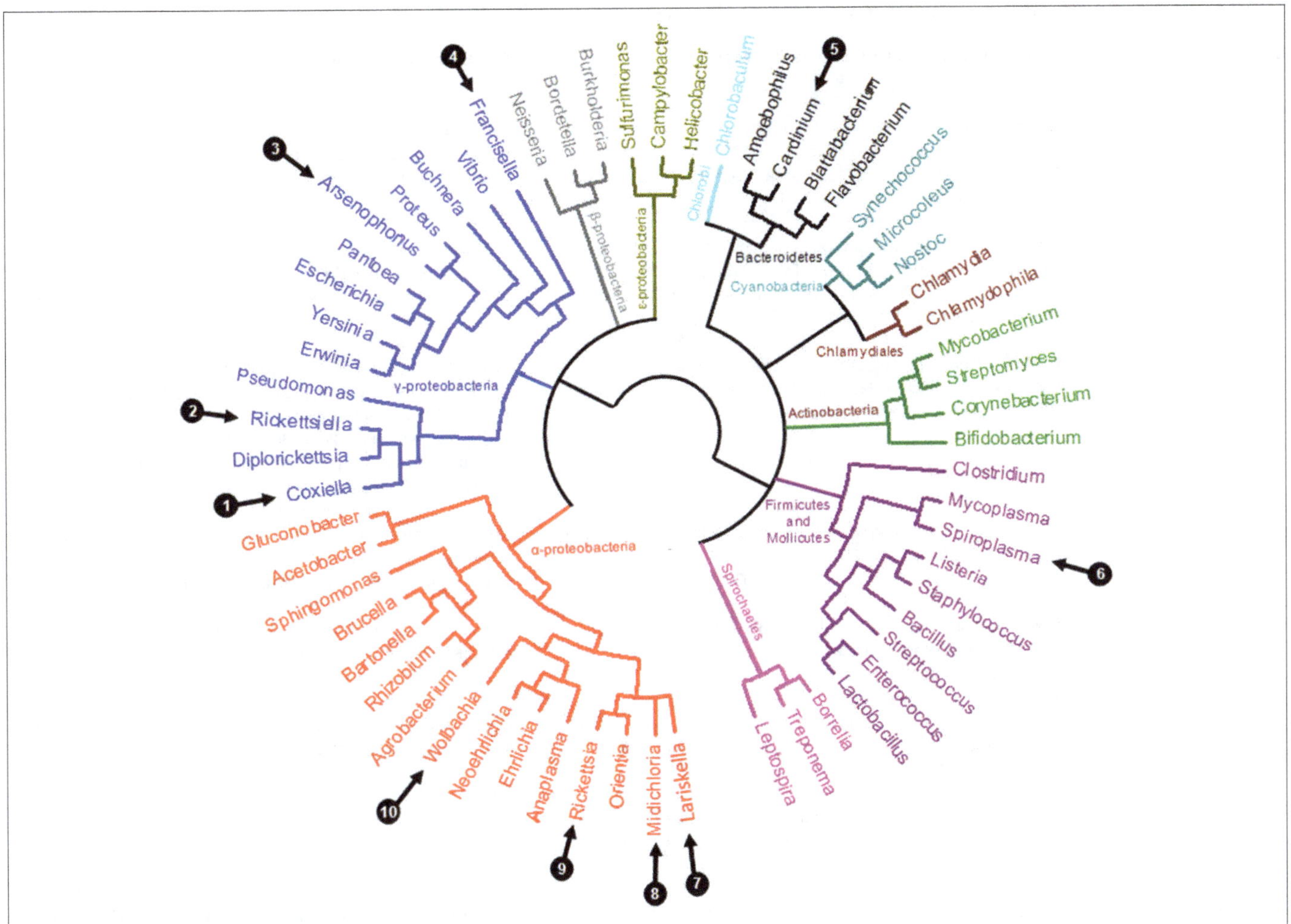

FIGURE 2 | Simplified eubacterial phylogeny showing the evolutionary relationships between the ten genera containing maternally inherited tick symbionts (labeled 1–10, as detailed in **Table 1**).

Duron et al., 2015a). Remarkably, the *Coxiella*-LE genome was shown to encode major B vitamin synthesizing pathways such as biotin (B7 vitamin), folic acid (B9), riboflavin (B2), and their cofactors, that are not usually obtainable in sufficient quantities from a uniquely blood-based diet (Gottlieb et al., 2015; Smith et al., 2015). By ensuring nutritional upgrading of the blood diet, *Coxiella*-LE has enabled ticks to utilize an unbalanced dietary resource and thus become hematophagy specialists.

Recent studies have suggested that alternative obligate symbionts other than *Coxiella*-LE may also exist. Around one third of examined tick species lack *Coxiella*-LE or harbor *Coxiella*-LE at much lower frequencies than expected for an obligate symbiont (Duron et al., 2014, 2015a, 2017). A large survey of 81 tick species showed that in almost all tick species without *Coxiella*-LE infection, another maternally-inherited symbiont was usually present (Duron et al., 2017). Among these alternative obligate symbionts were *Francisella*-LE, *Rickettsia*, and *Rickettsiella,* which are often present in all specimens of the infected tick species (Duron et al., 2017). Although formal testing with nutritional and physiological experiments is now required to validate their role as alternative obligate symbionts, recent bacterial genome data suggest that these bacteria have highly-evolved adaptive mechanisms enabling tick survival. Indeed, their genomes encode functions suggesting that they have—at least partially as for *Coxiella*-LE—a genetic capability for *de novo* B vitamin synthesis. Indeed, the *Francisella*-LE genomes from the fowl tick *Argas persicus* and the Gulf Coast tick *Amblyomma maculatum* contain complete genetic pathways for biotin, folic acid, and riboflavin biosynthesis (Sjodin et al., 2012; Gerhart et al., 2016). Similarly, recent metabolic reconstructions of *Rickettsia* genomes indicated that all genes required for folic acid biosynthesis are present in *Rickettsia* symbiont genomes obtained from both the black-legged tick *Ixodes scapularis* and the Western black-legged tick *I. pacificus* (Hunter et al., 2015). Worthy of note here is that laboratory findings directly corroborate the existence of beneficial *Rickettsia* symbionts since they exert a significant effect on larval motility of *A. americanum*, *Dermacentor variabilis*, and *I. scapularis* ticks (Kagemann and Clay, 2013). Overall, these maternally-inherited symbionts are thus of ecological and evolutionary importance to the tick species they infect, and potentially mediate tick adaptation to hematophagy. In addition, it should be notice

TABLE 1 | List of the ten maternally inherited bacteria found in ticks and relevant (non-exhaustive) references.

Maternally inherited bacteria	Distribution in ticks and other arthropods	Major properties (non-exhaustive references)
1-*Coxiella*-LE	Very common in ticks, not found in other arthropods (Noda et al., 1997; Jasinskas et al., 2007; Clay et al., 2008; Carpi et al., 2011; Machado-Ferreira et al., 2011; Almeida et al., 2012; Lalzar et al., 2012; Duron et al., 2014, 2015a, 2017)	Obligate symbiont in most tick species (Zhong et al., 2007; Gottlieb et al., 2015; Smith et al., 2015). Closely related to the agent of Q fever, *C. burnetii* (Duron et al., 2015a)
2-*Rickettsiella*	Scattered distribution in arthropods (Tsuchida et al., 2010, 2014; Bouchon et al., 2012; Iasur-Kruh et al., 2013), common in ticks (Kurtti et al., 2002; Vilcins et al., 2009; Anstead and Chilton, 2014; Duron et al., 2015a, 2016, 2017)	Unknown effect in ticks. Facultative mutualist in aphids (Tsuchida et al., 2010, 2014) and likely in other insects (Iasur-Kruh et al., 2013). Some strains are entomopathogenic (Bouchon et al., 2012)
3-*Arsenophonus*	Common in arthropods (Duron et al., 2008a; Novakova et al., 2009), present in ticks (Clay et al., 2008; Dergousoff and Chilton, 2010; Reis et al., 2011; Clayton et al., 2015; Duron et al., 2017)	Male-killer in parasitoid wasps (Werren et al., 1986; Duron et al., 2010), putative obligate symbiont in bat flies and louse flies (Duron et al., 2014), facultative symbiont in other insects (Novakova et al., 2009; Jousselin et al., 2013). In the sheep tick, *Ixodes ricinus*, detection of *Arsenophonus* may be due to contamination by a hymenopteran parasitoid (Bohacsova et al., 2016)
4-*Francisella*-LE	Rare in ticks, not found in other arthropods (Niebylski et al., 1997a; Noda et al., 1997; Scoles, 2004; Goethert and Telford, 2005; Clayton et al., 2015; Gerhart et al., 2016; Duron et al., 2017)	Unknown effect in most cases but alternative obligate symbiont in some tick species (Gerhart et al., 2016; Duron et al., 2017); closely related to the agent of tularaemia (*F. tularensis*) (Sjodin et al., 2012)
5-*Cardinium*	Common in arthropods (Zchori-Fein and Perlman, 2004; Duron et al., 2008a,b), present in ticks (Kurtti et al., 1996; Benson et al., 2004; Duron et al., 2017)	Unknown effect in ticks. Reproductive manipulator in diverse insect species (Engelstadter and Hurst, 2009)
6-*Spiroplasma*	Common in arthropods (Weinert et al., 2007; Duron et al., 2008a), present in ticks (Tully et al., 1981, 1995; Henning et al., 2006; Duron et al., 2017)	Unknown effect in ticks. Male-killer in diverse insect species (Engelstadter and Hurst, 2009)
7-*Lariskella*	Rare and with a scattered distribution in arthropods (Matsuura et al., 2012; Toju et al., 2013), rarely reported in ticks (Qiu et al., 2014; Duron et al., 2017)	Unknown effect
8-*Midichloria*	Present in ticks, not found in other arthropods (Lo et al., 2006; Epis et al., 2008; Venzal et al., 2008; Reis et al., 2011; Najm et al., 2012; Qiu et al., 2014; Williams-Newkirk et al., 2014; Paul et al., 2016; Bonnet et al., 2017; Duron et al., 2017)	Unknown effect; inhabits tick mitochondria (Epis et al., 2013)
9-*Rickettsia*	Common in arthropods (Perlman et al., 2006; Weinert et al., 2009), present in ticks (Niebylski et al., 1997b; Clayton et al., 2015; Kurtti et al., 2015; Duron et al., 2017)	Unknown effect in ticks. Reproductive manipulator in diverse insect species (Engelstadter and Hurst, 2009) and defensive symbiont in other insects (Lukasik et al., 2013) closely related to pathogenic strains, often tick-borne, infecting vertebrates (Perlman et al., 2006; Darby et al., 2007; Weinert et al., 2009)
10-*Wolbachia*	Very common in arthropods (Duron et al., 2008b; Zug and Hammerstein, 2012), present in ticks (Andreotti et al., 2011; Carpi et al., 2011; Reis et al., 2011; Duron et al., 2017)	Unknown effect in ticks. Reproductive manipulation in many arthropods (Engelstadter and Hurst, 2009), facultative mutualist (defensive symbiosis) in others such as mosquitoes (Brownlie and Johnson, 2009; Hamilton and Perlman, 2013), obligate symbiont in bed bugs (Hosokawa et al., 2010; Nikoh et al., 2014). At least in the case of the sheep tick, *Ixodes ricinus*, it has been demonstrated that the detection of *Wolbachia* was due to a contamination by a hymenopteran parasitoid (Plantard et al., 2012)

Adapted from Duron et al. (2017).

that some tick-borne pathogenic Anaplasmataceae bacteria (including *Anaplasma phagocytophilum, Ehrlichia chaffeensis,* and *Neorickettsia sennetsu*) are also able to synthetize all major vitamins, suggesting that they may also confer a beneficial role in ticks when present (Dunning Hotopp et al., 2006).

Many *Rickettsia* species are well-known TBP, therefore a comment on the true ecological diversity existing within the *Rickettsia* genus is appropriate. Indeed, most of the novel *Rickettsia* species or strains discovered in recent years are found exclusively in arthropods and never in vertebrates (Perlman et al., 2006; Darby et al., 2007; Weinert et al., 2009). In ticks, as for many other arthropods, these *Rickettsia* are not pathogenic but are actually maternally-inherited symbionts with poorly known effects on tick biology. This is the case for the *Rickettsia* species identified in the black-legged tick *I. scapularis* (*Rickettsia buchneri*, formerly known as *Rickettsia* REIS; Kurtti et al., 2015), the American dog tick *Dermacentor variabilis* (*Rickettsia peacockii*; Felsheim et al., 2009), and likely the tree-hole tick *Ixodes arboricola* (*Rickettsia vini*; Duron et al., 2017). The fact that ticks carry both pathogenic and non-pathogenic *Rickettsia* that may interact (as early reported by Burgdorfer et al., 1981), underscores the need to be able to clearly distinguish between the two in further studies on these bacteria.

Along with obligate symbionts, ticks commonly harbor facultative symbionts belonging to a variety of bacterial genera (listed in **Table 1**). Examination of a representative collection of 81 tick species (i.e., approximately 10% of known tick species and including both soft and hard ticks) illustrated facultative symbiont diversity, since it revealed the presence of maternally-inherited bacteria in almost all species (79 of 81) (Duron et al., 2017). Remarkably, many of these tick species (44) hosted more than one symbiont. In multi-infected tick species, symbionts assembled in communities which could reach high levels of complexity. Indeed, six distinct genera of maternally-inherited symbionts co-exist in sheep tick *I. ricinus* populations (*Midichloria*, *Spiroplasma*, *Coxiella*-LE, *Rickettsia*, *Wolbachia*, and *Rickettsiella*) and in African blue tick *Rhipicephalus decoloratus* populations (*Midichloria*, *Coxiella*-LE, *Francisella*-LE, *Rickettsia*, *Cardinium*, and *Spiroplasma*) (Duron et al., 2017). It should be noted that detecting a heritable bacterium can sometimes be due to cross-contamination as for several *I. ricinus* studies. Some recorded *Wolbachia* and *Arsenophonus* infections were actually due to the cryptic presence of a *Wolbachia*- and *Arsenophonus*-infected endoparasitoid wasp, *Ixodiphagus hookeri*, within tick tissues (Plantard et al., 2012; Bohacsova et al., 2016). As a result, the presence of at least some of these tick symbionts must be treated with caution.

Although the role of these facultative symbionts is not yet clearly elucidated, one study suggested that *Arsenophonus* sp. can affect host-seeking success by decreasing *A. americanum, I. scapularis,* and *D. variabilis* tick motility when *Rickettsia* symbionts increased such mobility (Kagemann and Clay, 2013). Recent sequencing and analysis of the *Midichloria mitochondrii* genome led to the hypothesis that the bacteria could serve as an additional ATP source for the host cell during oogenesis (Sassera et al., 2011). In addition, this symbiont has been ascribed a possible helper role in tick molting processes (Zchori-Fein and Bourtzis, 2011). As mentioned above, there is no evidence to date showing that the *Wolbachia* detected in ticks are "true" tick symbionts (Plantard et al., 2012). Interestingly, in insects, *Wolbachia* is known to act as defensive endosymbionts (reviewed by Brownlie and Johnson, 2009), or as manipulator of host reproduction (review in Engelstadter and Hurst, 2009; Cordaux et al., 2011), suggesting that similar effect may exist in ticks.

The same questioning are required regarding *Arsenophonus nasoniae*: known to be responsible for sex-ratio distortion in diverse arthropod species (Werren et al., 1986; Duron et al., 2010) but of unknown effect in ticks. Finally and interestingly, a *Rickettsiella* symbiont has been observed in a parthenogenetic laboratory colony of the tick *I. woodi* (Kurtti et al., 2002). This tick species is generally known to be bisexual, suggesting that *Rickettsiella* infection may induce asexuality which represents to date the only demonstration of sex ratio distortion in ticks possibly due to a symbiont.

High symbiont infection frequency is rarely observed within each tick species, and an intermediate infection frequency is much more common (Noda et al., 1997; Clay et al., 2008; Lalzar et al., 2012; Duron et al., 2017). Interestingly, infection frequencies of each maternally-inherited symbiont are often variable between geographic populations of a given tick species (Clay et al., 2008; Lalzar et al., 2012; Duron et al., 2017). This is the case for the soft tick *Ornithodoros sonrai*, with *Midichloria* and *Rickettsia* reaching high infection frequencies in some populations, but remaining absent from others (Duron et al., 2017). Similar geographical patterns were observed for many other tick species and for several symbionts such as *Rickettsiella* and *Spiroplasma* in the tree-hole tick *I. arboricola* and the polar seabird tick *I. uriae* (Duron et al., 2016, 2017). These patterns strongly suggest that maternally-inherited symbiont infection dynamics are variable across tick populations and species. Such infection frequency variations may be driven by costs and benefits associated with harboring maternally-inherited symbionts, and may maintain intermediate frequencies in tick populations, as is commonly observed in other arthropod species (Oliver et al., 2010). However, even if the nature of these costs and benefits has been well-studied in insects, they remain to be determined in ticks. Another important parameter in our understanding of this infection dynamics may be variation of biological features between tick males and females: indeed, adult males from *Ixodes* species do not blood-feed, contrary to females, which may imply that adult males do not need nutritional symbionts. The importance of this "sex" parameter to symbiont infection dynamics remains also to be demonstrated. Interestingly, this pattern was observed for *Midichloria* with males less commonly infected than females in *I. ricinus* (Lo et al., 2006). This suggests that *Midichloria* may be an important nutritional symbiont for *I. ricinus*, as recently proposed (Duron et al., 2017).

Along with maternally-inherited symbionts, other non-pathogenic microbes are present in ticks (Andreotti et al., 2011; Carpi et al., 2011; Narasimhan et al., 2014; Qiu et al., 2014; Williams-Newkirk et al., 2014; Abraham et al., 2017). Most are likely to inhabit the tick gut, while others may also colonize the tick surface cuticle. Overall, the biological effects of these non-pathogenic microbes on ticks remain entirely unknown, but it is likely that those inhabiting the tick gut could participate in blood meal digestion (Narasimhan and Fikrig, 2015) and complex interactions with TBP as we further detailed.

NON-PATHOGENIC MICROORGANISMS INTERACT WITH TBP IN DIFFERENT WAYS

An alternative fascinating aspect is that non-pathogenic microorganisms can also interfere with TBP replication and transmission by influencing TBP abundance and diversity in tick populations, as well as their transmission to vertebrate hosts. All aforementioned non-pathogenic bacteria present in ticks could have the potential to impact TBP infection processes in different ways. One can assume that TBP and non-pathogenic microorganisms may neutralize each other because they are in direct competition for limited resources, such as a particular nutrient or tissue, or because they stimulate the same immune system function. Alternatively, non-pathogenic microorganisms may excrete molecules directly inhibiting the growth of a TBP competitor, or, inversely, facilitate TBP development by immunosuppressing the tick host. As a result, non-pathogenic microorganisms may facilitate, limit, or block TBP transmission, depending on the nature of tick microbial interactions.

Equally pertinent in this regard is the role of the microbiota inhabiting the tick gut (Narasimhan et al., 2014; Abraham et al., 2017). The tick gut represents the TBP entry point, therefore gut microbiota can directly mediate TBP colonization and influence their early survival (Narasimhan and Fikrig, 2015). This finding has been perfectly illustrated in a recent study which manipulated the gut microbiota of the black-legged tick *I. scapularis*: specimens reared in sterile containers (i.e., thus preventing preventing external bacterial contamination) showed increased engorgement weights, and decreased colonization by the causative agent of Lyme disease, *Borrelia burgdorferi*, when compared to normal specimens (Narasimhan et al., 2014). Similarly, ticks fed on antibiotic-treated mice exhibited modified gut microbiota that also resulted in increased feeding and low *B. burgdorferi* colonization rates (Narasimhan et al., 2014). Altering the gut microbiota was actually found to decrease production of a glycoprotein from the tick peritrophic matrix, which separates the gut lumen from the epithelium. This peritrophic matrix is pivotal for *Borrelia* colonization success, as it protects *B. burgdorferi* colonizing the gut epithelial cells from toxic gut lumen compounds. Compromised peritrophic matrix due to altered gut microbiota will thus impede *B. burgdorferi* colonization. However, the reverse is true for another TBP, the anaplasmosis agent, *A. phagocytophilum* (Abraham et al., 2017). Remarkably, this bacterium manipulates the gut microbiota of *I. scapularis* to favor its establishment. By inducing tick glycoprotein production, *A. phagocytophilum* partially blocks bacterial biofilm formation, and thus reduces peritrophic matrix integrity, rendering the tick more susceptible to infection (Abraham et al., 2017). Altogether, these observations have uncovered a "Dr. Jekyll and Mr. Hyde"-like role of the tick gut microbiota, so that an unaltered gut microbiota will favor colonization by some TBP, such as *Borrelia*, whereas it may also block colonization by other TBP, such as *Anaplasma*. This antagonistic effect of tick gut microbiota on TBP may explain the rarity of *Borrelia-Anaplasma* co-infections in ticks collected from the field (Abraham et al., 2017).

Other interaction mechanisms may also exist. In well-studied animals, such as insects, antagonistic interactions arise when horizontally-transmitted parasites and vertically-transmitted microorganisms co-infecting the same host have conflicting evolutionary interests (Haine et al., 2005; reviewed by Haine, 2008; Ben-Ami et al., 2011; Hamilton and Perlman, 2013). Vertically-transmitted microorganisms, such as maternally-inherited symbionts, are under strong selection pressure to enhance the reproductive success of the hosts they infect (Moran et al., 2008). Conversely, parasites are typically transmitted between unrelated hosts and are therefore not directly affected by altered host fecundity. This conflict of interest has favored the emergence of defensive symbionts in insects, including maternally-inherited symbionts that protect their insect host against a variety of pathogens (reviewed by Haine, 2008; Brownlie and Johnson, 2009). For instance, some maternally-inherited symbionts such as *Wolbachia* may interfere with the replication and transmission of a wide range of pathogens (including viruses, bacteria, protozoa, nematodes, and parasitoids), and protect insects from parasite-induced mortality, possibly by up-regulating the insect's immune system (Brownlie and Johnson, 2009; Gross et al., 2009). Recently, some of these findings have been applied to the development of parasite control methods, where *Wolbachia* infection has been used to limit the vector competence of mosquitoes (Hoffmann et al., 2011). In comparison, very little was known about the existence of defensive symbionts in ticks. However, Burgdorfer et al. were the first to report the presence of defensive symbionts in the Rocky Mountain wood tick *Dermacentor andersoni*. In this tick, a maternally-inherited symbiont, *Rickettsia peacockii*, hampered the multiplication and transovarial transmission of the spotted fever agent, *Rickettsia rickettsii* (Burgdorfer et al., 1981). Similarly, resistance of the ovaries of *D. variabilis* to co-infection with *Ricketisia montana* and *Rickettsia rhipicephali* has been reported (Macaluso et al., 2002). Other experiments on *D. andersoni* further showed that *A. marginale* infection density was negatively correlated to the infection density of another maternally-inherited symbiont, *Rickettsia belli* (Gall et al., 2016). In *I. scapularis*, it has also been reported that male ticks infected by the maternally-inherited symbionts *Rickettsia buchneri* have significantly lower rates of *B. burgdorferi* infection than symbiont-free males (Steiner et al., 2008). Overall, these observations suggested that the maternally-inherited *Rickettsia* symbionts may be major defensive symbionts protecting ticks against TBP colonization. As a result, *Rickettsia* symbionts may be a key factor influencing TBP abundance and diversity in tick populations.

Conversely, maternally-inherited symbionts may not always protect ticks against pathogens: the presence of one maternally-inherited symbiont, *Francisella*-LE, in *D. andersoni* was positively associated with pathogenic *Francisella novicida* infection (Gall et al., 2016). Because these results were only obtained following laboratory manipulations, they should be treated with caution as *F. novicida* is not considered to be a TBP, as the majority of people infected with *F. novicida* contract the pathogen after ingesting infected water or ice, and not via tick bites. This study thus relies on an artificial *F. novicida* tick infection that is unlikely to happen in the field, and most importantly, using a pathogen that has not co-evolved with tick symbionts. This naturally raises the question of whether *Francisella*-LE can actually protect *D. andersoni* against TBPs that naturally occur in this tick species.

TICK SYMBIONTS CAN BE OPPORTUNISTIC VERTEBRATE PATHOGENS

Although biologists often classify host-microbe relationships as either "mutualism," "commensalism," or "parasitism," there are difficulties in defining the boundaries of these definitions. Rather, host-microbe relationships should be best described as a broad continuum, as intermediate states and transitions between states occur frequently. Several maternally-inherited tick symbionts are remarkable examples of this continuum, as recent literature has reported that certain symbionts may be transmitted to vertebrates following tick bite, as will be detailed further in this section (Shivaprasad et al., 2008; Woc-Colburn et al., 2008; Vapniarsky et al., 2012; Bazzocchi et al., 2013; Edouard et al., 2013; Angelakis et al., 2016; Seo et al., 2016a; Bonnet et al., 2017). Most importantly, some of these symbionts have the potential to opportunistically infect vertebrate hosts, including humans.

Maternally-inherited arthropod symbionts are commonly thought to be exclusively domesticated by their arthropod hosts: they cannot invade naïve hosts and have evolved to be dependent on arthropod-based transmission mechanisms through transovarial inheritance (Moran et al., 2008; Wernegreen, 2012). However, some tick symbionts, such as certain *Coxiella*, *Midichloria* and *Arsenophonus* strains, are not actually completely dependent on ticks. Rather than strictly maternal, their transmission may be partially horizontal, i.e., infectious, thus presenting a substantial infection risk to vertebrates (Shivaprasad et al., 2008; Woc-Colburn et al., 2008; Vapniarsky et al., 2012; Bazzocchi et al., 2013; Edouard et al., 2013; Angelakis et al., 2016; Seo et al., 2016a). Among these symbionts, *Coxiella*-LE are the most commonly found microorganisms in vertebrates. Indeed, tick-transmitted *Coxiella*-LE has recently been reported to cause mild infectious symptoms in humans from Europe (Angelakis et al., 2016). These microorganisms were notably detected in human skin biopsy samples and may be a common causative agent of scalp eschar and neck lymphadenopathy. *Coxiella*-LE infections have also been occasionally reported in pet birds such as psittacines and toucans reared in North America (Shivaprasad et al., 2008; Woc-Colburn et al., 2008; Vapniarsky et al., 2012). These latter *Coxiella*-LE can cause fatal disease: infected birds exhibited lethargy, weakness, emaciation, and progressive neurologic signs for several days prior to death. Conversely, another *Coxiella*-LE was identified in several South Korean horse blood samples, but none of the horses showed apparent symptoms of infection (Seo et al., 2016b).

The ability of *Coxiella*-LE to infect vertebrates through tick biting is at least partially explained by their tissue tropism within the tick body. Aside from tick ovaries and Malpighian tubules, examination of tick internal organs also revealed substantial *Coxiella*-LE concentrations within the salivary glands of some tick species (Klyachko et al., 2007; Machado-Ferreira et al., 2011; Qiu et al., 2014) but not in others (Liu et al., 2013; Lalzar et al., 2014). This tissue tropism may enable *Coxiella*-LE release into the vertebrate during tick bite, thus favoring opportunistic infections (Duron et al., 2015a). The overall likelihood of such *Coxiella*-LE tick-to-vertebrate transfers seems high since (i) ticks are found worldwide and feed on many different vertebrate species, (ii) at least two thirds of tick species are infected by *Coxiella*-LE, and (iii) when present in a given tick species, *Coxiella*-LE are usually present in almost all specimens (Duron et al., 2015a). Overall, these observations suggest that, through tick parasitism, vertebrates are often exposed to *Coxiella*-LE, and probably at a higher rate than TBP. However, despite this, *Coxiella*-LE infections are very rare in vertebrates, and most strains described to date have only been identified from ticks (Duron et al., 2015a). It is thus thought that these bacteria pose a low infection risk to vertebrates because their genome seems to be extremely reduced and is devoid of known virulence genes (Gottlieb et al., 2015; Smith et al., 2015). Nonetheless, *Coxiella*-LE have the potential to cause rare infections in vertebrates and should always be considered in future studies on tick-borne diseases.

In comparison, vertebrate infections by symbionts other than *Coxiella*-LE are clearly less common. This includes the maternally-inherited symbiont *Arsenophonus*, present in approximately 5% of terrestrial arthropods, including some tick species (Duron et al., 2008a, 2017). *Arsenophonus* is actually unique among maternally-inherited symbionts because it is able to grow outside arthropod cells, in extracellular environments (Huger et al., 1985; Werren et al., 1986). This ability enhances the likelihood of successful opportunistic *Arsenophonus* infection, as was recently observed in a woman who was bitten by a tick during a trip to Southeast Asia. This patient presenting with a rash and an eschar developed a co-infection with *Arsenophonus* and *Orientia tsutsugamushi* (the causative agent of scrub typhus) (Edouard et al., 2013). In this context, it is likely that rash and eschar development following *Orientia* infection may have favored a secondary, opportunistic, *Arsenophonus* infection.

In other cases, the identification of symbionts as opportunistic vertebrate pathogens is more difficult and remains speculative. This is the case for *Midichloria*, an intra-mitochondrial symbiont of the sheep tick *I. ricinus* and a few other tick species. Several lines of evidence have recently suggested that vertebrate hosts can be inoculated with *Midichloria* during a tick bite. Indeed, most *Midichloria* are localized in the tick ovaries, where they are transmitted to the progeny, but some have also been detected in the salivary glands and saliva of *I. ricinus* (Di Venere et al., 2015). In addition, *Midichloria* DNA, as well as antibodies against a *Midichloria* antigen, were detected in the blood of vertebrates exposed to tick bites (Bazzocchi et al., 2013). However, whether *Midichloria* can cause a true infection and pathological alteration in mammalian hosts remains to be determined.

PATHOGENS AND TICK SYMBIONTS ARE OFTEN PHYLOGENETICALLY RELATED

The vast range of intracellular bacteria in ticks is particularly illustrative of their propensity to evolve extreme and contrasting phenotypes. Certain species, such as *Rickettsia* spp. and *Coxiella* spp., have taken eukaryote associations to the extreme by completely abandoning any semblance of a free-living phase and replicating solely within the host cell. However, they do use a large panel of lifestyle strategies to spread and persist within host populations: while some are extremely virulent pathogens, others behave as subtle mutualistic symbionts (Perlman et al., 2006; Darby et al., 2007; Weinert et al., 2009; Sjodin et al., 2012; Duron et al., 2015a, 2017; Gerhart et al., 2016). Although both strategies require high degrees of lifestyle specialization, they are not fixed endpoints along the bacterium-eukaryote interaction spectrum;

rather, parasitism and mutualism may shift through repeated evolutionary transitions. This explains why both pathogenic and mutualistic forms of several major bacterial genera commonly hosted by ticks are abundantly represented.

The foremost examples of these transitions are found in three major intracellular bacteria genera: *Coxiella*, *Francisella*, and *Rickettsia* (**Figure 2**), which are all commonly identified in ticks. In medical and veterinary research, these intracellular bacteria are traditionally recognized as highly virulent vertebrate pathogens, as they have evolved specific mechanisms to penetrate into the host cytosol, appropriate nutrients for replication, subvert host immune responses, and ultimately enable infectious transmission to a new host individual (Darby et al., 2007; Celli and Zahrt, 2013; van Schaik et al., 2013; Jones et al., 2014). In humans, major intracellular pathogens have been identified from these bacterial groups, as exemplified by the agent of Q fever, *Coxiella burnetii*, the agent of tularaemia, *Francisella tularensis*, the agent of epidemic typhus, *Rickettsia prowazekii,* the agent of Rocky Mountain spotted fever, *Rickettsia rickettsia*, or the causative agent of Mediterranean spotted fever, *Rickettsia conorii* (**Figure 2**). All of these organisms are extremely infectious and some are currently classified as potential weapons for biological warfare (Darby et al., 2007; Celli and Zahrt, 2013; van Schaik et al., 2013; Jones et al., 2014). In addition, several species of tick-borne bacteria as typified by rickettsiae that were considered non-pathogenic for decades are now associated with human infections (Parola et al., 2013; Bonnet et al., 2017). However, as we have detailed above, novel intracellular bacteria engaged in endosymbiotic associations with arthropod hosts have also recently been discovered within each of these groups (**Figure 2**).

Phylogenetic investigations have revealed rapid and repeated evolutionary shifts within these three genera between pathogenic (associated with vertebrates and, in some cases, vectored by arthropods) and endosymbiotic forms (specifically linked to arthropods). However, the evolutionary shifting pattern varies among genera (**Figure 2**). In *Coxiella*, complementary lines of argument indicate a recent emergence of the Q fever agent, *C. burnetii*, from a *Coxiella*-LE strain hosted by soft ticks (Duron et al., 2015a). The *Coxiella* genus displays extensive genetic diversity, with at least four highly divergent clades (Duron et al., 2015a). While *Coxiella*-LE strains hosted by ticks are found in all these clades, all *C. burnetii* strains cluster within one of these clades, delineating an embedded group among soft tick *Coxiella*-LE (**Figure 3A**). This phylogenetic pattern indicates that the ancestor of *C. burnetii* was a tick-associated *Coxiella* which succeeded in infecting vertebrate cells (Duron et al., 2015a). The remarkably low genetic diversity of *C. burnetii* indicates unique and recent emergence of this highly infectious vertebrate pathogen (Duron et al., 2015a). Interestingly, this hypothesis was initially raised a decade ago from observations of the profound differences in *C. burnetii* genome content relative to other pathogenic intracellular bacteria (Seshadri et al., 2003).

Similarly, in *Rickettsia* spp., recent evidence revealed that human pathogens—vectored by blood feeding arthropods such as ticks—emerged relatively late in the evolution of this genus (**Figure 3C**; Perlman et al., 2006; Darby et al., 2007; Weinert et al., 2009). Phylogenetic investigations taking into account the entire *Rickettsial* diversity (i.e., including pathogenic and non-pathogenic forms) clearly indicate that switching between hosts (invertebrates, vertebrates, and even plants) has been a common feature of *Rickettsia* evolution (Perlman et al., 2006; Darby et al., 2007; Weinert et al., 2009). Based on current data, it is difficult to estimate how often vertebrate pathogenesis has evolved within *Rickettsia*. But as intracellular adaptation to arthropods is a feature of all current *Rickettsia*, it suggests that their most common recent ancestor was adapted to arthropod endosymbiosis. Surprisingly, comparing human pathogens with closely related non-pathogens showed no relationships between pathogenicity and the acquisition of novel virulence genes: vertebrate virulence seems to occur rather as result of lost or malfunctioning replication systems (Darby et al., 2007).

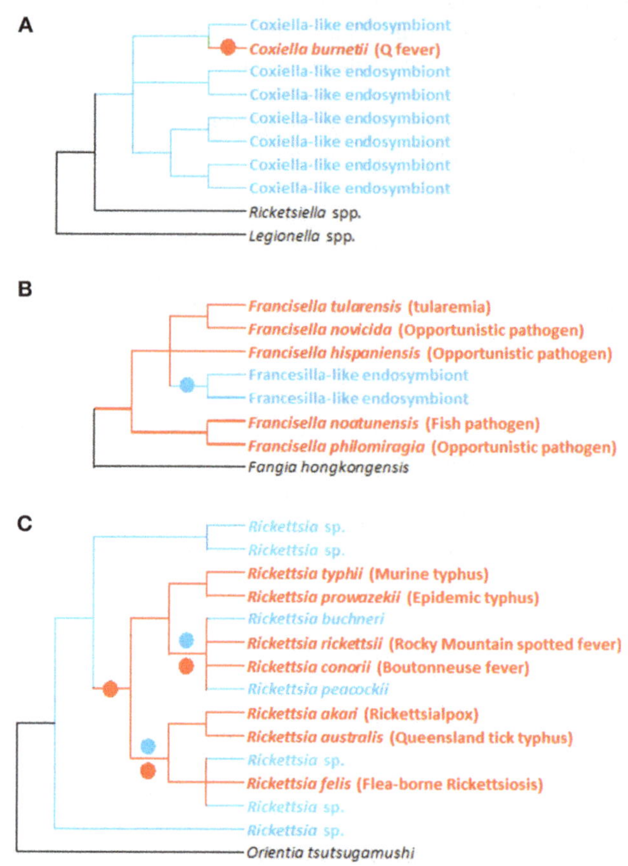

FIGURE 3 | Evolutionary relationships between pathogenic and non-pathogenic (symbiotic) forms within the *Francisella*, *Coxiellai,* and *Rickettsia* bacterial genera. **(A–C)** Simplified phylogenies of *Coxiella*, *Francisella*, and *Rickettsia*, respectively, adapted from Perlman et al. (2006), Weinert et al. (2009), Duron et al. (2015a), and Sjodin et al. (2012). Red: pathogenic forms; blue: endosymbiotic forms associated with arthropods (ticks for *Francisella* and *Coxiella*; ticks and other arthropods for *Rickettsia*); black: bacterial outgroups. Colored circles on tree branches indicate major evolutionary transitions from symbiotic ancestors to pathogenic descendants (red circles) and from pathogenic ancestors to symbiotic descendants (blue circles).

Conversely, in *Francisella*, the evolutionary pattern is substantially different, since most of the diversity found in this genus is due to pathogenic or opportunistic species (Sjodin et al., 2012). Very little is known about the evolution and origin of tick *Francisella*-LE (Michelet et al., 2013; Gerhart et al., 2016; Duron et al., 2017). However, the few *Francisella*-LE species identified to date delineate a unique monophyletic clade that clearly originates from pathogenic forms (**Figure 3B**; Duron et al., 2017). Interestingly, the *Francisella*-LE genome is similar in size to pathogenic *Francisella* species' genomes, but about one-third of the protein-coding genes are pseudogenized and are likely non-functional (Gerhart et al., 2016). This suggests that *Francisella*-LE is undergoing a global process of genome reduction, an evolutionary development typically observed in maternally-inherited symbionts (Moran et al., 2008). Interestingly, *Francisella*-LE has conserved intact most of its genes involved in B vitamin biosynthesis, highlighting the pivotal role these genes play in adaption to its current endosymbiotic lifestyle (Gerhart et al., 2016).

Overall, these two very different phenotypes (symbiosis vs. pathogenesis), along with two contrasting transmission modes (vertical vs. horizontal), and variable host specificity (ticks vs. vertebrates), make the *Coxiella*, *Francisella*, and *Rickettsia* genera especially fascinating. They thus offer an unusual opportunity to answer questions about the origins and mechanisms of symbiosis and pathogenesis. Further studies characterizing host range and infectivity of different genera members would be invaluable to obtaining such results, as would the characterization of tick symbiotic strain genomes. However, research efforts to date have invariably tended to concentrate on their medically important relatives, and so we know comparatively little about the biology of maternally-inherited symbionts. This neglect is unfortunate because fully understanding the whole scope of *Coxiella*, *Francisella*, and *Rickettsia* phenotypes linked to genome sequences, will provide an excellent system to test hypotheses on the importance of genome content and plasticity in the emergence and reversibility of extreme phenotypes such as symbiosis and pathogenesis.

CONCLUSION AND PERSPECTIVES

Extensive literature studies have now made it clear that TBP are not alone: an appreciable range of diverse non-pathogenic microorganisms has also been detected in almost all tick species examined so far. Perhaps the most important consideration for the future is not the incidence of these non-pathogenic microorganisms, but their phenotypes. The varied collection of non-pathogenic microorganisms includes intracellular maternally-inherited symbionts and microbes inhabiting the tick gut, and each could strongly influence—in very different ways—the biology of their tick hosts as well as TBP infection dynamics. Recent findings have shown that several maternally-inherited symbionts such as *Coxiella*-LE are important drivers of evolutionary change in ticks, as clearly shown by their role in driving their tick hosts to adapt to a strict hematophagous diet (Gottlieb et al., 2015; Smith et al., 2015; Duron et al., 2017). Other non-pathogenic microorganisms such as maternally-inherited *Rickettsia* symbionts and gut microbiota are also likely to substantially contribute to the acquisition of ecologically important traits, such as TBP resistance (Burgdorfer et al., 1981; Steiner et al., 2008; Narasimhan et al., 2014; Abraham et al., 2017). It is therefore vital to establish the nature of the interactions between non-pathogenic microorganisms, their tick hosts, and co-infecting TBP. To achieve this goal, it is essential to understand how ticks acquire their microbiota, and how microbial community structures are shaped by various environmental and host factors, and also by microbial interactions within these communities. This knowledge is a key step toward using non-pathogenic microorganisms to limit TBP transmission and persistence. Similarly, whether tick symbionts have the potential to opportunistically infect humans and other vertebrates should be investigated in depth. Lastly, we would like to emphasize that the study of some non-pathogenic microorganisms, such as members of the *Coxiella*, *Francisella*, and *Rickettsia* genera, can advance our understanding of many infectious diseases including Q fever, tularemia, and rickettsial diseases. The broad phenotypic diversity present in these three bacterial genera make them perfect models to study the evolutionary emergence of pathogenicity and adaptations to living in vertebrate cells. Owing to their medical importance, the pathogenic species of these genera have been the targets of several genome sequencing projects, which have provided insights into the mechanisms and consequences of their specialized lifestyles (Darby et al., 2007; van Schaik et al., 2013). Conversely, the symbiotic forms adapted to tick hosts have received much less attention and a lot of things remain to be elucidated (but see Gillespie et al., 2012, 2015; Clark et al., 2015 for genomics insights about *Rickettsia*). In this context, comparative genomic approaches will be highly valuable in enhancing our understanding of the evolutionary ecology of both pathogenic and non-pathogenic intracellular bacteria, and in identifying novel candidate genes contributing to virulence and persistence in vertebrate cells.

AUTHOR CONTRIBUTIONS

SB, AH, FB, and OD conducted the literature research, wrote the paper and prepared the figures and tables. All authors provided critical review and revisions.

ACKNOWLEDGMENTS

We thank members of our laboratories for fruitful discussions and especially the ≪ Tiques et Maladies à Tiques ≫ group (REID-Réseau Ecologie des Interactions Durables). We also acknowledge an Investissement d'Avenir grant of the Agence Nationale de la Recherche (CEBA: ANR-10-LABX-25-01).

REFERENCES

Abraham, N. M., Liu, L., Jutras, B. L., Yadav, A. K., Narasimhan, S., Gopalakrishnan, V., et al. (2017). Pathogen-mediated manipulation of arthropod microbiota to promote infection. *Proc. Natl. Acad. Sci. U.S.A.* 114, E781–E790. doi: 10.1073/pnas.1613422114

Akman, L., Yamashita, A., Watanabe, H., Oshima, K., Shiba, T., Hattori, M., et al. (2002). Genome sequence of the endocellular obligate symbiont of tsetse flies, *Wigglesworthia glossinidia*. *Nat. Genet.* 32, 402–407. doi: 10.1038/ng986

Almeida, A. P., Marcili, A., Leite, R. C., Nieri-Bastos, F. A., Domingues, L. N., Martins, J. R., et al. (2012). Coxiella symbiont in the tick Ornithodoros rostratus (*Acari*: *Argasidae*). *Ticks Tick Borne Dis.* 3, 203–206. doi: 10.1016/j.ttbdis.2012.02.003

Andreotti, R., Perez de Leon, A. A., Dowd, S. E., Guerrero, F. D., Bendele, K. G., and Scoles, G. A. (2011). Assessment of bacterial diversity in the cattle tick *Rhipicephalus* (Boophilus) microplus through tag-encoded pyrosequencing. *BMC Microbiol.* 11:6. doi: 10.1186/1471-2180-11-6

Angelakis, E., Mediannikov, O., Jos, S. L., Berenger, J. M., Parola, P., and Raoult, D. (2016). Candidatus Coxiella massiliensis infection. *Emerging Infect. Dis.* 22, 285–288. doi: 10.3201/eid2202.150106

Anstead, C. A., and Chilton, N. B. (2014). Discovery of novel *Rickettsiella* spp. in ixodid ticks from Western Canada. *Appl. Environ. Microbiol.* 80, 1403–1410. doi: 10.1128/AEM.03564-13

Bazzocchi, C., Mariconti, M., Sassera, D., Rinaldi, L., Martin, E., Cringoli, G., et al. (2013). Molecular and serological evidence for the circulation of the tick symbiont Midichloria (*Rickettsiales*: *Midichloriaceae*) in different mammalian species. *Parasit. Vectors* 6:350. doi: 10.1186/1756-3305-6-350

Ben-Ami, F., Rigaud, T., and Ebert, D. (2011). The expression of virulence during double infections by different parasites with conflicting host exploitation and transmission strategies. *J. Evol. Biol.* 24, 1307–1316. doi: 10.1111/j.1420-9101.2011.02264.x

Benson, M. J., Gawronski, J. D., Eveleigh, D. E., and Benson, D. R. (2004). Intracellular symbionts and other bacteria associated with deer ticks (*Ixodes scapularis*) from Nantucket and Wellfleet, Cape Cod, Massachusetts. *Appl. Environ. Microbiol.* 70, 616–620. doi: 10.1128/AEM.70.1.616-620.2004

Bohacsova, M., Mediannikov, O., Kazimirova, M., Raoult, D., and Sekeyova, Z. (2016). *Arsenophonus nasoniae* and Rickettsiae Infection of *Ixodes ricinus* due to parasitic wasp ixodiphagus hookeri. *PLoS ONE* 11:e0149950. doi: 10.1371/journal.pone.0149950

Bonnet, S. I., Paul, R. E., Bischoff, E., Cote, M., and Le Naour, E. (2017). First identification of *Rickettsia helvetica* in questing ticks from a French Northern Brittany Forest. *PLoS Negl. Trop. Dis.* 11:e0005416. doi: 10.1371/journal.pntd.0005416

Bouchon, D., Cordaux, R., and Grève, P. (2012). "Rickettsiella, intracellular pathogens of arthropods," in *Manipulative Tenants*, eds E. Zchori-Fein and K. Bourtzis. (Boca Raton, FL: CRC Press), 127–148.

Boyd, B. M., Allen, J. M., de Crecy-Lagard, V., and Reed, D. L. (2013). Genome sequence of Candidatus Riesia pediculischaeffi, endosymbiont of chimpanzee lice, and genomic comparison of recently acquired endosymbionts from human and chimpanzee lice. *G3 (Bethesda)* 4, 2189–2195. doi: 10.1534/g3.114.012567

Brownlie, J. C., and Johnson, K. N. (2009). Symbiont-mediated protection in insect hosts. *Trends Microbiol.* 17, 348–354. doi: 10.1016/j.tim.2009.05.005

Burgdorfer, W., Hayes, S., and MAvros, A. (1981). "Non-pathogenic rickettsiae in *Dermacentor andersoni*: a limiting factor for the distribution of *Rickettsia rickettsii*," in *Rickettsia and Rickettsial Disease*, ed W. A. A. Burgdorfer and R. L. Anacker (New York, NY: Academic), 585–594.

Carpi, G., Cagnacci, F., Wittekindt, N. E., Zhao, F., Qi, J., Tomsho, L. P., et al. (2011). Metagenomic profile of the bacterial communities associated with *Ixodes ricinus* ticks. *PLoS ONE* 6:e25604. doi: 10.1371/journal.pone.0025604

Celli, J., and Zahrt, T. C. (2013). Mechanisms of *Francisella tularensis* intracellular pathogenesis. *Cold Spring Harb. Perspect. Med.* 3:a010314. doi: 10.1101/cshperspect.a010314

Chauvin, A., Moreau, E., Bonnet, S., Plantard, O., and Malandrin, L. (2009). Babesia and its hosts: adaptation to long-lasting interactions as a way to achieve efficient transmission. *Vet. Res.* 40:37. doi: 10.1051/vetres/2009020

Clark, T. R., Noriea, N. F., Bublitz, D. C., Ellison, D. W., Martens, C., Lutter, E. I., et al. (2015). Comparative genome sequencing of *Rickettsia rickettsii* strains that differ in virulence. *Infect. Immun.* 83, 1568–1576. doi: 10.1128/IAI.03140-14

Clay, K., Klyachko, O., Grindle, N., Civitello, D., Oleske, D., and Fuqua, C. (2008). Microbial communities and interactions in the lone star tick, *Amblyomma americanum*. *Mol. Ecol.* 17, 4371–4381. doi: 10.1111/j.1365-294X.2008.03914.x

Clayton, K. A., Gall, C. A., Mason, K. L., Scoles, G. A., and Brayton, K. A. (2015). The characterization and manipulation of the bacterial microbiome of the Rocky Mountain wood tick, *Dermacentor andersoni*. *Parasit. Vectors* 8:632. doi: 10.1186/s13071-015-1245-z

Cordaux, R., Bouchon, D., and Greve, P. (2011). The impact of endosymbionts on the evolution of host sex-determination mechanisms. *Trends Genet.* 27, 332–341. doi: 10.1016/j.tig.2011.05.002

Dantas-Torres, F., Chomel, B. B., and Otranto, D. (2012). Ticks and tick-borne diseases: a one health perspective. *Trends Parasitol.* 28, 437–446. doi: 10.1016/j.pt.2012.07.003

Darby, A. C., Cho, N. H., Fuxelius, H. H., Westberg, J., and Andersson, S. G. (2007). Intracellular pathogens go extreme: genome evolution in the *Rickettsiales*. *Trends Genet.* 23, 511–520. doi: 10.1016/j.tig.2007.08.002

de la Fuente, J., Estrada-Pena, A., Venzal, J. M., Kocan, K. M., and Sonenshine, D. E. (2008). Overview: ticks as vectors of pathogens that cause disease in humans and animals. *Front. Biosci.* 13, 6938–6946. doi: 10.2741/3200

Dergousoff, S. J., and Chilton, N. B. (2010). Detection of a new Arsenophonus-type bacterium in Canadian populations of the Rocky Mountain wood tick, *Dermacentor andersoni*. *Exp. Appl. Acarol.* 52, 85–91. doi: 10.1007/s10493-010-9340-5

Di Venere, M., Fumagalli, M., Cafiso, A., De Marco, L., Epis, S., Plantard, O., et al. (2015). *Ixodes ricinus* and its endosymbiont midichloria mitochondrii: a comparative proteomic analysis of salivary glands and ovaries. *PLoS ONE* 10:e0138842. doi: 10.1371/journal.pone.0138842

Dunning Hotopp, J. C., Lin, M., Madupu, R., Crabtree, J., Angiuoli, S. V., Eisen, J. A., et al. (2006). Comparative genomics of emerging human ehrlichiosis agents. *PLoS Genet.* 2:e21. doi: 10.1371/journal.pgen.0020021

Duron, O., Binetruy, F., Noël, V., Cremaschi, J., McCoy, K. D., Arnathau, A., et al. (2017). Evolutionary changes in symbiont community structure in ticks. *Mol. Ecol.* 26, 2905–2921. doi: 10.1111/mec.14094

Duron, O., Bouchon, D., Boutin, S., Bellamy, L., Zhou, L., Engelstadter, J., et al. (2008a). The diversity of reproductive parasites among arthropods: wolbachia do not walk alone. *BMC Biol.* 6:27. doi: 10.1186/1741-7007-6-27

Duron, O., Cremaschi, J., and McCoy, K. D. (2016). The high diversity and global distribution of the intracellular bacterium *Rickettsiella* in the polar seabird tick Ixodes uriae. *Microb. Ecol.* 71, 761–770. doi: 10.1007/s00248-015-0702-8

Duron, O., Hurst, G. D., Hornett, E. A., Josling, J. A., and Engelstadter, J. (2008b). High incidence of the maternally inherited bacterium Cardinium in spiders. *Mol. Ecol.* 17, 1427–1437. doi: 10.1111/j.1365-294X.2008.03689.x

Duron, O., Jourdain, E., and McCoy, K. D. (2014). Diversity and global distribution of the *Coxiella* intracellular bacterium in seabird ticks. *Ticks Tick Borne Dis.* 5, 557–563. doi: 10.1016/j.ttbdis.2014.04.003

Duron, O., Noel, V., McCoy, K. D., Bonazzi, M., Sidi-Boumedine, K., Morel, O., et al. (2015a). The recent evolution of a maternally-inherited endosymbiont of ticks led to the emergence of the Q Fever pathogen, *Coxiella burnetii*. *PLoS Pathog.* 11:e1004892. doi: 10.1371/journal.ppat.1004892

Duron, O., Sidi-Boumedine, K., Rousset, E., Moutailler, S., and Jourdain, E. (2015b). The importance of ticks in q fever transmission: what has (and has not) been demonstrated? *Trends Parasitol.* 31, 536–552. doi: 10.1016/j.pt.2015.06.014

Duron, O., Wilkes, T. E., and Hurst, G. D. (2010). Interspecific transmission of a male-killing bacterium on an ecological timescale. *Ecol. Lett.* 13, 1139–1148. doi: 10.1111/j.1461-0248.2010.01502.x

Edouard, S., Subramanian, G., Lefevre, B., Dos Santos, A., Pouedras, P., Poinsignon, Y., et al. (2013). Co-infection with *Arsenophonus nasoniae* and *Orientia tsutsugamushi* in a traveler. *Vector Borne Zoonotic Dis.* 13, 565–571. doi: 10.1089/vbz.2012.1083

Engelstadter, J., and Hurst, G. D. D. (2009). The ecology and evolution of microbes that manipulate host reproduction. *Annu. Rev. Ecol. Evol. Syst.* 40, 127–149. doi: 10.1146/annurev.ecolsys.110308.120206

Epis, S., Mandrioli, M., Genchi, M., Montagna, M., Sacchi, L., Pistone, D., et al. (2013). Localization of the bacterial symbiont Candidatus Midichloria mitochondrii within the hard tick *Ixodes ricinus* by whole-mount FISH staining. *Ticks Tick Borne Dis.* 4, 39–45. doi: 10.1016/j.ttbdis.2012.06.005

Epis, S., Sassera, D., Beninati, T., Lo, N., Beati, L., Piesman, J., et al. (2008). Midichloria mitochondrii is widespread in hard ticks (Ixodidae) and resides in the mitochondria of phylogenetically diverse species. *Parasitology* 135, 485–494. doi: 10.1017/S0031182007004052

Felsheim, R. F., Kurtti, T. J., and Munderloh, U. G. (2009). Genome sequence of the endosymbiont *Rickettsia peacockii* and comparison with virulent *Rickettsia rickettsii*: identification of virulence factors. *PLoS ONE* 4:e8361. doi: 10.1371/journal.pone.0008361

Ferrari, J., and Vavre, F. (2011). Bacterial symbionts in insects or the story of communities affecting communities. *Philos. Trans. R. Soc. Lond. B Biol. Sci.* 366, 1389–1400. doi: 10.1098/rstb.2010.0226

Gall, C. A., Reif, K. E., Scoles, G. A., Mason, K. L., Mousel, M., Noh, S. M., et al. (2016). The bacterial microbiome of *Dermacentor andersoni* ticks influences pathogen susceptibility. *ISME J.* 10, 1846–1855. doi: 10.1038/ismej.2015.266

Gerhart, J. G., Moses, A. S., and Raghavan, R. (2016). A *Francisella*-like endosymbiont in the Gulf Coast tick evolved from a mammalian pathogen. *Sci. Rep.* 6:33670. doi: 10.1038/srep33670

Gillespie, J. J., Joardar, V., Williams, K. P., Driscoll, T., Hostetler, J. B., Nordberg, E., et al. (2012). A *Rickettsia* genome overrun by mobile genetic elements provides insight into the acquisition of genes characteristic of an obligate intracellular lifestyle. *J. Bacteriol.* 194, 376–394. doi: 10.1128/jb.06244-11

Gillespie, J. J., Kaur, S. J., Rahman, M. S., Rennoll-Bankert, K., Sears, K. T., Beier-Sexton, M., et al. (2015). Secretome of obligate intracellular *Rickettsia*. *FEMS Microbiol. Rev.* 39, 47–80. doi: 10.1111/1574-6976.12084

Gross, R., Vavre, F., Heddi, A., Hurst, G. D., Zchori-Fein, E., and Bourtzis, K. (2009). Immunity and symbiosis. *Mol. Microbiol.* 73, 751–759. doi: 10.1111/j.1365-2958.2009.06820.x

Goethert, H. K., and Telford, S. R. III. (2005). A new Francisella (*Beggiatiales: Francisellaceae*) inquiline within *Dermacentor variabilis* say (*Acari: Ixodidae*). *J. Med. Entomol.* 42, 502–505. doi: 10.1093/jmedent/42.3.502

Gottlieb, Y., Lalzar, I., and Klasson, L. (2015). Distinctive genome reduction rates revealed by genomic analyses of two *Coxiella*-like endosymbionts in ticks. *Genome Biol. Evol.* 7, 1779–1796. doi: 10.1093/gbe/evv108

Haine, E. R. (2008). Symbiont-mediated protection. *Proc. Biol. Sci.* 275, 353–361. doi: 10.1098/rspb.2007.1211

Haine, E. R., Boucansaud, K., and Rigaud, T. (2005). Conflict between parasites with different transmission strategies infecting an amphipod host. *Proc. Biol. Sci.* 272, 2505–2510. doi: 10.1098/rspb.2005.3244

Hamilton, P. T., and Perlman, S. J. (2013). Host defense via symbiosis in *Drosophila*. *PLoS Pathog.* 9:e1003808. doi: 10.1371/journal.ppat.1003808

Heise, S. R., Elshahed, M. S., and Little, S. E. (2010). Bacterial diversity in *Amblyomma americanum* (*Acari: Ixodidae*) with a focus on members of the genus *Rickettsia*. *J. Med. Entomol.* 47, 258–268. doi: 10.1093/jmedent/47.2.258

Henning, K., Greiner-Fischer, S., Hotzel, H., Ebsen, M., and Theegarten, D. (2006). Isolation of *Spiroplasma* sp. from an Ixodes tick. *Int. J. Med. Microbiol.* 296(Suppl. 40), 157–161. doi: 10.1016/j.ijmm.2006.01.012

Heyman, P., Cochez, C., Hofhuis, A., van der Giessen, J., Sprong, H., Porter, S. R., et al. (2010). A clear and present danger: tick-borne diseases in Europe. *Expert Rev. Anti Infect. Ther.* 8, 33–50. doi: 10.1586/eri.09.118

Hoffmann, A. A., Montgomery, B. L., Popovici, J., Iturbe-Ormaetxe, I., Johnson, P. H., Muzzi, F., et al. (2011). Successful establishment of Wolbachia in Aedes populations to suppress dengue transmission. *Nature* 476, 454–457. doi: 10.1038/nature10356

Hosokawa, T., Koga, R., Kikuchi, Y., Meng, X. Y., and Fukatsu, T. (2010). Wolbachia as a bacteriocyte-associated nutritional mutualist. *Proc. Natl. Acad. Sci. U.S.A.* 107, 769–774. doi: 10.1073/pnas.0911476107

Huger, A. M., Skinner, S. W., and Werren, J. H. (1985). Bacterial infections associated with the son-killer trait in the parasitoid wasp Nasonia (= Mormoniella) vitripennis (Hymenoptera: Pteromalidae). *J. Invertebr. Pathol.* 46, 272–280. doi: 10.1016/0022-2011(85)90069-2

Hunter, D. J., Torkelson, J. L., Bodnar, J., Mortazavi, B., Laurent, T., Deason, J., et al. (2015). The *Rickettsia* endosymbiont of ixodes pacificus contains all the genes of *De novo* folate biosynthesis. *PLoS ONE* 10:e0144552. doi: 10.1371/journal.pone.0144552

Iasur-Kruh, L., Weintraub, P. G., Mozes-Daube, N., Robinson, W. E., Perlman, S. J., and Zchori-Fein, E. (2013). Novel *Rickettsiella* bacterium in the leafhopper Orosius albicinctus (*Hemiptera: Cicadellidae*). *Appl. Environ. Microbiol.* 79, 4246–4252. doi: 10.1128/AEM.00721-13

Jasinskas, A., Zhong, J., and Barbour, A. G. (2007). Highly prevalent *Coxiella* sp. bacterium in the tick vector Amblyomma americanum. *Appl. Environ. Microbiol.* 73, 334–336. doi: 10.1128/AEM.02009-06

Jones, B. D., Faron, M., Rasmussen, J. A., and Fletcher, J. R. (2014). Uncovering the components of the *Francisella tularensis* virulence stealth strategy. *Front. Cell. Infect. Microbiol.* 4:32. doi: 10.3389/fcimb.2014.00032

Jousselin, E., Coeur d'Acier, A., Vanlerberghe-Masutti, F., and Duron, O. (2013). Evolution and diversity of *Arsenophonus endosymbionts* in aphids. *Mol. Ecol.* 22, 260–270. doi: 10.1111/mec.12092

Kagemann, J., and Clay, K. (2013). Effects of infection by *Arsenophonus* and *Rickettsia* bacteria on the locomotive ability of the ticks *Amblyomma americanum, Dermacentor variabilis,* and *Ixodes scapularis. J. Med. Entomol.* 50, 155–162. doi: 10.1603/ME12086

Klyachko, O., Stein, B. D., Grindle, N., Clay, K., and Fuqua, C. (2007). Localization and visualization of a *Coxiella*-type symbiont within the lone star tick, *Amblyomma americanum*. *Appl. Environ. Microbiol.* 73, 6584–6594. doi: 10.1128/AEM.00537-07

Kurtti, T. J., Felsheim, R. F., Burkhardt, N. Y., Oliver, J. D., Heu, C. C., and Munderloh, U. G. (2015). *Rickettsia buchneri* sp. nov., a rickettsial endosymbiont of the blacklegged tick *Ixodes scapularis*. *Int. J. Syst. Evol. Microbiol.* 65(Pt 3), 965–970. doi: 10.1099/ijs.0.000047

Kurtti, T. J., Munderloh, U. G., Andreadis, T. G., Magnarelli, L. A., and Mather, T. N. (1996). Tick cell culture isolation of an intracellular prokaryote from the tick *Ixodes scapularis*. *J. Invertebr. Pathol.* 67, 318–321. doi: 10.1006/jipa.1996.0050

Kurtti, T. J., Palmer, A. T., and Oliver, J. H. Jr. (2002). Rickettsiella-like bacteria in Ixodes woodi (*Acari: Ixodidae*). *J. Med. Entomol.* 39, 534–540. doi: 10.1603/0022-2585-39.3.534

Lalzar, I., Friedmann, Y., and Gottlieb, Y. (2014). Tissue tropism and vertical transmission of *Coxiella* in *Rhipicephalus sanguineus* and *Rhipicephalus turanicus* ticks. *Environ. Microbiol.* 16, 3657–3668. doi: 10.1111/1462-2920.12455

Lalzar, I., Harrus, S., Mumcuoglu, K. Y., and Gottlieb, Y. (2012). Composition and seasonal variation of *Rhipicephalus turanicus* and *Rhipicephalus sanguineus* bacterial communities. *Appl. Environ. Microbiol.* 78, 4110–4116. doi: 10.1128/AEM.00323-12

Liu, L. M., Liu, J. N., Liu, Z., Yu, Z. J., Xu, S. Q., Yang, X. H., et al. (2013). Microbial communities and symbionts in the hard tick *Haemaphysalis longicornis* (*Acari: Ixodidae*) from north China. *Parasit. Vectors* 6:310. doi: 10.1186/1756-3305-6-310

Lo, N., Beninati, T., Sassera, D., Bouman, E. A., Santagati, S., Gern, L., et al. (2006). Widespread distribution and high prevalence of an alpha-proteobacterial symbiont in the tick Ixodes ricinus. *Environ. Microbiol.* 8, 1280–1287. doi: 10.1111/j.1462-2920.2006.01024.x

Lukasik, P., Guo, H., van Asch, M., Ferrari, J., and Godfray, H. C. (2013). Protection against a fungal pathogen conferred by the aphid facultative endosymbionts *Rickettsia* and *Spiroplasma* is expressed in multiple host genotypes and species and is not influenced by co-infection with another symbiont. *J. Evol. Biol.* 26, 2654–2661. doi: 10.1111/jeb.12260

Macaluso, K. R., Sonenshine, D. E., Ceraul, S. M., and Azad, A. F. (2002). *Rickettsial* infection in *Dermacentor variabilis* (*Acari: Ixodidae*) inhibits transovarial transmission of a second *Rickettsia*. *J. Med. Entomol.* 39, 809–813. doi: 10.1603/0022-2585-39.6.809

Machado-Ferreira, E., Dietrich, G., Hojgaard, A., Levin, M., Piesman, J., Zeidner, N. S., et al. (2011). *Coxiella* symbionts in the Cayenne tick *Amblyomma cajennense*. *Microb. Ecol.* 62, 134–142. doi: 10.1007/s00248-011-9868-x

Matsuura, Y., Kikuchi, Y., Meng, X. Y., Koga, R., and Fukatsu, T. (2012). Novel clade of alphaproteobacterial endosymbionts associated with stinkbugs and other arthropods. *Appl. Environ. Microbiol.* 78, 4149–4156. doi: 10.1128/AEM.00673-12

Menchaca, A. C., Visi, D. K., Strey, O. F., Teel, P. D., Kalinowski, K., Allen, M. S., et al. (2013). Preliminary assessment of microbiome changes following blood-feeding and survivorship in the *Amblyomma americanum* nymph-to-adult transition using semiconductor sequencing. *PLoS ONE* 8:e67129. doi: 10.1371/journal.pone.0067129

Michelet, L., Bonnet, S., Madani, N., and Moutailler, S. (2013). Discriminating *Francisella tularensis* and Francisella-like endosymbionts in *Dermacentor reticulatus* ticks: evaluation of current molecular techniques. *Vet. Microbiol.* 163, 399–403. doi: 10.1016/j.vetmic.2013.01.014

Moran, N. A., McCutcheon, J. P., and Nakabachi, A. (2008). Genomics and evolution of heritable bacterial symbionts. *Annu. Rev. Genet.* 42, 165–190. doi: 10.1146/annurev.genet.41.110306.130119

Moreno, C. X., Moy, F., Daniels, T. J., Godfrey, H. P., and Cabello, F. C. (2006). Molecular analysis of microbial communities identified in different developmental stages of Ixodes scapularis ticks from Westchester and Dutchess Counties, New York. *Environ. Microbiol.* 8, 761–772. doi: 10.1111/j.1462-2920.2005.00955.x

Najm, N. A., Silaghi, C., Bell-Sakyi, L., Pfister, K., and Passos, L. M. (2012). Detection of bacteria related to Candidatus Midichloria mitochondrii in tick cell lines. *Parasitol. Res.* 110, 437–442. doi: 10.1007/s00436-011-2509-y

Nakao, R., Abe, T., Nijhof, A. M., Yamamoto, S., Jongejan, F., Ikemura, T., et al. (2013). A novel approach, based on BLSOMs (Batch Learning Self-Organizing Maps), to the microbiome analysis of ticks. *ISME J.* 7, 1003–1015. doi: 10.1038/ismej.2012.171

Narasimhan, S., and Fikrig, E. (2015). Tick microbiome: the force within. *Trends Parasitol.* 31, 315–323. doi: 10.1016/j.pt.2015.03.010

Narasimhan, S., Rajeevan, N., Liu, L., Zhao, Y. O., Heisig, J., Pan, J., et al. (2014). Gut microbiota of the tick vector Ixodes scapularis modulate colonization of the Lyme disease spirochete. *Cell Host Microbe* 15, 58–71. doi: 10.1016/j.chom.2013.12.001

Niebylski, M. L., Peacock, M. G., Fischer, E. R., Porcella, S. F., and Schwan, T. G. (1997a). Characterization of an endosymbiont infecting wood ticks, *Dermacentor andersoni*, as a member of the genus *Francisella*. *Appl. Environ. Microbiol.* 63, 3933–3940.

Niebylski, M. L., Schrumpf, M. E., Burgdorfer, W., Fischer, E. R., Gage, K. L., and Schwan, T. G. (1997b). *Rickettsia peacockii* sp. nov., a new species infecting wood ticks, *Dermacentor andersoni*, in western Montana. *Int. J. Syst. Bacteriol.* 47, 446–452. doi: 10.1099/00207713-47-2-446

Nikoh, N., Hosokawa, T., Moriyama, M., Oshima, K., Hattori, M., and Fukatsu, T. (2014). Evolutionary origin of insect-Wolbachia nutritional mutualism. *Proc. Natl. Acad. Sci. U.S.A.* 111, 10257–10262. doi: 10.1073/pnas.1409284111

Noda, H., Munderloh, U. G., and Kurtti, T. J. (1997). Endosymbionts of ticks and their relationship to *Wolbachia* spp. and tick-borne pathogens of humans and animals. *Appl. Environ. Microbiol.* 63, 3926–3932.

Novakova, E., Hypsa, V., and Moran, N. A. (2009). Arsenophonus, an emerging clade of intracellular symbionts with a broad host distribution. *BMC Microbiol.* 9:143. doi: 10.1186/1471-2180-9-143

Oliver, K. M., Degnan, P. H., Burke, G. R., and Moran, N. A. (2010). Facultative symbionts in aphids and the horizontal transfer of ecologically important traits. *Annu. Rev. Entomol.* 55, 247–266. doi: 10.1146/annurev-ento-112408-085305

Parola, P., Paddock, C. D., Socolovschi, C., Labruna, M. B., Mediannikov, O., Kernifd, T., et al. (2013). Update on tick-borne rickettsioses around the world: a geographic approach. *Clin. Microbiol. Rev.* 26, 657–702. doi: 10.1128/CMR.00032-13

Paul, R., Cote, M., Le Naour, E., and Bonnet, S. (2016). Environmental factors influencing tick densities over seven years in a French suburban forest. *Parasit. Vectors* 9:309. doi: 10.1186/s13071-016-1591-5

Perlman, S. J., Hunter, M. S., and Zchori-Fein, E. (2006). The emerging diversity of *Rickettsia*. *Proc. Biol. Sci.* 273, 2097–2106. doi: 10.1098/rspb.2006.3541

Plantard, O., Bouju-Albert, A., Malard, M. A., Hermouet, A., Capron, G., and Verheyden, H. (2012). Detection of Wolbachia in the tick *Ixodes ricinus* is due to the presence of the hymenoptera endoparasitoid *Ixodiphagus hookeri*. *PLoS ONE* 7:e30692. doi: 10.1371/journal.pone.0030692

Qiu, Y., Nakao, R., Ohnuma, A., Kawamori, F., and Sugimoto, C. (2014). Microbial population analysis of the salivary glands of ticks; a possible strategy for the surveillance of bacterial pathogens. *PLoS ONE* 9:e103961. doi: 10.1371/journal.pone.0103961

Reis, C., Cote, M., Paul, R. E., and Bonnet, S. (2011). Questing ticks in suburban forest are infected by at least six tick-borne pathogens. *Vector Borne Zoonotic Dis.* 11, 907–916. doi: 10.1089/vbz.2010.0103

Rizzoli, A., Silaghi, C., Obiegala, A., Rudolf, I., Hubalek, Z., Foldvari, G., et al. (2014). *Ixodes ricinus* and its transmitted pathogens in urban and peri-urban areas in Europe: new hazards and relevance for public health. *Front Public Health* 2:251. doi: 10.3389/fpubh.2014.00251

Rodriguez-Valle, M., Lew-Tabor, A., Gondro, C., Moolhuijzen, P., Vance, M., Guerrero, F. D., et al. (2010). Comparative microarray analysis of *Rhipicephalus* (Boophilus) microplus expression profiles of larvae pre-attachment and feeding adult female stages on *Bos indicus* and *Bos taurus cattle*. *BMC Genomics* 11:437. doi: 10.1186/1471-2164-11-437

Sassera, D., Beninati, T., Bandi, C., Bouman, E. A., Sacchi, L., Fabbi, M., et al. (2006). 'Candidatus Midichloria mitochondrii', an endosymbiont of the tick *Ixodes ricinus* with a unique intramitochondrial lifestyle. *Int. J. Syst. Evol. Microbiol.* 56(Pt 11), 2535–2540. doi: 10.1099/ijs.0.64386-0

Sassera, D., Lo, N., Epis, S., D'Auria, G., Montagna, M., Comandatore, F., et al. (2011). Phylogenomic evidence for the presence of a flagellum and cbb oxidase in the free-living mitochondrial ancestor. *Mol. Biol. Evol.* 28, 3285–3296. doi: 10.1093/molbev/msr159

Scoles, G. A. (2004). Phylogenetic analysis of the *Francisella*-like endosymbionts of *Dermacentor* ticks. *J. Med. Entomol.* 41, 277–286. doi: 10.1603/0022-2585-41.3.277

Seo, M. G., Lee, S. H., Ouh, I. O., Lee, G. H., Goo, Y. K., Kim, S., et al. (2016a). Molecular detection and genotyping of *Coxiella-like* endosymbionts in ticks that infest horses in South Korea. *PLoS ONE* 11:e0165784. doi: 10.1371/journal.pone.0165784

Seo, M. G., Lee, S. H., VanBik, D., Ouh, I. O., Yun, S. H., Choi, E., et al. (2016b). Detection and genotyping of *Coxiella burnetii* and *Coxiella-like* bacteria in horses in South Korea. *PLoS ONE* 11:e0156710. doi: 10.1371/journal.pone.0156710

Seshadri, R., Paulsen, I. T., Eisen, J. A., Read, T. D., Nelson, K. E., Nelson, W. C., et al. (2003). Complete genome sequence of the Q-fever pathogen *Coxiella burnetii*. *Proc. Natl. Acad. Sci. U.S.A.* 100, 5455–5460. doi: 10.1073/pnas.0931379100

Shivaprasad, H. L., Cadenas, M. B., Diab, S. S., Nordhausen, R., Bradway, D., Crespo, R., et al. (2008). *Coxiella-like* infection in psittacines and a toucan. *Avian Dis.* 52, 426–432. doi: 10.1637/8192-120707-Reg

Sjodin, A., Svensson, K., Ohrman, C., Ahlinder, J., Lindgren, P., Duodu, S., et al. (2012). Genome characterisation of the genus *Francisella* reveals insight into similar evolutionary paths in pathogens of mammals and fish. *BMC Genomics* 13:268. doi: 10.1186/1471-2164-13-268

Smith, T. A., Driscoll, T., Gillespie, J. J., and Raghavan, R. (2015). A *Coxiella-like* endosymbiont is a potential vitamin source for the Lone Star tick. *Genome Biol. Evol.* 7, 831–838. doi: 10.1093/gbe/evv016

Steiner, F. E., Pinger, R. R., Vann, C. N., Grindle, N., Civitello, D., Clay, K., et al. (2008). Infection and co-infection rates of Anaplasma phagocytophilum variants, *Babesia* spp., *Borrelia burgdorferi*, and the rickettsial endosymbiont in *Ixodes scapularis* (*Acari*: *Ixodidae*) from sites in Indiana, Maine, Pennsylvania, and Wisconsin. *J. Med. Entomol.* 45, 289–297. doi: 10.1093/jmedent/45.2.289

Toju, H., Tanabe, A. S., Notsu, Y., Sota, T., and Fukatsu, T. (2013). Diversification of endosymbiosis: replacements, co-speciation and promiscuity of bacteriocyte symbionts in weevils. *ISME J.* 7, 1378–1390. doi: 10.1038/ismej.2013.27

Tsuchida, T., Koga, R., Fujiwara, A., and Fukatsu, T. (2014). Phenotypic effect of "*Candidatus Rickettsiella viridis*," a facultative symbiont of the pea aphid (*Acyrthosiphon pisum*), and its interaction with a coexisting symbiont. *Appl. Environ. Microbiol.* 80, 525–533. doi: 10.1128/AEM.03049-13

Tsuchida, T., Koga, R., Horikawa, M., Tsunoda, T., Maoka, T., Matsumoto, S., et al. (2010). Symbiotic bacterium modifies aphid body color. *Science* 330, 1102–1104. doi: 10.1126/science.1195463

Tully, J. G., Rose, D. L., Yunker, C. E., Carle, P., Bove, J. M., Williamson, D. L., et al. (1995). Spiroplasrna *ixodetis* sp. nov., a new species from *Ixodes pacificus* ticks collected in Oregon. *Int. J. Syst. Bacteriol.* 45, 23–28. doi: 10.1099/00207713-45-1-23

Tully, J. G., Rose, D. L., Yunker, C. E., Cory, J., Whitcomb, R. F., and Williamson, D. L. (1981). Helical mycoplasmas (spiroplasmas) from *Ixodes* ticks. *Science* 212, 1043–1045. doi: 10.1126/science.7233197

van Overbeek, L., Gassner, F., van der Plas, C. L., Kastelein, P., Nunes-da Rocha, U., and Takken, W. (2008). Diversity of Ixodes ricinus tick-associated bacterial communities from different forests. *FEMS Microbiol. Ecol.* 66, 72–84. doi: 10.1111/j.1574-6941.2008.00468.x van Schaik, E. J., Chen, C., Mertens, K., Weber, M. M., and Samuel, J. E. (2013). Molecular pathogenesis of the obligate intracellular bacterium *Coxiella burnetii*. *Nat. Rev. Microbiol.* 11, 561–573. doi: 10.1038/nrmicro3049

Vapniarsky, N., Barr, B. C., and Murphy, B. (2012). Systemic *Coxiella-like* infection with myocarditis and hepatitis in an eclectus parrot (*Eclectus roratus*). *Vet. Pathol.* 49, 717–722. doi: 10.1177/0300985811409251

Vayssier-Taussat, M., Moutailler, S., Michelet, L., Devillers, E., Bonnet, S., Cheval, J., et al. (2013). Next generation sequencing uncovers unexpected bacterial pathogens in ticks in western Europe. *PLoS ONE* 8:e81439. doi: 10.1371/journal.pone.0081439

Venzal, J. M., Estrada-Pena, A., Portillo, A., Mangold, A. J., Castro, O., de Souza, C. G., et al. (2008). Detection of alpha and gamma-proteobacteria in *Amblyomma triste* (Acari: Ixodidae) from Uruguay. *Exp. Appl. Acarol.* 44, 49–56. doi: 10.1007/s10493-007-9126-6

Vilcins, I. M., Old, J. M., and Deane, E. (2009). Molecular detection of *Rickettsia, Coxiella* and *Rickettsiella* DNA in three native Australian tick species. *Exp. Appl. Acarol.* 49, 229–242. doi: 10.1007/s10493-009-9260-4

Weinert, L. A., Tinsley, M. C., Temperley, M., and Jiggins, F. M. (2007). Are we underestimating the diversity and incidence of insect bacterial symbionts? A case study in ladybird beetles. *Biol. Lett.* 3, 678–681. doi: 10.1098/rsbl.2007.0373

Weinert, L. A., Werren, J. H., Aebi, A., Stone, G. N., and Jiggins, F. M. (2009). Evolution and diversity of *Rickettsia* bacteria. *BMC Biol.* 7:6. doi: 10.1186/1741-7007-7-6

Weller, S. J., Baldridge, G. D., Munderloh, U. G., Noda, H., Simser, J., and Kurtti, T. J. (1998). Phylogenetic placement of rickettsiae from the ticks Amblyomma americanum and Ixodes scapularis. *J. Clin. Microbiol.* 36, 1305–1317.

Wernegreen, J. J. (2012). Endosymbiosis. *Curr. Biol.* 22, R555–R561. doi: 10.1016/j.cub.2012.06.010

Werren, J. H., Skinner, S. W., and Huger, A. M. (1986). Male-killing bacteria in a parasitic wasp. *Science* 231, 990–992. doi: 10.1126/science.3945814

Williams-Newkirk, A. J., Rowe, L. A., Mixson-Hayden, T. R., and Dasch, G. A. (2014). Characterization of the bacterial communities of life stages of free living lone star ticks (*Amblyomma americanum*). *PLoS ONE* 9:e102130. doi: 10.1371/journal.pone.0102130

Woc-Colburn, A. M., Garner, M. M., Bradway, D., West, G., D'Agostino, J., Trupkiewicz, J., et al. (2008). Fatal coxiellosis in Swainson's Blue Mountain Rainbow Lorikeets (*Trichoglossus haematodus moluccanus*). *Vet. Pathol.* 45, 247–254. doi: 10.1354/vp.45-2-247

Xia, H., Beck, A. S., Gargili, A., Forrester, N., Barrett, A. D., and Bente, D. A. (2016). Transstadial transmission and long-term association of crimean-congo hemorrhagic fever virus in ticks shapes genome plasticity. *Sci. Rep.* 6:35819. doi: 10.1038/srep35819

Zchori-Fein, E., and Bourtzis, K. (2011). *Manipulative Tenants: Bacteria Associated with Arthropods.* New York, NY: CRC press.

Zchori-Fein, E., and Perlman, S. J. (2004). Distribution of the bacterial symbiont Cardinium in arthropods. *Mol. Ecol.* 13, 2009–2016. doi: 10.1111/j.1365-294X.2004.02203.x

Zhang, X. C., Yang, Z. N., Lu, B., Ma, X. F., Zhang, C. X., and Xu, H. J. (2014). The composition and transmission of microbiome in hard tick, *Ixodes persulcatus*, during blood meal. *Ticks Tick Borne Dis.* 5, 864–870. doi: 10.1016/j.ttbdis.2014.07.009

Zhong, J., Jasinskas, A., and Barbour, A. G. (2007). Antibiotic treatment of the tick vector *Amblyomma americanum* reduced reproductive fitness. *PLoS ONE* 2:e405. doi: 10.1371/journal.pone.0000405

Zolnik, C. P., Prill, R. J., Falco, R. C., Daniels, T. J., and Kolokotronis, S. O. (2016). Microbiome changes through ontogeny of a tick pathogen vector. *Mol. Ecol.* 25, 4963–4977. doi: 10.1111/mec.13832

Zug, R., and Hammerstein, P. (2012). Still a host of hosts for Wolbachia: analysis of recent data suggests that 40% of terrestrial arthropod species are infected. *PLoS ONE* 7:e38544. doi: 10.1371/journal.pone.0038544

10

Arthropods Under Pressure: Stress Responses and Immunity at the Pathogen-Vector Interface

Kristin L. Rosche, Lindsay C. Sidak-Loftis[†], Joanna Hurtado[†], Elizabeth A. Fisk and Dana K. Shaw[*]

Program in Vector-borne Disease, Department of Veterinary Microbiology and Pathology, Washington State University, Pullman, WA, United States

***Correspondence:**
Dana K. Shaw
Dana.Shaw@wsu.edu

[†]These authors have contributed equally to this work

Understanding what influences the ability of some arthropods to harbor and transmit pathogens may be key for controlling the spread of vector-borne diseases. Arthropod immunity has a central role in dictating vector competence for pathogen acquisition and transmission. Microbial infection elicits immune responses and imparts stress on the host by causing physical damage and nutrient deprivation, which triggers evolutionarily conserved stress response pathways aimed at restoring cellular homeostasis. Recent studies increasingly recognize that eukaryotic stress responses and innate immunity are closely intertwined. Herein, we describe two well-characterized and evolutionarily conserved mechanisms, the Unfolded Protein Response (UPR) and the Integrated Stress Response (ISR), and examine evidence that these stress responses impact immune signaling. We then describe how multiple pathogens, including vector-borne microbes, interface with stress responses in mammals. Owing to the well-conserved nature of the UPR and ISR, we speculate that similar mechanisms may be occurring in arthropod vectors and ultimately impacting vector competence. We conclude this Perspective by positing that novel insights into vector competence will emerge when considering that stress-signaling pathways may be influencing the arthropod immune network.

Keywords: vector-borne diseases, vector competence, vector-borne pathogens, arthropod immunity, eukaryotic stress response, integrated stress response, unfolded protein response

INTRODUCTION

Among arthropods, the adaptation to blood-feeding is a life history trait that evolved independently at least 20 times (1). From the arthropod's perspective, a hematophageous lifestyle has both benefits and drawbacks. Blood is a good source of proteins and lipids, which are necessary for development and egg production (2–4). However, blood-feeding comes with a variety of risks and stressors (5) including long periods between nutrient supplementation (6–13), thermal stress associated with the influx of a hot blood meal (5, 14–16), heme toxicity (17–30) and excess amounts of ions and water (31). Cells respond to acute environmental changes by activating stress responses that temporarily increase tolerance limits in adverse conditions and/or eliminate stressful stimuli. Being able to respond to stressful stimuli is an evolutionary advantage, which explains the highly conserved nature of cellular stress responses across eukaryotes (32–40).

For arthropods that transmit disease, another stressor is the presence of pathogens with incoming blood meals (41–44). Although vector-borne pathogens do not typically kill their arthropod vectors (45), infection does impart stress on the host by parasitizing nutrients, secreting toxic by-products and/or causing physical damage (46). For this reason, arthropod immune processes responding to infection are a key factor influencing vector competence (47–53). From mammals, it is now recognized that innate immunity is tightly intertwined with cellular stress responses and may represent an ancient mode of host defense against infection (32–34, 54–60). Whether stress-responses also intersect with arthropod immunity and how this may influence vector competence of blood-feeding arthropods is not known. Herein we briefly outline current knowledge of two well-characterized cellular stress response mechanisms, the Unfolded Protein Response (UPR) and the Integrated Stress Response (ISR) and discuss evidence that stress signaling impacts immunity. We then cite examples of cellular stress responses mediating outcomes at the host-pathogen interface in mammals and conclude that, given the well-conserved nature of the UPR and the ISR, similar crosstalk may be occurring in arthropods that would fundamentally impact vector competence.

ARTHROPOD INNATE IMMUNE SIGNALING

Arthropod innate immune pathways are best characterized in the model organism *Drosophila* which are briefly summarized owing to space constraints. The Toll pathway is generally characterized as responding to Gram-positive bacteria and fungi, resulting in activation of Rel-family transcription factors Dorsal and Dif (Dorsal-related immunity factor) (61–64). The IMD (immune deficiency) pathway is analogous to the tumor necrosis factor receptor (TNFR) pathway in mammals (65) and is initiated by Gram-negative bacteria, although exceptions outside of *Drosophila* have been observed (66–71). The Janus Kinase (JAK)-signal transducers and activators of transcription (STAT) pathway, first described in mammals, is activated in the presence of bacterial or protozoan pathogens as well as more than 35 ligands, including interferons (IFN) and interleukins (IL) (72, 73). In arthropods, the JAK-STAT pathway is induced by the endogenous cytokine Unpaired (Upd) (74). Owing to space constraints, we refer readers to excellent reviews that comprehensively cover arthropod Toll, IMD and JAK-STAT signaling (65, 75, 76).

THE UNFOLDED PROTEIN RESPONSE

The UPR is a cellular stress response mechanism that is highly conserved across species, from single-celled eukaryotes to mammals (**Figure 1**). The UPR is triggered when the endoplasmic reticulum (ER) is under stress, which can result from a variety of stimuli such as oxidative stress, changes in temperature or pH, lack of nutrients or infection (32–34, 77–84). Such conditions can impart stress when protein-folding requirements exceed the processing capacity of the ER, causing an accumulation of unfolded proteins in the ER lumen. The UPR is activated through any combination of 3 transmembrane receptors: PERK (PKR-like ER kinase), ATF6 (activating transcription factor 6) or IRE1α (inositol-requiring enzyme 1α). In a non-stressed state, the negative regulator, BiP (binding immunoglobulin protein; also known as GRP78), keeps all three receptors in an inactive state by binding to them. Upon activation, BiP disassociates from the receptors, thereby activating signaling. Disassociation allows IRE1α and PERK to oligomerize and autophophorylate (85–87), whereas ATF6 is released for migration to the Golgi (88, 89). If homeostasis cannot be restored, the UPR will switch from pro-survival to proapoptotic outcomes (90).

PERK is a type I transmembrane protein kinase that has dual roles in the UPR as well as the ISR (91). When activated, PERK dimerizes, autophosphorylates and then also phosphorylates the regulatory molecule, eIF2α (eukaryotic translation initiation factor 2α). Phosphorylated eIF2α promotes cell survival by temporarily inhibiting protein translation, which decreases the amount of proteins entering the ER and alleviates the demand for protein folding. While inhibiting the translation of most mRNAs, eIF2α selectively induces the expression of some proteins including ATF4 (activating transcription factor 4). ATF4 can activate transcription of the growth arrest and DNA damage-inducible protein, GADD34, which negatively regulates eIF2α phosphorylation, or CHOP (C/EBP homologous protein), which is a proapoptotic factor (85, 92, 93).

ATF6 is a type II transmembrane protein that contains a bZIP transcription factor within the cytosolic domain. Once BiP disassociates from ATF6, it is transported to the Golgi compartment by COPII-containing vesicles (33, 94, 95). ATF6 is proteolytically processed by the Golgi-resident proteases S1P and S2P (site-1/2 proteases), which cleave the amino-terminal portion and allow the bZIP transcription factor to translocate to the nucleus (81, 94, 96). ATF6 upregulates the expression of GRP94 (endoplasmin) to increase the ER's folding capacity and p58IPK to induce the ER associated degradation pathway (ERAD). ATF6 also induces the expression of other UPR-associated proteins including BiP and XBP1 (X-box binding protein) (32, 60, 97, 98).

IRE1α is a type I transmembrane protein with a cytosolic serine/threonine kinase domain and an RNase (ribonuclease) domain. When the ER is stressed, IRE1α autophosphorylates and splices the inactive mRNA $xbp1^U$ into $xbp1^S$, which is then translated into a protein (33, 81, 99, 100). XBP1 translocates to the nucleus where it induces genes that are involved in lipid biosynthesis, ERAD and chaperone production (100, 101). IRE1α signaling also limits the amount of new proteins entering the ER through regulated IRE1α-dependent decay (RIDD), which degrades mRNA (102). With high levels of ER stress, IRE1α recruits the adaptor protein TRAF2 (TNF receptor-

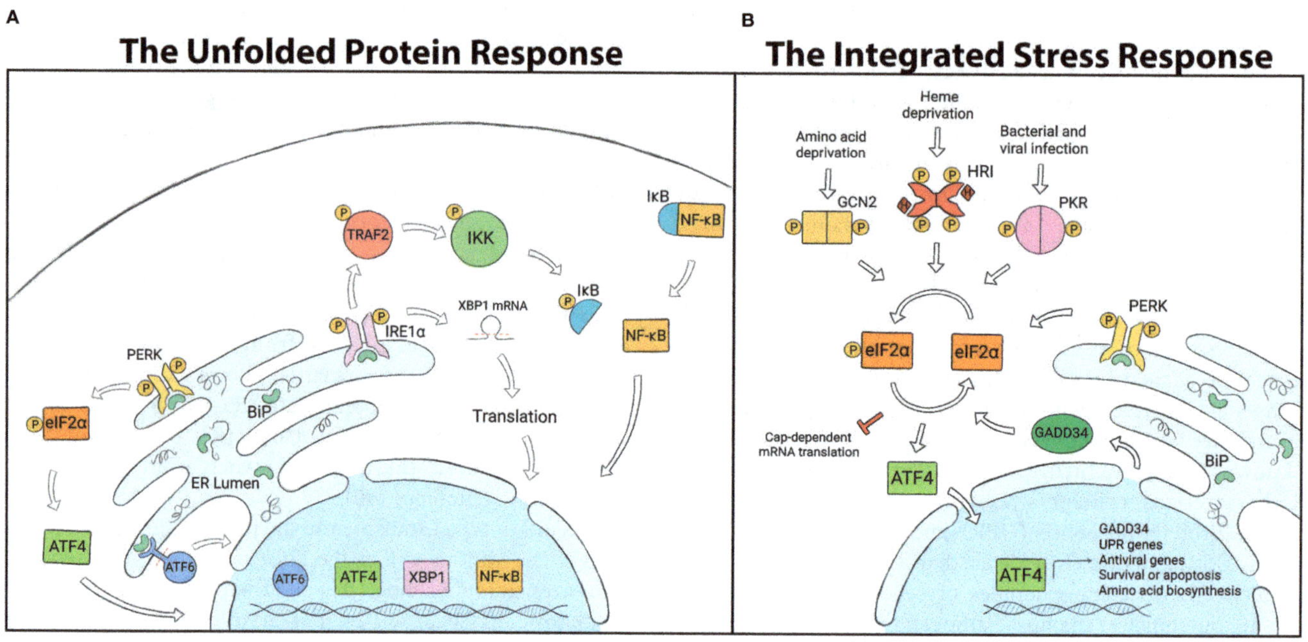

FIGURE 1 | **(A)** The Unfolded Protein Response (UPR) is regulated by three transmembrane endoplasmic reticulum (ER) receptors: PERK, ATF6 and IRE1α. BiP binds to and holds the receptors in an inactive state under non-stressed conditions. The accumulation of unfolded proteins in the ER leads to the disassociation of BiP from the receptors and UPR activation. PERK phosphorylates eIF2α and induces ATF4, which controls transcription of *chop* and *gadd34*. ATF6 is cleaved and translocated to the nucleus to regulate expression of GRP94, p58IPK, and UPR-associated proteins. IRE1α splices *xbp1*, which is translated into a protein that controls genes involved in lipid biosynthesis, ER associated degradation pathway (ERAD) and chaperone production. IRE1α can also recruit TRAF2, which leads to NF-κB, ASK1 and JNK signaling. **(B)** The Integrated Stress Response (ISR) is initiated by stress-specific stimuli that activate kinases GCN2, HRI, PKR and PERK, which all converge on the regulatory molecule eIF2α. Phosphorylation of eIF2α halts global protein translation and upregulates the transcription factor ATF4, which determines cell fate. To terminate the ISR, ATF4 induces GADD34 expression which dephosphorylates eIF2α and allows global protein translation to resume.

associated factor 2) a component of the TNFR pathway. IRE1α-TRAF2 association recruits the IKK complex, leading to NF-κB activation and proinflammatory responses (33, 103, 104). Alternatively, IRE1α-mediated signaling through TRAF2 can also lead to ASK1 (apoptosis signal regulating kinase 1; also known as mitogen-activated protein kinase 5, MAP3K5) activation and downstream JNK (JUN N-terminal kinase) signaling to induce apoptotic outcomes (33, 100, 104, 105). Less is known about UPR mechanisms in arthropods, but genome comparisons indicate that UPR-encoding genes are well-conserved between species, which may suggest similar mechanisms of action (**Table 1**).

THE INTEGRATED STRESS RESPONSE

The ISR is responsible for alleviating cellular stress and restoring homeostasis in eukaryotes (93, 106–109) (**Figure 1**). In mammalian cells, the ISR can be activated by one of four stress-sensing kinases: PKR (protein kinase double-stranded RNA-dependent), GCN2 (general control nonderepressible 2), HRI (heme-regulated inhibitor) and PERK (110, 111). These serine-threonine kinases are stimulated by pathological and physiological changes in the cellular environment. GCN2, a highly conserved cytoplasmic kinase, is stimulated by UV irradiation and nutrient deprivation (e.g. amino acid, glucose) (107, 108, 112). PERK is stimulated when misfolded proteins accumulate in the ER, causing ER stress (91, 113, 114). PKR is activated primarily in response to viral infections, as well as bacterial infections and oxidative stress (109, 115–117). Unlike the other kinases, HRI is mostly expressed in erythrocytes and acts as a heme sensor that is activated by iron deficiency (118).

All four stress-sensing kinases converge on a common regulatory factor: the phosphorylation of eIF2α (106, 110). Under non-stressed conditions, protein translation is initiated when the eIF2 complex (consisting of eIF2α, eIF2β and eIF2γ) binds with GTP and Met-tRNA (initiator methionyl tRNA). The ternary complex then associates with the 40S ribosome subunit to form the 43S pre-initiation complex that binds to the 5' end of mRNA and scans for start codons. Upon recognition, eIF2-GTP (active state) is hydrolyzed to eIF2-GDP (inactive state) and causes a conformational change to the pre-initiation complex, halting the mRNA scanning process and allowing protein translation to begin (119–123). eIF2B, a guanine nucleotide exchange factor, is essential for recycling GDP to GTP for new rounds of protein translation. Phosphorylated eIF2α attenuates protein synthesis owing to its increased affinity for eIF2B that prevents eIF2-GDP to eIF2-GTP exchange (110, 121–123).

As previously discussed in reference to PERK signaling, ATF4 is activated downstream of eIF2α phosphorylation and can act as

TABLE 1 | Distribution of Unfolded Protein Response (UPR) and Integrated Stress Response (ISR) genes across arthropod vectors.

Common Name	Genus	UPR and ISR genes									
		BiP	ATF6	IRE1α	XBP1	ATF4	eIF2α	PERK	GCN2	PKR	HRI
Fruit Flies	*Drosophila*	+	+	+	+	+	+	+	+	−	−
Mosquitoes	*Culex*	+	+	+	+	+	+	+	+	−	+
	Aedes	+	+	+	+	+	+	+	+	−	+
	Anopheles	+	+	+	+	+	+	+	+	−	+
Fleas	*Xenopsylla**	+	+	+	+	+	+	+	+	−	−
	Ctenocephalides	+	+	+	+	+	+	+	+	−	+
Lice	*Pediculus*	+	+	+	+	−	+	+	+	−	+
Triatome bugs	*Triatoma**	+	+	+	+	+	+	+	+	−	+
Ticks	*Ixodes*	+	+	+	+	+	+	+	+	−	+
	*Dermacentor**	+	+	+	+	−	+	+	+	−	+
	*Ornithodoros**	+	+	+	+	+	+	+	+	−	+
Mites	*Leptotrombidium*	+	−	+	+	−	+	+	+	−	+

NCBI's Basic Local Alignment Search Tool (BLAST) was used with query sequences from Homo sapiens to identify putative homologs. (+) homologs identified (–), homologous gene targets not found.
**homologs found in vector transcriptomes.*

both a transcriptional activator and repressor of genes important for determining cell fate, including *chop* and *gadd34* (124–126). In response to prolonged ER-stress, ATF4 interacts with CHOP to generate reactive oxygen species (ROS), a key signal for mediating cell death (125). Once cellular stress is resolved, ATF4 induces GADD34 which interacts with protein phosphatase 1 (PP1) to dephosphorylate eIF2α and terminate the ISR (126).

The ISR has known roles in regulating host immunity. In response to ISR activation, cells will form cytoplasmic aggregates of untranslated mRNA and proteins termed "stress granules" that influence immune signaling. Phosphorylated eIF2α induces stress granules, which become cell signaling hubs that can intercept molecules from other pathways to modulate processes such as immunity (35, 127, 128). For example, TRAF2 is sequestered into stress granules, which ultimately suppresses NF-κB-mediated inflammation (127). The ISR can also act as an antiviral defense mechanism (129–131). A stress granule-nucleating protein G3BP1 (Ras-GTPase-activating protein SH3 domain binding protein 1) recruits and activates PKR to suppress viral protein synthesis. It also activates innate immune responses through NF-κB and JNK pathways and promotes the expression of proinflammatory cytokines such as IL-17 (117). The arthropod ISR is less-studied when compared to mammals, but comparative genomic analyses demonstrate that many ISR genes are well-conserved in arthropod vectors (**Table 1**).

INTERSPECIES INTERACTIONS

UPR-Pathogen Interface

The UPR is increasingly implicated in host defense against infection (132–137). For example, mammalian macrophages limit methicillin resistant *Staphylococcus aureus* (MRSA) through IRE1α with sustained ROS production and concentrated delivery of ROS to bacteria-containing phagosomes (138). The foodborne pathogen *Camplyobacter jejuni* activates eIF2α and CHOP, while decreasing expression of *perk*, *ire1α* and *atf6* in human intestinal epithelial cells. Pharmacologically inducing the UPR prior to infection resulted in decreased *C. jejuni* invasion (139), highlighting the UPR as a host defense strategy.

Some pathogens manipulate or selectively induce the UPR to promote growth and survival. *Legionella pneumophila*, causative agent of Legionnaires' disease, inhibits UPR-induced apoptosis with secreted effector proteins Lgtl and Lgt2 that block IRE1α-mediated $xbp1^{U}$ splicing (140, 141). The intracellular pathogen *Brucella* manipulates the UPR in mammalian cells with secreted effectors TcpB and VceC (142–144), which induce IRE1α signaling and NF-κB to potentiate pro-inflammatory responses (81, 144–147). This effector-mediated manipulation appears to benefit the bacterium, with VceC providing an advantage for long-term *in vivo* colonization (144).

Vector-borne pathogens are also reported to cause ER stress and UPR activation in mammalian hosts. *Francisella tularensis*, causative agent of Tularemia vectored by ticks (*Dermacentor* spp. and *Amblyomma americanum*) and biting insects (148–151), alters the expression of *bip*, increases IRE1α phosphorylation and ATF6 activation, but decreases PERK phosphorylation and CHOP (152). IRE1α-XBP1 signaling is reported to limit *F. tularensis in vivo* with increased pathogen burdens in the liver, spleen and lungs of $xbp1^{-/-}$ mice (153). *Orientia tsutsugamushi*, the causative agent of Scrub Typhus transmitted by trombiculid mites (chiggers), induces the UPR and ERAD in HeLa cells to benefit bacterial growth, owing to the increase in available amino acids (154). The *Ixodes scapularis*-transmitted bacterium *Anaplasma phagocytophilum* induces all the three UPR branches in THP-1 cells (155).

Due to their very nature, viral replication requires host cells for protein production, which often engages the UPR. For example, herpesviruses activate one or more of the UPR receptors, but limit downstream signaling to ensure global protein translation, including viral proteins, is not halted (156–158). Many arthropod-transmitted viruses activate one or more UPR sensors in mammalian cells as well. Bluetongue virus, transmitted by *Culicoides* spp. (biting midges), induces autophagy to benefit viral replication by activating PERK-eIF2α signaling of the UPR (159). Mosquito-transmitted viruses Chikungunya (CHIKV), Dengue (DENV) and West Nile (WNV) all activate one or more UPR sensors in mammalian cells. CHIKV activates BiP and the ATF6 and IRE1α branches of the UPR, but blocks PERK signaling by suppressing eIF2α phosphorylation through the nonstructural viral protein nsP4 (160, 161). The flaviviruses DENV and WNV induce $xbp1^U$ splicing, ATF6 proteolysis, and eIF2α phosphorylation to benefit viral propagation in mammalian cells and, in the case of WNV, to inhibit type I IFN signaling (161–164). Tick-borne encephalitis virus (TBEV) and Langat virus (LGTV) are Ixodid-transmitted flaviviruses. TBEV infection activates the IRE1α and ATF6 pathways to facilitate viral replication (165). In contrast, while LGTV infection activates the UPR, PERK signaling restricts viral load (166), highlighting the importance of the UPR as a host defense mechanism.

Much less is known about the UPR-pathogen interface in arthropod vectors. Recent work shows differential regulation of ER-resident proteins involved in ERAD in *Borrelia burgdorferi*-infected adult *I. scapularis* (167). There is also evidence that arthropod-transmitted plant pathogens manipulate the UPR in their arthropod vectors. *Candidatus* Liberibacter asiaticus (CLas), causative agent of Asian citrus greening disease, is vectored by the Asian citrus psyllid *Diaphorina citri* Kuwayama (*D. citri*). Infection of *D. citri* with CLas upregulates expression of ERAD and UPR components. A related bacterium, *Candidatus* Liberibacter solanacerarum, also upregulates *ire1α* and multiple genes involved in ERAD in its arthropod vector, the potato psyllid (*Bactericera cockerelli*) (168). Although more work is required to understand what role the UPR and ERAD-mediated protein degradation have during arthropod infection, these studies demonstrate that vector-borne pathogens are interfacing with the UPR in arthropods.

ISR-Pathogen Interface

The ISR broadly responds to a variety of stress-inducing stimuli, including invasion and damage caused by infection. *Listeria monocytogenes*-infected mammalian cells activate PERK, ATF4, eIF2α, PKR and induce the expression of CHOP. *L. monocytogenes* secretes listeriolysin O (LLO), which is a pore-forming hemolysin required for phagosomal escape and bacterial survival. Cells treated with *L. monocytogenes* LLO resulted in a similar ISR activation phenotype as infection, indicating that this effector is partially responsible for inducing the ISR. Downstream production of type I IFN activates the ISR kinase PKR, increasing its expression and activation, and further stimulating eIF2α signaling (169). Epithelial cell infection with *Shigella flexneri* disrupts host cell membranes, causing GCN2-mediated eIF2α phosphorylation. This halts global protein translation, leading to stress granule formation and autophagy that eliminates bacteria (170).

These examples reflect the role of the ISR as a host-defense strategy against infection. In response, many pathogens have evolved methods to counteract ISR-mediated defenses. For example, the causative agent of Q fever, *Coxiella burnetii*, increases eIF2α phosphorylation in a Type IV Secretion System-dependent manner and induces ATF4 and CHOP in human macrophages. However, nuclear translocation of CHOP is blocked by *C. burnetii* to prevent ER stress-induced apoptosis (171). Coronavirus protein AcP10 and picornavirus protein AiVL promote viral protein synthesis by acting as competitive inhibitors for phosphorylated-eIF2 and eIF2B interactions (172). Excellent reviews summarizing ISR-mediated antiviral responses, including stress granules, and concurrent viral evasion strategies have been published in the past several years which readers are referred to (129, 173).

Interactions between vector-borne pathogens and ISR mechanisms have been reported, with several focusing on insect-borne viruses. In mammalian cells, the sandfly fever Sicilian phlebovirus evades PKR defense mechanisms by expressing a nonstructural protein that binds to eIF2B, blocking translation inhibition and promoting viral replication (174). Rift valley fever virus, transmitted by mosquitoes and sandflies, degrades host PKR and inhibits IFN induction (175–177). WNV inhibits PKR activation and downstream phosphorylation of eIF2α and stress granule formation (178). Zika virus likewise has evolved to evade stress granule formation in host cells by repurposing host proteins, including G3BP1, to facilitate viral replication and repress normal stress granule assembly (179, 180). Other flaviviruses such as WNV, DENV and Japanese encephalitis virus hijack or further inhibit stress granule machinery to benefit replication (181–184). These studies illustrate that vectored pathogens evade ISR signaling to facilitate replication and survival.

CONCLUDING REMARKS

Vector-borne pathogens selectively interface with the UPR and the ISR to promote survival and infection in mammals. Given the well-conserved nature of both the UPR and the ISR between evolutionarily distant species (**Table 1**), it is reasonable to speculate that vectored microbes may also be modulating the stress responses in their arthropod vectors. Moreover, this type of manipulation may be a common survival strategy used by vector-borne pathogens to suppress host defenses and create replicative niches.

Cellular stress responses are increasingly recognized as being closely intertwined with innate immunity (32–34, 54–60). For example, there are multiple reports that mammalian Toll-like receptors (TLRs) influence the UPR and the ISR. TLR2 and TLR4 in mammalian macrophages activate the IRE1α-XBP1 axis, which leads to proinflammatory TNFα and IL-6 cytokine production (153). MRSA induces $xbp1^U$ splicing in wildtype bone marrow-derived macrophages, but not in $TLR2/4/9^{-/-}$ or $myd88^{-/-}$ mutant cells, indicating that TLR signaling is required for IRE1α activation (138). The ISR kinase PKR is activated downstream from TLR3 and TLR4, which induces type I IFN (185, 186). Whether a similar phenomenon occurs in arthropods is not known, but considering the well-conserved nature of the Toll pathway between arthropods and mammals (70, 187) it is possible that this type of crosstalk is occurring across species.

Beyond TLR signaling, overlap between the UPR and ISR with other innate immunity components has also been noted. During infection, the mammalian UPR is capable of initiating an immune response by crosstalking with the TNFR pathway (33, 56–58, 188–190). IRE1α can produce proinflammatory responses by signaling through TRAF2, a component of the TNFR pathway, recruiting the IKK complex for phosphorylation and releasing NF-κB for nuclear translocation (32–34). Arthropod immunity may similarly be influenced by the UPR, as the arthropod IMD pathway is analogous to the mammalian TNFR network. PERK was shown to interact with JAK-STAT signaling in mammalian glial cells (191) and several examples of IFN production being influenced by the ISR and UPR have been reported, which could potentially influence JAK-STAT signaling in an indirect manner (169, 175–177, 185, 186, 192). Similar crosstalk between JAK-STAT and cellular stress responses may also be occurring in arthropod vectors.

Since one of the major factors determining vector competence is arthropod immunity (47–53), it is feasible that cellular stress responses may be influencing vector competence. With this in mind, understanding how stress responses may interface with arthropod immunity and conversely how vector-borne pathogens may be inducing or manipulating cellular stress responses could be important for opening new avenues in vector-borne disease control. This knowledge could be leveraged for the future design of disease transmission-blocking strategies to reduce the global burden of vector-borne diseases.

AUTHOR CONTRIBUTIONS

KR, LS-L, JH, and DS wrote this perspective. EF designed and constructed **Figure 1** and contributed to intellectual discussions. All authors contributed to the article and approved the submitted version.

FUNDING

This work was supported by National Institute of Health grants GM008336 to JH and R21AI139772, R21AI148578 and Washington State University to DKS. The content is solely the responsibility of the authors and does not necessarily represent the official views of the National Institute of Allergy and Infectious Diseases or the National Institutes of Health.

REFERENCES

Dantas-Torres F, Fernandes Martins T, Munoz-Leal S, Onofrio VC, Barros-Battesti DM. Ticks (Ixodida: Argasidae, Ixodidae) of Brazil: Updated species checklist and taxonomic keys. *Ticks Tick Borne Dis* (2019) 10:101252. doi: 10.1016/j.ttbdis.2019.06.012

Mans BJ. Evolution of vertebrate hemostatic and inflammatory control mechanisms in blood-feeding arthropods. *J Innate Immun* (2011) 3:41–51. doi: 10.1159/000321599

Lehane MJ. *The Biology of Blood-Sucking in Insects. 2nd ed.* Cambridge: Cambridge University Press (2005). doi: 10.1017/CBO9780511610493

Coast GM. Neuroendocrine control of ionic homeostasis in blood-sucking insects. *J Exp Biol* (2009) 212:378–86. doi: 10.1242/jeb.024109

Sterkel M, Oliveira JHM, Bottino-Rojas V, Paiva-Silva GO, Oliveira PL. The Dose Makes the Poison: Nutritional Overload Determines the Life Traits of Blood-Feeding Arthropods. *Trends Parasitol* (2017) 33:633–44. doi: 10.1016/j.pt.2017.04.008

Benoit JB, Denlinger DL. Bugs battle stress from hot blood. *eLife* (2017) 6: e33035. doi: 10.7554/eLife.33035

Philip CB, Burgdorfer W. Arthropod Vectors as Reservoirs of Microbial Disease Agents. *Annu Rev Entomol* (1961) 6:391–412. doi: 10.1146/annurev.en.06.010161.002135

Fritz GN. Biology and Ecology of Bat Flies (Diptera: Streblidae) on Bats in the Genus Carollia. *J Med Entomol* (1983) 20:1–10. doi: 10.1093/jmedent/ 20.1.1

Zhao YO, Kurscheid S, Zhang Y, Liu L, Zhang L, Loeliger K, et al. Enhanced Survival of Plasmodium-Infected Mosquitoes during Starvation. *PloS One* (2012) 7:e40556. doi: 10.1371/journal.pone.0040556

McCue MD, Boardman L, Clusella-Trullas S, Kleynhans E, Terblanche JS. The speed and metabolic cost of digesting a blood meal depends on temperature in a major disease vector. *J Exp Biol* (2016) 219:1893–902. doi: 10.1242/jeb.138669

Krasnov BR, Khokhlova IS, Fielden LJ, Burdelova NI. Time of survival under starvation in two flea species (Siphonaptera: Pulicidae) at different air temperatures and relative humidities. *J Vector Ecol J Soc Vector Ecol* (2002) 27:70–81.

Cabello DR. Resistance to starvation of Rhodnius neivai Lent, 1953 (Hemiptera: Reduviidae: Triatominae) under experimental conditions. *Mem Inst Oswaldo Cruz* (2001) 96:587–91. doi: 10.1590/S0074-02762001000400023

Polanco AM, Miller DM, Brewster CC. Survivorship During Starvation for Cimex lectularius L. *Insects* (2011) 2:232–42. doi: 10.3390/insects2020232

Oliver JH. Biology and Systematics of Ticks (Acari:Ixodida). *Annu Rev Ecol Syst* (1989) 20:397–430. doi: 10.1146/annurev.es.20.110189.002145

Benoit JB, Lopez-Martinez G, Patrick KR, Phillips ZP, Krause TB, Denlinger DL. Drinking a hot blood meal elicits a protective heat shock response in mosquitoes. *Proc Natl Acad Sci* (2011) 108:8026–9. doi: 10.1073/pnas.1105195108

Lahondère C, Lazzari CR. Mosquitoes Cool Down during Blood Feeding to Avoid Overheating. *Curr Biol* (2012) 22:40–5. doi: 10.1016/j.cub.2011.11.029

Lahondère C, Lazzari CR. Thermal effect of blood feeding in the telmophagous fly Glossina morsitans morsitans. *J Therm Biol* (2015) 48:45–50. doi: 10.1016/j.jtherbio.2014.12.009

Lane NJ, Harrison JB. An unusual cell surface modification: a double plasma membrane. *J Cell Sci* (1979) 39:355–72.

Silva CP, Silva JR, Vasconcelos FF, Petretski MDA, Damatta RA, Ribeiro AF, et al. Occurrence of midgut perimicrovillar membranes in paraneopteran insect orders with comments on their function and evolutionary significance. *Arthropod Struct Dev* (2004) 33:139–48. doi: 10.1016/j.asd.2003.12.002

Gutiérrez-Cabrera AE, Córdoba-Aguilar A, Zenteno E, Lowenberger C, Espinoza B. Origin, evolution and function of the hemipteran perimicrovillar membrane with emphasis on Reduviidae that transmit Chagas disease. *Bull Entomol Res* (2016) 106:279–91. doi: 10.1017/S0007485315000929

Oliveira MF, Silva JR, Dansa-Petretski M, de Souza W, Lins U, Braga CM, et al. Haem detoxification by an insect. *Nature* (1999) 400:517–8. doi: 10.1038/22910

Oliveira MF, Silva JR, Dansa-Petretski M, de Souza W, Braga CM, Masuda H, et al. Haemozoin formation in the midgut of the blood-sucking insect Rhodnius prolixus. *FEBS Lett* (2000) 477:95–8. doi: 10.1016/s0014-5793(00)01786-5

Oliveira MF, Kycia SW, Gomez A, Kosar AJ, Bohle DS, Hempelmann E, et al. Structural and morphological characterization of hemozoin produced by Schistosoma mansoni and Rhodnius prolixus. *FEBS Lett* (2005) 579:6010–6. doi: 10.1016/j.febslet.2005.09.035

Pagola S, Stephens PW, Bohle DS, Kosar AD, Madsen SK. The structure of malaria pigment beta-haematin. *Nature* (2000) 404:307–10. doi: 10.1038/35005132

Silva JR, Mury FB, Oliveira MF, Oliveira PL, Silva CP, Dansa-Petretski M. Perimicrovillar membranes promote hemozoin formation into Rhodnius prolixus midgut. *Insect Biochem Mol Biol* (2007) 37:523–31. doi: 10.1016/j.ibmb.2007.01.001

Braz GR, Coelho HS, Masuda H, Oliveira PL. A missing metabolic pathway in the cattle tick Boophilus microplus. *Curr Biol CB* (1999) 9:703–6. doi: 10.1016/s0960-9822(99)80312-1

Lara FA, Lins U, Paiva-Silva G, Almeida IC, Braga CM, Miguens FC, et al. A new intracellular pathway of haem detoxification in the midgut of the cattle tick Boophilus microplus: aggregation inside a specialized organelle, the hemosome. *J Exp Biol* (2003) 206:1707–15. doi: 10.1242/jeb.00334

Narasimhan S, Rajeevan N, Liu L, Zhao YO, Heisig J, Pan J, et al. Gut microbiota of the tick vector Ixodes scapularis modulate colonization of the lyme disease spirochete. *Cell Host Microbe* (2014) 15:58–71. doi: 10.1016/ j.chom.2013.12.001

Rose C, Belmonte R, Armstrong SD, Molyneux G, Haines LR, Lehane MJ, et al. An investigation into the protein composition of the teneral Glossina morsitans morsitans peritrophic matrix. *PloS Negl Trop Dis* (2014) 8:e2691. doi: 10.1371/journal.pntd.0002691

Graça-Souza AV, Maya-Monteiro C, Paiva-Silva GO, Braz GRC, Paes MC, Sorgine MHF, et al. Adaptations against heme toxicity in blood-feeding arthropods. *Insect Biochem Mol Biol* (2006) 36:322–35. doi: 10.1016/j.ibmb.2006.01.009

Solyman M, Brayton KA, Shaw DK, Omsland A, McGeehan S, Scoles GA, et al. Predicted iron metabolism genes in hard ticks and their response to iron reduction in Dermacentor andersoni cells. *Ticks Tick-Borne Dis* (2021) 12:101584. doi: 10.1016/j.ttbdis.2020.101584

Beyenbach KW, Piermarini PM. Transcellular and paracellular pathways of transepithelial fluid secretion in Malpighian (renal) tubules of the yellow fever mosquito Aedes aegypti. *Acta Physiol* (2011) 202:387–407. doi: 10.1111/j.1748- 1716.2010.02195.x

Grootjans J, Kaser A, Kaufman RJ, Blumberg RS. The unfolded protein response in immunity and inflammation. *Nat Rev Immunol* (2016) 16:469–84. doi: 10.1038/nri.2016.62

Hetz C. The unfolded protein response: controlling cell fate decisions under ER stress and beyond. *Nat Rev Mol Cell Biol* (2012) 13:89–102. doi: 10.1038/nrm3270

Schröder M, Kaufman RJ. The mammalian unfolded protein response. *Annu Rev Biochem* (2005) 74:739–89. doi: 10.1146/annurev.biochem.73.011303.074134

Kedersha N, Ivanov P, Anderson P. Stress granules and cell signaling: more than just a passing phase? *Trends Biochem Sci* (2013) 38:494–506. doi: 10.1016/j.tibs.2013.07.004

Protter DSW, Parker R. Principles and Properties of Stress Granules. *Trends Cell Biol* (2016) 26:668–79. doi: 10.1016/j.tcb.2016.05.004

Mahboubi H, Stochaj U. Cytoplasmic stress granules: Dynamic modulators of cell signaling and disease. *Biochim Biophys Acta BBA Mol Basis Dis* (2017) 1863:884–95. doi: 10.1016/j.bbadis.2016.12.022

Zhou Y, Fang L, Wang D, Cai K, Chen H, Xiao S. Porcine Reproductive and Respiratory Syndrome Virus Infection Induces Stress Granule Formation Depending on Protein Kinase R-like Endoplasmic Reticulum Kinase (PERK) in MARC-145 Cells. *Front Cell Infect Microbiol* (2017) 7:111. doi: 10.3389/ fcimb.2017.00111

Kültz D. Evolution of the cellular stress proteome: from monophyletic origin to ubiquitous function. *J Exp Biol* (2003) 206:3119–24. doi: 10.1242/jeb.00549

Kültz D. Molecular and evolutionary basis of the cellular stress response. *Annu Rev Physiol* (2004) 67:225–57. doi: 10.1146/annurev.physiol.67.040403.103635

Dostálová A, Volf P. Leishmania development in sand flies: parasite-vector interactions overview. *Parasit Vectors* (2012) 5:276–6. doi: 10.1186/1756-3305-5-276

Maier WA, Becker-Feldman H, Seitz HM. Pathology of malaria-infected mosquitoes. *Parasitol Today Pers Ed* (1987) 3:216–8. doi: 10.1016/0169-4758(87)90063-9

Bacot AW. LXXXI. Further notes on the mechanism of the transmission of plague by fleas. *J Hyg (Lond)* (1915) 14:774–6.

Bacot AW, Martin CJ. LXVII. Observations on the mechanism of the transmission of plague by fleas. *J Hyg (Lond)* (1914) 13:423–39.

Shaw DK, Tate AT, Schneider DS, Levashina EA, Kagan JC, Pal U, et al. Vector Immunity and Evolutionary Ecology: The Harmonious Dissonance. *Trends Immunol* (2018) 39:862–73. doi: 10.1016/j.it.2018.09.003

Casadevall A, Pirofski L. Host-Pathogen Interactions: The Attributes of Virulence. *J Infect Dis* (2001) 184:337–44. doi: 10.1086/322044

Hillyer JF, Schmidt SL, Christensen BM. Hemocyte-mediated phagocytosis and melanization in the mosquito Armigeres subalbatus following immune challenge by bacteria. *Cell Tissue Res* (2003) 313:117–27. doi: 10.1007/s00441-003-0744-y

Garver LS, Dong Y, Dimopoulos G. Caspar Controls Resistance to Plasmodium falciparum in Diverse Anopheline Species. *PloS Pathog* (2009) 5:e1000335. doi: 10.1371/journal.ppat.1000335

Blumberg BJ, Trop S, Das S, Dimopoulos G. Bacteria- and IMD pathway-independent immune defenses against Plasmodium falciparum in Anopheles gambiae. *PloS One* (2013) 8:e72130. doi: 10.1371/journal.pone.0072130

Oliva Chávez AS, Shaw DK, Munderloh UG, Pedra JHF. Tick Humoral Responses: Marching to the Beat of a Different Drummer. *Front Microbiol* (2017) 8:223. doi: 10.3389/fmicb.2017.00223

de la Fuente J, Antunes S, Bonnet S, Cabezas-Cruz A, Domingos AG, Estrada-Peña A, et al. Tick-Pathogen Interactions and Vector Competence: Identification of Molecular Drivers for Tick-Borne Diseases. *Front Cell Infect Microbiol* (2017) 7:114. doi: 10.3389/fcimb.2017.00114

Lane RS. "Competence of ticks as vectors of microbial agents with an emphasis on Borrelia burgdorferi. In: DE Sonenshine, TN Mather, editors. *Ecological dynamics of tick-borne zoonoses*. New York, NY: Oxford University Press (1994). p. 45–67.

Goddard J. *Infectious Diseases and Arthropods*. Totowa, NJ: Humana Press (2000). Available at: http://www.springer.com/us/book/9781603273992 (Accessed September 28, 2017).

Byndloss MX, Keestra-Gounder AM, Bäumler AJ, Tsolis RM. NOD1 and NOD2: New Functions Linking Endoplasmic Reticulum Stress and Inflammation. *DNA Cell Biol* (2016) 35:311–3. doi: 10.1089/dna.2016.3396

Keestra-Gounder AM, Byndloss MX, Seyffert N, Young BM, Chávez-Arroyo A, Tsai AY, et al. NOD1 and NOD2 signalling links ER stress with inflammation. *Nature* (2016) 532:394–7. doi: 10.1038/nature17631

Hu P, Han Z, Couvillon AD, Kaufman RJ, Exton JH. Autocrine tumor necrosis factor alpha links endoplasmic reticulum stress to the membrane death receptor pathway through IRE1alpha-mediated NF-kappaB activation and down-regulation of TRAF2 expression. *Mol Cell Biol* (2006) 26:3071–84. doi: 10.1128/MCB.26.8.3071-3084.2006

Yamazaki H, Hiramatsu N, Hayakawa K, Tagawa Y, Okamura M, Ogata R, et al. Activation of the Akt-NF-kappaB pathway by subtilase cytotoxin through the ATF6 branch of the unfolded protein response. *J Immunol Baltim Md 1950* (2009) 183:1480–7. doi: 10.4049/jimmunol.0900017

Nakajima S, Kitamura M. Bidirectional regulation of NF-*k*B by reactive oxygen species: A role of unfolded protein response. *Free Radic Biol Med* (2013) 65:162–74. doi: 10.1016/j.freeradbiomed.2013.06.020

Moretti J, Blander JM. Cell-autonomous stress responses in innate immunity. *J Leukoc Biol* (2017) 101:77–86. doi: 10.1189/jlb.2MR0416-201R

Janssens S, Pulendran B, Lambrecht BN. Emerging functions of the unfolded protein response in immunity. *Nat Immunol* (2014) 15:910–9. doi: 10.1038/ni.2991

Valanne S, Wang J-H, Rämet M. The Drosophila Toll Signaling Pathway. *J Immunol* (2011) 186:649–56. doi: 10.4049/jimmunol.1002302

Engström Y. Induction and regulation of antimicrobial peptides in Drosophila. *Dev Comp Immunol* (1999) 23:345–58. doi: 10.1016/S0145-305X(99)00016-6

Dushay MS, Asling B, Hultmark D. Origins of immunity: Relish, a compound Rel-like gene in the antibacterial defense of Drosophila. *Proc Natl Acad Sci* (1996) 93:10343–7. doi: 10.1073/pnas.93.19.10343

Meng X, Khanuja BS, Ip YT. Toll receptor-mediated Drosophila immune response requires Dif, an NF-*k*B factor. *Genes Dev* (1999) 13:792–7.

Kleino A, Silverman N. The Drosophila IMD pathway in the activation of the humoral immune response. *Dev Comp Immunol* (2014) 42:25–35. doi: 10.1016/j.dci.2013.05.014

Kaneko T, Yano T, Aggarwal K, Lim J-H, Ueda K, Oshima Y, et al. PGRP-LC and PGRP-LE have essential yet distinct functions in the drosophila immune response to monomeric DAP-type peptidoglycan. *Nat Immunol* (2006) 7:715–23. doi: 10.1038/ni1356

Lu Y, Su F, Li Q, Zhang J, Li Y, Tang T, et al. Pattern recognition receptors in Drosophila immune responses. *Dev Comp Immunol* (2020) 102:103468. doi: 10.1016/j.dci.2019.103468

Hedengren-Olcott M, Olcott MC, Mooney DT, Ekengren S, Geller BL, Taylor BJ. Differential Activation of the NF-*k*B-like Factors Relish and Dif in Drosophila melanogaster by Fungi and Gram-positive Bacteria. *J Biol Chem* (2004) 279:21121–7. doi: 10.1074/jbc.M313856200

Christophides GK, Zdobnov E, Barillas-Mury C, Birney E, Blandin S, Blass C, et al. Immunity-Related Genes and Gene Families in Anopheles gambiae. *Science* (2002) 298:159–65. doi: 10.1126/science.1077136

Palmer WJ, Jiggins FM. Comparative Genomics Reveals the Origins and Diversity of Arthropod Immune Systems. *Mol Biol Evol* (2015) 32:2111–29. doi: 10.1093/molbev/msv093

Gulia-Nuss M, Nuss AB, Meyer JM, Sonenshine DE, Roe RM, Waterhouse RM, et al. Genomic insights into the Ixodes scapularis tick vector of Lyme disease. *Nat Commun* (2016) 7:10507. doi: 10.1038/ncomms10507

Rawlings JS, Rosler KM, Harrison DA. The JAK/STAT signaling pathway. *J Cell Sci* (2004) 117:1281–3. doi: 10.1242/jcs.00963

Darnell JE. STATs and Gene Regulation. *Science* (1997) 277:1630–5. doi: 10.1126/science.277.5332.1630

Harrison DA, McCoon PE, Binari R, Gilman M, Perrimon N. Drosophila unpaired encodes a secreted protein that activates the JAK signaling pathway. *Genes Dev* (1998) 12:3252–63.

Buchon N, Silverman N, Cherry S. Immunity in Drosophila melanogaster–from microbial recognition to whole-organism physiology. *Nat Rev Immunol* (2014) 14:796–810. doi: 10.1038/nri3763

Lemaitre B, Hoffmann J. The Host Defense of Drosophila melanogaster. *Annu Rev Immunol* (2007) 25:697–743. doi: 10.1146/annurev.immunol.25.022106.141615

Tsunoda S, Avezov E, Zyryanova A, Konno T, Mendes-Silva L, Pinho Melo E, et al. Intact protein folding in the glutathione-depleted endoplasmic reticulum implicates alternative protein thiol reductants. *eLife* (2014) 3:e03421. doi: 10.7554/eLife.03421

Malhotra JD, Miao H, Zhang K, Wolfson A, Pennathur S, Pipe SW, et al. Antioxidants reduce endoplasmic reticulum stress and improve protein secretion. *Proc Natl Acad Sci USA* (2008) 105:18525–30. doi: 10.1073/pnas.0809677105

Lerner AG, Upton J-P, Praveen PVK, Ghosh R, Nakagawa Y, Igbaria A, et al. IRE1*a* induces thioredoxin-interacting protein to activate the NLRP3 inflammasome and promote programmed cell death under irremediable ER stress. *Cell Metab* (2012) 16:250–64. doi: 10.1016/j.cmet.2012.07.007

Oslowski CM, Hara T, O'Sullivan-Murphy B, Kanekura K, Lu S, Hara M, et al. Thioredoxin-interacting protein mediates ER stress-induced *b* cell death through initiation of the inflammasome. *Cell Metab* (2012) 16:265–73. doi: 10.1016/j.cmet.2012.07.005

Celli J, Tsolis RM. Bacteria, the ER and the Unfolded Protein Response: Friends or Foes? *Nat Rev Microbiol* (2015) 13:71–82. doi: 10.1038/nrmicro3393

Fu S, Yang L, Li P, Hofmann O, Dicker L, Hide W, et al. Aberrant lipid metabolism disrupts calcium homeostasis causing liver endoplasmic reticulum stress in obesity. *Nature* (2011) 473:528–31. doi: 10.1038/nature09968

Schröder M, Clark R, Liu CY, Kaufman RJ. The unfolded protein response represses differentiation through the RPD3-SIN3 histone deacetylase. *EMBO J* (2004) 23:2281–92. doi: 10.1038/sj.emboj.7600233

Schröder M, Chang JS, Kaufman RJ. The unfolded protein response represses nitrogen-starvation induced developmental differentiation in yeast. *Genes Dev* (2000) 14:2962–75. doi: 10.1101/gad.852300

Bertolotti A, Zhang Y, Hendershot LM, Harding HP, Ron D. Dynamic interaction of BiP and ER stress transducers in the unfolded-protein response. *Nat Cell Biol* (2000) 2:326–32. doi: 10.1038/35014014

Adams CJ, Kopp MC, Larburu N, Nowak PR, Ali MMU. Structure and Molecular Mechanism of ER Stress Signaling by the Unfolded Protein Response Signal Activator IRE1. *Front Mol Biosci* (2019) 6:11. doi: 10.3389/fmolb.2019.00011

Pincus D, Chevalier MW, Aragón T, van Anken E, Vidal SE, El-Samad H, et al. BiP binding to the ER-stress sensor Ire1 tunes the homeostatic behavior of the unfolded protein response. *PloS Biol* (2010) 8:e1000415. doi: 10.1371/journal.pbio.1000415

Shen J, Chen X, Hendershot L, Prywes R. ER stress regulation of ATF6 localization by dissociation of BiP/GRP78 binding and unmasking of Golgi localization signals. *Dev Cell* (2002) 3:99–111. doi: 10.1016/s1534-5807(02)00203-4

Nadanaka S, Okada T, Yoshida H, Mori K. Role of disulfide bridges formed in the luminal domain of ATF6 in sensing endoplasmic reticulum stress. *Mol Cell Biol* (2007) 27:1027–43. doi: 10.1128/MCB.00408-06

Medigeshi GR, Lancaster AM, Hirsch AJ, Briese T, Lipkin WI, DeFilippis V, et al. West Nile Virus Infection Activates the Unfolded Protein Response, Leading to CHOP Induction and Apoptosis. *J Virol* (2007) 81:10849–60. doi: 10.1128/JVI.01151-07

Harding HP, Zhang Y, Ron D. Protein translation and folding are coupled by an endoplasmic-reticulum-resident kinase. *Nature* (1999) 397:271–4. doi: 10.1038/16729

Connor JH, Weiser DC, Li S, Hallenbeck JM, Shenolikar S. Growth Arrest and DNA Damage-Inducible Protein GADD34 Assembles a Novel Signaling Complex Containing Protein Phosphatase 1 and Inhibitor 1. *Mol Cell Biol* (2001) 21:6841–50. doi: 10.1128/MCB.21.20.6841-6850.2001

Harding HP, Zhang Y, Zeng H, Novoa I, Lu PD, Calfon M, et al. An Integrated Stress Response Regulates Amino Acid Metabolism and Resistance to Oxidative Stress. *Mol Cell* (2003) 11:619–33. doi: 10.1016/ S1097-2765(03)00105-9

Ye J, Rawson RB, Komuro R, Chen X, Davé UP, Prywes R, et al. ER Stress Induces Cleavage of Membrane-Bound ATF6 by the Same Proteases that Process SREBPs. *Mol Cell* (2000) 6:1355–64. doi: 10.1016/S1097-2765(00) 00133-7

Schindler AJ, Schekman R. In vitro reconstitution of ER-stress induced ATF6 transport in COPII vesicles. *Proc Natl Acad Sci* (2009) 106:17775–80. doi: 10.1073/pnas.0910342106

Wu H, Ng BSH, Thibault G. Endoplasmic reticulum stress response in yeast and humans. *Biosci Rep* (2014) 34:321–30. doi: 10.1042/BSR20140058

Adachi Y, Yamamoto K, Okada T, Yoshida H, Harada A, Mori K. ATF6 Is a Transcription Factor Specializing in the Regulation of Quality Control Proteins in the Endoplasmic Reticulum. *Cell Struct Funct* (2008) 33:75–89. doi: 10.1247/csf.07044

Oslowski CM, Urano F. Measuring ER stress and the unfolded protein response using mammalian tissue culture system. *Methods Enzymol* (2011) 490:71–92. doi: 10.1016/B978-0-12-385114-7.00004-0

Yoshida H, Matsui T, Yamamoto A, Okada T, Mori K. XBP1 mRNA Is Induced by ATF6 and Spliced by IRE1 in Response to ER Stress to Produce a Highly Active Transcription Factor. *Cell* (2001) 107:881–91. doi: 10.1016/ S0092-8674(01)00611-0

Calfon M, Zeng H, Urano F, Till JH, Hubbard SR, Harding HP, et al. IRE1 couples endoplasmic reticulum load to secretory capacity by processing the XBP-1 mRNA. *Nature* (2002) 415:92–6. doi: 10.1038/415092a

Shoulders MD, Ryno LM, Genereux JC, Moresco JJ, Tu PG, Wu C, et al. Stress-Independent Activation of XBP1s and/or ATF6 Reveals Three Functionally Diverse ER Proteostasis Environments. *Cell Rep* (2013) 3:1279–92. doi: 10.1016/j.celrep.2013.03.024

Hollien J, Lin JH, Li H, Stevens N, Walter P, Weissman JS. Regulated Ire1-dependent decay of messenger RNAs in mammalian cells. *J Cell Biol* (2009) 186:323–31. doi: 10.1083/jcb.200903014

Hu P, Han Z, Couvillon AD, Kaufman RJ, Exton JH. Autocrine Tumor Necrosis Factor Alpha Links Endoplasmic Reticulum Stress to the Membrane Death Receptor Pathway through IRE1*a*-Mediated NF-*k*B Activation and Down-Regulation of TRAF2 Expression. *Mol Cell Biol* (2006) 26:3071–84. doi: 10.1128/MCB.26.8.3071-3084.2006

Zhu X, Zhang J, Sun H, Jiang C, Dong Y, Shan Q, et al. Ubiquitination of Inositol-requiring Enzyme 1 (IRE1) by the E3 Ligase CHIP Mediates the IRE1/TRAF2/JNK Pathway. *J Biol Chem* (2014) 289:30567–77. doi: 10.1074/ jbc.M114.562868

Urano F, Wang X, Bertolotti A, Zhang Y, Chung P, Harding HP, et al. Coupling of Stress in the ER to Activation of JNK Protein Kinases by Transmembrane Protein Kinase IRE1. *Science* (2000) 287:664–6. doi: 10.1126/science.287.5453.664

Pakos-Zebrucka K, Koryga I, Mnich K, Ljujic M, Samali A, Gorman AM. The integrated stress response. *EMBO Rep* (2016) 17:1374–95. doi: 10.15252/embr.201642195

Ye J, Kumanova M, Hart LS, Sloane K, Zhang H, De Panis DN, et al. The GCN2-ATF4 pathway is critical for tumour cell survival and proliferation in response to nutrient deprivation. *EMBO J* (2010) 29:2082–96. doi: 10.1038/ emboj.2010.81

Natarajan K, Meyer MR, Jackson BM, Slade D, Roberts C, Hinnebusch AG, et al. Transcriptional Profiling Shows that Gcn4p Is a Master Regulator of Gene Expression during Amino Acid Starvation in Yeast. *Mol Cell Biol* (2001) 21:4347–68. doi: 10.1128/MCB.21.13.4347-4368.2001

Webster SJ, Ellis L, O'Brien LM, Tyrrell B, Fitzmaurice TJ, Elder MJ, et al. IRE1*a* mediates PKR activation in response to Chlamydia trachomatis infection. *Microbes Infect* (2016) 18:472–83. doi: 10.1016/j.micinf.2016.03.010

Donnelly N, Gorman AM, Gupta S, Samali A. The eIF2*a* kinases: their structures and functions. *Cell Mol Life Sci* (2013) 70:3493–511. doi: 10.1007/s00018-012-1252-6

Taniuchi S, Miyake M, Tsugawa K, Oyadomari M, Oyadomari S. Integrated stress response of vertebrates is regulated by four eIF2*a* kinases. *Sci Rep* (2016) 6:32886. doi: 10.1038/srep32886

Deng J, Harding HP, Raught B, Gingras A-C, Berlanga JJ, Scheuner D, et al. Activation of GCN2 in UV-Irradiated Cells Inhibits Translation. *Curr Biol* (2002) 12:1279–86. doi: 10.1016/S0960-9822(02)01037-0

Harding HP, Zhang Y, Bertolotti A, Zeng H, Ron D. Perk Is Essential for Translational Regulation and Cell Survival during the Unfolded Protein Response. *Mol Cell* (2000) 5:897–904. doi: 10.1016/S1097-2765(00)80330-5

Szegezdi E, Logue SE, Gorman AM, Samali A. Mediators of endoplasmic reticulum stress-induced apoptosis. *EMBO Rep* (2006) 7:880–5. doi: 10.1038/sj.embor.7400779

Lemaire PA, Anderson E, Lary J, Cole JL. Mechanism of PKR Activation by dsRNA. *J Mol Biol* (2008) 381:351–60. doi: 10.1016/j.jmb.2008.05.056

Chukwurah E, Patel RC. Stress-induced TRBP phosphorylation enhances its interaction with PKR to regulate cellular survival. *Sci Rep* (2018) 8:1020. doi: 10.1038/s41598-018-19360-8

Reineke LC, Lloyd RE. The Stress Granule Protein G3BP1 Recruits Protein Kinase R To Promote Multiple Innate Immune Antiviral Responses. *J Virol* (2015) 89:2575–89. doi: 10.1128/JVI.02791-14

Han A-P, Yu C, Lu L, Fujiwara Y, Browne C, Chin G, et al. Heme-regulated eIF2*a* kinase (HRI) is required for translational regulation and survival of erythroid precursors in iron deficiency. *EMBO J* (2001) 20:6909–18. doi: 10.1093/emboj/20.23.6909

Aitken CE, Lorsch JR. A mechanistic overview of translation initiation in eukaryotes. *Nat Struct Mol Biol* (2012) 19:568–76. doi: 10.1038/nsmb.2303

Sonenberg N, Hinnebusch AG. Regulation of Translation Initiation in Eukaryotes: Mechanisms and Biological Targets. *Cell* (2009) 136:731–45. doi: 10.1016/j.cell.2009.01.042

Krishnamoorthy T, Pavitt GD, Zhang F, Dever TE, Hinnebusch AG. Tight Binding of the Phosphorylated *a* Subunit of Initiation Factor 2 (eIF2*a*) to the Regulatory Subunits of Guanine Nucleotide Exchange Factor eIF2B Is Required for Inhibition of Translation Initiation. *Mol Cell Biol* (2001) 21:5018–30. doi: 10.1128/MCB.21.15.5018-5030.2001

Pavitt GD, Ramaiah KVA, Kimball SR, Hinnebusch AG. eIF2 independently binds two distinct eIF2B subcomplexes that catalyze and regulate guanine-nucleotide exchange. *Genes Dev* (1998) 12:514–26.

Adomavicius T, Guaita M, Zhou Y, Jennings MD, Latif Z, Roseman AM, et al. The structural basis of translational control by eIF2 phosphorylation. *Nat Commun* (2019) 10:2136. doi: 10.1038/s41467-019-10167-3

Ohoka N, Yoshii S, Hattori T, Onozaki K, Hayashi H. TRB3, a novel ER stress-inducible gene, is induced via ATF4–CHOP pathway and is involved in cell death. *EMBO J* (2005) 24:1243–55. doi: 10.1038/sj.emboj.7600596

Han J, Back SH, Hur J, Lin Y-H, Gildersleeve R, Shan J, et al. ER-stress-induced transcriptional regulation increases protein synthesis leading to cell death. *Nat Cell Biol* (2013) 15:481–90. doi: 10.1038/ncb2738

Ma Y, Hendershot LM. Delineation of a Negative Feedback Regulatory Loop That Controls Protein Translation during Endoplasmic Reticulum Stress. *J Biol Chem* (2003) 278:34864–73. doi: 10.1074/jbc.M301107200

Kim WJ, Back SH, Kim V, Ryu I, Jang SK. Sequestration of TRAF2 into Stress Granules Interrupts Tumor Necrosis Factor Signaling under Stress Conditions. *Mol Cell Biol* (2005) 25:2450–62. doi: 10.1128/MCB.25.6.2450-2462.2005

Arimoto K, Fukuda H, Imajoh-Ohmi S, Saito H, Takekawa M. Formation of stress granules inhibits apoptosis by suppressing stress-responsive MAPK pathways. *Nat Cell Biol* (2008) 10:1324–32. doi: 10.1038/ncb1791

Hoang H-D, Graber TE, Alain T. Battling for Ribosomes: Translational Control at the Forefront of the Antiviral Response. *J Mol Biol* (2018) 430:1965–92. doi: 10.1016/j.jmb.2018.04.040

Won S, Eidenschenk C, Arnold CN, Siggs OM, Sun L, Brandl K, et al. Increased Susceptibility to DNA Virus Infection in Mice with a GCN2 Mutation. *J Virol* (2012) 86:1802–8. doi: 10.1128/JVI.05660-11

Berlanga JJ, Ventoso I, Harding HP, Deng J, Ron D, Sonenberg N, et al. Antiviral effect of the mammalian translation initiation factor 2*a* kinase GCN2 against RNA viruses. *EMBO J* (2006) 25:1730–40. doi: 10.1038/sj.emboj.7601073

Amen OM, Sarker SD, Ghildyal R, Arya A. Endoplasmic Reticulum Stress Activates Unfolded Protein Response Signaling and Mediates Inflammation, Obesity, and Cardiac Dysfunction: Therapeutic and Molecular Approach. *Front Pharmacol* (2019) 10:977. doi: 10.3389/fphar.2019.00977

Meyerovich K, Ortis F, Allagnat F, Cardozo AK. Endoplasmic reticulum stress and the unfolded protein response in pancreatic islet inflammation. *J Mol Endocrinol* (2016) 57:R1–R17. doi: 10.1530/jme-15-0306

Ghosh R, Colon-Negron K, Papa FR. Endoplasmic reticulum stress, degeneration of pancreatic islet *b*-cells, and therapeutic modulation of the unfolded protein response in diabetes. *Mol Metab* (2019) 27:S60–8. doi: 10.1016/j.molmet.2019.06.012

Coope A, Pascoal LB, Botezelli JD, da Silva FAR, de LS Ayrizono M, Rodrigues BL, et al. ER stress activation in the intestinal mucosa but not in mesenteric adipose tissue is associated with inflammation in Crohn's disease patients. *PloS One* (2019) 14:e0223105. doi: 10.1371/journal.pone.0223105

Fougeray S, Bouvier N, Beaune P, Legendre C, Anglicheau D, Thervet E, et al. Metabolic stress promotes renal tubular inflammation by triggering the unfolded protein response. *Cell Death Dis* (2011) 2:e143–3. doi: 10.1038/cddis.2011.26

Yang W, Sheng F, Sun B, Fischbach S, Xiao X. The role of ORMDL3/ATF6 in compensated beta cell proliferation during early diabetes. *Aging* (2019) 11:2787–96. doi: 10.18632/aging.101949

Abuaita BH, Burkholder KM, Boles BR, O'Riordan MX. The Endoplasmic Reticulum Stress Sensor Inositol-Requiring Enzyme 1*a* Augments Bacterial Killing through Sustained Oxidant Production. *mBio* (2015) 6. doi: 10.1128/mBio.00705-15

Tentaku A, Shimohata T, Hatayama S, Kido J, Nguyen AQ, Kanda Y, et al. Host cellular unfolded protein response signaling regulates Campylobacter jejuni invasion. *PloS One* (2018) 13:e0205865. doi: 10.1371/journal.pone.0205865

Treacy-Abarca S, Mukherjee S. Legionella suppresses the host unfolded protein response via multiple mechanisms. *Nat Commun* (2015) 6. doi: 10.1038/ncomms8887

Hempstead AD, Isberg RR. Inhibition of host cell translation elongation by Legionella pneumophila blocks the host cell unfolded protein response. *Proc Natl Acad Sci* (2015) 112:E6790–7. doi: 10.1073/pnas.1508716112

Smith JA, Khan M, Magnani DD, Harms JS, Durward M, Radhakrishnan GK, et al. Brucella Induces an Unfolded Protein Response via TcpB That Supports Intracellular Replication in Macrophages. *PloS Pathog* (2013) 9: e1003785. doi: 10.1371/journal.ppat.1003785

Myeni S, Child R, Ng TW, Iii JJK, Wehrly TD, Porcella SF, et al. Brucella Modulates Secretory Trafficking via Multiple Type IV Secretion Effector Proteins. *PloS Pathog* (2013) 9:e1003556. doi: 10.1371/journal.ppat.1003556

de Jong MF, Starr T, Winter MG, den Hartigh AB, Child R, Knodler LA, et al. Sensing of Bacterial Type IV Secretion via the Unfolded Protein Response. *mBio* (2013) 4. doi: 10.1128/mBio.00418-12

Zhou D, Zhi F-J, Qi M-Z, Bai F-R, Zhang G, Li J-M, et al. Brucella induces unfolded protein response and inflammatory response via GntR in alveolar macrophages. *Oncotarget* (2017) 9:5184–96. doi: 10.18632/oncotarget.23706

Taguchi Y, Imaoka K, Kataoka M, Uda A, Nakatsu D, Horii-Okazaki S, et al. Yip1A, a Novel Host Factor for the Activation of the IRE1 Pathway of the Unfolded Protein Response during Brucella Infection. *PloS Pathog* (2015) 11: e1004747. doi: 10.1371/journal.ppat.1004747

Keestra-Gounder AM, Byndloss MX, Seyffert N, Young BM, Chávez-Arroyo A, Tsai AY, et al. NOD1/NOD2 signaling links ER stress with inflammation. *Nature* (2016) 532:394–7. doi: 10.1038/nature17631

Zellner B, Huntley JF. Ticks and Tularemia: Do We Know What We Don't Know? *Front Cell Infect Microbiol* (2019) 9:146. doi: 10.3389/fcimb.2019.00146

Petersen JM, Schriefer ME. Tularemia: emergence/re-emergence. *Vet Res* (2005) 36:455–67. doi: 10.1051/vetres:2005006

Calhoun EL. Natural Occurrence of Tularemia in the Lone Star Tick, Amblyomma Americanum (Linn.), and in Dogs in Arkansas. *Am J Trop Med Hyg* (1954) 3:360–6. doi: 10.4269/ajtmh.1954.3.360

Goethert HK, Shani I, Telford SR. Genotypic Diversity of Francisella tularensis Infecting Dermacentor variabilis Ticks on Martha's Vineyard, Massachusetts. *J Clin Microbiol* (2004) 42:4968–73. doi: 10.1128/JCM.42.11.4968-4973.2004

Barel M, Harduin-Lepers A, Portier L, Slomianny M-C, Charbit A. Host glycosylation pathways and the unfolded protein response contribute to the infection by Francisella. *Cell Microbiol* (2016) 18:1763–81. doi: 10.1111/cmi.12614

Martinon F, Chen X, Lee A-H, Glimcher LH. Toll-like receptor activation of XBP1 regulates innate immune responses in macrophages. *Nat Immunol* (2010) 11:411–8. doi: 10.1038/ni.1857

Rodino KG, VieBrock L, Evans SM, Ge H, Richards AL, Carlyon JA. Orientia tsutsugamushi Modulates Endoplasmic Reticulum-Associated Degradation To Benefit Its Growth. *Infect Immun* (2018) 86. doi: 10.1128/IAI.00596-17

Yoshikawa Y, Sugimoto K, Ochiai Y, Ohashi N. Intracellular proliferation of Anaplasma phagocytophilum is promoted via modulation of endoplasmic reticulum stress signaling in host cells. *Microbiol Immunol* (2020) 64:270–9. doi: 10.1111/1348-0421.12770

Isler JA, Skalet AH, Alwine JC. Human Cytomegalovirus Infection Activates and Regulates the Unfolded Protein Response. *J Virol* (2005) 79:6890–9. doi: 10.1128/JVI.79.11.6890-6899.2005

Stahl S, Burkhart JM, Hinte F, Tirosh B, Mohr H, Zahedi RP, et al. Cytomegalovirus Downregulates IRE1 to Repress the Unfolded Protein Response. *PloS Pathog* (2013) 9:e1003544. doi: 10.1371/journal.ppat.1003544

Johnston BP, McCormick C. Herpesviruses and the Unfolded Protein Response. *Viruses* (2020) 12:17. doi: 10.3390/v12010017

Lv S, Sun E-C, Xu Q-Y, Zhang J-K, Wu D-L. Endoplasmic reticulum stress-mediated autophagy contributes to bluetongue virus infection via the PERK- eIF2*a* pathway. *Biochem Biophys Res Commun* (2015) 466:406–12. doi: 10.1016/j.bbrc.2015.09.039

Rathore APS, Ng M-L, Vasudevan SG. Differential unfolded protein response during Chikungunya and Sindbis virus infection: CHIKV nsP4 suppresses eIF2*a* phosphorylation. *Virol J* (2013) 10:36. doi: 10.1186/1743-422X-10-36

Li S, Kong L, Yu X. The expanding roles of endoplasmic reticulum stress in virus replication and pathogenesis. *Crit Rev Microbiol* (2015) 41:150–64. doi: 10.3109/1040841X.2013.813899

Lee Y-R, Kuo S-H, Lin C-Y, Fu P-J, Lin Y-S, Yeh T-M, et al. Dengue virus-induced ER stress is required for autophagy activation, viral replication, and pathogenesis both in vitro and in vivo. *Sci Rep* (2018) 8:489. doi: 10.1038/s41598-017-18909-3

Ambrose RL, Mackenzie JM. ATF6 Signaling Is Required for Efficient West Nile Virus Replication by Promoting Cell Survival and Inhibition of Innate Immune Responses. *J Virol* (2013) 87:2206–14. doi: 10.1128/JVI.02097-12

Ambrose RL, Mackenzie JM. West Nile Virus Differentially Modulates the Unfolded Protein Response To Facilitate Replication and Immune Evasion. *J Virol* (2011) 85:2723–32. doi: 10.1128/JVI.02050-10

Yu C, Achazi K, Niedrig M. Tick-borne encephalitis virus triggers inositol-requiring enzyme 1 (IRE1) and transcription factor 6 (ATF6) pathways of unfolded protein response. *Virus Res* (2013) 178:471–7. doi: 10.1016/j.virusres.2013.10.012

Lewy TG, Offerdahl DK, Grabowski JM, Kellman E, Mlera L, Chiramel A, et al. PERK-Mediated Unfolded Protein Response Signaling Restricts Replication of the Tick-Borne Flavivirus Langat Virus. *Viruses* (2020) 12:328. doi: 10.3390/v12030328

Kumar D, Embers M, Mather TN, Karim S. Is selenoprotein K required for Borrelia burgdorferi infection within the tick vector Ixodes scapularis? *Parasit Vectors* (2019) 12:289. doi: 10.1186/s13071-019-3548-y

Ghosh S, Jassar O, Kontsedalov S, Lebedev G, Wang C, Turner D, et al. Ghanim M. A Transcriptomics Approach Reveals Putative Interaction of Candidatus Liberibacter Solanacearum with the Endoplasmic Reticulum of Its Psyllid Vector. *Insects* (2019) 10:279. doi: 10.3390/insects10090279

Valderrama C, Clark A, Urano F, Unanue ER, Carrero JA. Listeria monocytogenes induces an interferon-enhanced activation of the integrated stress response that is detrimental for resolution of infection in mice. *Eur J Immunol* (2017) 47:830–40. doi: 10.1002/eji.201646856

Tattoli I, Sorbara MT, Vuckovic D, Ling A, Soares F, Carneiro LAM, et al. Amino Acid Starvation Induced by Invasive Bacterial Pathogens Triggers an Innate Host Defense Program. *Cell Host Microbe* (2012) 11:563–75. doi: 10.1016/j.chom.2012.04.012

Brann KR, Fullerton MS, Voth DE. Coxiella burnetii Requires Host Eukaryotic Initiation Factor 2*a* Activity for Efficient Intracellular Replication. *Infect Immun* (2020) 88. doi: 10.1128/IAI.00096-20

Rabouw HH, Visser LJ, Passchier TC, Langereis MA, Liu F, Giansanti P, et al. Inhibition of the integrated stress response by viral proteins that block p- eIF2–eIF2B association. *Nat Microbiol* (2020) 5:1361–73. doi: 10.1038/s41564-020-0759-0

McCormick C, Khaperskyy DA. Translation inhibition and stress granules in the antiviral immune response. *Nat Rev Immunol* (2017) 17:647–60. doi: 10.1038/nri.2017.63

Wuerth JD, Habjan M, Kainulainen M, Berisha B, Bertheloot D, Superti-Furga G, et al. eIF2B as a Target for Viral Evasion of PKR-Mediated Translation Inhibition. *mBio* (2020) 11. doi: 10.1128/mBio.00976-20

Ikegami T, Narayanan K, Won S, Kamitani W, Peters CJ, Makino S. Rift Valley Fever Virus NSs Protein Promotes Post-Transcriptional Downregulation of Protein Kinase PKR and Inhibits eIF2*a* Phosphorylation. *PloS Pathog* (2009) 5:e1000287. doi: 10.1371/journal.ppat.1000287

Kainulainen M, Habjan M, Hubel P, Busch L, Lau S, Colinge J, et al. Virulence Factor NSs of Rift Valley Fever Virus Recruits the F-Box Protein FBXO3 To Degrade Subunit p62 of General Transcription Factor TFIIH. *J Virol* (2014) 88:3464–73. doi: 10.1128/JVI.02914-13

Kainulainen M, Lau S, Samuel CE, Hornung V, Weber F. NSs Virulence Factor of Rift Valley Fever Virus Engages the F-Box Proteins FBXW11 and *b*-TRCP1 To Degrade the Antiviral Protein Kinase PKR. *J Virol* (2016) 90:6140–7. doi: 10.1128/JVI.00016-16

Courtney SC, Scherbik SV, Stockman BM, Brinton MA. West Nile Virus Infections Suppress Early Viral RNA Synthesis and Avoid Inducing the Cell Stress Granule Response. *J Virol* (2012) 86:3647–57. doi: 10.1128/JVI.06549-11

Hou S, Kumar A, Xu Z, Airo AM, Stryapunina I, Wong CP, et al. Zika Virus Hijacks Stress Granule Proteins and Modulates the Host Stress Response. *J Virol* (2017) 91. doi: 10.1128/JVI.00474-17

Bonenfant G, Williams N, Netzband R, Schwarz MC, Evans MJ, Pager CT. Zika Virus Subverts Stress Granules To Promote and Restrict Viral Gene Expression. *J Virol* (2019) 93. doi: 10.1128/JVI.00520-19

Emara MM, Brinton MA. Interaction of TIA-1/TIAR with West Nile and dengue virus products in infected cells interferes with stress granule formation and processing body assembly. *Proc Natl Acad Sci* (2007) 104:9041–6. doi: 10.1073/pnas.0703348104

Roth H, Magg V, Uch F, Mutz P, Klein P, Haneke K, et al. Flavivirus Infection Uncouples Translation Suppression from Cellular Stress Responses. *mBio* (2017) 8. doi: 10.1128/mBio.02150-16

Katoh H, Okamoto T, Fukuhara T, Kambara H, Morita E, Mori Y, et al. Japanese Encephalitis Virus Core Protein Inhibits Stress Granule Formation through an Interaction with Caprin-1 and Facilitates Viral Propagation. *J Virol* (2013) 87:489–502. doi: 10.1128/JVI.02186-12

Tu Y-C, Yu C-Y, Liang J-J, Lin E, Liao C-L, Lin Y-L. Blocking Double-Stranded RNA-Activated Protein Kinase PKR by Japanese Encephalitis Virus Nonstructural Protein 2A. *J Virol* (2012) 86:10347–58. doi: 10.1128/JVI.00525-12

Hsu L-C, Park JM, Zhang K, Luo J-L, Maeda S, Kaufman RJ, et al. The protein kinase PKR is required for macrophage apoptosis after activation of Toll-like receptor 4. *Nature* (2004) 428:341–5. doi: 10.1038/nature02405

Diebold SS, Montoya M, Unger H, Alexopoulou L, Roy P, Haswell LE, et al. Viral infection switches non-plasmacytoid dendritic cells into high interferon producers. *Nature* (2003) 424:324–8. doi: 10.1038/nature01783

Hoffmann JA, Reichhart J-M. Drosophila innate immunity: an evolutionary perspective. *Nat Immunol* (2002) 3:121–6. doi: 10.1038/ni0202-121

Nakajima S, Hiramatsu N, Hayakawa K, Saito Y, Kato H, Huang T, et al. Selective abrogation of BiP/GRP78 blunts activation of NF-*k*B through the ATF6 branch of the UPR: involvement of C/EBP*b* and mTOR-dependent dephosphorylation of Akt. *Mol Cell Biol* (2011) 31:1710–8. doi: 10.1128/MCB.00939-10

Naudé PJW, den Boer JA, Luiten PGM, Eisel ULM. Tumor necrosis factor receptor cross-talk. *FEBS J* (2011) 278:888–98. doi: 10.1111/j.1742-4658.2011.08017.x

Oeckinghaus A, Hayden MS, Ghosh S. Crosstalk in NF-*k*B signaling pathways. *Nat Immunol* (2011) 12:695–708. doi: 10.1038/ni.2065

Meares GP, Liu Y, Rajbhandari R, Qin H, Nozell SE, Mobley JA, et al. PERK-dependent activation of JAK1 and STAT3 contributes to endoplasmic reticulum stress-induced inflammation. *Mol Cell Biol* (2014) 34:3911–25. doi: 10.1128/MCB.00980-14

Överby AK, Popov VL, Niedrig M, Weber F. Tick-Borne Encephalitis Virus Delays Interferon Induction and Hides Its Double-Stranded RNA in Intracellular Membrane Vesicles. *J Virol* (2010) 84:8470–83. doi: 10.1128/JVI.00176-10

11

Protease Inhibitors in Tick Saliva: The Role of Serpins and Cystatins in Tick-Host-Pathogen Interaction

Jindřich Chmelař[1†], Jan Kotál[1,2†], Helena Langhansová[1,2] and Michail Kotsyfakis[2*]*

[1] Faculty of Science, University of South Bohemia in České Budějovice, České Budějovice, Czechia, [2] Institute of Parasitology, Biology Center, Czech Academy of Sciences, České Budějovice, Czechia

***Correspondence:**
Jindřich Chmela
chmelar@jcu.cz
Michail Kotsyfakis
mich_kotsyfakis@yahoo.com*

[†] These authors have contributed equally to this work.

The publication of the first tick sialome (salivary gland transcriptome) heralded a new era of research of tick protease inhibitors, which represent important constituents of the proteins secreted via tick saliva into the host. Three major groups of protease inhibitors are secreted into saliva: Kunitz inhibitors, serpins, and cystatins. Kunitz inhibitors are anti-hemostatic agents and tens of proteins with one or more Kunitz domains are known to block host coagulation and/or platelet aggregation. Serpins and cystatins are also anti-hemostatic effectors, but intriguingly, from the translational perspective, also act as pluripotent modulators of the host immune system. Here we focus especially on this latter aspect of protease inhibition by ticks and describe the current knowledge and data on secreted salivary serpins and cystatins and their role in tick-host-pathogen interaction triad. We also discuss the potential therapeutic use of tick protease inhibitors.

Keywords: tick-host interaction, immunomodulation, protease inhibitors, serpins, cystatins

SERPINS AND CYSTATINS AS HOMEOSTATIC REGULATORS

Proteases (also proteinases or peptidases) are ubiquitous enzymes that cleave proteins to smaller peptides and amino acids. Proteases participate in a range of physiological processes including extracellular digestion, protein degradation, and tissue development (Rawlings and Salvesen, 2013). Relevant to this review, however, is the fact that many proteases, in particular highly substrate-specific endopeptidases, mediate defense and homeostatic processes in both vertebrates and invertebrates. Proteolytic pathways rely on the precise and tightly regulated activation and inhibition of these endopeptidases. As a result of this evolutionary need, many crucial pathophysiological processes are regulated via proteolytic cascades, with notable examples being coagulation of plasma (or haemolymph in arthropods), bacterial wall perforation with complement, or melanization in arthropods (Amara et al., 2008; Tang, 2009; Gulley et al., 2013). Each step involves proteolytic activation of another downstream protease, and all proteases in such cascades usually have their own endogenous inhibitors that balance the system. The role of arthropod protease inhibitors in the defense is supported by the fact that the expression of serpins and cystatins in *Ixodes scapularis* nymphs was attenuated upon infection with *Anaplasma phagocytophilum*, as seen in the transcriptomic data (Ayllon et al., 2015). On the other hand, the expression of protease inhibitors in salivary glands and midguts of adult females differed among individual inhibitors, i.e., some cystatins and serpins were upregulated upon the infection and vice versa (Ayllon et al., 2015). Similar data were collected from *Ixodes ricinus* infected with *Bartonella henselae* (Liu et al., 2014). Therefore, precise involvement of every individual inhibitor in tick infection would have to be evaluated experimentally.

Other intracellular and extracellular processes, such as cytokine activation, phagocytosis, intracellular signaling, and antigen processing, are also dependent on proteolysis (Muller et al., 2012). Serpins and cystatins are the two main superfamilies of endogenous serine and cysteine protease inhibitors involved in the regulation of these processes. It is therefore unsurprising that both groups of inhibitors are well represented in parasites and are important in their interactions with hosts (Schwarz et al., 2012; Meekins et al., 2017). In order to obtain a blood meal, ticks secrete hundreds of different pharmacoactive molecules into the host via their saliva. These molecules have anti-hemostatic, anti-inflammatory, anti-complement and immunomodulatory properties and their function is to overcome or evade host defense mechanisms including immune response (Brossard and Wikel, 2004; Chmelar et al., 2012). Moreover, tick saliva and also several salivary compounds were found to facilitate and enhance the establishment of tick-borne pathogens in the host (Anguita et al., 2002; Pal et al., 2004; Kazimirova and Stibraniova, 2013; Wikel, 2013). Inhibitors of proteases represent the most prominent protein families in tick salivary secretion that are responsible for alteration of many different host defense pathways.

SERINE PROTEASE INHIBITORS IN TICKS

Four groups of serine protease inhibitors have been described in ticks: Kunitz domain inhibitors, Kazal domain inhibitors, trypsin inhibitor-like cysteine rich domain (TIL) inhibitors, and serpins. Inhibitors with 1–7 Kunitz domains mostly act as anti-hemostatic proteins and form a large multigenic family of secreted salivary proteins in ticks that have probably played a crucial role in the development of tick hematophagy (Corral-Rodriguez et al., 2009; Dai et al., 2012; Schwarz et al., 2014). Moreover, single Kunitz-domain inhibitors in other organisms are involved in ion channel blockade and may play a similar role in ticks (Frazao et al., 2012; Valdes and Moal, 2014). Kazal domain inhibitors are described in hematophagous insects such as mosquitoes and triatomine bugs (Rimphanitchayakit and Tassanakajon, 2010), but they are only rarely reported in ticks, in which their function is still unknown (Zhou et al., 2006a; Mulenga et al., 2007a, 2008). TIL-domain inhibitors represent an interesting group of small inhibitors with a conserved 5-disulphide bridge structure that were first reported in *Apis melifera* (Bania et al., 1999) and have also been detected in ticks (Fogaca et al., 2006; Sasaki et al., 2008). The sequences of over 80 TIL-domain inhibitors have been found in arthropod genomes (Zeng et al., 2014), and the unique features of TIL-domain proteins make them an excellent model for designing novel serine protease inhibitors and antimicrobial peptides (Li et al., 2007).

Serpins

Serpins form the largest superfamily of protease inhibitors, and they are ubiquitously distributed in nature including viruses and prokaryotes. With over 1,500 members, serpins are the most studied protease inhibitors (Law et al., 2006), also helped by their unique and highly intriguing mechanism of inhibition (Whisstock et al., 2010) and the evolutionary changes that turned inhibitory serpins into non-inhibitory proteins with completely different functions (Law et al., 2006; Silverman et al., 2010). For example, there are 29 inhibitory and seven non-inhibitory serpins in humans and 60 functional serpin genes in mice (Heit et al., 2013). Angiotensinogen is a non-inhibitory serpin that is proteolytically activated by renin into several oligopeptides (angiotensins) that regulate vasoconstriction and blood pressure (Lu et al., 2016). Cortisol and thyroxine-binding proteins (human *SERPINA6* and *SERPINA7*) are also notable serpins that act as major transport proteins for glucocorticoids and progesterone (Carrell and Read, 2016). Inhibitory serpins have very diverse functions depending on their specificity, but their importance is highlighted by the serpinopathies—diseases caused by serpin dysfunction or deficiency (Belorgey et al., 2007). Emphysema, cirrhosis, angioedema, hypertension, and even familial dementia are caused at least in part by serpin dysfunction (Kim et al., 1995; Davis et al., 1999; Ekeowa et al., 2009; Huntington and Li, 2009; Lomas et al., 2016).

Arthropod serpins have mostly immunological and hemostatic functions. Serpins have been shown to regulate haemolymph coagulation, are involved in phenoloxidase system activation in insects, and regulate an immune toll pathway in haemolymph (Kanost, 1999; Gulley et al., 2013; Meekins et al., 2017). Furthermore, in bloodfeeding arthropods, serpins can act as modulators of host hemostasis and/or immune responses. Indeed, several insect serpins act as anti-coagulants, anti-complement proteins and immunosuppressors (Stark and James, 1995, 1998; Colinet et al., 2009; Calvo et al., 2011; Ooi et al., 2015). Serpins are abundant in ticks, and one of their functions is to modulate host immune system. Recent advances in this area have been facilitated by the publication of *I. scapularis* genome (Gulia-Nuss et al., 2016) and several next-generation sequencing transcriptome studies that added tens of unique sequences from different tick species to already existing and long list of tick serpins. In 2009, Mulenga and colleagues found 45 serpins in the genome of *I. scapularis* (Mulenga et al., 2009). Two years earlier, the same group described 17 serpins (Lospins) in *Amblyomma americanum* (Mulenga et al., 2007b). This number was, however, substantially broadened by the combination of several approaches up to approximately 120 serpins (Karim and Ribeiro, 2015; Porter et al., 2015, 2017). In the work of Porter and colleagues (Porter et al., 2015), the authors compare homologous serpins across tick species, showing both conserved and species-specific inhibitors. The conservation seems to be higher in serpins with basic or polar uncharged amino acid residues at P1 site (Porter et al., 2015). Other 32 serpin transcripts from the *Amblyomma* genus were found in *Amblyomma maculatum* (Karim et al., 2011) and 50 in *Amblyomma sculptum* (Moreira et al., 2017). Two groups described 18 and 22 serpins in *R. microplus*, respectively (Tirloni et al., 2014b; Rodriguez-Valle et al., 2015) and at least 36 serpins were found in several published trancriptomes from *I. ricinus* (our own unpublished data based on the analysis of transcriptomes) (Schwarz et al., 2013; Kotsyfakis et al., 2015a,b; Perner et al., 2016). Another recent publication described 10 different serpin transcripts in the sialotranscriptome of the tick *Hyalomma excavatum* (Ribeiro et al., 2017). Despite high number of identified transcripts, only small portion was characterized functionally.

Tick Serpins with Known Function

To date, almost 20 tick serpins from different tick species have been functionally validated by *in vitro* assays, *in vivo* experimental models, vaccination and by RNA interference (RNAi) experiments (**Table 1**). These are detailed below.

AamS6 (A. americanum)

Only two serpins (AamS6 and AAS19) have been characterized thus far in *A. americanum*, despite the overall high number of serpins identified in this tick (Porter et al., 2015). *A. americanum* serpin 6 (AamS6) is upregulated during first 3 days of feeding and is likely to be injected into the host during feeding; however, RNAi did not affect tick feeding ability (Chalaire et al., 2011). Recombinant AamS6 inhibited the serine proteases trypsin, chymotrypsin, elastase, and chymase and the cysteine protease papain in a dose-dependent manner (Chalaire et al., 2011). AamS6 also reduced platelet aggregation and delayed plasma clotting time, suggesting that this serpin facilitates blood feeding by ticks (Mulenga et al., 2013). The complement activation pathway, however, was not affected (Mulenga et al., 2013).

AAS19 (A. americanum)

AAS19 is an anti-coagulant that was shown to inhibit five of the eight serine protease blood clotting factors. AAS19 inhibited thrombin—but not ADP—and cathepsin G-activated platelet aggregation and delayed clotting in re-calcification and thrombin time assays (Kim et al., 2015). AAS19 RNAi halved the blood intake and resulted in morphological deformation of ticks (Kim et al., 2016). In rabbits, immunized with AAS19, tick feeding was faster, but smaller blood volumes were ingested, and tick ability to lay eggs was impaired (Kim et al., 2016).

HLS-1 and 2 (Haemaphysalis longicornis)

Sugino and colleagues isolated a serpin from *H. longicornis* in 2003 (HLS1) (Sugino et al., 2003). Recombinant HLS1 displayed anticoagulant activity, and nymph and adult tick feeding on immunized rabbits resulted in 43.9 and 11.2% tick mortality, respectively. Antibodies raised against tick saliva did not react with recombinant HSL1, suggesting that the serpin was not secreted (Sugino et al., 2003). Moreover, HLS1 expression was detected in the midgut rather than the salivary glands, and HLS1 was therefore considered a concealed antigen, similar to the first commercially used anti-tick vaccine based on the Bm86 tick protein (Willadsen et al., 1995). HLS1 does not contain a signal peptide. Therefore, it is likely that HLS1 is not a secreted protein playing an immunomodulatory or anti-hemostatic role in the host during tick feeding.

A second serpin from *H. longicornis* (HLS2) possesses a signal sequence and seems to be secreted by hemocytes into the haemolymph but not by the salivary glands or midgut (Imamura et al., 2005). HLS2 prolonged the coagulation time in a dose-dependent manner (Imamura et al., 2005), and rabbit vaccination with HLS2 resulted in greater immunization than with HLS1 and almost 50% mortality of feeding nymphs and adults (Imamura et al., 2005). This might be explained by better accessibility and inactivation of extracellular HLS2 in the haemolymph by antibodies from the ingested blood of immunized animals.

Ipis-1 (Ixodes persulcatus)

To date, Ipis-1 is the only characterized salivary serpin from tick *I. persulcatus* (Toyomane et al., 2016). Ipis-1 transcripts were detected only in salivary glands of ticks at same level throughout all phases of feeding. It significantly reduced IFN-γ production and the proliferation of bovine PBMC cells after ConA stimulation. Authors suggest that Ipis-1 could inhibit T cells function by direct interaction with this cell population (Toyomane et al., 2016).

Iris (I. ricinus)

The first tick serpin to be described that had an effect on host defense mechanisms was named Iris (Ixodes ricinus immunosuppressor) (Leboulle et al., 2002a,b). Iris displayed several notable and important features. First, Iris was noted to inhibit T cell and splenocyte proliferation and altered peripheral blood mononuclear cell (PBMC)-derived cytokine levels (Leboulle et al., 2002a). Second, Iris showed anti-hemostatic properties including suppression of coagulation and fibrinolysis (Prevot et al., 2006). Finally, Iris was shown to bind to monocytes/macrophages and suppress the secretion of TNF (Prevot et al., 2009). Interestingly, these activities were independent on the protease inhibitory function of Iris. Of note, Iris, together with HLS1 and several other proteins, belongs to a group of serpins in *Ixodes* spp. that have methionine and cysteine in their reactive center loop (RCL) and lack a signaling peptide, suggesting intracellular rather than extracellular function. However, Iris has been detected in tick saliva using a polyclonal serum raised against recombinant protein (Leboulle et al., 2002a; Prevot et al., 2007), and vaccination of rabbits with recombinant Iris increased the mortality of feeding ticks and lowered weight after engorgement (Prevot et al., 2007). This contradictory observation might be explained by cross-reactivity with another secreted serpin or by the action of another, non-classical secretory mechanism (Nickel, 2003). Nevertheless, Iris represents a pleiotropic protein that affects multiple processes simultaneously via independent mechanisms.

IRS-2 (I. ricinus)

IRS-2 (Ixodes ricinus serpin-2) was the second serpin to be characterized in *I. ricinus*. IRS-2 has tryptophan in its P1 site, confirmed by its resolved crystal structure (Kovarova et al., 2010; Chmelar et al., 2011). IRS-2 displayed inhibitory specificity against mast cell chymase and cathepsin G, two proteases involved in inflammatory responses (Chmelar et al., 2011), with its anti-inflammatory function evidenced by *in vivo* paw edema experiments, in which IRS-2 significantly decreased paw swelling and neutrophil recruitment in treated animals (Chmelar et al., 2011). Moreover, IRS-2 inhibited the production of proinflammatory cytokine IL-6 in dendritic cells (DC) and impaired IL-6-dependent JAK/STAT3 signaling in T-helper (Th) cells, inhibiting the maturation of proinflammatory Th17 lymphocytes (Palenikova et al., 2015). IRS-2 also inhibited

TABLE 1 | Tick serpins with known function.

Serpin	Tick species	Secreted	Effect (where known)	Tissue/stage	Target enzyme	References
AamS6	*A. americanum*	Yes	Reduced platelet aggregation and delayed plasma clotting time	SG, MG, OVA, CA	Plasmin, papain, elastase, chymase	Chalaire et al., 2011; Mulenga et al., 2013
AAS19	*A. americanum*	Yes	Anti-coagulant protein, delayed clotting in recalcification and thrombin time assays		Trypsin, plasmin, fIXa, fXa, fXIa, fXIIa, thrombin, tryptase, chymotrypsin	Kim et al., 2015; Porter et al., 2015
			RNAi led to smaller blood meals and deformed ticks	SG, MG, OVA, SYN, CA, MT		Kim et al., 2016
			Feeding on immunized rabbits led to smaller blood meals and disrupted egg laying			
HLS1	*H. longicornis*	No	Feeding on immunized animals increased tick mortality rate	MG		Sugino et al., 2003
HLS2	*H. longicornis*	No	Prolonged coagulation, Immunization of rabbits increased tick mortality	LY		Imamura et al., 2005
Ipis-1	*I. persulcatus*	Yes	Inhibited proliferation and IFN-γ production of bovine PBMCs	SG		Toyomane et al., 2016
Iris	*I. ricinus*	Yes	Disrupted blood coagulation and fibrinolysis	SG, saliva	Elastase, thrombin, t-PA, fXa, trypsin	Prevot et al., 2006
			Suppressed T cell and splenocyte proliferation			Leboulle et al., 2002a
			Altered cytokine secretion by PBMC			Prevot et al., 2009
			Bound monocytes/macrophages and inhibited TNF secretion			Prevot et al., 2007
			Vaccination resulted in higher mortality and lower engorgement			
IRS-2	*I. ricinus*	Yes	Inflammation inhibitor, bound mast cell protease-4, blocked induced platelet aggregation	SG, OVA, MG	Cathepsin G, chymase, thrombin, trypsin, a-chymotrypsin	Chmelar et al., 2011
			Inhibited Th17 differentiation by reduced production of IL-6 in DC			Palenikova et al., 2015
IxscS-1E1	*I. scapularis*	Yes	Inhibited platelet aggregation and plasma clotting	SG, MG	Thrombin, trypsin, cathepsin G, fXa	Mulenga et al., 2009; Ibelli et al., 2014
RAS-1, 2	*R. appendiculatus*	No	Feeding on immunized animals increased tick mortality rate			Imamura et al., 2006
RAS-3, 4	*R. appendiculatus*	Yes	Feeding on immunized animals increased tick mortality rate and delayed *Theleria* infection			Imamura et al., 2008
RHS-1	*R. haemaphysaloides*	Yes	Anticoagulation activity, RNAi disrupted tick feeding	SG	Chymotrypsin, thrombin, fXa	Yu et al., 2013
RHS-2	*R. haemaphysaloides*	No	RNAi disrupted tick feeding	MG	Chymotrypsin, thrombin, fXa	Yu et al., 2013
RmS-3	*R. microplus*	Yes	Reduced platelet aggregation Feeding of ticks with RMS-3 antibodies impaired reproduction	SG, MG, CA	Chymotrypsin, cathepsin G, elastase, chymase	Tirloni et al., 2014b, 2016; Rodriguez-Valle et al., 2012, 2015
RmS-6	*R. microplus*	Yes		SG, MG, OVA, CA	Trypsin, plasmin, fXa, fXIa, chymotrypsin	Tirloni et al., 2014b, 2016
RmS-15	*R. microplus*	Yes	Delayed plasma clotting	SG, OVA, CA	Thrombin	Tirloni et al., 2014b; Xu et al., 2016
RmS-17	*R. microplus*	Yes	Delayed plasma clotting, reduced platelet aggregation	SG, MG, OVA, CA	Trypsin, plasmin, cythepsin G, chymotrypsin, fXIa	Tirloni et al., 2014b, 2016
rSerpin	*R. microplus*	Yes	Feeding on immunized animals increased feeding time and tick mortality and reduced tick engorgement and egg mass	SG		Kaewhom et al., 2007; Jittapalapong et al., 2010

SG, salivary glands; MG, midgut; OVA, ovaries; FB, fat body; HE, hemocytes; MAL, Malpighian tubules; DC, dendritic cells.

platelet aggregation induced by cathepsin G but not other inducers such as collagen or arachidonic acid derivatives (Chmelar et al., 2011).

IxscS-1E1 (I. scapularis)

A blood meal-induced salivary serpin IxscS-1E1 from *I. scapularis* has been shown to trap thrombin and trypsin in SDS- and heat-stable complexes, reduce their activity and inhibit the activities of cathepsin G and factor Xa, although protease/inhibitor complexes were not detected (Ibelli et al., 2014). Furthermore, IxscS-1E1 inhibited adenosine diphosphate- and thrombin-activated platelet aggregation and delayed plasma clotting time, suggesting an anti-hemostatic role (Ibelli et al., 2014). IxscS-1E1 had no effect on the classical complement activation pathway (Ibelli et al., 2014).

RAS-1, 2, 3, 4 (Rhipicephalus appendiculatus)

Four serpin cDNAs, two putatively secreted (RAS-3 and RAS-4) and two putatively intracellular (RAS-1 and RAS-2), were identified in and isolated from the salivary glands of *R. appendiculatus* (Mulenga et al., 2003). Although RAS-1 and RAS-2 are expressed in the salivary glands, antibodies against them were not found at the bite site as determined by the reactivity of anti-tick saliva sera to recombinant RAS-1 and RAS-2 (Imamura et al., 2006). This finding is, however, consistent with their predicted intracellular location (Imamura et al., 2006). Vaccination of cattle with a RAS-1/RAS-2 cocktail resulted in a 61.4% reduction in nymph engorgement rate and a 28 and 43% increase in mortality rate in female and male adult ticks, respectively (Imamura et al., 2006). Similar results were obtained when cattle were vaccinated with a mixture of two secreted serpins RAS-3 and RAS-4 and a 36-kDa immunodominant cement protein RIM36 (Imamura et al., 2008): immunization resulted in 40% mortality rate for *R. appendiculatus* ticks and almost 50% for *Theileria parva*-infected female ticks (Imamura et al., 2008). However, no significant protective effect against infection with *T. parva* was observed in spite of a 1–2 day delay in the detection of pathogens in the host peripheral blood after immunization (Imamura et al., 2008).

RHS-1 and 2 (Rhipicephalus haemaphysaloides)

Two serpins (RHS-1 and RHS-2) have been identified and characterized from *R. haemaphysaloides* (Yu et al., 2013), both of which were expressed in the salivary glands and midguts of ticks fed for 4 days. Both inhibited chymotrypsin, and RHS-1 also inhibited thrombin (Yu et al., 2013). Consistent with their inhibitory activity, only RHS-1 exhibited anticoagulation activity based on the activated partial thrombin time assay (Yu et al., 2013). Only RHS-1 seems to be secreted into the saliva and the host, as only RHS-1 was detected by serum from rabbits that were exposed to ticks and only RHS-1 possesses a signal peptide sequence (Yu et al., 2013). Nevertheless, RNAi of both serpins negatively affected the attachment rate after 24 h and decreased the engorgement rate (Yu et al., 2013).

RmS-3, 6, 15, 17 (R. microplus)

Serpin RmS-3 from *R. microplus* displayed anti-elastase and anti-chymotrypsin inhibitory activities (Rodriguez-Valle et al., 2015). Tirloni and colleagues subsequently confirmed this specificity (albeit with much lower inhibitory activity), tested more proteases, and found the highest inhibitory activity against chymase and cathepsin G (Tirloni et al., 2016). RmS-3 is likely to be secreted into the saliva and the host as evidenced by differential antibody responses of tick-resistant and tick-susceptible cattle (Rodriguez-Valle et al., 2012). RmS-3 is expressed in nymphs and in the salivary glands of adult ticks, data on RmS-3 transcription in ovaries differ between the two studies (Tirloni et al., 2014b; Rodriguez-Valle et al., 2015). Capillary feeding of ticks with a RmS-3 antibody reduced tick reproductive capacity (Rodriguez-Valle et al., 2012, 2015).

In addition to RmS-3, three other recombinant *R. microplus* serpins were produced for enzymatic and functional characterization (Tirloni et al., 2014a,b; Xu et al., 2016). RmS-6 inhibited factor Xa, factor XIa and plasmin, suggesting an anticoagulant function, while RmS-17 showed weaker inhibitory activity against chymotrypsin, cathepsin G, trypsin, and plasmin (Tirloni et al., 2016). Both RmS-3 and RmS-17 inhibited cathepsin G-induced platelet aggregation. Interestingly, RmS-3, -6, and -17 from *R. microplus* were recognized by antibodies raised by the saliva of *A. americanum*, *I. scapularis*, and *Rhipicephalus sanguineus*, suggesting a potential use for these proteins as an universal tick vaccine (Tirloni et al., 2016) but also highlighting the pitfall of false-positive detection of serpins in tick saliva. RmS-15 was identified as a thrombin inhibitor and, together with RmS-17, delayed plasma clotting in a re-calcification time assay (Tirloni et al., 2016; Xu et al., 2016). Moreover, RmS-15 is an immunogen, as the infestation of cattle with *R. microplus* resulted in increased anti-RmS-15 IgG titers (Xu et al., 2016).

rSerpin (R. microplus)

Rabbits immunized with putatively secreted serpin (rSerpin) from *R. microplus* (Kaewhom et al., 2007) led to extended feeding time, an 83% reduction in adult engorgement, 67% mortality of engorged females and a 34% reduction in egg mass weight (Jittapalapong et al., 2010).

Cystatins

Cystatins form a superfamily of tight-binding reversible inhibitors of papain-like cysteine proteases and legumains and, similar to serpins, they are present in all organisms including prokaryotes (Kordis and Turk, 2009). Cystatins regulate many physiological processes including immunity-related mechanisms such as antigen presentation, phagocytosis, and cytokine expression (Zavasnik-Bergant, 2008). There are four cystatin subgroups: type 1 (stefins), type 2, type 3 (kininogens), and type 4 cystatins (fetuins) (Rawlings and Barrett, 1990). Cystatins' target proteases are usually lysosomal cathepsins involved in protein degradation, but they also target those involved in degradation of antigens presented via MHCII to lymphocytes or in the activation of caspase 1 and thus inflammasome regulation (Jin and Flavell, 2010; Turk et al., 2012).

Cystatins with Known Function

Similarly to serpins, there are around 20 tick cystatins described in the literature and only type 1 and type 2 cystatins have thus far been reported in ticks. While stefins lack a secretory signal and are most likely involved in the intracellular digestion of hemoglobin or in developmental processes, type 2 cystatins are secreted and expressed in both the midgut and salivary glands (Schwarz et al., 2012). Tick cystatins either regulate hemoglobin digestion, which is driven by cathepsins (Horn et al., 2009), or they can be secreted as immunomodulators into the host with saliva. The majority (84%) of tick cystatin transcripts that are conserved across tick species, belong to the extracellular group, suggesting predominantly immunomodulatory role (Ibelli et al., 2013) Tick cystatins with experimentally validated functions are listed in **Table 2** and detailed below.

Bmcystatin (R. microplus)

Bmcystatin from *R. microplus* is specifically expressed in the salivary glands, ovaries, and fat bodies. Bmcystatin did not inhibit papain but inhibited human cathepsin L and tick vitellin-degrading cysteine endopeptidase (VDTCE), suggesting a role in regulating tick embryogenesis (Lima et al., 2006).

BrBmcys2a, b, c, d, e, (R. microplus)

In addition to Bmcystatin, another five cystatins (BrBmcys2a, b, c, d, e) were identified in the cattle tick *R. microplus*. Their expression differs among various developmental stages and tissues, but since their presence has only been assessed by immunodetection methods, cross reactivity between antibodies is possible and has indeed been reported (Imamura et al., 2013). This study also examined the inhibitory specificity of two cystatins: while BrBmcys2b targeted cathepsins B, C, and L, BrBmcys2c only inhibited cathepsins C and L (Parizi et al., 2015). Antibodies raised against recombinant proteins detected BrBmcys2b in all tick tissues, while anti-BrBmcys2c serum only recognized the protein in the gut from partially engorged females and in the ovaries, salivary glands, and fat bodies from fully engorged females (Parizi et al., 2015). The expression patterns suggest rather homeostatic function of these cystatins in ticks than immunomodulatory activity in the host (Imamura et al., 2013).

Cystatin (A. americanum)

One cystatin was detected in the salivary glands and midguts of unfed and partially fed *A. americanum* ticks (Karim et al., 2005). RNAi of this cystatin led to a 90 and 50% reduction in transcript abundance in the early and late phases of feeding, respectively. RNAi knockdown decreased tick body weight, killed ticks during feeding, and disrupted feeding to full engorgement. Rabbits pre-exposed to dsRNA-injected ticks were re-exposed to naïve ticks, which led to detachment of 34% ticks after 1 day and over 50% mortality of attached ticks (Karim et al., 2005). No such effect was observed in the control group, in which rabbits were pre-exposed to normal ticks. Such a strong immune response indicates an important immunomodulatory function for silenced cystatin that impairs responses to salivary antigens and leads to an overall less intense immune reaction (Karim et al., 2005).

HISC-1 (H. longicornis)

HISC-1 is a type 2 cystatin detected in *H. longicornis* (Yamaji et al., 2009b). It is found mainly in the acinar cells of the tick salivary glands and is therefore likely to be secreted into the host. The number of transcripts was found to be approximately 5-fold higher in the salivary glands than in the midgut, with strong upregulation in early phase of blood feeding and with a pattern suggestive of importance in the feeding process. HISC-1 inhibited cathepsins L and papain but not cathepsin B (Yamaji et al., 2009b).

Hlcyst-1, 2 and 3 (H. longicornis)

While Hlcyst-1 is a type 1 intracellular cystatin with specificity against papain and cathepsin L (Zhou et al., 2009), Hlcyst-2 and Hlcyst-3 are secreted type 2 cystatins (Zhou et al., 2006b, 2010). Hlcyst-2 has been shown to inhibit cathepsin L and cathepsin B, with transcripts found mainly in the midgut and hemocytes of all tick developmental stages. Expression increased with tick development and was induced by blood feeding (Zhou et al., 2006b). Moreover, Hlcyst-2 expression was induced by injecting ticks with LPS or *Babesia gibsoni*, suggesting a role in tick immunity. *In vitro* cultivation of *B. gibsoni* in the presence of Hlcyst-2 significantly inhibited pathogen growth (Zhou et al., 2006b). Hlcyst-1 and Hlcyst-2 also inhibited cysteine protease HlCPL-A with hemoglobinase activity, isolated from *H. longicornis*, which can act as natural target of these cystatins, suggesting an involvement of both the protease and its inhibitors in blood digestion (Yamaji et al., 2009a). Hlcyst-3 inhibited papain and cathepsin L, and its expression was detected preferentially in the midgut (Zhou et al., 2010).

JpIocys2 (Ixodes ovatum)

JpIocys2 was isolated from *I. ovatum* and was shown to modulate the enzymatic activity of cathepsins B, C, and L with cathepsin L as the preferred target (Parizi et al., 2015). Similar to BrBmcys2b and BrBmcys2c, JpIocys2 is considered to be involved in tick homeostasis and egg development.

JpIpcys2a, b, c (I. persulcatus)

Three novel cystatins from *I. persulcatus*, JpIpcys2a, b, and c, have recently been described in terms of sequence and structural analysis and expression profile (Rangel et al., 2017). All three possess a signal peptide and two disulfide bridges in their mature form. Although varying in their tertiary structure, all three *I. persulcatus* cystatins should bind human cathepsin L and papain, based on *in silico* analyses. Transcripts of all three cystatins were detected in almost all tissues (salivary glands, midgut, carcass) and stages (larvae, nymphs, adults) of tick development. The only exception was absence of JpIpcys2c transcripts in unfed larvae. Furthermore, vaccination of hamsters with a structurally similar BrBmcys2c cystatin from *R. microplus* did not show any cross-reactivity and did not lead to impaired *I. persulcatus* feeding or reproduction (Rangel et al., 2017).

Om-cystatin 1 and 2 (Ornithodoros moubata)

Om-cystatin 1 and 2 were described in a soft tick *O. moubata* (Grunclova et al., 2006). While Om-cystatin 1 transcripts were found only in the midguts of unfed ticks, Om-cystatin 2 mRNA was present in all tissues. Transcript levels were rapidly suppressed after tick feeding. Both possessed inhibitory activity against cathepsins B, C, and H and papain (Grunclova et al.,

TABLE 2 | Tick cystatins with known function.

Cystatin	Tick species	Secreted	Effect (where known)	Tissue/stage	Target enzyme	References
Bmcystatin	*R. microplus*	No		SG, OVA, FB	Cathepsin L, VDTCE	Lima et al., 2006
BrBmcys2a	*R. microplus*	Yes		MG, OVA, FB		Imamura et al., 2013
BrBmcys2b	*R. microplus*	Yes		MG	Cathepsin B, C, L	Imamura et al., 2013; Parizi et al., 2015
BrBmcys2c	*R. microplus*	Yes		MG	Cathepsin C, L	Imamura et al., 2013; Parizi et al., 2015
BrBmcys2d, e	*R. microplus*	Yes		larvae		Imamura et al., 2013
Cystatin	*A. americanum*	Yes	RNAi caused decreased tick body weight, dying of ticks during feeding or disrupted feeding to the fully engorged state	MG, SG		Karim et al., 2005
HISC-1	*H. longicornis*	Yes		SG	Cathepsin L, papain	Yamaji et al., 2009b
Hlcyst-1	*H. longicornis*	No	Regulated hemoglobin degradation	MG	Cathepsin B, H, L, papain, HICPL-A	Zhou et al., 2006b, 2009; Yamaji et al., 2009a, 2010
Hlcyst-2	*H. longicornis*	Yes	Regulated hemoglobin degradation, inhibited *Babesia* growth *in vitro*	MG, SG, OVA, HE, FB	Cathepsin L, papain, HICPL-A	Zhou et al., 2006b; Yamaji et al., 2009a, 2010
Hlcyst-3	*H. longicornis*	Yes		MG, SG, OVA, HE, FB	Cathepsin L, papain	Zhou et al., 2006b, 2010
Jplocys2	*I. ovatum*	Yes		Assumed MG	Cathepsin B, C, L	Parizi et al., 2015
Jplpcys2a, b, c	*I. persulcatus*	Yes		SG, MG / larvae, nymphs, adult	Cathapsin L, papain	Rangel et al., 2017
Om cystatin 1	*O. moubata*	Yes		MG	Cathepsin B, C, H	Grunclova et al., 2006
Om cystatin 2	*O. moubata*	Yes	Inhibited TNF-α and IL-12 production by DC and proliferation of CD4+ T cells, immunization decreased tick feeding success	SG, OVA, MAL, MG	Cathepsin B, C, H, L, S, papain	Grunclova et al., 2006; Kotsyfakis et al., 2010
RHcyst-1	*R. haemaphysaloides*	No	Inhibitors, RNAi of RHcyst-1 impaired tick attachment rate and decreased hatching rate	Egg, larvae	Cathepsin B, C, H, L, S, papain	Wang et al., 2015b
RHcyst-2	*R. haemaphysaloides*	Yes		Egg, adult MG, SG, OVA, FB	Cathepsin B, C, H, L, S, papain	Wang et al., 2015a
Rmcystatin3	*R. microplus*	Yes		FB, HE	Cathepsin B, L, BmCl1	Lu et al., 2014
Sialostatin L	*I. scapularis*	Yes	Inhibited CTL proliferation, anti-inflammatory effects	SG	Cathepsin C, L, V, X, papain	Valenzuela et al., 2002
			Impaired DC maturation and differentiation and T cells proliferation		Binds cathepsin S	Kotsyfakis et al., 2006
			Prevented experimental asthma, inhibited IL-9 production by Th9 cells and mast cells by targeting IRF-4			Sa-Nunes et al., 2009
			Decreased IFN-β production in DC and DC maturation			Horka et al., 2012; Klein et al., 2015
			Attenuated IFN-β-triggered JAK/STAT signaling pathway in dendritic cells			Lieskovska et al., 2015a
						Lieskovska et al., 2015b
Sialostatin L2	*I. scapularis*	Yes	RNAi caused tick mortality, reduced weight and less eggs	SG, MG	Cathepsin C, L, S, V	Kotsyfakis et al., 2007
			Immunization caused decreased feeding ability of nymphs			Kotsyfakis et al., 2008
			Enhanced establishment of *Borrelia* infection			Kotsyfakis et al., 2010
			Inhibited caspase-1 maturation and diminished IL-1β and IL-18 secretion by macrophages during *Anaplasma phagocytophilum* infection			Chen et al., 2014
			Attenuated IFN-β-triggered JAK/STAT signaling in DC and promotes TBEV replication, decreases MIP-a and IP-10 production by DC			Lieskovska et al., 2015a,b

SG, salivary glands; MG, midgut; OVA, ovaries; FB, fat body; HE, hemocytes; MAL, Malpighian tubules; VDTCE, vitellin-degrading cysteine endopeptidases; DC, dendritic cell; TBEV, tick-borne encephalitis virus.

2006). Om-cystatin 2 was further functionally and structurally characterized under the name OmC2 (Salát et al., 2010). OmC2 inhibited the secretion of pro-inflammatory cytokines TNF and IL-12 by DC after LPS stimulation and reduced antigen-specific $CD4^+$ T cell proliferation induced by DC (Salát et al., 2010). Exposing OmC2 immunized mice to *O. moubata* nymphs reduced feeding ability and increased mortality during nymphal development to the next stage. Interestingly, nymphs mortality was positively correlated with higher titers of anti-OmC2 antibodies in the serum (Salát et al., 2010).

RHcyst-1 and RHcyst-2 (R. haemaphysaloides)

Two cystatins have been described in *R. haemaphysaloides*, RHcyst-1 and RHcyst-2. RHcyst-1 is an intracellular type 1 cystatin that inhibited cathepsins L, B, C, H, and S and papain, with strongest affinity to cathepsin S (Wang et al., 2015b). RHcyst-1 was expressed at all developmental stages but was most abundant in tick eggs, and its expression decreased throughout the development. RNAi of RHcyst-1 reduced the attachment rate of adult ticks and decreased hatching rate (Wang et al., 2015b). RHcyst-2 is a secreted type 2 cystatin that inhibited the same cathepsins as RHcyst-1 (Wang et al., 2015a) and was again present at all developmental stages with highest expression in eggs. However, RHcyst-2 expression increased during blood feeding, and RHcyst-2 was secreted to the host during tick feeding according to immunodetection methods (Wang et al., 2015a).

Rmcystatin3 (R. microplus)

Rmcystatin3 inhibited cathepsins L and B and *Boophilus microplus* cathepsin L-1 (BmCl1) (Lu et al., 2014). Bmcystatin3 transcripts were found in tick hemocytes, fat bodies, and salivary glands, but protein was only detected in hemocytes and the fat bodies by western blotting. Infection of ticks with *E. coli* significantly downregulated Bmcystatin3 expression (Lu et al., 2014) but increased efficacy of pathogen clearance, suggesting that Rmcystatin3 may be a negative regulator of tick immune responses, probably by regulating cysteine proteases responsible for the production of antimicrobial effectors in hemocytes (Lu et al., 2014).

Sialostatin L (I. scapularis)

One of the best studied tick cystatins is sialostatin L, a type 2 cystatin detected in *I. scapularis*. Sialostatin L has preferential specificity for cathepsin L; however, cathepsins V, C, X, S, and papain were also inhibited in enzymatic assays (Kotsyfakis et al., 2006). In the same study, sialostatin L inhibited the proliferation of the cytotoxic T lymphocyte cell line CTLL-2, suggesting its effect on adaptive immunity. Moreover, the anti-inflammatory activity of sialostatin L was confirmed in a mouse model of carrageenan-induced paw edema, in which sialostatin L reduced edema and neutrophil myeloperoxidase activity (Kotsyfakis et al., 2006).

Sialostatin L has been shown to inhibit IL-2 and IL-9 production by Th9 lymphocytes (Horka et al., 2012). IL-9 production by Th cells is IL-2 dependent (Schmitt et al., 1994), but the addition of exogenous IL-2 did not rescue IL-9 synthesis, suggesting that mechanisms other than IL-2 reduction may be involved in IL-9 inhibition (Horka et al., 2012). Nevertheless, the impairment of Th9 cells by sialostatin L abrogated the eosinophilia and airway hyperresponsiveness of mice challenged with OVA antigen (Horka et al., 2012). The inhibition of IL-9 production together with reduced expression of IL-1β and IRF4 (interferon regulating factor 4) was also observed in mast cells, with IL-9 production rescued by the application of exogenous IL-1β (Klein et al., 2015). The inhibition of IL-9 was IRF4 or IL-1β dependent, as proven by the fact that IRF4-deficient or IL-1 receptor-deficient mast cells failed to produce IL-9. The transcription factor IRF4 binds to IL-1β and IL-9 promoters, implying that sialostatin L inhibits IL-9 production via its effect on IRF4 (Klein et al., 2015). Furthermore, mice with IRF4 knockdown in mast cells or mice administered with sialostatin L showed a strong reduction in eosinophilia and airway hyperresponsiveness, important symptoms of asthma. Conversely, sialostatin L did not affect mast cell degranulation or IL-6 expression (Klein et al., 2015).

Sialostatin L inhibits cathepsin S, resulting in reduced antigen-specific $CD4^+$ T cell proliferation *in vitro* and *in vivo*; sialostatin L treatment during OVA immunization impaired early T cell expansion of splenocytes in OT-II mice and late recall immune responses by impairing the proliferation of lymph node cells (Sa-Nunes et al., 2009). Sialostatin L also potently prevented symptoms of experimental autoimmune encephalomyelitis in mice accompanied by impaired IFN-γ and IL-17 production and specific T cell proliferation (Sa-Nunes et al., 2009).

In addition to modulating T cells, sialostatin L inhibited DC maturation and reduced the production of IL-12 and TNF by DC (Sa-Nunes et al., 2009). These effects on DC can also be attributed to anti-cathepsin S activity, as cathepsin S plays a role in an invariant chain processing (Pierre and Mellman, 1998) and its inhibition thus leads to poor antigen presentation by DC (Sa-Nunes et al., 2009). Similar to another *I. scapularis* cystatin Sialostatin L2 (Lieskovska et al., 2015b), sialostatin L attenuated IFN-β-triggered JAK/STAT signaling in DC (Lieskovska et al., 2015a). However, unlike Sialostatin L2, it did not suppress expression of the IP-10 chemokine or IRF-7, suggesting that these two cystatins can produce the same phenotype by impairing different pathways in the same cell (Chmelar et al., 2016). It also decreased IFN-β production in DC activated by either *Borrelia* or TLR-7 ligand (Lieskovska et al., 2015a).

Sialostatin L2 (I. scapularis)

Sialostatin L2 is an *I. scapularis* cystatin similar in sequence to sialostatin L but with different anti-protease potency, antigenicity, and expression pattern. Unlike sialostatin L, sialostatin L2 transcripts accumulate in the salivary glands during tick feeding (Kotsyfakis et al., 2007). Its target proteases are cathepsins L, V, S, and C with preferential affinity for cathepsins L and V (Kotsyfakis et al., 2007). Sialostatin L2 was shown to inhibit inflammasome formation during infection with *A. phagocytophilum* (Chen et al., 2014) via sialostatin L2-driven inhibition of caspase-1 maturation, leading to diminished IL-1β and IL-18 secretion by macrophages after stimulation with *A. phagocytophilum* (Chen et al., 2014). However, the mechanism was not due to direct caspase-1 or cathepsin L inhibition, but was instead dependent on reactive oxygen species (ROS) production by NADPH oxidase that was affected by the Loop2 domain of the cystatin (Chen et al., 2014). As mentioned above, sialostatin L2 interfered with JAK/STAT signaling in DC (Lieskovska et al., 2015b), attenuating STAT phosphorylation upon IFN-β treatment and thus inhibiting the IFN-β stimulated IP-10 and IRF7 chemokine genes (Lieskovska et al., 2015b). No interference with the IFN-β receptor was observed, so the downstream components of the pathway were most likely affected. Moreover, this activity enhanced the replication of tick borne encephalitis virus in DC (Lieskovska et al., 2015b). Sialostatin L2 decreased the production of specific DC chemokines MIP-1α and IP-10 in response to *Borrelia* (Lieskovska et al., 2015a). Upon LTA/TLR2 stimulation of DC, sialostatin L2 attenuated Erk1/2 phosphorylation, inhibited the PI3K pathway by reducing Akt phosphorylation, and also reduced NF-κB phosphorylation. Impaired Erk1/2 phosphorylation was the only effect observed for sialostatin L2 after stimulation of DC with *Borrelia* spirochetes (Lieskovska et al., 2015a).

The role of sialostatin L2 in *Borrelia* transmission and tick feeding has also been addressed. RNAi of sialostatin L2 led to 40% mortality in tick feeding, reduced tick size, and reduced the number of eggs by about 70% (Kotsyfakis et al., 2007). Similar effects were seen when *I. scapularis* nymphs were exposed to guinea pigs immunized with sialostatin L2 (Kotsyfakis et al., 2008). The rejection rate of nymphs fed on immunized animals was three times higher compared to controls, and the time needed to finish a blood meal was prolonged by approximately 1 day (Kotsyfakis et al., 2008). Moreover, IgG isolated from immunized animals reduced sialostatin L2 inhibitory activity against cathepsin L (Kotsyfakis et al., 2008). Of note, sialostatin L2 has been referred to as a "silent antigen," meaning that corresponding antibodies cannot be found in naïve animals exposed to ticks despite an increased titer of specific antibodies in animals pre-immunized with recombinant protein. This can be explained by the amount of sialostatin L2 injected via the saliva into the host being too small to elicit a response (Kotsyfakis et al., 2008). Sialostatin L2 has also been shown to play an important role in *Borrelia* infection (Kotsyfakis et al., 2010). The skin of mice simultaneously injected with *Borrelia* and sialostatin L2 contained six-times more spirochetes than controls. Sialostatin L2 does not appear to bind spirochetes directly and had no effect on *Borrelia* growth *in vitro*, so the mechanism of *Borrelia* growth boost in skin remains unknown (Kotsyfakis et al., 2010).

PROTEASE INHIBITORS AT THE TICK-HOST INTERFACE

Tick cystatins and serpins can obviously affect many intracellular pathways and thus impair the functions of host immune cells. Moreover, they can also interfere with extracellular proteolysis, thereby inhibiting hemostasis (**Figure 1**). These activities take place at the site of attachment, where they cause local immunosuppression and inhibition of blood clotting. Of note, different inhibitors can cause similar phenotypes by targeting different pathways or even different components of the same pathway. Their actions are therefore redundant. Conversely, more than one effect is usually observed for a single inhibitor. Such concept of redundancy and pluripotency is probably a strategy developed by ticks during long-term co-evolution with their hosts (Chmelar et al., 2016). There is no doubt that salivary secretion at the tick-host interface is beneficial for the tick and deleterious for the host. From this perspective, tick inhibitors represent an important and interesting research field for the development of anti-tick vaccines and tick control strategies.

As shown on vaccination experiments, tick serpins and cystatins can contribute to the establishment of pathogens in the host (Imamura et al., 2008; Kotsyfakis et al., 2010). Such role of serpins is in accordance with observed positive effect of activated plasminogen activation system (PAS) with upregulated serpin PAI-2 on the establishment of *Borrelia burgdorferi* infection. The facilitation of infection resulted from direct enhancement of *Borrelia* dissemination and from the inhibition of inflammatory infiltration to the site of exposure (Haile et al., 2006). *Borrelia recurrentis* was shown to bind host serpin—C1 inhibitor—on its surface and thus inhibit complement activation (Grosskinsky et al., 2010). On contrary, mammalian cystatins were shown as regulators of cysteine proteases like cathepsin S and L, which contribute to the establishment of several viral infections (Kopitar-Jerala, 2012). Thus, the involvement of cystatins in the establishment of microbial and viral infection is not clear and cannot be easily addressed without experimental evidence.

TICK PROTEASE INHIBITORS AS NOVEL DRUGS

Cystatins

The inhibition of target proteases with tick-derived inhibitors can, however, be beneficial in different scenarios. Almost all the mammalian serine and cysteine proteases that are targets of tick inhibitors described in this review play important roles in various human diseases and pathologies. For a long time, the functions of lysosomal cysteine cathepsins (B, C, F, H, K, L, O, S, V, X, and W) were thought to be strictly limited to intracellular protein degradation and cellular metabolism. Recently, many cathepsins have been shown to be involved in multiple pathological processes. For example, increased serum levels of cathepsin L are associated with metastatic stage of different cancer types and poor patient prognosis (Tumminello et al., 1996; Chen et al., 2011). Tumor cells can produce high amounts of cathepsin L, leading to high serum level, which is considered as blood marker of cancer (Denhardt et al., 1987). High concentration of cathepsin L in tumor and its vicinity leads to extracellular matrix degradation, higher tumor invasiveness, and several cancer-related health complications (Sudhan and Siemann, 2015). Other cysteine cathepsins may also participate in tumor invasion and metastasis (Kuester et al., 2008; Tan et al., 2013), so cystatins are considered possible effectors that could block the deleterious activity of cysteine cathepsins in cancer (Cox, 2009; Hap et al., 2011). Cysteine cathepsins also contribute to neurodegenerative disorders such as Alzheimer's, Parkinson's, and Huntington's disease and amyotrophic lateral

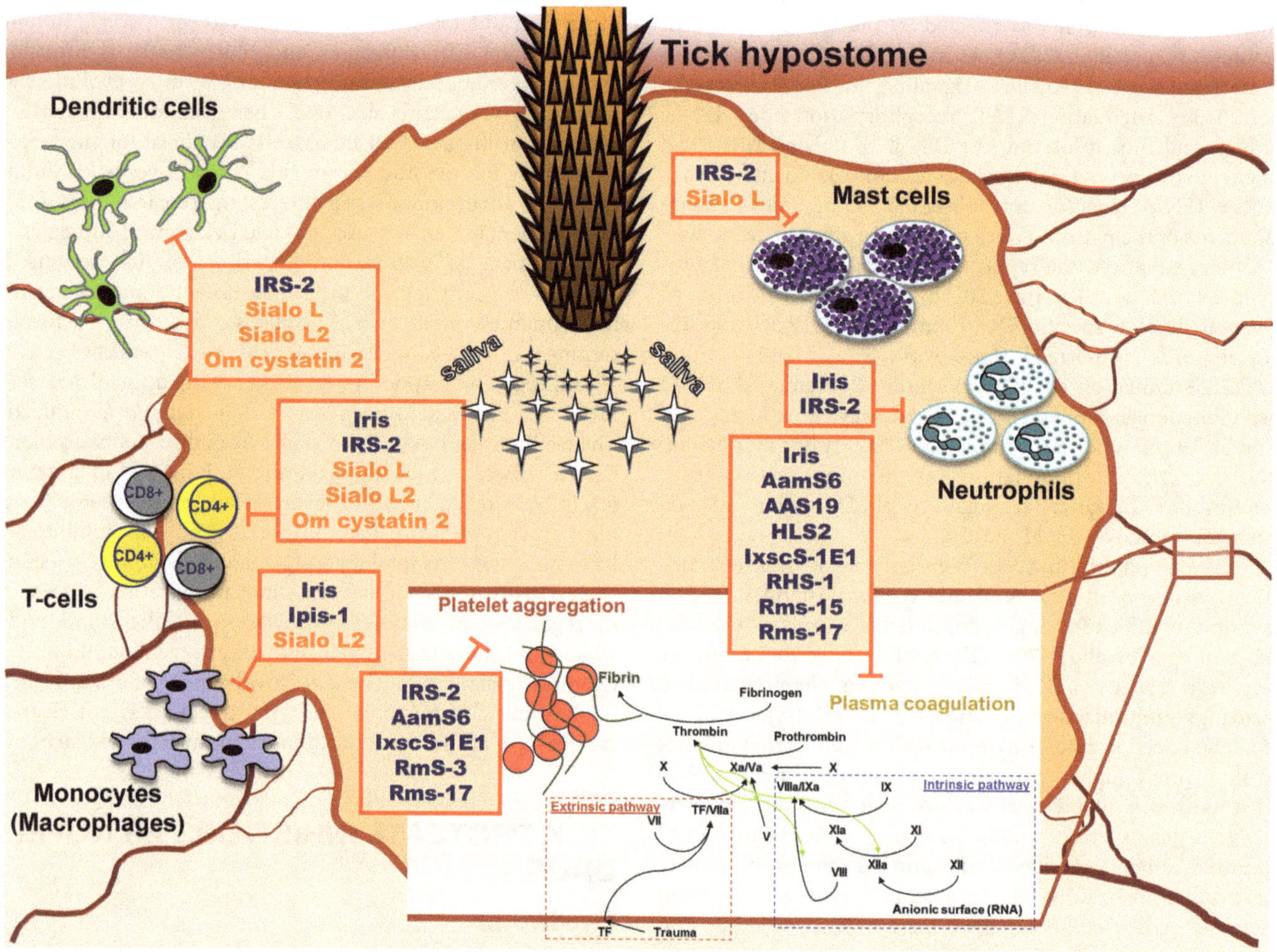

FIGURE 1 | Tick serpins and cystatins and their targets at the site of tick attachment.

sclerosis (**Figure 2A**; Pislar and Kos, 2014). The leakage of lysosomal cathepsins induces neuronal apoptosis and can also increase the inflammatory milieu in the central nervous system (Pislar and Kos, 2014). Cysteine cathepsins are also implicated in the pathogenesis of psoriasis (Kawada et al., 1997), muscular dystrophy (Takeda et al., 1992), abdominal aortic aneurysm and atherosclerosis (Liu et al., 2006), osteoporosis and rheumatoid arthritis (Yasuda et al., 2005), and acute pancreatitis (Halangk et al., 2000). Relatively recent data are accumulating to suggest that cysteine cathepsins are promising therapeutic targets (Kos et al., 2014; Sudhan and Siemann, 2015). The wide spectrum of tick cystatins with varying specificities provides an opportunity to take advantage of this rich source of natural cathepsin inhibitors.

Serpins

Serine proteases are best known as the building blocks of proteolytic cascades in the blood such as coagulation (**Figure 1**) or complement activation. The portfolio of their activities, however, is much wider. Neutrophils, mast cells, natural killer cells, and cytotoxic T cells all produce serine proteases responsible for extracellular matrix remodeling, microbe killing, cytokine activation, signaling via protease-activated receptors (PARs), or chemoattraction of leukocytes. As regulators of many processes, serine proteases often contribute to disease pathologies. Some diseases, in which serine proteases are implicated, are shown in **Figure 2B**. Signaling via PARs and the activation of coagulation in the tumor microenvironment link coagulation proteases with some of the complications seen in cancer (Shi et al., 2004; Han et al., 2011; Lima and Monteiro, 2013). Neutrophil proteases from azurophilic granules, namely cathepsin G, elastase, and protease 3 (PR3), play crucial roles in neutrophil anti-microbial activity and are indispensable for the clearance of some pathogens (Hahn et al., 2011; Steinwede et al., 2012). Many studies have also described neutrophil proteases as important regulators of inflammatory and immune processes (Pham, 2006, 2008), albeit with deleterious effects in some cases. For instance, due to the large amounts of elastin present in the lung connective tissue, lungs are very sensitive to dysregulation and/or increased levels of elastolytic proteases such as neutrophil elastase (Sandhaus and Turino,

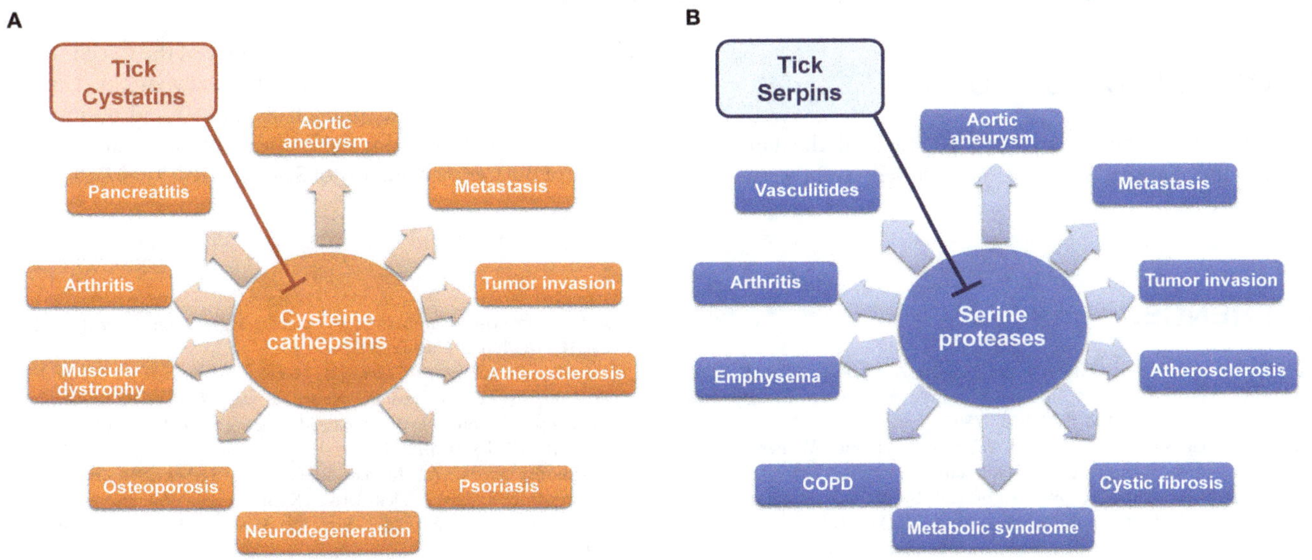

FIGURE 2 | The therapeutic potential of tick cystatins (A) and serpins **(B)** by inhibiting cysteine and serine proteases in various diseases.

2013), which results in several lung diseases. Elastase and cathepsin G facilitate the spreading of metastases to the lungs due to the degradation of antitumorigenic factor thrombospondin-1 (El Rayes et al., 2015). Furthermore, neutrophil proteases have been implicated in the pathogenesis of cystic fibrosis (Twigg et al., 2015; Wagner et al., 2016), chronic obstructive pulmonary disease (COPD) (Shapiro, 2002; Owen, 2008), and emphysema (Ekeowa et al., 2009). In anti-neutrophil cytoplasmic autoantibody (ANCA)-associated vasculitides such as Wegener's granulomatosis, neutrophils are activated by auto-antibodies against PR3 (Niles et al., 1989), leading to the production of neutrophil extracellular traps (NETs) containing PR3 and to necrosis (Kessenbrock et al., 2009). Cathepsin G is chemotactic for monocytes in rheumatoid arthritis (Miyata et al., 2007), and the inhibition of neutrophil elastase improved some of the symptoms of this disease (Di Cesare Mannelli et al., 2016). Interestingly, obesity and metabolic syndrome also seem to be affected by neutrophil proteases (Talukdar et al., 2012; Mansuy-Aubert et al., 2013). Mast cells are another significant source of several serine proteases, mainly chymases and tryptases, which are involved in extracellular matrix remodeling, chemoattraction of neutrophils, and protein processing and activation (Pejler et al., 2010). Mast cell chymase and tryptase have been shown to be involved in the pathogenesis of abdominal aortic aneurysm (Sun et al., 2009; Zhang et al., 2011) and atherosclerosis (Sun et al., 2007; Bot et al., 2015).

Due to these diverse and clinically relevant effects of serine proteases, their potential use as therapeutic targets is being thoroughly discussed by scientific community (Guay et al., 2006; Quinn et al., 2010; Caughey, 2016). Tick salivary glands express a large number of serine protease inhibitors with different specificities that could be used as novel drugs against malfunctioning proteases.

CONCLUDING REMARKS

Novel pharmacoactive compounds are being developed either by artificial synthesis or by isolating potential candidates from various organisms including parasites (Cherniack, 2011). For instance, hirudin (a thrombin inhibitor from leeches) and its congener bivalrudin have been useful in the treatment of blood coagulation disorders (Kennedy et al., 2012). Ticks are parasites that have evolved multiple ways to evade or manipulate host immune and hemostatic systems (Chmelar et al., 2012). Tick saliva contains hundreds of proteins not only with anti-hemostatic features (Maritz-Olivier et al., 2007) but also with anti-complement, anti-inflammatory, and immunomodulatory effects on the host (Kazimirova and Stibraniova, 2013).

As discussed in this review, salivary cystatins and serpins display such features and their functions have been studied thoroughly. Moreover, both superfamilies are represented in the vertebrate host and the functions of their members are often known. Therefore, we can predict at least to some degree, which processes or pathways will be targeted by tick proteins. An important advantage of cystatins and serpins is their functional specificity; for example, sialostatins L and L2 cause similar phenotypes (inhibition of IFN-β signaling) either by inhibiting the IFN-β production (sialostatin L) or by inhibiting STAT3 phosphorylation downstream from IFN-β (sialostatin L2) (Lieskovska et al., 2015a,b). The possibility of targeting specific processes is crucial for the development of "patient-tailored" immunotherapeutic strategies (Scherer et al., 2010; Stephenson et al., 2016). Furthermore, tick cystatins and serpins are not the only families in ticks that deserve attention, since there are many tick-specific proteins secreted into the saliva of unknown function. Characterizing ticks using the transcriptomic approach has created a broad field and data repository, which we can search for novel drugs and potential therapeutics.

AUTHOR CONTRIBUTIONS

JC and JK wrote the manuscript, JK prepared the tables, JC prepared the figures, HL and MK edited and revised the manuscript.

FUNDING

This work was supported by Grant agency of the Czech Republic (grant 16-07117Y to JC), by Grant agency of the University of South Bohemia to JK (grant 038/2016/P) and by intramural institutional support from the Institute of Parasitology, Biology Center of the Czech Academy of Sciences [RVO 60077344] to MK and JK.

REFERENCES

Amara, U., Rittirsch, D., Flierl, M., Bruckner, U., Klos, A., Gebhard, F., et al. (2008). Interaction between the coagulation and complement system. *Adv. Exp. Med. Biol.* 632, 71–79. doi: 10.1007/978-0-387-78952-1_6

Anguita, J., Ramamoorthi, N., Hovius, J. W., Das, S., Thomas, V., Persinski, R., et al. (2002). Salp15, an ixodes scapularis salivary protein, inhibits CD4(+) T cell activation. *Immunity* 16, 849–859. doi: 10.1016/S1074-7613(02)00325-4

Ayllon, N., Villar, M., Galindo, R. C., Kocan, K. M., Sima, R., Lopez, J. A., et al. (2015). Systems biology of tissue-specific response to *Anaplasma phagocytophilum* reveals differentiated apoptosis in the tick vector Ixodes scapularis. *PLoS Genet.* 11:e1005120. doi: 10.1371/journal.pgen.1005120

Bania, J., Stachowiak, D., and Polanowski, A. (1999). Primary structure and properties of the cathepsin G/chymotrypsin inhibitor from the larval hemolymph of *Apis mellifera*. *Eur. J. Biochem.* 262, 680–687. doi: 10.1046/j.1432-1327.1999.00406.x

Belorgey, D., Hagglof, P., Karlsson-Li, S., and Lomas, D. A. (2007). Protein misfolding and the serpinopathies. *Prion* 1, 15–20. doi: 10.4161/pri.1.1.3974

Bot, I., Shi, G. P., and Kovanen, P. T. (2015). Mast cells as effectors in atherosclerosis. *Arterioscler. Thromb. Vasc. Biol.* 35, 265–271. doi: 10.1161/ATVBAHA.114.303570

Brossard, M., and Wikel, S. K. (2004). Tick immunobiology. *Parasitology* 129 (Suppl.), S161–S176. doi: 10.1017/S0031182004004834

Calvo, E., Mizurini, D. M., Sa-Nunes, A., Ribeiro, J. M., Andersen, J. F., Mans, B. J., et al. (2011). Alboserpin, a factor Xa inhibitor from the mosquito vector of yellow fever, binds heparin and membrane phospholipids and exhibits antithrombotic activity. *J. Biol. Chem.* 286, 27998–28010. doi: 10.1074/jbc.M111.247924

Carrell, R. W., and Read, R. J. (2016). How serpins transport hormones and regulate their release. *Semin. Cell Dev. Biol.* 62, 133–141. doi: 10.1016/j.semcdb.2016.12.007

Caughey, G. H. (2016). Mast cell proteases as pharmacological targets. *Eur. J. Pharmacol.* 778, 44–55. doi: 10.1016/j.ejphar.2015.04.045

Chalaire, K. C., Kim, T. K., Garcia-Rodriguez, H., and Mulenga, A. (2011). *Amblyomma americanum* (L.) (Acari: Ixodidae) tick salivary gland serine protease inhibitor (serpin) 6 is secreted into tick saliva during tick feeding. *J. Exp. Biol.* 214, 665–673. doi: 10.1242/jeb.052076

Chen, G., Wang, X., Severo, M. S., Sakhon, O. S., Sohail, M., Brown, L. J., et al. (2014). The tick salivary protein sialostatin L2 inhibits caspase-1-mediated inflammation during *Anaplasma phagocytophilum* infection. *Infect. Immun.* 82, 2553–2564. doi: 10.1128/IAI.01679-14

Chen, Q., Fei, J., Wu, L., Jiang, Z., Wu, Y., Zheng, Y., et al. (2011). Detection of cathepsin B, cathepsin L, cystatin C, urokinase plasminogen activator and urokinase plasminogen activator receptor in the sera of lung cancer patients. *Oncol. Lett.* 2, 693–699. doi: 10.3892/ol.2011.302

Cherniack, E. P. (2011). Bugs as drugs, part two: worms, leeches, scorpions, snails, ticks, centipedes, and spiders. *Altern. Med. Rev.* 16, 50–58.

Chmelar, J., Calvo, E., Pedra, J. H., Francischetti, I. M., and Kotsyfakis, M. (2012). Tick salivary secretion as a source of antihemostatics. *J. Proteomics* 75, 3842–3854. doi: 10.1016/j.jprot.2012.04.026

Chmelar, J., Kotal, J., Kopecky, J., Pedra, J. H., and Kotsyfakis, M. (2016). All for one and one for all on the tick-host battlefield. *Trends Parasitol.* 32, 368–377. doi: 10.1016/j.pt.2016.01.004

Chmelar, J., Oliveira, C. J., Rezacova, P., Francischetti, I. M., Kovarova, Z., Pejler, G., et al. (2011). A tick salivary protein targets cathepsin G and chymase and inhibits host inflammation and platelet aggregation. *Blood* 117, 736–744. doi: 10.1182/blood-2010-06-293241

Colinet, D., Dubuffet, A., Cazes, D., Moreau, S., Drezen, J. M., and Poirie, M. (2009). A serpin from the parasitoid wasp *Leptopilina boulardi* targets the Drosophila phenoloxidase cascade. *Dev. Comp. Immunol.* 33, 681–689. doi: 10.1016/j.dci.2008.11.013

Corral-Rodriguez, M. A., Macedo-Ribeiro, S., Barbosa Pereira, P. J., and Fuentes-Prior, P. (2009). Tick-derived Kunitz-type inhibitors as antihemostatic factors. *Insect Biochem. Mol. Biol.* 39, 579–595. doi: 10.1016/j.ibmb.2009.07.003

Cox, J. L. (2009). Cystatins and cancer. *Front. Biosci. (Landmark Ed)* 14, 463–474. doi: 10.2741/3255

Dai, S. X., Zhang, A. D., and Huang, J. F. (2012). Evolution, expansion and expression of the Kunitz/BPTI gene family associated with long-term blood feeding in Ixodes Scapularis. *BMC Evol. Biol.* 12:4. doi: 10.1186/1471-2148-12-4

Davis, R. L., Shrimpton, A. E., Holohan, P. D., Bradshaw, C., Feiglin, D., Collins, G. H., et al. (1999). Familial dementia caused by polymerization of mutant neuroserpin. *Nature* 401, 376–379. doi: 10.1038/43894

Denhardt, D. T., Greenberg, A. H., Egan, S. E., Hamilton, R. T., and Wright, J. A. (1987). Cysteine proteinase cathepsin L expression correlates closely with the metastatic potential of H-ras-transformed murine fibroblasts. *Oncogene* 2, 55–59.

Di Cesare Mannelli, L., Micheli, L., Cinci, L., Maresca, M., Vergelli, C., Pacini, A., et al. (2016). Effects of the neutrophil elastase inhibitor EL-17 in rat adjuvant-induced arthritis. *Rheumatology (Oxford)* 55, 1285–1294. doi: 10.1093/rheumatology/kew055

Ekeowa, U. I., Gooptu, B., Belorgey, D., Hagglof, P., Karlsson-Li, S., Miranda, E., et al. (2009). alpha1-Antitrypsin deficiency, chronic obstructive pulmonary disease and the serpinopathies. *Clin. Sci.* 116, 837–850. doi: 10.1042/CS20080484

El Rayes, T., Catena, R., Lee, S., Stawowczyk, M., Joshi, N., Fischbach, C., et al. (2015). Lung inflammation promotes metastasis through neutrophil protease-mediated degradation of Tsp-1. *Proc. Natl. Acad. Sci. U.S.A.* 112, 16000–16005. doi: 10.1073/pnas.1507294112

Fogaca, A. C., Almeida, I. C., Eberlin, M. N., Tanaka, A. S., Bulet, P., and Daffre, S. (2006). Ixodidin, a novel antimicrobial peptide from the hemocytes of the cattle tick Boophilus microplus with inhibitory activity against serine proteinases. *Peptides* 27, 667–674. doi: 10.1016/j.peptides.2005.07.013

Frazao, B., Vasconcelos, V., and Antunes, A. (2012). Sea anemone (Cnidaria, Anthozoa, Actiniaria) toxins: an overview. *Mar. Drugs* 10, 1812–1851. doi: 10.3390/md10081812

Grosskinsky, S., Schott, M., Brenner, C., Cutler, S. J., Simon, M. M., and Wallich, R. (2010). Human complement regulators C4b-binding protein and C1 esterase inhibitor interact with a novel outer surface protein of *Borrelia recurrentis*. *PLoS Negl. Trop. Dis.* 4:e698. doi: 10.1371/journal.pntd.0000698

Grunclova, L., Horn, M., Vancova, M., Sojka, D., Franta, Z., Mares, M., et al. (2006). Two secreted cystatins of the soft tick *Ornithodoros moubata*: differential expression pattern and inhibitory specificity. *Biol. Chem.* 387, 1635–1644. doi: 10.1515/BC.2006.204

Guay, C., Laviolette, M., and Tremblay, G. M. (2006). Targeting serine proteases in asthma. *Curr. Top. Med. Chem.* 6, 393–402. doi: 10.2174/156802606776287054

Gulia-Nuss, M., Nuss, A. B., Meyer, J. M., Sonenshine, D. E., Roe, R. M., Waterhouse, R. M., et al. (2016). Genomic insights into the Ixodes scapularis tick vector of Lyme disease. *Nat. Commun.* 7:10507. doi: 10.1038/ncomms10507

Gulley, M. M., Zhang, X., and Michel, K. (2013). The roles of serpins in mosquito immunology and physiology. *J. Insect Physiol.* 59, 138–147. doi: 10.1016/j.jinsphys.2012.08.015

Hahn, I., Klaus, A., Janze, A. K., Steinwede, K., Ding, N., Bohling, J., et al. (2011). Cathepsin G and neutrophil elastase play critical and nonredundant roles in lung-protective immunity against *Streptococcus pneumoniae* in mice. *Infect. Immun.* 79, 4893–4901. doi: 10.1128/IAI.05593-11

Haile, W. B., Coleman, J. L., and Benach, J. L. (2006). Reciprocal upregulation of urokinase plasminogen activator and its inhibitor, PAI-2, by *Borrelia burgdorferi* affects bacterial penetration and host-inflammatory response. *Cell. Microbiol.* 8, 1349–1360. doi: 10.1111/j.1462-5822.2006.00717.x

Halangk, W., Lerch, M. M., Brandt-Nedelev, B., Roth, W., Ruthenbuerger, M., Reinheckel, T., et al. (2000). Role of cathepsin B in intracellular trypsinogen activation and the onset of acute pancreatitis. *J. Clin. Invest.* 106, 773–781. doi: 10.1172/JCI9411

Han, N., Jin, K., He, K., Cao, J., and Teng, L. (2011). Protease-activated receptors in cancer: a systematic review. *Oncol. Lett.* 2, 599–608. doi: 10.3892/ol.2011.291

Hap, A., Kielan, W., Grzebieniak, Z., Siewinski, M., Rudnicki, J., Tarnawa, R., et al. (2011). Control of active B and L cathepsins in tissues of colorectal cancer using cystatins isolated from chicken egg proteins: *in vitro* studies. *Folia Histochem. Cytobiol.* 49, 670–676. doi: 10.5603/FHC.2011.0075

Heit, C., Jackson, B. C., Mcandrews, M., Wright, M. W., Thompson, D. C., Silverman, G. A., et al. (2013). Update of the human and mouse SERPIN gene superfamily. *Hum. Genomics* 7:22. doi: 10.1186/1479-7364-7-22

Horka, H., Staudt, V., Klein, M., Taube, C., Reuter, S., Dehzad, N., et al. (2012). The tick salivary protein sialostatin L inhibits the Th9-derived production of the asthma-promoting cytokine IL-9 and is effective in the prevention of experimental asthma. *J. Immunol.* 188, 2669–2676. doi: 10.4049/jimmunol.1100529

Horn, M., Nussbaumerova, M., Sanda, M., Kovarova, Z., Srba, J., Franta, Z., et al. (2009). Hemoglobin digestion in blood-feeding ticks: mapping a multipeptidase pathway by functional proteomics. *Chem. Biol.* 16, 1053–1063. doi: 10.1016/j.chembiol.2009.09.009

Huntington, J. A., and Li, W. (2009). Structural insights into the multiple functions of protein C inhibitor. *Cell. Mol. Life Sci.* 66, 113–121. doi: 10.1007/s00018-008-8371-0

Ibelli, A. M., Hermance, M. M., Kim, T. K., Gonzalez, C. L., and Mulenga, A. (2013). Bioinformatics and expression analyses of the Ixodes scapularis tick cystatin family. *Exp. Appl. Acarol.* 60, 41–53. doi: 10.1007/s10493-012-9613-2

Ibelli, A. M., Kim, T. K., Hill, C. C., Lewis, L. A., Bakshi, M., Miller, S., et al. (2014). A blood meal-induced Ixodes scapularis tick saliva serpin inhibits trypsin and thrombin, and interferes with platelet aggregation and blood clotting. *Int. J. Parasitol.* 44, 369–379. doi: 10.1016/j.ijpara.2014.01.010

Imamura, S., Da Silva Vaz Junior, I., Sugino, M., Ohashi, K., and Onuma, M. (2005). A serine protease inhibitor (serpin) from *Haemaphysalis longicornis* as an anti-tick vaccine. *Vaccine* 23, 1301–1311. doi: 10.1016/j.vaccine.2004.08.041

Imamura, S., Konnai, S., Vaz Ida, S., Yamada, S., Nakajima, C., Ito, Y., et al. (2008). Effects of anti-tick cocktail vaccine against *Rhipicephalus appendiculatus*. *Jpn. J. Vet. Res.* 56, 85–98. doi: 10.14943/jjvr.56.2.85

Imamura, S., Konnai, S., Yamada, S., Parizi, L. F., Githaka, N., Vaz Ida, S. Jr., et al. (2013). Identification and partial characterization of a gut *Rhipicephalus appendiculatus* cystatin. *Ticks Tick Borne Dis.* 4, 138–144. doi: 10.1016/j.ttbdis.2012.11.001

Imamura, S., Namangala, B., Tajima, T., Tembo, M. E., Yasuda, J., Ohashi, K., et al. (2006). Two serine protease inhibitors (serpins) that induce a bovine protective immune response against *Rhipicephalus appendiculatus* ticks. *Vaccine* 24, 2230–2237. doi: 10.1016/j.vaccine.2005.10.055

Jin, C., and Flavell, R. A. (2010). Molecular mechanism of NLRP3 inflammasome activation. *J. Clin. Immunol.* 30, 628–631. doi: 10.1007/s10875-010-9440-3

Jittapalapong, S., Kaewhom, P., Pumhom, P., Canales, M., De La Fuente, J., and Stich, R. W. (2010). Immunization of rabbits with recombinant serine protease inhibitor reduces the performance of adult female *Rhipicephalus microplus*. *Transbound. Emerg. Dis.* 57, 103–106. doi: 10.1111/j.1865-1682.2010.01108.x

Kaewhom, P., Sirinarumitr, T., Chantakru, S., and Jittapalapong, S. (2007). Cloning and characterization of cDNA encoding a serine protease inhibitor from salivary glands of thai cattle tick (*Boophilus microplus*). *Kasetsart J. (Nat. Sci.)* 41, 74–80.

Kanost, M. R. (1999). Serine proteinase inhibitors in arthropod immunity. *Dev. Comp. Immunol.* 23, 291–301. doi: 10.1016/S0145-305X(99)00012-9

Karim, S., Miller, N. J., Valenzuela, J., Sauer, J. R., and Mather, T. N. (2005). RNAi-mediated gene silencing to assess the role of synaptobrevin and cystatin in tick blood feeding. *Biochem. Biophys. Res. Commun.* 334, 1336–1342. doi: 10.1016/j.bbrc.2005.07.036

Karim, S., and Ribeiro, J. M. (2015). An Insight into the Sialome of the Lone Star Tick, *Amblyomma americanum*, with a Glimpse on its time dependent gene expression. *PLoS ONE* 10:e0131292. doi: 10.1371/journal.pone.0131292

Karim, S., Singh, P., and Ribeiro, J. M. (2011). A deep insight into the sialotranscriptome of the gulf coast tick, *Amblyomma maculatum*. *PLoS ONE* 6:e28525. doi: 10.1371/journal.pone.0028525

Kawada, A., Hara, K., Kominami, E., Hiruma, M., Noguchi, H., and Ishibashi, A. (1997). Processing of cathepsins L, B and D in psoriatic epidermis. *Arch. Dermatol. Res.* 289, 87–93. doi: 10.1007/s004030050160

Kazimirova, M., and Stibraniova, I. (2013). Tick salivary compounds: their role in modulation of host defences and pathogen transmission. *Front. Cell. Infect. Microbiol.* 3:43. doi: 10.3389/fcimb.2013.00043

Kennedy, B., Gargoum, F. S., Kennedy, L., Khan, F., Curran, D. R., and O'connor, T. M. (2012). Emerging anticoagulants. *Curr. Med. Chem.* 19, 3388–3416. doi: 10.2174/092986712801215847

Kessenbrock, K., Krumbholz, M., Schonermarck, U., Back, W., Gross, W. L., Werb, Z., et al. (2009). Netting neutrophils in autoimmune small-vessel vasculitis. *Nat. Med.* 15, 623–625. doi: 10.1038/nm.1959

Kim, H. S., Krege, J. H., Kluckman, K. D., Hagaman, J. R., Hodgin, J. B., Best, C. F., et al. (1995). Genetic control of blood pressure and the angiotensinogen locus. *Proc. Natl. Acad. Sci. U.S.A.* 92, 2735–2739. doi: 10.1073/pnas.92.7.2735

Kim, T. K., Radulovic, Z., and Mulenga, A. (2016). Target validation of highly conserved *Amblyomma americanum* tick saliva serine protease inhibitor 19. *Ticks Tick Borne Dis.* 7, 405–414. doi: 10.1016/j.ttbdis.2015.12.017

Kim, T. K., Tirloni, L., Radulovic, Z., Lewis, L., Bakshi, M., Hill, C., et al. (2015). Conserved *Amblyomma americanum* tick Serpin19, an inhibitor of blood clotting factors Xa and XIa, trypsin and plasmin, has anti-haemostatic functions. *Int. J. Parasitol.* 45, 613–627. doi: 10.1016/j.ijpara.2015.03.009

Klein, M., Bruhl, T. J., Staudt, V., Reuter, S., Grebe, N., Gerlitzki, B., et al. (2015). Tick salivary sialostatin L represses the initiation of immune responses by targeting IRF4-dependent transcription in murine mast cells. *J. Immunol.* 195, 621–631. doi: 10.4049/jimmunol.1401823

Kopitar-Jerala, N. (2012). The role of cysteine proteinases and their inhibitors in the host-pathogen cross talk. *Curr. Protein Pept. Sci.* 13, 767–775. doi: 10.2174/138920312804871102

Kordis, D., and Turk, V. (2009). Phylogenomic analysis of the cystatin superfamily in eukaryotes and prokaryotes. *BMC Evol. Biol.* 9:266. doi: 10.1186/1471-2148-9-266

Kos, J., Mitrovic, A., and Mirkovic, B. (2014). The current stage of cathepsin B inhibitors as potential anticancer agents. *Future Med. Chem.* 6, 1355–1371. doi: 10.4155/fmc.14.73

Kotsyfakis, M., Anderson, J. M., Andersen, J. F., Calvo, E., Francischetti, I. M., Mather, T. N., et al. (2008). Cutting edge: immunity against a "silent" salivary antigen of the Lyme vector Ixodes scapularis impairs its ability to feed. *J. Immunol.* 181, 5209–5212. doi: 10.4049/jimmunol.181.8.5209

Kotsyfakis, M., Horka, H., Salat, J., and Andersen, J. F. (2010). The crystal structures of two salivary cystatins from the tick *Ixodes scapularis* and the effect of these inhibitors on the establishment of Borrelia burgdorferi infection in a murine model. *Mol. Microbiol.* 77, 456–470. doi: 10.1111/j.1365-2958.2010.07220.x

Kotsyfakis, M., Karim, S., Andersen, J. F., Mather, T. N., and Ribeiro, J. M. (2007). Selective cysteine protease inhibition contributes to blood-feeding success of the tick *Ixodes scapularis*. *J. Biol. Chem.* 282, 29256–29263. doi: 10.1074/jbc.M703143200

Kotsyfakis, M., Kopacek, P., Franta, Z., Pedra, J. H., and Ribeiro, J. M. (2015a). Deep Sequencing Analysis of the Ixodes ricinus Haemocytome. *PLoS Negl. Trop. Dis.* 9:e0003754. doi: 10.1371/journal.pntd.0003754

Kotsyfakis, M., Sa-Nunes, A., Francischetti, I. M., Mather, T. N., Andersen, J. F., and Ribeiro, J. M. (2006). Antiinflammatory and immunosuppressive activity of sialostatin L, a salivary cystatin from the tick Ixodes scapularis. *J. Biol. Chem.* 281, 26298–26307. doi: 10.1074/jbc.M513010200

Kotsyfakis, M., Schwarz, A., Erhart, J., and Ribeiro, J. M. (2015b). Tissue- and time-dependent transcription in Ixodes ricinus salivary glands and midguts when blood feeding on the vertebrate host. *Sci. Rep.* 5:9103. doi: 10.1038/srep09103

Kovarova, Z., Chmelar, J., Sanda, M., Brynda, J., Mares, M., and Rezacova, P. (2010). Crystallization and diffraction analysis of the serpin IRS-2 from the hard tick Ixodes ricinus. *Acta Crystallogr. Sect. F Struct. Biol. Cryst. Commun.* 66, 1453–1457. doi: 10.1107/S1744309110032343

Kuester, D., Lippert, H., Roessner, A., and Krueger, S. (2008). The cathepsin family and their role in colorectal cancer. *Pathol. Res. Pract.* 204, 491–500. doi: 10.1016/j.prp.2008.04.010

Law, R. H., Zhang, Q., Mcgowan, S., Buckle, A. M., Silverman, G. A., Wong, W., et al. (2006). An overview of the serpin superfamily. *Genome Biol.* 7:216. doi: 10.1186/gb-2006-7-5-216

Leboulle, G., Crippa, M., Decrem, Y., Mejri, N., Brossard, M., Bollen, A., et al. (2002a). Characterization of a novel salivary immunosuppressive protein from Ixodes ricinus ticks. *J. Biol. Chem.* 277, 10083–10089. doi: 10.1074/jbc.M111391200

Leboulle, G., Rochez, C., Louahed, J., Ruti, B., Brossard, M., Bollen, A., et al. (2002b). Isolation of Ixodes ricinus salivary gland mRNA encoding factors induced during blood feeding. *Am. J. Trop. Med. Hyg.* 66, 225–233. doi: 10.4269/ajtmh.2002.66.225

Li, J., Zhang, C., Xu, X., Wang, J., Yu, H., Lai, R., et al. (2007). Trypsin inhibitory loop is an excellent lead structure to design serine protease inhibitors and antimicrobial peptides. *FASEB J.* 21, 2466–2473. doi: 10.1096/fj.06-7966com

Lieskovska, J., Palenikova, J., Langhansova, H., Campos Chagas, A., Calvo, E., Kotsyfakis, M., et al. (2015a). Tick sialostatins L and L2 differentially influence dendritic cell responses to Borrelia spirochetes. *Parasit. Vectors* 8:275. doi: 10.1186/s13071-015-0887-1

Lieskovska, J., Palenikova, J., Sirmarova, J., Elsterova, J., Kotsyfakis, M., Campos Chagas, A., et al. (2015b). Tick salivary cystatin sialostatin L2 suppresses IFN responses in mouse dendritic cells. *Parasite Immunol.* 37, 70–78. doi: 10.1111/pim.12162

Lima, C. A., Sasaki, S. D., and Tanaka, A. S. (2006). Bmcystatin, a cysteine proteinase inhibitor characterized from the tick *Boophilus microplus*. *Biochem. Biophys. Res. Commun.* 347, 44–50. doi: 10.1016/j.bbrc.2006.06.018

Lima, L. G., and Monteiro, R. Q. (2013). Activation of blood coagulation in cancer: implications for tumour progression. *Biosci. Rep.* 33:pii: e00064. doi: 10.1042/BSR20130057

Liu, J., Sukhova, G. K., Yang, J. T., Sun, J., Ma, L., Ren, A., et al. (2006). Cathepsin L expression and regulation in human abdominal aortic aneurysm, atherosclerosis, and vascular cells. *Atherosclerosis* 184, 302–311. doi: 10.1016/j.atherosclerosis.2005.05.012

Liu, X. Y., De La Fuente, J., Cote, M., Galindo, R. C., Moutailler, S., Vayssier-Taussat, M., et al. (2014). IrSPI, a tick serine protease inhibitor involved in tick feeding and Bartonella henselae infection. *PLoS Negl. Trop. Dis.* 8:e2993. doi: 10.1371/journal.pntd.0002993

Lomas, D. A., Hurst, J. R., and Gooptu, B. (2016). Update on alpha-1 antitrypsin deficiency: new therapies. *J. Hepatol.* 65, 413–424. doi: 10.1016/j.jhep.2016.03.010

Lu, H., Cassis, L. A., Kooi, C. W., and Daugherty, A. (2016). Structure and functions of angiotensinogen. *Hypertens. Res.* 39, 492–500. doi: 10.1038/hr.2016.17

Lu, S., Soares, T. S., Vaz Junior, I. S., Lovato, D. V., and Tanaka, A. S. (2014). Rmcystatin3, a cysteine protease inhibitor from Rhipicephalus microplus hemocytes involved in immune response. *Biochimie* 106, 17–23. doi: 10.1016/j.biochi.2014.07.012

Mansuy-Aubert, V., Zhou, Q. L., Xie, X., Gong, Z., Huang, J. Y., Khan, A. R., et al. (2013). Imbalance between neutrophil elastase and its inhibitor alpha1-antitrypsin in obesity alters insulin sensitivity, inflammation, and energy expenditure. *Cell Metab.* 17, 534–548. doi: 10.1016/j.cmet.2013.03.005

Maritz-Olivier, C., Stutzer, C., Jongejan, F., Neitz, A. W., and Gaspar, A. R. (2007). Tick anti-hemostatics: targets for future vaccines and therapeutics. *Trends Parasitol.* 23, 397–407. doi: 10.1016/j.pt.2007.07.005

Meekins, D. A., Kanost, M. R., and Michel, K. (2017). Serpins in arthropod biology. *Semin. Cell Dev. Biol.* 62, 105–119. doi: 10.1016/j.semcdb.2016.09.001

Miyata, J., Tani, K., Sato, K., Otsuka, S., Urata, T., Lkhagvaa, B., et al. (2007). Cathepsin G: the significance in rheumatoid arthritis as a monocyte chemoattractant. *Rheumatol Int.* 27, 375–382. doi: 10.1007/s00296-006-0210-8

Moreira, H. N., Barcelos, R. M., Vidigal, P. M., Klein, R. C., Montandon, C. E., Maciel, T. E., et al. (2017). A deep insight into the whole transcriptome of midguts, ovaries and salivary glands of the *Amblyomma sculptum* tick. *Parasitol. Int.* 66, 64–73. doi: 10.1016/j.parint.2016.10.011

Mulenga, A., Blandon, M., and Khumthong, R. (2007a). The molecular basis of the *Amblyomma americanum* tick attachment phase. *Exp. Appl. Acarol.* 41, 267–287. doi: 10.1007/s10493-007-9064-3

Mulenga, A., Khumthong, R., and Blandon, M. A. (2007b). Molecular and expression analysis of a family of the *Amblyomma americanum* tick Lospins. *J. Exp. Biol.* 210, 3188–3198. doi: 10.1242/jeb.006494

Mulenga, A., Khumthong, R., and Chalaire, K. C. (2009). Ixodes scapularis tick serine proteinase inhibitor (serpin) gene family; annotation and transcriptional analysis. *BMC Genomics* 10:217. doi: 10.1186/1471-2164-10-217

Mulenga, A., Khumthong, R., Chalaire, K. C., Strey, O., and Teel, P. (2008). Molecular and biological characterization of the *Amblyomma americanum* organic anion transporter polypeptide. *J. Exp. Biol.* 211, 3401–3408. doi: 10.1242/jeb.022376

Mulenga, A., Kim, T., and Ibelli, A. M. (2013). *Amblyomma americanum* tick saliva serine protease inhibitor 6 is a cross-class inhibitor of serine proteases and papain-like cysteine proteases that delays plasma clotting and inhibits platelet aggregation. *Insect. Mol. Biol.* 22, 306–319. doi: 10.1111/imb.12024

Mulenga, A., Tsuda, A., Onuma, M., and Sugimoto, C. (2003). Four serine proteinase inhibitors (serpin) from the brown ear tick, Rhiphicephalus appendiculatus; cDNA cloning and preliminary characterization. *Insect Biochem. Mol. Biol.* 33, 267–276. doi: 10.1016/S0965-1748(02)00240-0

Muller, S., Dennemarker, J., and Reinheckel, T. (2012). Specific functions of lysosomal proteases in endocytic and autophagic pathways. *Biochim. Biophys. Acta* 1824, 34–43. doi: 10.1016/j.bbapap.2011.07.003

Nickel, W. (2003). The mystery of nonclassical protein secretion. A current view on cargo proteins and potential export routes. *Eur. J. Biochem.* 270, 2109–2119. doi: 10.1046/j.1432-1033.2003.03577.x

Niles, J. L., Mccluskey, R. T., Ahmad, M. F., and Arnaout, M. A. (1989). Wegener's granulomatosis autoantigen is a novel neutrophil serine proteinase. *Blood* 74, 1888–1893.

Ooi, C. P., Haines, L. R., Southern, D. M., Lehane, M. J., and Acosta-Serrano, A. (2015). Tsetse GmmSRPN10 has anti-complement activity and is important for successful establishment of trypanosome infections in the fly midgut. *PLoS Negl. Trop. Dis.* 9:e3448. doi: 10.1371/journal.pntd.0003448

Owen, C. A. (2008). Roles for proteinases in the pathogenesis of chronic obstructive pulmonary disease. *Int. J. Chron. Obstruct. Pulmon. Dis.* 3, 253–268. doi: 10.2147/COPD.S2089

Pal, U., Li, X., Wang, T., Montgomery, R. R., Ramamoorthi, N., Desilva, A. M., et al. (2004). TROSPA, an Ixodes scapularis receptor for *Borrelia burgdorferi*. *Cell* 119, 457–468. doi: 10.1016/j.cell.2004.10.027

Palenikova, J., Lieskovska, J., Langhansova, H., Kotsyfakis, M., Chmelar, J., and Kopecky, J. (2015). Ixodes ricinus salivary serpin IRS-2 affects Th17 differentiation via inhibition of the interleukin-6/STAT-3 signaling pathway. *Infect. Immun.* 83, 1949–1956. doi: 10.1128/IAI.03065-14

Parizi, L. F., Sabadin, G. A., Alzugaray, M. F., Seixas, A., Logullo, C., Konnai, S., et al. (2015). *Rhipicephalus microplus* and *Ixodes ovatus* cystatins in tick blood digestion and evasion of host immune response. *Parasit. Vectors* 8:122. doi: 10.1186/s13071-015-0743-3

Pejler, G., Ronnberg, E., Waern, I., and Wernersson, S. (2010). Mast cell proteases: multifaceted regulators of inflammatory disease. *Blood* 115, 4981–4990. doi: 10.1182/blood-2010-01-257287

Perner, J., Provaznik, J., Schrenkova, J., Urbanova, V., Ribeiro, J. M., and Kopacek, P. (2016). RNA-seq analyses of the midgut from blood- and serum-fed Ixodes ricinus ticks. *Sci. Rep.* 6:36695. doi: 10.1038/srep36695

Pham, C. T. (2006). Neutrophil serine proteases: specific regulators of inflammation. *Nat. Rev. Immunol.* 6, 541–550. doi: 10.1038/nri1841

Pham, C. T. (2008). Neutrophil serine proteases fine-tune the inflammatory response. *Int. J. Biochem. Cell Biol.* 40, 1317–1333. doi: 10.1016/j.biocel.2007.11.008

Pierre, P., and Mellman, I. (1998). Developmental regulation of invariant chain proteolysis controls MHC class II trafficking in mouse dendritic cells. *Cell* 93, 1135–1145. doi: 10.1016/S0092-8674(00)81458-0

Pislar, A., and Kos, J. (2014). Cysteine cathepsins in neurological disorders. *Mol. Neurobiol.* 49, 1017–1030. doi: 10.1007/s12035-013-8576-6

Porter, L. M., Radulovic, Z. M., and Mulenga, A. (2017). A repertoire of protease inhibitor families in *Amblyomma americanum* and other tick species: inter-species comparative analyses. *Parasit. Vectors* 10:152. doi: 10.1186/s13071-017-2080-1

Porter, L., Radulovic, Z., Kim, T., Braz, G. R., Da Silva Vaz, I. Jr., and Mulenga, A. (2015). Bioinformatic analyses of male and female *Amblyomma americanum* tick expressed serine protease inhibitors (serpins). *Ticks Tick Borne Dis.* 6, 16–30. doi: 10.1016/j.ttbdis.2014.08.002

Prevot, P. P., Adam, B., Boudjeltia, K. Z., Brossard, M., Lins, L., Cauchie, P., et al. (2006). Anti-hemostatic effects of a serpin from the saliva of the tick Ixodes ricinus. *J. Biol. Chem.* 281, 26361–26369. doi: 10.1074/jbc.M604197200

Prevot, P. P., Beschin, A., Lins, L., Beaufays, J., Grosjean, A., Bruys, L., et al. (2009). Exosites mediate the anti-inflammatory effects of a multifunctional serpin from the saliva of the tick *Ixodes ricinus*. *FEBS J.* 276, 3235–3246. doi: 10.1111/j.1742-4658.2009.07038.x

Prevot, P. P., Couvreur, B., Denis, V., Brossard, M., Vanhamme, L., and Godfroid, E. (2007). Protective immunity against Ixodes ricinus induced by a salivary serpin. *Vaccine* 25, 3284–3292. doi: 10.1016/j.vaccine.2007.01.008

Quinn, D. J., Weldon, S., and Taggart, C. C. (2010). Antiproteases as therapeutics to target inflammation in cystic fibrosis. *Open Respir. Med. J.* 4, 20–31. doi: 10.2174/1874306401004010020

Rangel, C. K., Parizi, L. F., Sabadin, G. A., Costa, E. P., Romeiro, N. C., Isezaki, M., et al. (2017). Molecular and structural characterization of novel cystatins from the taiga tick Ixodes persulcatus. *Ticks Tick Borne Dis.* 8, 432–441. doi: 10.1016/j.ttbdis.2017.01.007

Rawlings, N. D., and Barrett, A. J. (1990). Evolution of proteins of the cystatin superfamily. *J. Mol. Evol.* 30, 60–71. doi: 10.1007/BF02102453

Rawlings, N. D., and Salvesen, G. (2013). *Handbook of Proteolytic Enzymes, 3rd Edn.* London; Boston: Academic Press.

Ribeiro, J. M., Slovak, M., and Francischetti, I. M. (2017). An insight into the sialome of *Hyalomma excavatum*. *Ticks Tick Borne Dis.* 8, 201–207. doi: 10.1016/j.ttbdis.2016.08.011

Rimphanitchayakit, V., and Tassanakajon, A. (2010). Structure and function of invertebrate Kazal-type serine proteinase inhibitors. *Dev. Comp. Immunol.* 34, 377–386. doi: 10.1016/j.dci.2009.12.004

Rodriguez-Valle, M., Vance, M., Moolhuijzen, P. M., Tao, X., and Lew-Tabor, A. E. (2012). Differential recognition by tick-resistant cattle of the recombinantly expressed Rhipicephalus microplus serine protease inhibitor-3 (RMS-3). *Ticks Tick Borne Dis.* 3, 159–169. doi: 10.1016/j.ttbdis.2012.03.002

Rodriguez-Valle, M., Xu, T., Kurscheid, S., and Lew-Tabor, A. E. (2015). *Rhipicephalus microplus* serine protease inhibitor family: annotation, expression and functional characterisation assessment. *Parasit. Vectors* 8:7. doi: 10.1186/s13071-014-0605-4

Salát, J., Paesen, G. C., Rezácová, P., Kotsyfakis, M., Kovárová, Z., Sanda, M., et al. (2010). Crystal structure and functional characterization of an immunomodulatory salivary cystatin from the soft tick Ornithodoros moubata. *Biochem. J.* 429, 103–112. doi: 10.1042/BJ20100280

Sandhaus, R. A., and Turino, G. (2013). Neutrophil elastase-mediated lung disease. *COPD* 10 (Suppl. 1), 60–63. doi: 10.3109/15412555.2013.764403

Sa-Nunes, A., Bafica, A., Antonelli, L. R., Choi, E. Y., Francischetti, I. M., Andersen, J. F., et al. (2009). The immunomodulatory action of sialostatin L on dendritic cells reveals its potential to interfere with autoimmunity. *J. Immunol.* 182, 7422–7429. doi: 10.4049/jimmunol.0900075

Sasaki, S. D., De Lima, C. A., Lovato, D. V., Juliano, M. A., Torquato, R. J., and Tanaka, A. S. (2008). BmSI-7, a novel subtilisin inhibitor from *Boophilus microplus*, with activity toward Pr1 proteases from the fungus *Metarhizium anisopliae*. *Exp. Parasitol.* 118, 214–220. doi: 10.1016/j.exppara.2007.08.003

Scherer, H. U., Dorner, T., and Burmester, G. R. (2010). Patient-tailored therapy in rheumatoid arthritis: an editorial review. *Curr. Opin. Rheumatol.* 22, 237–245. doi: 10.1097/BOR.0b013e328337b832

Schmitt, E., Germann, T., Goedert, S., Hoehn, P., Huels, C., Koelsch, S., et al. (1994). IL-9 production of naive CD4+ T cells depends on IL-2, is synergistically enhanced by a combination of TGF-beta and IL-4, and is inhibited by IFN-gamma. *J. Immunol.* 153, 3989–3996.

Schwarz, A., Cabezas-Cruz, A., Kopecky, J., and Valdes, J. J. (2014). Understanding the evolutionary structural variability and target specificity of tick salivary Kunitz peptides using next generation transcriptome data. *BMC Evol. Biol.* 14:4. doi: 10.1186/1471-2148-14-4

Schwarz, A., Valdes, J. J., and Kotsyfakis, M. (2012). The role of cystatins in tick physiology and blood feeding. *Ticks Tick Borne Dis.* 3, 117–127. doi: 10.1016/j.ttbdis.2012.03.004

Schwarz, A., Von Reumont, B. M., Erhart, J., Chagas, A. C., Ribeiro, J. M., and Kotsyfakis, M. (2013). *De novo* Ixodes ricinus salivary gland transcriptome analysis using two next-generation sequencing methodologies. *FASEB J.* 27, 4745–4756. doi: 10.1096/fj.13-232140

Shapiro, S. D. (2002). Proteinases in chronic obstructive pulmonary disease. *Biochem. Soc. Trans.* 30, 98–102. doi: 10.1042/bst0300098

Shi, X., Gangadharan, B., Brass, L. F., Ruf, W., and Mueller, B. M. (2004). Protease-activated receptors (PAR1 and PAR2) contribute to tumor cell motility and metastasis. *Mol. Cancer Res.* 2, 395–402. Available online at: http://mcr.aacrjournals.org/content/2/7/395.article-info

Silverman, G. A., Whisstock, J. C., Bottomley, S. P., Huntington, J. A., Kaiserman, D., Luke, C. J., et al. (2010). Serpins flex their muscle: I. Putting the clamps on proteolysis in diverse biological systems. *J. Biol. Chem.* 285, 24299–24305. doi: 10.1074/jbc.R110.112771

Stark, K. R., and James, A. A. (1995). A factor Xa-directed anticoagulant from the salivary glands of the yellow fever mosquito *Aedes aegypti*. *Exp. Parasitol.* 81, 321–331. doi: 10.1006/expr.1995.1123

Stark, K. R., and James, A. A. (1998). Isolation and characterization of the gene encoding a novel factor Xa-directed anticoagulant from the yellow fever mosquito, *Aedes aegypti*. *J. Biol. Chem.* 273, 20802–20809. doi: 10.1074/jbc.273.33.20802

Steinwede, K., Maus, R., Bohling, J., Voedisch, S., Braun, A., Ochs, M., et al. (2012). Cathepsin G and neutrophil elastase contribute to lung-protective immunity against mycobacterial infections in mice. *J. Immunol.* 188, 4476–4487. doi: 10.4049/jimmunol.1103346

Stephenson, E., Savvatis, K., Mohiddin, S. A., and Marelli-Berg, F. M. (2016). T-cell immunity in myocardial inflammation: pathogenic role and therapeutic manipulation. *Br. J. Pharmacol.* doi: 10.1111/bph.13613

Sudhan, D. R., and Siemann, D. W. (2015). Cathepsin L targeting in cancer treatment. *Pharmacol. Ther.* 155, 105–116. doi: 10.1016/j.pharmthera.2015.08.007

Sugino, M., Imamura, S., Mulenga, A., Nakajima, M., Tsuda, A., Ohashi, K., et al. (2003). A serine proteinase inhibitor (serpin) from ixodid tick *Haemaphysalis longicornis*; cloning and preliminary assessment of its suitability as a candidate for a tick vaccine. *Vaccine* 21, 2844–2851. doi: 10.1016/S0264-410X(03)00167-1

Sun, J., Sukhova, G. K., Wolters, P. J., Yang, M., Kitamoto, S., Libby, P., et al. (2007). Mast cells promote atherosclerosis by releasing proinflammatory cytokines. *Nat. Med.* 13, 719–724. doi: 10.1038/nm1601

Sun, J., Zhang, J., Lindholt, J. S., Sukhova, G. K., Liu, J., He, A., et al. (2009). Critical role of mast cell chymase in mouse abdominal aortic aneurysm formation. *Circulation* 120, 973–982. doi: 10.1161/CIRCULATIONAHA.109.849679

Takeda, A., Jimi, T., Wakayama, Y., Misugi, N., Miyake, S., and Kumagai, T. (1992). Demonstration of cathepsins B, H and L in xenografts of normal and Duchenne-muscular-dystrophy muscles transplanted into nude mice. *Biochem. J.* 288 (Pt 2), 643–648. doi: 10.1042/bj2880643

Talukdar, S., Oh, D. Y., Bandyopadhyay, G., Li, D., Xu, J., Mcnelis, J., et al. (2012). Neutrophils mediate insulin resistance in mice fed a high-fat diet through secreted elastase. *Nat. Med.* 18, 1407–1412. doi: 10.1038/nm.2885

Tan, G. J., Peng, Z. K., Lu, J. P., and Tang, F. Q. (2013). Cathepsins mediate tumor metastasis. *World J. Biol. Chem.* 4, 91–101. doi: 10.4331/wjbc.v4.i4.91

Tang, H. (2009). Regulation and function of the melanization reaction in Drosophila. *Fly (Austin)* 3, 105–111. doi: 10.4161/fly.3.1.7747

Tirloni, L., Kim, T. K., Coutinho, M. L., Ali, A., Seixas, A., Termignoni, C., et al. (2016). The putative role of *Rhipicephalus microplus* salivary serpins in the tick-host relationship. *Insect. Biochem. Mol. Biol.* 71, 12–28. doi: 10.1016/j.ibmb.2016.01.004

Tirloni, L., Reck, J., Terra, R. M., Martins, J. R., Mulenga, A., Sherman, N. E., et al. (2014a). Proteomic analysis of cattle tick Rhipicephalus (Boophilus) microplus saliva: a comparison between partially and fully engorged females. *PLoS ONE* 9:e94831. doi: 10.1371/journal.pone.0094831

Tirloni, L., Seixas, A., Mulenga, A., Vaz Ida, S. Jr., and Termignoni, C. (2014b). A family of serine protease inhibitors (serpins) in the cattle tick Rhipicephalus (Boophilus) microplus. *Exp. Parasitol.* 137, 25–34. doi: 10.1016/j.exppara.2013.12.001

Toyomane, K., Konnai, S., Niwa, A., Githaka, N., Isezaki, M., Yamada, S., et al. (2016). Identification and the preliminary *in vitro* characterization of IRIS homologue from salivary glands of *Ixodes persulcatus* Schulze. *Ticks Tick Borne Dis.* 7, 119–125. doi: 10.1016/j.ttbdis.2015.09.006

Tumminello, F. M., Leto, G., Pizzolanti, G., Candiloro, V., Crescimanno, M., Crosta, L., et al. (1996). Cathepsin D, B and L circulating levels as prognostic markers of malignant progression. *Anticancer Res.* 16, 2315–2319.

Turk, V., Stoka, V., Vasiljeva, O., Renko, M., Sun, T., Turk, B., et al. (2012). Cysteine cathepsins: from structure, function and regulation to new frontiers. *Biochim. Biophys. Acta* 1824, 68–88. doi: 10.1016/j.bbapap.2011.10.002

Twigg, M. S., Brockbank, S., Lowry, P., Fitzgerald, S. P., Taggart, C., and Weldon, S. (2015). The Role of Serine Proteases and Antiproteases in the Cystic Fibrosis Lung. *Mediators Inflamm.* 2015:293053. doi: 10.1155/2015/293053

Valdes, J. J., and Moal, I. H. (2014). Prediction of Kunitz ion channel effectors and protease inhibitors from the Ixodes ricinus sialome. *Ticks Tick Borne Dis.* 5, 947–950. doi: 10.1016/j.ttbdis.2014.07.016

Valenzuela, J. G., Francischetti, I. M., Pham, V. M., Garfield, M. K., Mather, T. N., and Ribeiro, J. M. (2002). Exploring the sialome of the tick *Ixodes scapularis. J. Exp. Biol.* 205, 2843–2864. Available online at: http://jeb.biologists.org/content/205/18/2843.article-info

Wagner, C. J., Schultz, C., and Mall, M. A. (2016). Neutrophil elastase and matrix metalloproteinase 12 in cystic fibrosis lung disease. *Mol Cell Pediatr* 3:25. doi: 10.1186/s40348-016-0053-7

Wang, Y., Yu, X., Cao, J., Zhou, Y., Gong, H., Zhang, H., et al. (2015a). Characterization of a secreted cystatin from the tick *Rhipicephalus haemaphysaloides. Exp. Appl. Acarol.* 67, 289–298. doi: 10.1007/s10493-015-9946-8

Wang, Y., Zhou, Y., Gong, H., Cao, J., Zhang, H., Li, X., et al. (2015b). Functional characterization of a cystatin from the tick Rhipicephalus haemaphysaloides. *Parasit. Vectors* 8:140. doi: 10.1186/s13071-015-0725-5

Whisstock, J. C., Silverman, G. A., Bird, P. I., Bottomley, S. P., Kaiserman, D., Luke, C. J., et al. (2010). Serpins flex their muscle: II. Structural insights into target peptidase recognition, polymerization, and transport functions. *J. Biol. Chem.* 285, 24307–24312. doi: 10.1074/jbc.R110.141408

Wikel, S. (2013). Ticks and tick-borne pathogens at the cutaneous interface: host defenses, tick countermeasures, and a suitable environment for pathogen establishment. *Front. Microbiol.* 4:337. doi: 10.3389/fmicb.2013.00337

Willadsen, P., Bird, P., Cobon, G. S., and Hungerford, J. (1995). Commercialisation of a recombinant vaccine against *Boophilus microplus. Parasitology* 110 (Suppl.), S43–S50. doi: 10.1017/S0031182000001487

Xu, T., Lew-Tabor, A., and Rodriguez-Valle, M. (2016). Effective inhibition of thrombin by Rhipicephalus microplus serpin-15 (RmS-15) obtained in the yeast *Pichia pastoris. Ticks Tick Borne Dis.* 7, 180–187. doi: 10.1016/j.ttbdis.2015.09.007

Yamaji, K., Tsuji, N., Miyoshi, T., Hatta, T., Alim, M. A., Anisuzzaman, et al. (2010). Hlcyst-1 and Hlcyst-2 are potential inhibitors of HlCPL-A in the midgut of the ixodid tick *Haemaphysalis longicornis. J. Vet. Med. Sci.* 72, 599–604. doi: 10.1292/jvms.09-0561

Yamaji, K., Tsuji, N., Miyoshi, T., Islam, M. K., Hatta, T., Alim, M. A., et al. (2009a). Hemoglobinase activity of a cysteine protease from the ixodid tick *Haemaphysalis longicornis. Parasitol. Int.* 58, 232–237. doi: 10.1016/j.parint.2009.05.003

Yamaji, K., Tsuji, N., Miyoshi, T., Islam, M. K., Hatta, T., Alim, M. A., et al. (2009b). A salivary cystatin, HlSC-1, from the ixodid tick *Haemaphysalis longicornis* play roles in the blood-feeding processes. *Parasitol. Res.* 106, 61–68. doi: 10.1007/s00436-009-1626-3

Yasuda, Y., Kaleta, J., and Bromme, D. (2005). The role of cathepsins in osteoporosis and arthritis: rationale for the design of new therapeutics. *Adv. Drug Deliv. Rev.* 57, 973–993. doi: 10.1016/j.addr.2004.12.013

Yu, Y., Cao, J., Zhou, Y., Zhang, H., and Zhou, J. (2013). Isolation and characterization of two novel serpins from the tick *Rhipicephalus haemaphysaloides. Ticks Tick Borne Dis.* 4, 297–303. doi: 10.1016/j.ttbdis.2013.02.001

Zavasnik-Bergant, T. (2008). Cystatin protease inhibitors and immune functions. *Front. Biosci.* 13, 4625–4637. doi: 10.2741/3028

Zeng, X. C., Liu, Y., Shi, W., Zhang, L., Luo, X., Nie, Y., et al. (2014). Genome-wide search and comparative genomic analysis of the trypsin inhibitor-like cysteine-rich domain-containing peptides. *Peptides* 53, 106–114. doi: 10.1016/j.peptides.2013.08.012

Zhang, J., Sun, J., Lindholt, J. S., Sukhova, G. K., Sinnamon, M., Stevens, R. L., et al. (2011). Mast cell tryptase deficiency attenuates mouse abdominal aortic aneurysm formation. *Circ. Res.* 108, 1316–1327. doi: 10.1161/CIRCRESAHA.111.243758

Zhou, J., Liao, M., Gong, H., Xuan, X., and Fujisaki, K. (2010). Characterization of Hlcyst-3 as a member of cystatins from the tick *Haemaphysalis longicornis. Exp. Appl. Acarol.* 51, 327–333. doi: 10.1007/s10493-010-9336-1

Zhou, J., Liao, M., Hatta, T., Tanaka, M., Xuan, X., and Fujisaki, K. (2006a). Identification of a follistatin-related protein from the tick *Haemaphysalis longicornis* and its effect on tick oviposition. *Gene* 372, 191–198. doi: 10.1016/j.gene.2005.12.020

Zhou, J., Liao, M., Ueda, M., Gong, H., Xuan, X., and Fujisaki, K. (2009). Characterization of an intracellular cystatin homolog from the tick *Haemaphysalis longicornis. Vet. Parasitol.* 160, 180–183. doi: 10.1016/j.vetpar.2008.10.086

Zhou, J., Ueda, M., Umemiya, R., Battsetseg, B., Boldbaatar, D., Xuan, X., et al. (2006b). A secreted cystatin from the tick *Haemaphysalis longicornis* and its distinct expression patterns in relation to innate immunity. *Insect Biochem. Mol. Biol.* 36, 527–535. doi: 10.1016/j.ibmb.2006.03.003

12

Emerging Tick-Borne Viruses in the Twenty-First Century

Karen L. Mansfield[1,2], Lv Jizhou[1,3], L. Paul Phipps[1] and Nicholas Johnson[1,4*]

[1] Animal and Plant Health Agency, Addlestone, United Kingdom, [2] Institute of Infection and Global Health, University of Liverpool, Liverpool, United Kingdom, [3] Chinese Academy of Inspection and Quarantine, Beijing, China, [4] Faculty of Health and Medicine, University of Surrey, Guildford, United Kingdom

***Correspondence:**
Nicholas Johnson
nick.johnson@apha.gsi.gov.uk

Ticks, as a group, are second only to mosquitoes as vectors of pathogens to humans and are the primary vector for pathogens of livestock, companion animals, and wildlife. The role of ticks in the transmission of viruses has been known for over 100 years and yet new pathogenic viruses are still being detected and known viruses are continually spreading to new geographic locations. Partly as a result of their novelty, tick-virus interactions are at an early stage in understanding. For some viruses, even the principal tick-vector is not known. It is likely that tick-borne viruses will continue to emerge and challenge public and veterinary health long into the twenty-first century. However, studies focusing on tick saliva, a critical component of tick feeding, virus transmission, and a target for control of ticks and tick-borne diseases, point toward solutions to emerging viruses. The aim of this review is to describe some currently emerging tick-borne diseases, their causative viruses, and to discuss research on virus-tick interactions. Through focus on this area, future protein targets for intervention and vaccine development may be identified.

Keywords: tick, virus, emerging, transmission

INTRODUCTION

Many arthropods, including ticks, transmit diseases that cause morbidity, and mortality amongst humans, livestock, companion animals, and/or wildlife. This in turn can cause major economic costs particularly to the owners of livestock affected by disease. The relationship between the tick, its host and pathogens has been shown to be complex and each may benefit or suffer detrimental effects due to the combination of physiological and immune mediated processes each elicits during infestation and infection (de la Fuente et al., 2016). Viruses form a major constituency of the pathogens transmitted by ticks (for review see Labuda and Nuttall, 2004). Although, the presence of microorganisms in ticks appears to have little impact on the tick, presumably there is an energetic cost to harboring them and studies have demonstrated that ticks do respond in a coordinated fashion to infection with bacterial (Mercado-Curiel et al., 2011; Ayllón et al., 2015) and protozoal (Antunes et al., 2012) pathogens. Recent studies using *in vitro* models are beginning to identify transcriptional responses in ticks cell during infection with viruses (Mansfield et al., 2017).

Viruses that are transmitted by ticks belong to a range of virus families with different characteristics and tick vectors. One of the first tick-borne viruses identified was the flavivirus, louping ill virus, the causative agent of encephalitis in sheep and grouse, a disease recognized in livestock for hundreds of years. The demonstration that ticks were the source of infection for the virus was described almost 100 years ago (Stockman, 1918). Since this time, many more pathogenic viruses have been identified around the world. However, new examples of emerging tick-borne viral diseases that affect man are constantly being reported. Another striking feature that favors pathogen transmission by ticks is the multi-stage lifecycle of ticks. Most species of *Ixodid* ticks have three states, larva, nymph and adult that each requires a blood-meal, sometimes requiring days to complete, in order to develop to the next stage. *Argasid* ticks, such as *Ornithodoros* sp. by contrast only require minutes to feed but each stage may feed multiple times. This ensures that the tick can become infected at any stage of its lifecycle and that infection persists through each developmental stage via transstadial transmission (Karbowiak et al., 2016) and then has the opportunity to transmit that virus back to a mammalian host (**Figure 1**). When blood feeding requires attachment to the host for a number of days, this provides ample opportunity for transfer of virus from tick to host within infected saliva. Horizontal transmission occurs following consumption of blood from an infected mammalian host, whilst co-feeding is a form of transmission that occurs when multiple ticks feed in close proximity enabling virus to transfer between ticks without infection in the host (Jones et al., 1987). Vertical transmission of pathogens between generations of ticks has been observed (transovarial transmission) for viruses such as tick-borne encephalitis virus (Reháček, 1962) and African swine fever virus (Rennie et al., 2001).

Currently, there are no effective therapeutic agents or vaccines for many tick-borne viruses with the exception of vaccines for louping ill virus, tick-borne encephalitis virus, and Kyasanur Forest disease virus, thus avoidance or control of the vector are the principal means of preventing disease. Emerging tick-borne diseases that affect humans and livestock will continue to challenge public and veterinary health. Most current research is limited to a small number of *Ixodid* tick species, mainly *Ixodes scapularis* and *Ixodes ricinus*, vectors of pathogens such as *Borrelia burgdorferi (sensu stricto* and *sensu lato)*, *Anaplasma phagocytophilum*, and tick-borne encephalitis virus, a virus that is currently increasing in range across Europe (Mansfield et al., 2009). However, with over 900 species of ticks in the world (Horak et al., 2002), many capable of transmitting viruses, future research on the interactions between the pathogen, its vector and the mammalian host will need to consider a greater number of virus-tick associations. This article provides an overview of some of the emerging tick-borne viruses (summarized in **Table 1** and located in **Figure 2**) that have arisen in the twenty-first century.

EMERGING TICK–BORNE BUNYAVIRUSES

Emergence of Severe Fever with Thrombocytopenia Syndrome Virus in China

Severe fever with thrombocytopenia syndrome (SFTS) was first documented in humans in 2007 when three patients were admitted to a hospital in Henan Province, China, with acute fever and severe leucopenia (Liu et al., 2014). Further cases were reported in Henan and Hubei provinces between 2008 and 2010

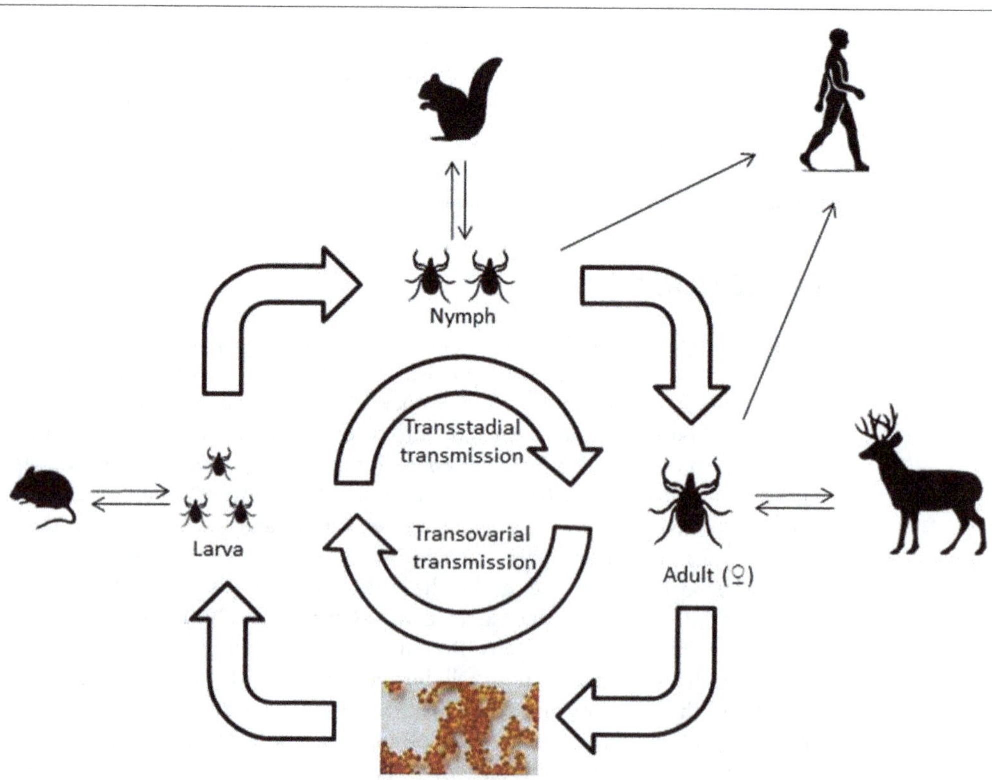

FIGURE 1 | A schematic of the three host *Ixodid* tick lifecycle illustrating the type of vertebrate hosts involved in each life stage of the tick.

TABLE 1 | Summary of emerging viruses discussed in this review.

Virus	Abbreviation	Classification (family, genus)	Description of genome	Distribution	Primary tick vector
Severe Fever with Thrombocytopenia syndrome virus	SFTSV	Bunyaviridae, *Phlebovirus*	Tri-segmented negative strand RNA	East Asia, North America	*Haemaphysalis longicornis*[a]
Heartland virus	HRTV	Bunyaviridae, *Phlebovirus*	Tri-segmented negative strand RNA	North America	*Amblyomma americanum*
Crimean congo haemorrhagic fever virus	CCHFV	Bunyaviridae, *Nairovirus*	Tri-segmented negative strand RNA	Africa, Central Asia, Mediterranean Basin	*Hyalomma marginatum*
Powassan virus	POWV	Flaviviridae, *Flavivirus*	Positive strand RNA	North America, Russian Federation	*Ixodes scapularis, Ixodes cookei*[b]
Deer tick virus	DTV	Flaviviridae, *Flavivirus*	Positive strand RNA	North America	*Ixodes scapularis*
Kyasunar forest disease virus	KFDV	Flaviviridae, *Flavivirus*	Positive strand RNA	India	*Haemaphysalis spinigera*
Alkhurma haemorrhagic fever virus	AHFV	Flaviviridae, *Flavivirus*	Positive strand RNA	Saudi Arabia	*Ornithidoros savigny*
African swine fever virus	ASFV	Asfarviridae, *Asfivirus*	Double-stranded DNA	Africa, Central Europe, Sardinia	*Ornithodoros moubata*[c]

[a] *In China.*
[b] *In North America.*
[c] *In Africa.*

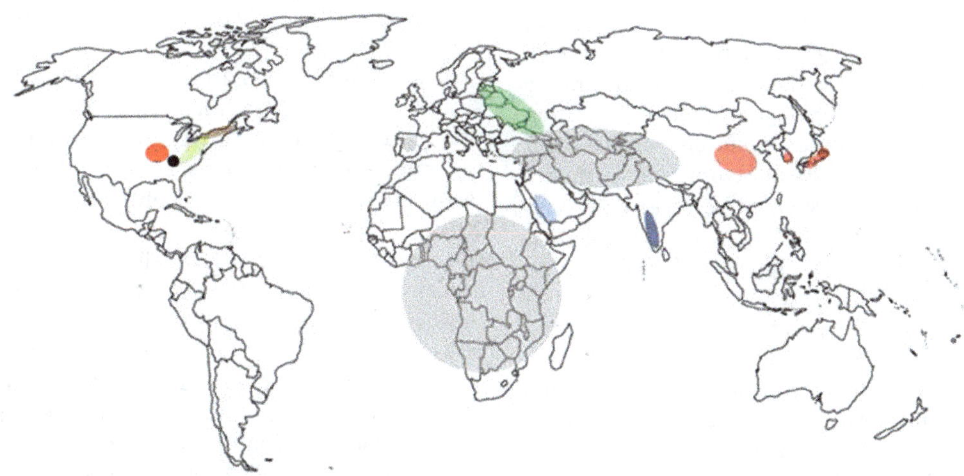

FIGURE 2 | Map of the world showing location of tick-borne disease outbreaks caused by emerging viruses. The regions marked are severe fever and thrombocytopenia syndrome virus (pale red), Heartlands virus (red), Crimean-Congo haemorrhagic fever virus (gray), Kysanur Forest disease virus (blue), Alkurma haemorrhagic fever virus (light blue), Powassan virus (brown), deer tick virus (pale green), Bourbon virus (black), Tofla virus (brown), and African swine fever virus (green).

with a similar clinical presentation and a case-fatality rate of over 10%. In 2009, the etiological agent of these infections was isolated from a patient's blood during the outbreaks of SFTS in Xinyang City in Henan province and identified as a bunyavirus related to viruses in the genus *Phlebovirus* (Zhang et al., 2012a,b; Lam et al., 2013). The virus was subsequently named severe fever with thrombocytopenia syndrome virus (SFTSV). Phleboviruses belong to the family Bunyaviridae, characterized by viruses with a segmented single-stranded negative sense genome divided into three segments, a small (S), medium (M), and large (L) segment coding for the nucleoprotein (N), surface glycoproteins (Gn/Gc), and RNA-dependent RNA polymerase (L), respectively. Related viruses include the mosquito-borne Rift Valley fever virus (Mansfield et al., 2015), the sandfly-borne Toscana virus (Charrel et al., 2012), and the tick-borne Uukuniemi virus (Matsuno et al., 2015). At present, infections with SFTSV have been reported in at least 13 provinces in China, including Henan, Hubei, Anhui, Shandong, Jiangsu, and Zhejiang (Li, 2013). Preliminary investigation of the first outbreak revealed that patients with SFTS were predominantly individuals who worked outdoors such as farmers indicating a rural source for the infection. Numerous patients presented with a history of tick bites (Zhang et al., 2012a). Subsequently, cases of SFTS were reported in North Korea, South Korea, and Japan (Liu et al., 2014).

In order to identify the reservoir of SFTSV, ticks were collected from livestock around the localities where patients originated and SFTSV was detected in *Haemaphysalis longicornis* (Zhang and Xu, 2016). Further surveys of *H. longicornis* provided strong evidence that this tick species was the definitive reservoir and vector responsible for SFTSV transmission to humans working in rural locations (Zhang et al., 2012b). Experimental studies also demonstrated transstadial transmission of the virus between the different life stages of *H. longicornis* and transmission to mice during feeding (Luo et al., 2015). With *H. longicornis* being the source of infection and associated with feeding on livestock, it was highly likely that domestic animals would be exposed to infection and seroprevalence studies in China have now confirmed this (Zhang and Xu, 2016). However, disease in livestock has not been reported suggesting that humans are particularly susceptible to infection with SFTSV.

Emergence of Heartland Virus in the USA

Heartland virus (HRTV) was first reported in 2009 from North America when two farmers from Missouri with a clinical presentation similar to SFTS were admitted to hospital (McMullan et al., 2012). Symptoms included fever, fatigue, headache, myalgia, arthralgia, anorexia and diarrhea. The source of the infection was identified as likely resulting from tick bites, and the isolated virus shared 73% sequence identity with SFTSV by alignment of the polymerase gene. Diagnosis of HRTV infection may be challenging but can be achieved through detection of viral RNA in blood or tissue or by demonstrating a four-fold or greater increase in virus-specific plaque reduction neutralization antibody titre between acute and convalescent serum specimens (McMullan et al., 2012). Seroprevalence studies of livestock in Minnesota State reported seropositivity rates ranging from 10 to 18%, for example 15.5% in cattle, suggesting widespread exposure to infected ticks (Xing et al., 2013).

Surveillance for HRTV in Missouri has identified virus in the lone star tick *Amblyomma americanum* (Savage et al., 2016), an abundant tick species in many regions of the United States. Transmission of virus to a vertebrate host, transstadial and transovarial transmission between lifecycle stages has been demonstrated in *A. americanum* (Godsey et al., 2016). Both SFTSV and HRTV are related phleboviruses and have emerged in the past 10 years. However, the viruses exist in different tick species and have emerged in different continents. Human encroachment, probably combined with environmental conditions that influence both tick abundance and behavior may have led to the simultaneous emergence of these viruses.

The Spread of Crimean Congo Haemorrhagic Fever Virus around the Mediterranean Basin

The virus now known as Crimean Congo Haemorrhagic fever virus (CCHFV) was first described during an outbreak of haemorrhagic fever in Red Army soldiers in the Crimea during the final years of the Second World War (Ergönül, 2006). This virus was shown to be antigenically similar to a second virus isolated from a human in what is now the Democratic Republic of the Congo (Simpson et al., 1967). Worldwide, many tick species have been found infected with CCHFV and could be implicated in transmission of this virus (Mertens et al., 2013). The virus is primarily transmitted by ticks of the genus *Hyalomma* (Morikawa et al., 2007). By the late twentieth century, CCHFV had one of the most extensive distributions of any tick-borne virus with infections being reported from the Middle East, Asia, and sub-Saharan Africa. However, during the late twentieth and early twenty-first century, cases of CCHFV have been reported in new geographical locations around the Mediterranean Basin. CCHFV belongs to the family Bunyaviridae, genus *Nairovirus*. Other members of this genus include Hazara virus and Nairobi sheep disease virus. The virus genome is a tri-segmented negative sense RNA genome that encodes four structural proteins, the nucleoprotein (N), glycoproteins (GN and GC), and the RNA-dependent RNA polymerase (L). The virus is particularly virulent for humans but has little or no pathogenic effect on livestock. Infection following a tick bite is followed by a short incubation period of between 3 and 7 days leading to a brief febrile illness characterized by fever, headache and myalgia. Haemorrhagic manifestations of disease develop 4–5 days after the development of fever and include bleeding from the nose, gastrointestinal system and urinary tract. The fatality rate ranges from 3 to 30%. Treatment is supportive, including replacement of fluids and blood constituents. There is no licensed antiviral treatment or licensed vaccine for CCHF.

Reports of infection around the Mediterranean Basin began around 2002 with cases reported in Turkey (Karti et al., 2004) and the Balkans (Papa et al., 2005). In Europe, the main tick vector is *Hy. marginatum*, a species found throughout the Iberian Peninsula, southern France, Italy, the Balkans, and Turkey. In 2010, the virus was detected in *Hy. lusitanicum* ticks in Spain (Estrada-Peña et al., 2012), followed 6 years later with two human cases of autochthonous transmission (Garcia Rada, 2016). Phylogenetic analysis of virus detected in ticks indicated that the virus present in Spain shared greater identity with CCHFV in West Africa than that spreading in the Balkans. This suggested that it was a separate introduction into Europe with the most likely mechanism of entry being by tick-infested migrating birds (Estrada-Peña et al., 2012; Palomar et al., 2016). *Hy. marginatum* have been detected on birds migrating into Europe on numerous occasions (Capek et al., 2014) including as far north as the United Kingdom (Jameson et al., 2012). It is likely that the severity of the winters prevents establishment of this tick species in countries of northern Europe. However, the existence of populations of *Hyalomma* spp. in Spain, Portugal, France, and Italy puts these countries at greater risk of CCHFV persisting if introduced.

EMERGING TICK-BORNE FLAVIVIRUSES

Interstate Spread of Kyasanur Forest Virus in India

Kyasanur Forest disease virus (KFDV) was isolated following an outbreak of haemorrhagic fever amongst villagers living in the Kyasanur Forest area in 1957 (Work and Trapido, 1957). The Forest is found in the Shimoga distict of Karnataka State in the south-west of India and has been the epicenter of the disease ever since with between 400 and 500 human cases reported annually (Holbrook, 2012). Initial studies demonstrated that the virus shared similar properties to Russian spring summer encephalitis virus (RRSEV), a variant of tick-borne encephalitis virus. However, the main clinical manifestation of disease is haemorrhagic fever unlike the encephalitis associated with RSSEV. KFDV is a member of the genus *Flavivirus*, family Flaviviridae. The flaviruses consist of a positive-sense single-stranded RNA genome that codes for three structural and seven non-structural proteins. Virion particles are enveloped with a single envelope protein projecting from the virus. KFDV is closely related to Alkhurma virus (AHFV) (Charrel et al., 2007) and a virus isolated in Yunnan Province, China (Wang et al., 2009). Phylogenetic studies on KFDV and AHFV suggest that they diverged over 700 years ago (Dodd et al., 2011) and that the virus has spread slowly within Karnataka Forest, reflecting dissemination by the tick vector that primarily feeds on small to medium sized mammals. Long distance movement that has separated the progenitors of both viruses could have been mediated by infected ticks attaching to migrating birds (Mehla et al., 2009).

The association with tick-borne viruses suggested a tick vector as the source of infection. Another early observation was mortality of non-human primates such as macaques and langurs in the area where human cases were reported. *Haemaphysalis* spp. ticks were collected from primate carcases and KFDV was isolated from *Haemaphysalis spinigera* (Trapido et al., 1959). Following the detection of KFDV, a second virus, Kaisodi virus, was isolated from *H. spinigera* sampled in India (Bhatt et al., 1966; Pavri and Casals, 1966). *Haemaphysalis* spp. are three-host ticks with a larval, nymphal and adult stage, each taking a blood meal prior to metamorphosis into the next stage, or egg development in the case of adult females. Although transovarial transmission of KFDV has been demonstrated in *H. spinigera* (Singh et al., 1963), it is the nymph and adult stages that are critical for the transmission of virus to small mammals and humans as these are the hosts favored by these life stages of the tick.

In recent years there have been reports of KFDV infections in both Karnataka province (Mourya et al., 2013; Yadav et al., 2014) and in the neighboring provinces of Kerala (Tandale et al., 2015; Sadanandane et al., 2017), Tamil Nadu and Maharashtra (Mourya and Yadav, 2016). As in previous reports, outbreaks are often preceded by disease in monkeys, and contact with carcases can lead to infection (Mourya et al., 2013).The appearance of dead monkeys, particularly target species such as the red-face bonnet monkey (*Macaca radiata*) and the black-faced langur (*Semnopithecus entellus*) are considered sentinels for the presence of KFDV at a site (Murhekar et al., 2015). The spread of KFDV in recent years could reflect further gradual spread of the virus by the tick vector, improvements in diagnosis (Mourya et al., 2012) and surveillance leading to increased frequency of reporting. Increased human exploitation of the environment leading to greater contact between humans and ticks could also contribute to this apparent spread. All of the affected regions form part of the Western Ghats, a mountain range running north-south parallel to the west coast of India. This in turn suggests that the areas affected share climatic features that are favorable to the tick vector, currently poorly studied, and that its presence could indicate a risk of KFDV. Further surveillance assessing the distribution and abundance of *H. spinigera* could reveal the true extent of KFDV in India.

Emergence of Alkhurma Haemorrhagic Fever in Saudi Arabia

Alkhurma haemorrhagic fever virus (AHFV) is a recently described tick-borne virus within the genus *Flavivirus* and family Flaviviridae (Horton et al., 2016). AHFV was first isolated in 1995 from a patient with haemorrhagic manifestations and fever in the city of Alkhurma in Saudi Arabia (Zaki, 1997). The whole genome of AHFV has been derived, and shares 89% sequence identity with KFDV (Charrel et al., 2001). This suggests that AHFV is a variant genotype of KFDV but with a distinct geographical distribution. AHFV is classified as biosafety level 3 agent (Charrel et al., 2007).

To investigate the tick-borne nature of AHFV, ticks were collected in both western and southern Saudi Arabia and assessed by reverse transcriptase PCR (Eraksoy, 2015). At present, AHFV has been identified in both the *Argasid* tick *Ornithodoros savignyi* and the *Ixodid* tick *Hyalomma dromedarii* (Charrel et al., 2007). As a recently emerged virus, the geographic range of AHFV is poorly understood. The wide distribution of *Ornithodoros* and *Hyalomma* spp. ticks suggests that the geographic limits of AHFV may be larger than presently assumed. The clinical case from Najran and report of AHFV in ticks from the Horn of Africa supports this view (Memish et al., 2005; Horton et al., 2016).

Increased Human Incidence of Powassan Virus in New England

Powassan virus (POWV) causes fatal encephalitis in a proportion of humans that become infected with it. Between 2013 and 2015, 8 cases of POWV encephalitis were reported from hospitals in Massachusetts and New Hampshire (Piantadosi et al., 2016). This represented the most recent evidence of an increasing trend for human cases of POWV in the United States where 9 cases were reported between 1999 and 2005 (Hinten et al., 2008). Similar trends were observed for other tick-borne diseases such as Lyme borreliosis (Bacon et al., 2008) and infection with *Babesia microti* (Vannier et al., 2015). POWV is a flavivirus, causing a febrile disease that can develop into severe meningoencephalitis. The virus was first reported from a fatal case in a 5 year old child in Powassan, Ontario in 1958 (McLean and Donohue, 1959).

Preliminary virological analysis suggested an association with tick-borne viruses such as (RSSEV) pointed researchers in the direction of ticks as the vector. Subsequent field surveillance detected POWV in pools of *Ixodes cookei* ticks and provided evidence that small mammals such as groundhogs (*Marmota monax*) contribute to the maintenance of virus (McLean et al., 1967). Surveillance by groups in the United States detected POWV in Colorado (Thomas et al., 1960) and New York State (Whitney and Jamnback, 1965). Numerous examples of POWV have now been isolated from the black-legged tick *I. scapularis* (Anderson and Armstrong, 2012) indicating that this tick species may be the most abundant vector of the virus across the eastern states of the US and southern states of Canada. In a further twist, POWV has been reported from the eastern province of Russia, Primorsky Krai, and is suspected of being established across a larger geographical area (Leonova et al., 2009; Deardorff et al., 2013). Here, the tick vector includes *Ixodes* spp. such as

I. persulcatus. Phylogenetic analysis of North American POWV strains indicates that POWV diverged from a common ancestor present ~500 years ago (Pesko et al., 2010). The viruses in Russia could be an introduction due to their similarity with American isolates. One possible means of introduction of the virus could be the importation of North American species such as mink (*Neovison vison*) with infected ticks during the expansion of the Russian fur trade.

The number of human cases of Powassan virus infection across its range has increased in recent years. The underlying cause is unclear but could be due to an increased awareness amongst clinicians and diagnosticians. Alternatively, the increase could be related to ecological factors that lead to the increase in abundance of the tick population driven in turn by increases in the number and range of mammalian hosts such as deer. This is believed to have been behind the increase in Lyme disease, caused by *B. burgdorferi*, across many States in the USA (Barbour and Fish, 1993). However, the nymphal form of the tick is suspected of being responsible for most cases of transmission and abundance of this life stage is more dependent on the availability of small mammals such as rodents, for example the white-footed mouse (*Peromyscus leucopus*). Therefore, factors that influence rodent abundance such as predator decline, mediated by the red fox (*Vulpes vulpes*) for example, may have greater impact on disease transmission by ticks (Levi et al., 2012).

The Spread of the Deer Tick Virus in North America

Deer tick virus (DTV), a flavivirus in the tick-borne encephalitis group, is a genetically distinct lineage (subtype) of POWV that can cause neuroinvasive infection in humans in parts of North America. DTV was originally isolated from the Rocky Mountain wood tick, *Dermacentor andersoni,* but is mainly found in *I. scapularis* collected from states in the north-east of the US (Telford et al., 1997; Aliota et al., 2014) and has since been responsible for a human case of encephalitis (Tavakoli et al., 2009). Although the first recognized human case of DTV encephalitis occurred in 1997, evidence of the causative virus, based on sequence data, was not available until 2001 (Gholam et al., 1999; Kuno et al., 2001). The DTV genome shares 84% sequence identity with POWV and 94% amino acid identity between the virus polyproteins. However, DTV and POWV are regarded as antigenically indistinguishable and the infecting virus cannot be determined by serological testing, and genotypic analysis is needed to make a definitive diagnosis. DTV is maintained in an enzootic cycle between *I. scapularis* and the white-footed mouse (*Peromycus leucopus*) (Ebel et al., 2000). Until now there have been a small number of published cases of proven DTV induced encephalitis (Kuno et al., 2001), one from Canada and three from USA. Based on detection of virus genome, prevalence with DTV ranged up to 5% in *I. scapularis* from several geographic areas including Hudson Valley, Nantucket Island and Prudence Island (Aliota et al., 2014). The increase in the number of human cases of Powassan virus encephalitis that have been reported since 2010 is remarkable. Most of these cases were diagnosed by serological assays (Khoury et al., 2013) and it is possible that DTV could be responsible for some of these cases.

THE EMERGENCE OF ASFARVIRUS IN EUROPE

Establishment of African Swine Fever Virus in Eastern Europe

African swine fever virus (ASFV) is the causative agent of African swine fever (ASF), an acute haemorrhagic fever that causes severe morbidity and high mortality in domestic pigs. ASFV is classified within the genus *Asfivirus* and family Asfarviridae, and consists of a double-stranded DNA genome coding for ~150 proteins. The genome is surrounded by a protein capsid and a host-derived envelope. Virus particles are very robust and can survive for days in the environment or months within pork meat. ASF was first described in Kenya and is found across sub-Saharan Africa (Thomson, 1985). The epidemiology of ASF in Africa is driven by two cycles. The first is sylvatic with bush pigs (*Potamochoerus larvatus*) and warthogs (*Phacochoerus africanus*) being infected following infestation with *Argasid* ticks of the genus *Ornithodorus*, particularly *O. moubata*. Infections in wild species do not result in clinical signs of disease. The second cycle involves infection of domestic pigs (*Sus scrofa*) that are highly susceptible to infection and shed virus in excreta. Initial infection is by tick bite but is then amplified by pig-to-pig transmission, either through contact or consumption of contaminated food. ASF is a notifiable disease in Europe (http://www.oie.int/animal-health-in-the-world/oie-listed-diseases-2016/) and significant effort is directed at preventing its introduction through import control of livestock and food stuffs. Outbreaks resulting from importation have occurred in domestic pigs on a number of occasions across Europe. Significantly in the case of Sardinia, following introduction in the late 1970s. Repeated attempt to eliminate the disease have failed and the disease is endemic (Mur et al., 2016). More recently, ASFV was introduced into the Caucasus region in 2007 (Rowlands et al., 2008) and led to extensive spread into neighboring countries including Armenia, Azerbaijan, and Russia. By 2016, ASFV has been detected throughout Eastern Europe and the Baltic region. Pig-to-pig transmission appears to be the main driver for the spread of the epidemic but wild boar, a species which is also susceptible to infection, could also contribute to spread (Guinat et al., 2016). A further concern for Europe is the infection of indigenous *Argasid* ticks such as *O. erraticus* that are present throughout the Mediterranean Basin and Balkans, and feed preferentially on domestic pigs, although less so on wild boar (Pietschmann et al., 2016). ASFV infects and replicates in *O. erraticus* (Basto et al., 2006; Ribeiro et al., 2015) and has been shown to experimentally transmit ASFV to pigs (Boinas et al., 2011). Widely distributed *Ixodid* ticks in Europe such as *I. ricinus* and *Dermacentor reticulatus* are unable to support ASFV replication and presumably do not contribute to disease spread (de Carvalho Ferreira et al., 2014). The spread of ASFV has been primarily caused by human activities including long distance transport of livestock. The presence of a susceptible wildlife host, wild boar, has further complicated efforts to control the disease and it is likely that it will continue to spread across the continent.

TICK SALIVA-ASSISTED TRANSMISSION AND POTENTIAL ANTIGENIC TARGETS FOR CONTROL

The components of saliva are critical to the successful completion of a blood meal by all life stages of ticks. As a result, tick saliva is a highly complex mixture of proteins, peptides, and other bioactive compounds. Transcriptomic analysis suggests that tick feeding leads to the upregulation of thousands of protein transcripts (Karim and Ribiero, 2015; Ribeiro et al., 2017) that when secreted promote attachment to the host, inhibit host responses such as blood clotting and inhibit microbial growth (Hovius et al., 2008). Tick saliva has also been shown to promote transmission of tick-borne viruses to the mammalian host. Early studies demonstrated that salivary gland extracts (SGE) from a range of tick species enhanced transmission of Thogoto virus and TBEV to guinea-pigs (Jones et al., 1989, 1992; Labuda et al., 1993). Recent studies have shown a similar enhancement by *O. porcinus* SGE of ASFV infection in pigs (Bernard et al., 2015) and *I. scapularis* SGE of POWV infection in mice (Hermance and Thangamani, 2015). One mechanism suggested for this enhancement is the increased attraction of macrophages and other antigen presenting cells to the site of tick attachment. These appear to rapidly disseminate the virus throughout the mammalian host. It is also possible that rather than being passively transmitted by the tick, viruses actively modulate tick salivary gland transcripts. In a study investigating feeding by *I. scapularis* nymphs, infection with Langat virus modulated tick salivary gland transcriptional responses during 3 days of feeding (McNally et al., 2012). Further analysis of virus-induced transcripts could lead to the identification of those proteins that promote virus transmission and in turn could be molecular targets for tick control and prevention of virus transmission. The concept of a tick vaccine has been discussed for decades and has led to a number of approaches based on specific tick salivary proteins that have been used as vaccine formulations that inhibit tick feeding (Labuda et al., 2006; Garcia-Varas et al., 2010). The advent of "omics" technologies using both the sialotranscriptome (Maruyama et al., 2017) and the proteome (Villar et al., 2017) have dramatically expanded the number of targets available for vaccine development. The application of such vaccines to livestock or even key wildlife species could provide an opportunity to suppress tick abundance and reduce the frequency of pathogen transmission in order to suppress incidence of disease.

CONCLUSIONS

The emergence of tick-borne viruses is driven by a range of factors, often inter-related, that lead to the appearance and/or increase in human or veterinary cases of disease. *Ixodid* tick species have multiple life stages (**Figure 1**) with each feeding off a different host, and often a different host species. Factors that influence each life stage will affect their ability to transmit pathogens. Key amongst these factors are those associated with the tick vector, including its presence in an area, feeding behavior, abundance, and contact with humans or livestock. Studies on TBEV suggest that co-feeding favors virus transmission between immature tick stages (larva/nymphs) and environmental factors that promote co-feeding will drive infection rates up via horizontal transmission and increase the risk of transmission to humans (Randolph et al., 1999). This leads to the paradoxical situation whereby decreases in numbers of mammalian hosts can lead to an increase in disease transmission. Seasonal variation in temperatures can also dramatically affect transmission to humans. Low temperatures in winter and warm summer temperatures between 2009 and 2012 have been identified as the reason for the increased incidence of TBEV in Sweden enhanced by co-feeding by *I. ricinus* on small mammals (Jaenson et al., 2012). Warm summer temperatures also encourage humans to spend more time outdoors and wear less clothing, both factors that could increase the risk of encountering ticks. The presence of large ruminants such as deer can increase the abundance of ticks and indirectly indicate risk of virus transmission (Carpi et al., 2008). Conversely, activities that reduce tick abundance will reduce virus transmission.

The distribution of a tick-borne disease is usually dictated by that of the tick vector. This appears to be the case for viruses such as CCHFV. However, when driven by anthropomorphic factors, such viruses can emerge in new locations, enabled by an alternative mechanism of transmission. This appears to have led to the emergence of ASFV in Central Europe where tick-borne transmission has been replaced by contact transmission between pigs, driven in part by the presence of wild boar (Guinat et al., 2016).

Human factors are a major influence on disease emergence. The paradigmatic example of this is the emergence of Omsk haemorrhagic fever virus in central Russia due to the importation of muskrats (*Ondatra zibethicus*) from North America in the nineteenth century (Růžek et al., 2010). The virus existed in the area within the *D. reticulatus* tick population but was rarely, if ever, encountered by humans. By introducing an exotic mammalian host that was highly susceptible to infection and regularly handled by humans, clusters of haemorrhagic disease occurred. A similar scenario appears to have resulted in the introduction of POWV in Eastern Russia and the activities of the farming industry in Eastern Europe has propelled the spread of ASFV. A further human factor that can increase detection rates of emerging tick-borne diseases is awareness by clinicians. Once a cluster of cases of disease have been reported, further cases come to light. However, a lack of disease awareness among clinicians and veterinarians can hamper the control of a disease epidemic, which could potentially be the case for ASFV where clinical signs can be similar to those observed with other diseases of swine (Guinat et al., 2016). Therefore, an increase in awareness and data sharing of new and emerging tick-borne diseases among medical and veterinary professionals is essential. Trans-national bodies such as the World Health Organization and the World Organization for Animal Health (OIE) play a key role in information sharing and setting standards for disease detection and reporting.

Tick-borne diseases continue to cause a burden to both animal and human health. As the twenty-first century progresses there will certainly be more examples of tick-borne virus spread and novel virus emergence. New viruses associated with ticks are being discovered as a result of human infection, such as Bourbon virus (Kosoy et al., 2015) or before there is any association with disease such as Tofla virus (Shimada et al., 2016; de Figueiredo et al., 2017). Early recognition of those that are pathogens will be critical to their control in addition to measures to control potential tick vectors. Understanding the interactions between these emerging viruses and the tick species that transmit them to vertebrate hosts represents both a colossal challenge and a great opportunity to identify targets for future control of tick-borne diseases. A greater understanding of tick feeding has identified both the complexity of the feeding process and its role in promoting pathogen transmission (Randolph, 2009). This understanding has also resulted in the identification of protein components within tick saliva that can act as antigens for vaccines that suppress tick infestation and protect against tick-borne virus transmission (Labuda et al., 2006). Such generic approaches may assist in protecting humans and livestock from emerging tick-borne viruses.

AUTHOR CONTRIBUTIONS

NJ conceived the review. KM, LJ, LP, and NJ wrote the paper. All authors reviewed the final version of the manuscript.

FUNDING

This work was funded by the European Commission Seventh Framework Programme under the "Anticipating the Global Onset of Novel Epidemics—ANTIGONE" project (#278976).

ACKNOWLEDGMENTS

The authors would like to thank Professors Trevor Drew and Tony Fooks for constructive criticism of this manuscript.

REFERENCES

Aliota, M. T., Wilczek, M. P., Peters, R. J., Ostfeld, R. S., and Kramer, L. D. (2014). The prevalence of zoonotic tick-borne pathogens in *Ixodes scapularis* collected in the Hudson Valley, New York State. *Vector Borne Zoonotic Dis.* 14, 245–250. doi: 10.1089/vbz.2013.1475

Anderson, J. F., and Armstrong, P. M. (2012). Prevalence and genetic characterisation of Powassan virus strains infecting *Ixodes scapularis* in Conneticut. *Am. J. Trop. Med. Hyg.* 87, 754–759. doi: 10.4269/ajtmh.2012.12-0294

Antunes, S., Galindo, R. C., Almazán, C., Rudenko, N., Golovchenko, M., Grubhoffer, L., et al. (2012). Functional genomics studies of *Rhipicephalus (Boophilus) annulatus* in response to infection with the cattle parasite, *Babesia bigemina*. *Int. J. Parasitol.* 42, 187–195. doi: 10.1016/j.ijpara.2011.12.003

Ayllón, N., Villar, M., Galindo, R. C., Kocan, K. M., Šima, R., López, R., et al. (2015). Systems biology of tissue-specific response to *Anaplasma phagocytophilum* reveals differentiated apoptosis in the tick vector Ixodes scapularis. *PLoS Genet.* 11:e1005120. doi: 10.1371/journal.pgen.1005120

Bacon, R. M., Kugeler, K. J., and Mead, P. S.(2008). Centers for Disease Control and Prevention (CDC). Surveillance for Lyme disease—United States, 1992–2006. *MMWR Surveill. Sum.* 57, 1–9.

Barbour, A. G., and Fish, D. (1993). The biological and social phenomenom of Lyme disease. *Science* 260, 1610–1616. doi: 10.1126/science.8503006

Basto, A. P., Nix, R. J., Boinas, F., Mendes, S., Silva, M. J., Cartaxeira, C., et al. (2006). Kinetics of African swine fever virus infection in *Ornithodoros erraticus* ticks. *J. Gen. Virol.* 87, 1863–1871. doi: 10.1099/vir.0.81765-0

Bernard, J., Hutet, E., Paboeuf, F., Randriamparany, T., Holzmuller, P., Lancelot, R., et al. (2015). Effect of *O. porcinus* tick salivary gland extract on the African swine fever virus infection in domestic pig. *PLoS ONE* 11:e0147869. doi: 10.1371/journal.pone.0147869

Bhatt, P. N., Kulkarni, K. G., Boshell, J., Rajagopalan, P. K., Patil, A. P., Goverdhan, M. K., et al. (1966). Kaisodi virus, a new agent isolated from *Haemaphysalis spinigera* in Mysore state, south India. *Am. J. Trop. Med. Hyg.* 15, 958–960. doi: 10.4269/ajtmh.1966.15.958

Boinas, F. S., Wilson, A. J., Hutchings, G. H., Martins, C., and Dixon, L. J. (2011). The persistence of African swine fever virus in field-infected *Ornithodoros erraticus* during the ASF endemic period in Portugal. *PLoS ONE* 6:e20383. doi: 10.1371/journal.pone.0020383

Capek, M., Literak, I., Kocianova, E., Sychra, O., Najer, T., Trnka, A., et al. (2014). Ticks of the *Hyalomma marginatum* complex transported by migratory birds into Central Europe. *Ticks Tick Borne Dis.* 5, 489–493. doi: 10.1016/j.ttbdis.2014.03.002

Carpi, G., Cagnacci, F., Neteler, M., and Rizzoli, A. (2008). Tick infestation on roe deer in relation to geographic and remotely sensed climatic variables in a tick-borne encephalitis endemic area. *Epidemiol. Infect.* 136, 1416–1424. doi: 10.1017/S0950268807000039

Charrel, R. N., Bichaud, L., and de Lamballerie, X. (2012). Emergence of Toscana virus in the Mediterranean area. *World J. Virol.* 1, 135–141. doi: 10.5501/wjv.v1.i5.135

Charrel, R. N., Fagbo, S., Moureau, G., Alqahtani, M. H., Temmam, S., and de Lamballerie, X. (2007). Alkhurma hemorrhagic fever virus in *Ornithodoros savigny* ticks. *Emerg. Infect. Dis.* 13, 153–155. doi: 10.3201/eid1301.061094

Charrel, R. N., Zaki, A. M., Attoui, H., Fakeeh, M., Billoir, F., Yousef, A. I., et al. (2001). Complete coding sequence of the alkhurma virus, a tick-borne flavivirus causing severe hemorrhagic fever in humans in Saudi Arabia. *Biochem. Biophys. Res. Comm.* 287, 455–461. doi: 10.1006/bbrc.2001.5610

Deardorff, E. R., Nofchissey, R. A., Cook, J. A., Hope, A. G., Tsvetkova, A., Talbot, S. L., et al. (2013). Powassan virus in mammals, Alaska and New Mexico, USA, and Russia, 2004–2007. *Emerg. Infect. Dis.* 12, 2012–2016. doi: 10.3201/eid1912.130319

de Carvalho Ferreira, H. C., Tudela Zúquete, S., Wijnveld, M., Weesendorp, E., Jongejan, F., Stegeman, A., et al. (2014). No evidence of African swine fever virus replication in hard ticks. *Ticks Tick Borne Dis.* 5, 582–589. doi: 10.1016/j.ttbdis.2013.12.012

de Figueiredo, G. G., Amarilla, A. A., de Souza, W. M., Fumagalli, M. J., de Figueiredo, M. L., Szabó, M. P., et al. (2017). Genetic characterization of Cacipacoré virus from ticks collected in São Paulo State, Brazil. *Arch. Virol.* 162, 1783–1786. doi: 10.1007/s00705-017-3279-3

de la Fuente, J., Villar, M., Cabezas-Cruz, A., Estrada-Peña, A., Ayllón, N., and Alberdi, P. (2016). Tick-host-pathogen interactions: conflict and cooperation. *PLoS Pathog.* 12:e1005488. doi: 10.1371/journal.ppat.1005488

Dodd, K. A., Bird, B. H., Khristova, M. L., Albariño, C. G., Carroll, S. A., Comer, J. A., et al. (2011). Ancient ancestry of KFDV and AHFV revealed by complete genome analysis of viruses isolated from ticks and mammalian hosts. *PLoS Negl. Trop. Dis.* 5:e1352. doi: 10.1371/journal.pntd.0001352

Ebel, G. D., Campbell, E. N., Goethert, H. K., Spielman, A., and Telford, S. R. III. (2000). Enzootic transmission of deer tick virus in New England and Wisconsin. *Am. J. Trop. Med. Hyg.* 63, 36–42. doi: 10.4269/ajtmh.2000.63.36

Eraksoy, H. (2015). Al-khurma haemorrhagic fever. *Klimik Dergisi* 27, 84–94. doi: 10.5152/kd.2014.22

Ergönül, O. (2006). Crimean-congo haemorrhagic fever. *Lancet Infect. Dis.* 6, 203–214. doi: 10.1016/S1473-3099(06)70435-2

Estrada-Peña, A., Palomar, A. M., Santibáñez, P., Sánchez, N., Habela, M. A., Portillo, A., et al. (2012). Crimean-Congo hemorrhagic fever virus in ticks, Southwestern Europe, 2010. *Emerg. Infect. Dis.* 18, 179–180. doi: 10.3201/eid1801.111040

Garcia Rada, A. (2016). First outbreak of Crimean-Congo haemorrhagic fever in western Europe kills one man in Spain. *BMJ* 354:i4891. doi: 10.1136/bmj.i4891

Garcia-Varas, G., Manzano-Román, R., Fernández-Soto, P., Encinas-Grandes, A., Oleaga, A., and Pérez-Sánchez, R. (2010). Purification and characterisation of a P-selectin-binding molecule from the salivary glands of *Ornithodoros moubata* that induces protective anti-tick immune responses in pigs. *Int. J. Parasitol.* 40, 313–326. doi: 10.1016/j.ijpara.2009.08.011

Gholam, B. I., Puksa, S., and Provias, J. P. (1999). Powassan encephalitis: a case report with neuropathology and literature review. *Can. Med. Assoc. J.* 161, 1419–1422.

Godsey M. S. Jr., Savage, H. M., Burkhalter, K. L., Bosco-Lauth, A. M., and Delorey, M. J. (2016). Transmission of Heartland virus (Bunyaviridae: Phlebovirus) by experimentally infected Ambylomma americanum (Acari: Ixodidae). *J. Med. Entomol.* 53, 1226–1233. doi: 10.1093/jme/tjw080

Guinat, C., Gogin, A., Blome, S., Keil, G., Pollin, R., Pfeiffer, D. U., et al. (2016). Transmission routes of African swine fever virus to domestic pigs: current knowledge and future direction. *Vet. Rec.* 178, 262–267. doi: 10.1136/vr.103593

Hermance, M. E., and Thangamani, S. (2015). Tick saliva enhances Powassan virus transmission to the host, influencing its dissemination and the course of disease. *J. Virol.* 89, 7852–7860. doi: 10.1128/JVI.01056-15

Hinten, S. R., Beckett, G. A., Gensheimer, K. F., Prichard, E., Courtney, T. M., Sears, S. D., et al. (2008). Increased recognition of Powassan encephalitis in the United States, 1999–2005. *Vector Borne Zoonotic Dis.* 8, 733–740. doi: 10.1089/vbz.2008.0022

Holbrook, M. R. (2012). Kyasanur forest disease. *Antiviral Res.* 96, 353–362. doi: 10.1016/j.antiviral.2012.10.005

Horak, I. G., Camicas, J. L., and Keirans, J. E. (2002). The Argasidae, Ixodidae and Nuttalliellidae (Acari: Ixodida): a world list of valid tick names. *Exp. Appl. Acarol.* 28, 27–54. doi: 10.1023/A:1025381712339

Horton, K. C., Fahmy, N. T., Watany, N., Zayed, A., Mohamed, A., Ahmed, A. A., et al. (2016). Crimean congo hemorrhagic fever virus and alkhurma (alkhumra) virus in ticks in Djibouti. *Vector Borne Zoonotic Dis.* 16, 680–682. doi: 10.1089/vbz.2016.1951

Hovius, J. W., Levi, M., and Fikrig, E. (2008). Salivating for knowledge: potential pharmacological agents in tick saliva. *PLoS Med.* 5:e43. doi: 10.1371/journal.pmed.0050043

Jaenson, T. G. T., Hjertqvist, M., Bergstrom, T., and Lundkvist, Å. (2012). Why is tick-borne encephalitis increasing? A review of the key factors causing the increasing incidence of human TBE in Sweden. *Parasit. Vectors* 5:184. doi: 10.1186/1756-3305-5-184

Jameson, L. J., Morgan, P. J., Medlock, J. M., Watola, G., and Vaux, A. G. (2012). Importation of *Hyalomma marginatum*, vector of Crimean-Cong haemorrhagic fever virus, into the United Kingdom by migratory birds. *Ticks Tick Borne Dis.* 3, 95–99. doi: 10.1016/j.ttbdis.2011.12.002

Jones, L. D., Davies, C. R., Steele, G. M., and Nuttall, P. A. (1987). A novel mode of arbovirus transmission involving a nonviraemic host. *Science* 237, 775–777. doi: 10.1126/science.3616608

Jones, L. D., Hodgson, E., and Nuttall, P. A. (1989). Enhancement of virus transmission by tick salivary glands. *J. Gen. Virol.* 70, 1895–1898. doi: 10.1099/0022-1317-70-7-1895

Jones, L. D., Matthewson, M., and Nuttall, P. A. (1992). Saliva-activated transmission (SAT) of Thogoto virus: dynamics of SAT factor activity in the salivary glands of *Rhipicephalus appendiculatus*, *Amblyomma variegatum*, and *Boophilus microplus* ticks. *Exp. Appl. Acarol.* 13, 241–248. doi: 10.1007/BF01195081

Karbowiak, G., Biernat, B., Werszko, J., and Rychlik, L. (2016). The transstadial persistence of tick-borne encephalitis virus in *Dermacentor reticulatus* ticks in natural conditions. *Acta Parasitol.* 61, 201–203. doi: 10.1515/ap-2016-0028

Karim, S., and Ribiero, J. M. (2015). An insight into the sialome of the lone star tick, *Ambylomma americanum*, with a glimpse on its time dependent gene expression. *PLoS ONE* 10:e0131292. doi: 10.1371/journal.pone.0131292

Karti, S. S., Odabasi, Z., Korten, V., Yilmaz, M., Sonmez, M., Caylan, R., et al. (2004). Crimean-congo hemorrhagic fever in Turkey. *Emerg. Infect. Dis.* 10, 1379–1384. doi: 10.3201/eid1008.030928

Khoury, M. Y., Hull, R. C., Bryant, P. W., Escuyer, K. L., George, K. S., Wong, S. J., et al. (2013). Diagnosis of acute deer tick virus encephalitis. *Clin. Infect. Dis.* 56, e40–e47. doi: 10.1093/cid/cis938

Kosoy, O. I., Lambert, A. J., Hawkinson, D. J., Patula, D. M., Goldsmith, C. S., Hunt, D. C., et al. (2015). Novel thogotovirus associated with febrile illness and death, United States, 2014. *Emerg. Infect. Dis.* 21, 760–764. doi: 10.3201/eid2105.150150

Kuno, G., Artsob, H., Karabatsos, N., Tsuchiya, K. R., and Chang, G. J. (2001). Genomic sequencing of deer tick virus and phylogeny of powassan-related viruses of North America. *Am. J. Trop. Med. Hyg.* 65, 671–676. doi: 10.4269/ajtmh.2001.65.671

Labuda, M., Jones, L. D., Williams, T., and Nuttall, P. A. (1993). Enhancement of tick-borne encephalitis virus transmission by tick salivary gland extracts. *Med. Vet. Entomol.* 7, 193–196. doi: 10.1111/j.1365-2915.1993.tb00674.x

Labuda, M., and Nuttall, P. A. (2004). Tick-borne viruses. *Parasitology* 129, S221–S245. doi: 10.1017/S0031182004005220

Labuda, M., Trimnell, A. R., Licková, M., Kazimirová, M., Davies, G. M., Lissina, O., et al. (2006). An antivector vaccine protects against a lethal vector-borne pathogen. *PLoS Pathog.* 2:e27. doi: 10.1371/journal.ppat.0020027

Lam, T. T., Liu, W., Bowden, T. A., Cui, N., Zhuang, L., Liu, K., et al. (2013). Evolutionary and molecular analysis of the emergent severe fever with thrombocytopenia syndrome virus. *Epidemics* 1, 1–10. doi: 10.1016/j.epidem.2012.09.002

Leonova, G. N., Kondratov, I. G., Ternovoi, V. A., Romanova, E. V., Protopopova, E. V., Chausov, E. V., et al. (2009). Characterisation of Powassan viruses from Far Eastern Russia. *Arch. Virol.* 154, 811–820. doi: 10.1007/s00705-009-0376-y

Levi, T., Kilpatrick, A. M., Mangel, M., and Wilmers, C. C. (2012). Deer, predators, and the emergence of Lyme disease. *Proc. Natl. Acad. Sci. U.S.A.* 109, 10942–10947. doi: 10.1073/pnas.1204536109

Li, D. X. (2013). A highly pathogenic new bunyavirus emerged in China. *Emerg. Microb. Infect.* 2:e1. doi: 10.1038/emi.2013.1

Liu, Q., He, B., Huang, S.-Y., Wei, F., and Zhu, X.-Q. (2014). Severe fever with thrombocytopenia syndrome, an emerging tick-borne zoonosis. *Lancet Infect. Dis.* 14, 763–772. doi: 10.1016/S1473-3099(14)70718-2

Luo, L. M., Zhao, L., Wen, H. L., Zhang, Z. T., Liu, J. W., Fang, L. Z., et al (2015). *Haemaphysalis longicornis* ticks as reservoir and vector of severe fever with thrombocytopenia syndrome in China. *Emerg. Infect. Dis.* 21, 1770–1776. doi: 10.3201/eid2110.150126

Mansfield, K. L., Banyard, A. C., McElhinney, L. M., Johnson, N., Horton, D. L., Hernández-Triana, L. M., et al. (2015). Rift valley fever virus: a review of diagnosis and vaccination, and implications for emergence in Europe. *Vaccine* 33, 5520–5531. doi: 10.1016/j.vaccine.2015.08.020

Mansfield, K. L., Cook, C., Ellis, R., Bell-Sakyi, L., Johnson, N., Alberdi, P., et al. (2017). Tick-borne pathogens induce differential expression of genes promoting cell survival and host resistence in *Ixodes ricinus* cells. *Parasit. Vectors* 10:81. doi: 10.1186/s13071-017-2011-1

Mansfield, K. L., Johnson, N., Phipps, L. P., Stephenson, J. R., Fooks, A. R., and Solomon, T. (2009). Tick-borne encephalitis virus – a review of an emerging zoonosis. *J. Gen. Virol.* 90, 1781–1794. doi: 10.1099/vir.0.011437-0

Maruyama, S. R., Garcia, G. R., Teixeira, F. R., Brandão, L. G., Anderson, J. M., Ribiero, J., et al. (2017). Mining a differential sialotranscriptome of *Rhipicephalus microplus* guides antigen discovery to formulate a vaccine that reduces tick infestations. *Parasit. Vectors* 10:206. doi: 10.1186/s13071-017-2136-2

Matsuno, K., Weisend, C., Kajihara, M., Williamson, B. N., Simuunza, M., Mweene, A. S., et al. (2015). Comprehensive molecular detection of tick-borne phleboviruses leads to the retrospective identification of taxonomically unassigned bunyaviruses and the discovery of a novel member of the genus phlebovirus. *J. Virol.* 89, 594–604. doi: 10.1128/jvi.02704-14

McLean, D. M., and Donohue, L. (1959). Powassan virus: isolation of virus from a fatal case of enecephalitis. *Can. Med. J.* 80, 708–711.

McLean, D. M., Cobb, C., Gooderham, S. E., Smart, C. A., Wilson, A. G., and Wilson, W. E. (1967). Powassan virus: persistence of virus activity during 1966. *Can. Med. J.* 96, 660–664.

McMullan, L. K., Folk, S. M., Kelly, A. J., MacNeil, A., Goldsmith, C. S., Metcalfe, M. G., et al. (2012). A new phlebovirus associated with severe febrile illness in Missouri. *N. Engl. J. Med.* 367, 834–841. doi: 10.1056/NEJMoa1203378

McNally, K. L., Mitzel, D. N., Anderson, J. M., Ribeiro, J. M. C., Valenzuela, J. G., Myers, T. G., et al. (2012). Differential salivary gland transcript expression profile in *Ixodes scapularis* nymphs upon feeding or flavivirus infection. *Tick Tick Borne Dis.* 3, 18–26. doi: 10.1016/j.ttbdis.2011.09.003

Mehla, R., Kumar, S. R. P., Yadav, P., Barde, P. V., Yergolkar, P. N., Erickson, B. R., et al. (2009). Recent ancestry of Kyasanur Forest disease virus. *Emerg. Infect. Dis.* 15, 1431–1437. doi: 10.3201/eid1509.080759

Memish, Z. A., Balkhy, H. H., Francis, C., Cunningham, G., Hajeer, A. H., and Almuneef, M. A. (2005). Alkhumra haemorrhagic fever: case report and infection control details. *Br. J. Biomed. Sci.* 62, 37–39.

Mercado-Curiel, R. F., Palmer, G. H., Guerro, F. D., and Brayton, K. A. (2011). Temporal characterisation of the organ-specific *Rhipicephalus microplus* transcriptional response to *Anaplasma marginale* infection. *Int. J. Parasitol.* 41, 851–860. doi: 10.1016/j.ijpara.2011.03.003

Mertens, M., Schmidt, K., Ozkul, A., and Groschup, M. H. (2013). The impact of Crimean-Congo hemorrhagic fever virus on public health. *Antiviral Res.* 98, 248–260. doi: 10.1016/j.antiviral.2013.02.007

Morikawa, S., Saijo, M., and Kurane, I. (2007). Recent progress in molecular biology of Crimean-Congo hemorrhagic fever. *Comp. Immunol. Microbiol. Infect. Dis.* 30, 375–389. doi: 10.1016/j.cimid.2007.07.001

Mourya, D. T., and Yadav, P. D. (2016). Recent scenario of emergence of Kyasanur Forest disease in India and public health importance. *Curr. Trop. Med. Rep.* 3, 7–13. doi: 10.1007/s40475-016-0067-1

Mourya, D. T., Yadav, P. D., Mehla, R., Barde, P. V., Yergolkar, P. N., Kumar, S. R., et al. (2012). Diagnosis of Kyasanur Forest disease by nested RT-PCR, real-time RT-PCR and IgM capture ELISA. *J. Virol. Methods* 186, 49–54. doi: 10.1016/j.jviromet.2012.07.019

Mourya, D. T., Yadav, P. D., Sandhya, V. K., and Reddy, S. (2013). Spread of kyasanur forest disease, Bandipur Tiger Reserve, India, 2012–2013. *Emerg. Infect. Dis.* 19, 1540–1541. doi: 10.3201/eid1909.121884

Mur, L., Atzeni, M., Marinez-López, B., Felizani, F., Rolescu, S., and Sanchez-Vizcaino, J. M. (2016). Thirty-five year presence of African swine fever in Sardinia: history, evolution and risk factors for disease maintenance. *Transbound Emerg. Dis.* 63, e165–e177. doi: 10.1111/tbed.12264

Murhekar, M. V., Kasabi, G. S., Mehendale, S. M., Mourya, D. T., Yadav, P. D., and Tandale, B. V. (2015). On the transmission pattern of Kyasanur Forest disease (KFD) in India. *Infect. Dis. Pov.* 4:37. doi: 10.1186/s40249-015-0066-9

Palomar, A. M., Portillo, A., Mazuelas, D., Roncero, L., Arizaga, J., Crespo, A., et al. (2016). Molecular analysis of Crimean-Congo hemorrhagic fever virus and Rickettsia in *Hyalomma marginatum* ticks removed from patients (Spain) and birds (Spain and Morocco), 2009–2015. *Ticks Tick Borne Dis.* 7, 983–987. doi: 10.1016/j.ttbdis.2016.05.004

Papa, A., Papadimitriou, E., Bozvić, B., and Antoniadis, A. (2005). Genetic characterization of the M RNA segment of a Balkan Crimean-Congo hemorrhagic fever virus strain. *J. Med. Virol.* 75, 466–469. doi: 10.1002/jmv.20290

Pavri, K. M., and Casals, J. (1966). Kaisodi virus, a new agent isolated from *Haemaphysalis spinigera* in Mysore state, South India. *Am J. Trop. Med. Hyg.* 15, 961–963. doi: 10.4269/ajtmh.1966.15.961

Pesko, K. N., Torres-Perez, F., Hjelle, B. L., and Ebel, G. D. (2010). Molecular epidemiology of Powassan virus in North America. *J. Gen. Virol.* 91, 2698–2705. doi: 10.1099/vir.0.024232-0

Piantadosi, A., Rubin, D. B., McQuillen, D. P., Hsu, L., Lederer, P. A., Ashbaugh, C. D., et al. (2016). Emerging cases of Powassan virus encephalitis in New England: clinical presentation, imaging and review of the literature. *Clin. Infect. Dis.* 62, 707–713. doi: 10.1093/cid/civ1005

Pietschmann, J., Mur, L., Blome, S., Beer, M., Pérez-Sánchez, R., Oleaga, A., et al. (2016). African swine fever virus transmission cycles in Central Europe: evaluation of wild boar-soft tick contacts through detection of antibodies against *Ornithodoros erraticus* saliva antigen. *BMC Vet. Res.* 12:1. doi: 10.1186/s12917-015-0629-9

Randolph, S. E. (2009). Tick-borne disease systems emerge from the shadows: the beauty lies in molecular detail, the message in epidemiology. *Parasitology* 136, 1403–1413. doi: 10.1017/S0031182009005782

Randolph, S. E., Mikloisová, D., Lysy, J., Rogers, D. J., and Labuda, M. (1999). Incidence from coincidence: patterns of tick infestations on rodents facilitate transmission of tick-borne encephalitis. *Parasitology* 118, 177–186. doi: 10.1017/S0031182098003643

Reháček, J. (1962). Transovarial transmission of tick-borne encephalitis virus by ticks. *Acta Virol.* 6, 220–226.

Rennie, L., Wilkinson, P. J., and Mellor, P. S. (2001). Transovarial transmission of African swine fever virus in the argasid tick *Ornithodoros moubata*. *Med. Vet. Entomol.* 15, 140–146. doi: 10.1046/j.1365-2915.2001.00282.x

Ribeiro, J. M., Slovák, M., and Francischetti, I. M. (2017). An insight into the sialome of *Hyalomma excavatum*. *Ticks Tick Borne Dis.* 8, 201–207. doi: 10.1016/j.ttbdis.2016.08.011

Ribeiro, R., Otte, J., Madeira, S., Hutchings, G. H., and Boinas, F. (2015). Experimental infection of *Ornithodoros erraticus* sensu stricto with two Portuguese African swine fever virus strains. Study of factors involved in the dynamics of infection in ticks. *PLoS ONE* 10:e0137718. doi: 10.1371/journal.pone.0137718

Rowlands, R. J., Michaud, V., Heath, L., Hutchings, G., Oura, C., Vosloo, W., et al. (2008). African swine fever virus isolate, Georgia, 2007. *Emerg. Infect. Dis.* 14, 1870–1874. doi: 10.3201/eid1412.080591

Růžek, D., Yakimenko, V. V., Karan, L. S., and Tkachev, D. E. (2010). Omsk haemorrhagic fever. *Lancet* 376, 2104–2113. doi: 10.1016/S0140-6736(10)61120-8

Sadanandane, C., Elango, A., Marja, N., Sasidharan, P. V., Raju, K. H., and Jamblingam, P. (2017). An outbreak of Kyasanur Forest disease in the Wayanad and Malappuram districts of Kerala, India. *Ticks Tick Borne Dis.* 8, 25–30. doi: 10.1016/j.ttbdis.2016.09.010

Savage, H. M., Godsey, M. S. Jr., Panella, N. A., Burkhalter, K. L., Ashley, D. C., Lash, R. R., et al. (2016). Surveillance for Heartland virus (Bunyaviridae: Phlebovirus) in Missouri during 2013: first detection of virus in adults of *Ambylomma americanum* (Acari: Ixodidae). *J. Med. Entomol.* 53, 607–612. doi: 10.1093/jme/tjw028

Shimada, S., Aoki, K., Nabeshima, T., Fuxun, Y., Kurosaki, Y., Shiogama, K., et al. (2016). Tofla virus: a newly identified Nairovirus of the Crimean-Congo hemorrhagic fever group isolated from ticks in Japan. *Sci. Rep.* 6:20213. doi: 10.1038/srep20213

Simpson, D. I., Knight, E. M., Courtois, G., Williams, M. C., Weinbern, M. P., and Kibukamusoke, J. W. (1967). Congo virus: a hitherto undescribed virus occurring in Africa. Human isolations-clinical notes. *East Afr. Med. J.* 44:87.

Singh, K. R., Pavri, K., and Anderson, C. R. (1963). Experimental transovarial transmission of Kyasanur forest disease virus in *Haemaphysalis spinigera*. *Nature* 199:513. doi: 10.1038/199513a0

Stockman, S. (1918). Louping-ill. *J. Comp. Pathol. Ther.* 31, 137–193. doi: 10.1016/S0368-1742(18)80019-4

Tandale, B. V., Balakrishnan, A., Yadav, P. D., Marja, N., and Mourya, D. T. (2015). New focus of Kyasanur Forest disease virus activity in a tribal area in Keral, India, 2014. *Infect. Dis. Pov.* 4:12. doi: 10.1186/s40249-015-0044-2

Tavakoli, N. P., Wang, H., Dupuis, M., Hull, R., Ebel, G. D., Gilmore, E. J., et al. (2009). Fatal case of deer tick virus encephalitis. *N. Engl. J. Med.* 360, 2099–2107. doi: 10.1056/NEJMoa0806326

Telford, S. R., Armstrong, P. M., Katavolos, P., Foppa, I., Garcia, A. S. O., Wilson, M. L., et al. (1997). A new tick-borne encephalitis-like virus infecting New England deer ticks, *Ixodes dammini*. *Emerg. Infect. Dis.* 3, 165–170. doi: 10.3201/eid0302.970209

Thomas, L. A., Kennedy, R. C., and Eklund, C. M. (1960). Isolation of a virus closely related to Powasson virus from *Dermacentor andersoni* collected along North Cache la Poudre River, Colorado. *Proc. Soc. Exp. Biol. Med.* 104, 355–359. doi: 10.3181/00379727-104-25836

Thomson, G. R. (1985). The epidemiology of African swine fever: the role of free-living hosts in Africa. Ondestepoort *J. Vet. Res.* 52, 201–209.

Trapido, H., Rajagopalan, P. K., Work, R. H., and Varma, M. G. (1959). Kayasanur Forest disease. VIII. Isolation of Kayasanur Forest disease virus from naturally infected ticks of the genus Haemaphysalis. *Indian J. Med. Res.* 47, 133–138.

Vannier, E. G., Diuk-Wasser, M. A., Ben Mamoun, C., and Krause, P. J. (2015). Babesiosis. *Infect. Dis. Clin. North Am.* 29, 358–370. doi: 10.1016/j.idc.2015.02.008

Villar, M., Marina, A., and de la Fuente, J. (2017). Applying proteomics to tick vaccine development: where are we? *Expert Rev. Proteomics* 14, 211–221. doi: 10.1080/14789450.2017.1284590

Wang, J., Zhang, H., Fu, S., Wang, H., Ni, D., Nasci, R., et al. (2009). Isolation of Kyasanur forest disease virus from febrile patient, Yannan, China. *Emerg. Infect. Dis.* 15, 326–328. doi: 10.3201/eid1502.080979

Whitney, E., and Jamnback, H. (1965). The first isolations of Powassan virus in New York State. *Proc. Soc. Exp. Biol. Med.* 119, 432–435. doi: 10.3181/00379727-119-30202

Work, T. H., and Trapido, H. (1957). Summary of preliminary report of investigations of the virus research centre on an epidemic disease affecting forest villagers and wild monkeys in Shimoga district, Mysore. *Indian J. Med. Sci.* 11, 340–341.

Xing, Z., Schefers, J., Schwabenlander, M., Jiao, Y., Liang, M., Qi, X., et al. (2013). Novel bunyavirus in domestic and captive animals, Minnesota, USA. *Emerg. Infect. Dis.* 19, 1487–1489. doi: 10.3201/eid1908.130165

Yadav, P. D., Shete, A. M., Patil, D. Y., Sandhya, V. K., Prakash, K. S., Surgihalli, R., et al. (2014). Outbreak of Kyasanur Forest disease in Thirthahalli, Karnataka, India, 2014. *Int. J. Infect. Dis.* 26, 132–134. doi: 10.1016/j.ijid.2014.05.013

Zaki, A. M. (1997). Isolation of a flavivirus related to the tick-borne encephalitis complex from human cases in saudi arabia. *Trans. R. Soc. Trop. Med. Hyg.* 91, 179–181. doi: 10.1016/S0035-9203(97)90215-7

Zhang, Y. Z., He, Y. W., Dai, Y. A., Xiong, Y., Zheng, H., Zhou, D. J., et al. (2012a). Hemorrhagic fever caused by a novel Bunyavirus in China: pathogenesis and correlates of fatal outcome. *Clin. Infect. Dis.* 54, 527–533. doi: 10.1093/cid/cir804

Zhang, Y. Z., and Xu, J. (2016). The emergence and cross species transmission of newly discovered tick-borne bunyavirus in China. *Curr. Opin. Virol.* 16, 126–131. doi: 10.1016/j.coviro.2016.02.006

Zhang, Y. Z., Zhou, D. J., Qin, X. C., Tian, J. H., Xiong, Y., Wang, J. B., et al. (2012b). The ecology, genetic diversity, and phylogeny of Huaiyangshan virus in China. *J. Virol.* 86, 2864–2868. doi: 10.1128/JVI.061 92-11

13

Modeling Modulation of the Tick Regulome in Response to *Anaplasma phagocytophilum* for the Identification of New Control Targets

Sara Artigas-Jerónimo[1†], Agustín Estrada-Peña[2†], Alejandro Cabezas-Cruz[3], Pilar Alberdi[1], Margarita Villar[1] and José de la Fuente[1,4*]

[1] SaBio, Instituto de Investigación en Recursos Cinegéticos IREC-CSIC-UCLM-JCCM, Ciudad Real, Spain, [2] Facultad de Veterinaria, Universidad de Zaragoza, Zaragoza, Spain, [3] UMR BIPAR, INRA, ANSES, Ecole Nationale Vétérinaire d'Alfort, Université Paris-Est, Maisons-Alfort, France, [4] Department of Veterinary Pathobiology, Center for Veterinary Health Sciences, Oklahoma State University, Stillwater, OK, United States

***Correspondence:**
José de la Fuente
jose_delafuente@yahoo.com

† These authors have contributed equally to this work

Ticks act as vectors of pathogens affecting human and animal health worldwide, and recent research has focused on the characterization of tick-pathogen interactions using omics technologies to identify new targets for developing novel control interventions. The regulome (transcription factors-target genes interactions) plays a critical role in cell response to pathogen infection. Therefore, the application of regulomics to tick-pathogen interactions would advance our understanding of these molecular interactions and contribute to the identification of novel control targets for the prevention and control of tick infestations and tick-borne diseases. However, limited information is available on the role of tick regulome in response to pathogen infection. In this study, we applied complementary *in silico* approaches to modeling how *Anaplasma phagocytophilum* infection modulates tick vector regulome. This proof-of-concept research provided support for the use of network analysis in the study of regulome response to infection, resulting in new information on tick-pathogen interactions and potential targets for developing interventions for the control of tick infestations and pathogen transmission. Deciphering the precise nature of circuits that shape the tick regulome in response to pathogen infection is an area of research that in the future will advance our knowledge of tick-pathogen interactions, and the identification of new antigens for the control of tick infestations and pathogen infection/transmission.

Keywords: regulome, transcription, tick, *Ixodes scapularis*, *Anaplasma phagocytophilum*, ISE6 cells, vaccine

INTRODUCTION

Ticks (Acari: Ixodida) are major vectors of pathogens affecting human and animal health worldwide, and consequently the focus of research for developing novel control interventions (de la Fuente, 2018). Among tick-transmitted pathogens, *Anaplasma phagocytophilum* (Alphaproteobacteria: Rickettsiales) is mainly transmitted by *Ixodes* spp. and the causative agent of human and animal anaplasmosis and tick-borne fever in small ruminants (Severo et al., 2015).

Recent developments in tick genomics have advanced research using latest omics technologies for the characterization of tick-host-pathogen interactions and the identification of candidate protective antigens (de la Fuente et al., 2016c,a, 2017; Gulia-Nuss et al., 2016; Shaw et al., 2017; de la Fuente, 2018). Vaccinomics, a holistic perspective based on the use of omics technologies and bioinformatics in a systems biology approach for the characterization of tick-host-pathogen molecular interactions is our platform for the identification of candidate vaccine antigens (de la Fuente and Merino, 2013; de la Fuente et al., 2016a, 2018; Contreras et al., 2017). In this context, tick cell lines constitute a valuable resource because it is a proven model for the study of tick-pathogen and particularly tick-*A. phagocytophilum* interactions, easy manipulation without animal experimentation, and the fact that *A. phagocytophilum* infects mainly one cell type in vertebrates (neutrophils) but multiple cell types in ticks better resembled by these cell lines (Munderloh et al., 1994; Severo et al., 2015; Villar et al., 2015; Bell-Sakyi et al., 2018).

The regulome (transcription factors-target genes interactions) and interactome (protein-protein physical and functional interactions) play a critical role in cell response to different stimuli including pathogen infection. Both regulome and interactome are implicated in transcriptional regulation, which is one of the most fundamental mechanisms for controlling the amount of protein produced by cells under different environmental and physiological conditions and developmental stages (Gronostajski et al., 2011; Vaquerizas et al., 2012; Shih et al., 2016; Rioualen et al., 2017). Therefore, the application of regulomics and interactomics to host/tick-pathogen interactions would advance our understanding of these molecular interactions and contribute to the identification of new control targets for the prevention and control of tick infestations and tick-borne diseases (de la Fuente et al., 2018; Artigas-Jerónimo et al., 2018a,b; Estrada-Peña et al., 2018).

Few studies have addressed the role of the regulome or regulon (part of the regulome including a set of genes that share a common regulatory element binding site) in the interaction between tick-borne pathogens and vertebrate hosts (i.e., Bugrysheva et al., 2015; Boyle et al., 2019). However, limited information is available on the role of tick regulome in response to pathogen infection (Artigas-Jerónimo et al., 2018b).

In this study, we applied complementary *in silico* approaches to modeling how *A. phagoctophilum* infection modulates tick vector regulome, and the possibilities for the identification of new control target antigens. This proof-of-concept research provided new information on tick-pathogen interactions and potential targets for developing interventions for the control of tick infestations and pathogen infection.

MATERIALS AND METHODS

Datasets

The RNA sequencing (RNAseq) datasets of differential expression of *I. scapularis* transcription factors (TF) and target genes (TG) in response to *A. phagocytophilum* infection was obtained from previously published transcriptomics analyses in ISE6 cells, and fed adult female midguts and salivary glands (Ayllón et al., 2015; Villar et al., 2015). Gene ontology (GO) level-3 annotations for biological processes (BP) were conducted using Blast2GO software (version 3.0)[1] (Villar et al., 2014; **Supplementary Dataset 1**). The RNAseq data is available at http://dx.doi.org/10.5061/dryad.50kt0 and http://www.ncbi.nlm.nih.gov/geo/query/acc.cgi?acc=GSE68881.

Network Analysis of the Tick Regulome in Response to Infection

A network of interactions followed by a co-correspondence analysis (CoCA) was used for the integration of TF and TG interactions (regulome) of *I. scapularis* tick response to *A. phagocytophilum* infection. The methodology to build the network of interactions between proteins and functional metabolic processes has been previously described and validated (Estrada-Peña et al., 2018). This network consists of a set of nodes that are connected by edges where nodes are the interacting items, and links between nodes represent the strength with which they interact. In this development, a TF or TG is the source node and the cell metabolic process(es) in which it is involved are the target(s). The edge linking both nodes has a weight, which is the expression of either TF or TG. Networks were built separately for infected and uninfected *I. scapularis* ISE6 cells, salivary glands and midguts. Only TF and TG with GO functional annotations were included in the networks (**Supplementary Dataset 1**). Centrality is a fundamental property of a network because it refers to nodes that connect high score nodes (Opsahl et al., 2010; Estrada-Peña et al., 2018). In this context, "high score" applies to other nodes with high importance in the network. We calculated the importance of a node in the "traffic" between different nodes of the network using Betweenness Centrality (BNC), giving a higher score to a node that sits on many shortest paths of other node pairs (Barthelemy, 2004; Estrada-Peña et al., 2018). In our context, it is an indicator of the relative importance of a TF/TG in the links between two or more processes. Other calculated indexes included the PageRank (PR), a measure of the importance of the nodes linking with a given node, and the Weighted Degree (WD), which was calculated from the expression profile of each TF/TG linking to a cell process (Estrada-Peña et al., 2018).

The interactions between TF and TG were demonstrated using CoCA. Only TF/TG with values of BNC or PR higher than zero were included. We did the CoCA using the indexes of centrality obtained from the network explained above. The function "coca" of the package "cocorresp" was used for the R programming environment (Simpson, 2016). Data on BNC, PR and WD of each infected and uninfected datasets from ISE6 cells, salivary glands and midguts were entered into separate CoCAs. The analysis aimed to relate two different datasets from uninfected and infected samples to find patterns that are common to both and associating the TF and TG that are close in the reduced multivariate space and establishing correspondences. The plotting of the scores in the two first axes of the reduced space gives the interaction between TF and TG, i.e., the closer

[1] www.blast2go.com

they are in the space, the higher is the expected interaction. The method produces a cloud of interacting TF and TG. To improve the resolution of the charts, we plotted only TF/TG that were at a maximum of two score units of distance. We assumed that other TG separated by more than 2 score units from the values of TF were not interacting with these TF.

In silico Prediction of TF-TG Interactions

Putative DNA binding sites in TG for TF present only in infected tick ISE6 cells were predicted based on published information for TF-interacting sequences in other species, and the *I. scapularis* genomic scaffold whole genome shotgun sequence using cisTargetX[2] and direct search for TF binding sequences in the predicted 5′ gene regulatory regions of the *I. scapularis* genome (**Supplementary Dataset 2**; Potier et al., 2012; Rougemont and Naef, 2012; Vaquerizas et al., 2012). The BP with higher representation in the upregulated than in downregulated regulome (peptidase inhibitor and stress response) in response to infection were selected for further characterization of TF-TG interactions.

RNA Interference (RNAi) for Gene Knockdown in Tick ISE6 Cells

The *I. scapularis* ISE6 cells (provided by U.G. Munderloh, University of Minnesota, United States) was maintained in L-15B300 medium as described previously (Munderloh et al., 1994). Four different TF (HSF, Ap-2, Arx and Hox; **Supplementary Dataset 2**) were silenced using two siRNAs for each TF (HSF: 5′ GCA CUC AGG GCC AGG AUU A 3′ and 5′ CCU CGG AAG CAG ACA GGA A 3′; Ap-2: 5′ AGA AAG AGG ACA CGA AGA A 3′ and 5′ CCA AGA AAG AGG ACA CGA A 3′; Arx: 5′ CCA AGA AAG AGG ACA CGA A 3′ and 5′ GAC CGA AGC CAG AGU GCA A 3′; Hox: 5′ CCU CCA GCU UCA ACA CAU A 3′ and 5′ ACG CCA CGG CCG AGC UUA A 3′) provided by Dharmacon (GE Healthcare Dharmacon Inc., Lafayette, CO, United States). As control, two *Rs86* siRNAs (5′ CGG UAA AUG UCG AAG CAA A 3′ and 5′ GCG AAU AUG AAG UCG GUA A 3′) were used. The siRNA experiments were conducted by incubating ISE6 tick cells with 100 nM of each siRNA diluted in 100 μl of serum-free medium in 24-well plates using four wells per treatment. To facilitate siRNA transfection, DharmaFECT (GE Healthcare Dharmacon Inc.) was used following manufacturer's recommendations. After 24 h, 0.5 ml/well of fresh medium was added. After 48 h of siRNA exposure, medium containing siRNA was removed and replaced with 1 ml fresh medium alone or containing cell free *A. phagocytophilum* NY18 obtained as previously reported (de la Fuente et al., 2005). Cells were incubated for a total of 72 h, and then collected for DNA and RNA extraction.

Determination of Gene Knockdown and TG mRNA Levels by RT-qPCR

Total RNA was extracted from ISE6 cells using All Prep DNA/RNA/PROTEIN Mini Kit (Qiagen, Hilden, Germany) following manufacturer's recommendations. Gene knockdown levels after TF RNAi were assessed for TF and TG by RT-qPCR on RNA samples using gene-specific oligonucleotide primers (**Supplementary Table 1**), the Kapa SYBR Fast One-Step RT-qPCR Kit (Kapa Biosystems, Roche Holding AG, Basel, Switzerland), and the QIAGEN Rotor-Gene Real-Time PCR Detection System (Qiagen). A dissociation curve was run at the end of the reaction to ensure that only one amplicon was formed and that the amplicons denatured consistently in the same temperature range for every sample. The mRNA levels were normalized against tick *rps4* using the genNorm method [Delta-Delta-Ct (ddCt) method] as described previously (Ayllón et al., 2013). Normalized Ct values were compared between test siRNAs-treated tick cells and controls treated with *Rs86* siRNA by Chi^2-test ($p = 0.05$; $n = 4$ biological replicates).

Determination of *A. phagocytophilum* DNA Levels by qPCR

Total DNA was extracted from infected cells using an All Prep DNA/RNA/Protein Mini Kit (Qiagen, Hilden, Germany). DNA samples were analyzed by qPCR using gene-specific primers for *A. phagocytophilum msp4* as previously described (Ayllón et al., 2013). Normalized against tick *rps4* Ct values were compared between test siRNAs-treated tick cells and controls treated with *Rs86* siRNA by Chi^2-test ($p = 0.001$; $n = 2$–4 biological replicates).

RESULTS AND DISCUSSION

Rationale and Experimental Design

The tick regulome in response to *A. phagocytophilum* infection was characterized in the *I. scapularis* tick vector to provide insights into tissue-specific regulome profiles, and the identification of potential targets for the control of tick infestations and pathogen infection/transmission. The experimental design included two independent methods for the *in silico* characterization of the tick regulome in response to *A. phagocytophilum* using transcriptomics data previously obtained from infected *I. scapularis* ISE6 cells, and fed female midguts and salivary glands (**Supplementary Figure 1A**). The first approach was based on a network analysis in which the nodes were either TF or TG together with their corresponding GO BP annotations, and the link between two nodes represented the expression of the gene (**Supplementary Figure 1B**). The indexes of centrality were calculated separately for each network of uninfected and infected samples, and only nodes of TF and TG with indexes of centrality higher than zero were used for co-correspondence CoCA analysis (**Supplementary Figure 1B**). The second approach was used in parallel with network analysis, and consisted in the *in silico* prediction of TF-TG interactions based on described TF recognition sequences by searching in the *I. scapularis* genomic scaffold whole genome shotgun sequence (**Supplementary Figure 1C**). This analysis was focused on TF present only in infected ISE6 cells, and TG in BP overrepresented in the upregulated than in the downregulated regulome in response to infection as a proof-of-concept to facilitate the

[2]https://omictools.com/cistargetx-tool

identification of candidate target antigens for development of vaccines and other control measures. The results of the network analysis were then plotted with TF and TG together in the reduced space to demonstrate that the position of the TF correlates with the TG that are near to these TF after the CoCA (**Supplementary Figure 1D**). Finally, the results of both approaches were compared, and the TF-TG interactions predicted by both methods were functionally characterized by RNAi in *A. phagocytophilum*-infected and uninfected tick ISE6 cells (**Supplementary Figure 1E**).

The *I. scapularis* Regulome Shows Tissue-Specific Signatures in Response to *A. phagocytophilum* Infection

For the construction of networks, a total of 144, 86, and 93 TF (**Supplementary Dataset 3**), and 5225, 3919, and 4341 TG (**Supplementary Dataset 4**) were used derived from tick ISE6 cells, salivary glands and midguts, respectively. Tick midgut did not show detectable differences in the network indexes of TF BP between uninfected and infected samples (close to 100% BNC; **Figure 1A**). However, the TF multicell development and anatomical structure development processes increased to near 200% in infected versus uninfected ISE6 cells (**Figure 1A**). The network centrality of all the TF processes showed a clear increase in infected salivary glands when compared to unifected controls (**Figure 1A**). The multicell development process was represented in TF from ISE6 cells only (**Figure 1A**).

Other than minor variations in the network indexes of the TF, each test showed different TF that were present or absent in either uninfected or infected samples. Four TF were detected only in uninfected ISE6 cells, and other 4 were recorded only in infected ISE6 cells (**Figure 1B**). The most prominent TF in ISE6 cells (ISCW01819) was completely inhibited in infected ISE6 cells (**Figure 1B**). The pattern was more complex in the salivary glands showing up to 17 TF recorded only in infected, and 4 in uninfected samples (**Figure 1C**). Nine TF were recorded only in uninfected and 8 only in infected midgut (**Figure 1D**). As in ISE6 cells, the three most highly represented TF in uninfected midgut were not recorded in infected samples (**Figure 1D**). The number of TG detected only in uninfected or infected samples varied from 197 (uninfected) to 206 (infected) ISE6 cells, 159 (uninfected) to 585 (infected) salivary glands, and 360 (uninfected) to 129 (infected) midgut.

Every detected TF that was unique for uninfected or infected samples was included in CoCA. Based on the values of network indexes of TG, 70 TG in uninfected and 88 TG in infected ISE6 cells, 5 TG in uninfected and 58 TG in infected salivary glands, and 43 TG in uninfected and 25 TG in infected midgut were included in the analysis. The results from multivariate analyses showed a clear correspondence between TF and TG recorded only in uninfected or infected samples while the origin of the first correspondence axis (value = 0) separated completely TF and TG occurring only in either uninfected or infected samples (**Figures 2A–C** and **Supplementary Figures 2A–C**). These analyses suggested that the TF closer to individual TG are likely to regulate the expression of these genes (**Figures 2A–C** and **Supplementary Figures 2A–C**).

These results evidenced tissue-specific differences between infected and uninfected cells, thus supporting previous findings at the mRNA, protein and metabolic levels in *I. scapularis* ISE6 cells, a model for hemocytes, midgut and salivary glands, which are involved in *A. phagocytophilum* life cycle in the tick vector (Ayllón et al., 2015; Villar et al., 2015; reviewed by de la Fuente et al., 2017). These results evidenced that the regulome regulates various BP involved in tick-*A. phagocytophilum* interactions (**Figures 1A, 3A** and **Supplementary Dataset 2**), a finding previously reported in other organisms (Shih et al., 2016; Casella et al., 2017).

A. phagocytophilum Modulates the Tick Regulome to Upregulate Biological Processes That Facilitate Pathogen Infection

To complement the network analysis approach to tick regulome study, the putative DNA binding sites were characterized *in silico* for TF and TG in the upregulated regulome in response to infection in tick vector ISE6 cells (**Figures 3A,B** and **Supplementary Dataset 2**). In particular, the peptidase inhibitor and stress response BP with higher representation in the upregulated than in downregulated regulome (**Figure 3A**) were selected for further characterization of TF-TG interactions (**Figure 3B**).

The results showed a correlation between complementary *in silico* approaches (**Figure 4A**), therefore providing support for the network analysis of the regulome to predict at the transcriptomics level the most significant TF-TG interactions in response to stimuli such as pathogen infection.

To characterize the functional implications of selected TF-TG interactions predicted by both methodological approaches (**Figures 3B, 4A**), RNAi was used in ISE6 cells to knockdown the expression of TF and characterize the effect on TG mRNA and *A. phagocytophilum* DNA levels (**Figures 4B–D**). The results showed that after 77–87% (average ± S.D., 81 ± 4%) TF silencing (**Figure 4B**), the levels of all predicted TG except for ISCW011771 and ISCW012363 decreased when compared to *Rs86* siRNA-treated controls (**Figure 4C**). The two TG that were not downregulated after TF knockdown had the lowest mRNA levels (**Figure 4C**), which could affect the possibility of detecting differences between test and control cells. Alternatively, other TF or interacting proteins could be involved in the regulation of these genes. Nevertheless, except for ISCW011771 and ISCW012363 the results supported the prediction that these TF are implicated in the regulation of TG. Nevertheless, these TF-TG interactions should be corroborated in future experiments using different *in vitro* protein-DNA binding assays (Yang, 1998; Forde and McCutchen-Maloney, 2002; Deplancke and Gheldof, 2012; Ogawa and Biggin, 2012).

Regarding *A. phagocytophilum* infection, the results showed a 96–97% decrease in pathogen DNA levels after TF knockdown (**Figure 4D**). These results suggested that the TF

A

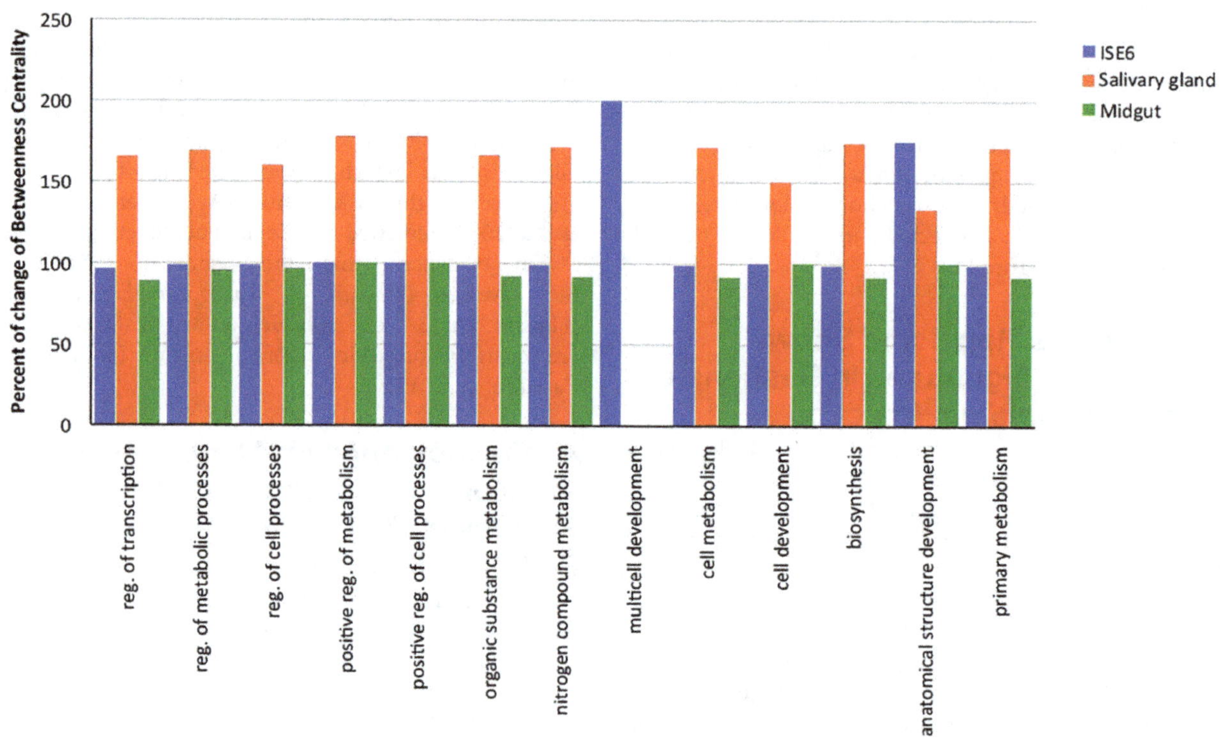

B

TF	BNC (u)	BNC (i)
ISCW006446	0.0	39.1
ISCW007820	0.0	19.7
ISCW021026	0.0	38.7
ISCW021207	0.0	39.1
ISCW008705	17.2	0.0
ISCW010324	17.2	0.0
ISCW012614	17.2	0.0
ISCW015819	93.5	0.0

C

TF	BNC (u)	BNC (i)
ISCW017832	0.0	99.0
ISCW011969	0.0	57.2
ISCW021026	0.0	56.9
ISCW023660	0.0	55.3
ISCW011796	0.0	55.3
ISCW000140	0.0	55.3
ISCW010324	0.0	15.8
ISCW018799	0.0	15.8
ISCW002484	0.0	15.8
ISCW017749	0.0	15.8
ISCW019692	0.0	15.8
ISCW019283	0.0	15.8
ISCW019280	0.0	15.8
ISCW021939	0.0	15.8
ISCW017821	0.0	15.8
ISCW020382	0.0	15.8
ISCW012211	0.0	10.8
ISCW020450	16.5	0.0
ISCW020450	16.5	0.0
ISCW024501	93.9	0.0
ISCW024501	93.9	0.0

D

TF	BNC (u)	BNC (i)
ISCW019692	0.0	15.1
ISCW024501	0.0	92.0
ISCW019280	0.0	15.1
ISCW004287	0.0	89.4
ISCW009030	0.0	15.1
ISCW015741	0.0	15.1
ISCW019283	0.0	15.1
ISCW013477	0.0	15.1
ISCW012211	15.1	0.0
ISCW012211	15.1	0.0
ISCW018799	21.8	0.0
ISCW019287	21.8	0.0
ISCW003117	21.8	0.0
ISCW008179	99.6	0.0
ISCW017832	102.3	0.0
ISCW017832	102.3	0.0
ISCW020382	279.1	0.0

FIGURE 1 | Changes in the expression of TF in tick ISE6 cells, salivary gland and midgut in response to *A. phagocytophilum* infection. **(A)** The percentage change of the index Betweenness Centrality (BNC) infection among uninfected and infected target organs in the 13 BP GO annotations. **(B)** Values of BNC of the 8 TF that showed the highest changes between uninfected BNC (u) and infected BNC (i) ISE6 cells. **(C)** Values of BNC of the 21 TF that showed the highest changes between uninfected BNC (u) and infected BNC (i) salivary glands. **(D)** Values of BNC of the 17 TF that showed the highest changes between uninfected BNC (u) and infected BNC (i) midgut. Abbreviations: reg., regulation; (u), uninfected; (i), infected.

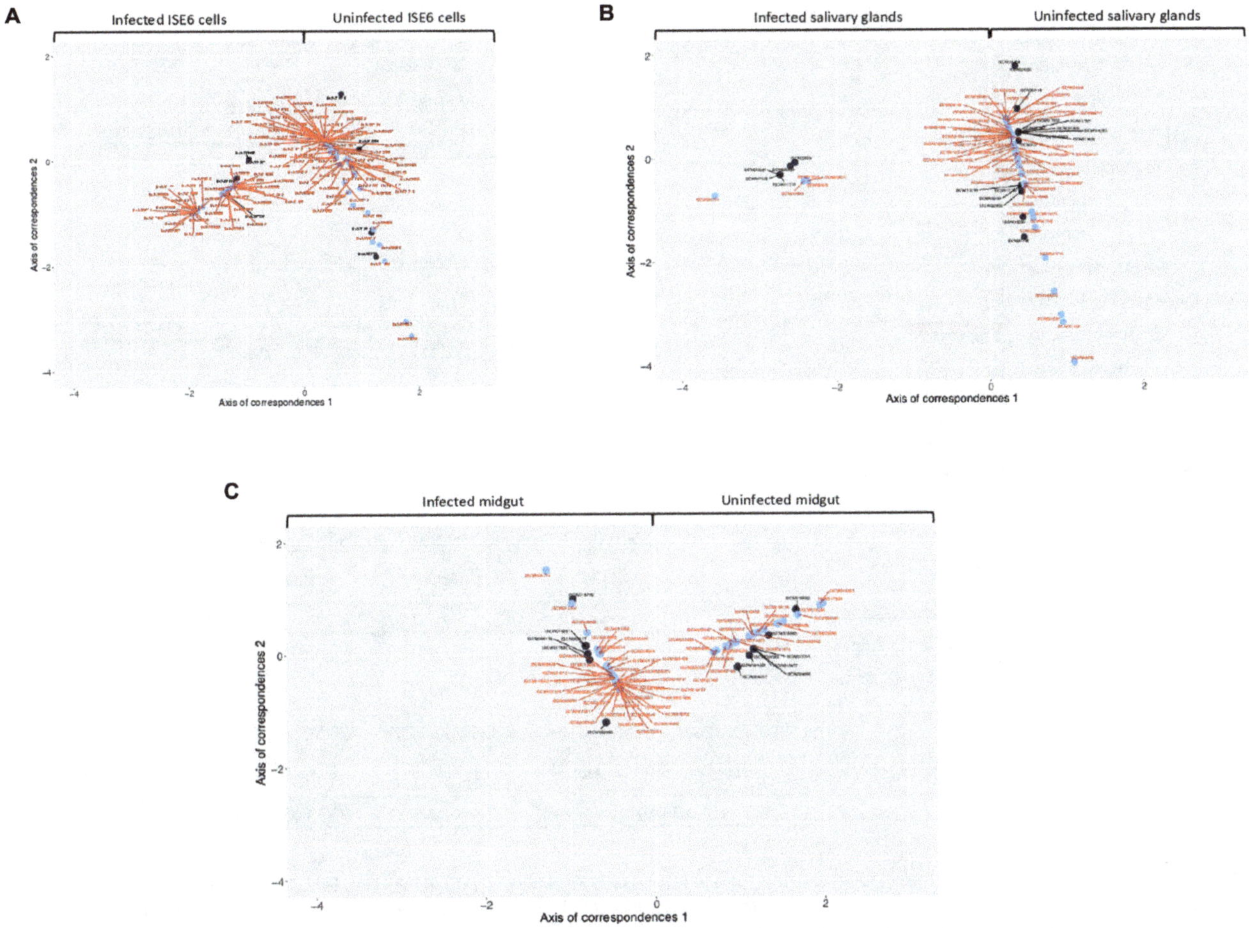

FIGURE 2 | Co-correspondence analysis (CoCA) of TF and TG in uninfected and *A. phagocytophilum*-infected samples. CoCA was conducted in *I. scapularis* **(A)** ISE6 cells, **(B)** salivary glands and **(C)** midgut. The charts show the position of TF (black symbol and label) and TG (blue symbol and red label) after the CoCA of the indexes of centrality. The TF and associated TG with highest values of centrality in the network of infected cells appear together at negative values of the Axis 1 (*n* = 4, 4, and 9 in ISE6 cells, salivary glands and midgut, respectively). The TF and the associated TG with highest values of centrality in the network of uninfected cells appear together at positive values of the Axis 1 (*n* = 4, 17, and 8 in ISE6 cells, salivary glands and midgut, respectively). High-resolution images are shown in **Supplementary Figures 2A–C**.

and corresponding TG are upregulated by *A. phagocytophilum* to facilitate pathogen infection.

Characterization of TF and Upregulated TG in Response to Infection as Putative Control Targets

The TF implicated in the regulation of selected TG included heat shock transcription factor (HSF), Ap-2, Aristaless-related homeobox gene (Arx) and Hox (**Figure 3B**). These TF has been described before to function in different transcriptionally regulated processes in other species. The mammalian Ap-2 TF has been shown to be involved in transcriptional activation and DNA binding/dimerization (Williams and Tjian, 1991). The HSF family has been implicated in the regulation of different physiological processes including cell response to stress and infection (Gomez-Pastor et al., 2018). Hox and Arx are members of a family of essential developmental regulators that bind to homeodomains target DNA sequences to regulate embryogenesis and neuronal processes in different organisms (Pellerin et al., 1994; Cho et al., 2012).

Few studies in other host-pathogen models have shown that some of these TF facilitate pathogen infection and therefore has been proposed as potential targets for control interventions. In primary peripheral blood monocytes, HSF1 is upregulated by human cytomegalovirus (HCMV) for pathogen survival, and has been suggested as a potential control target (Peppenelli et al., 2018). The tick-borne pathogen, *Ehrlichia chaffeensis*, upregulates the expression of certain Hox genes to facilitate infection through epigenetic mechanisms in human monocytic leukemia cells (THP-1) (Mitra et al., 2018). However, the role of these TF during pathogen infection in ticks has not been investigated before.

The BP modulated by the regulome of selected TF-TG interactions with a putative role in facilitating *A. phagocytophilum* infection included peptidase inhibitor

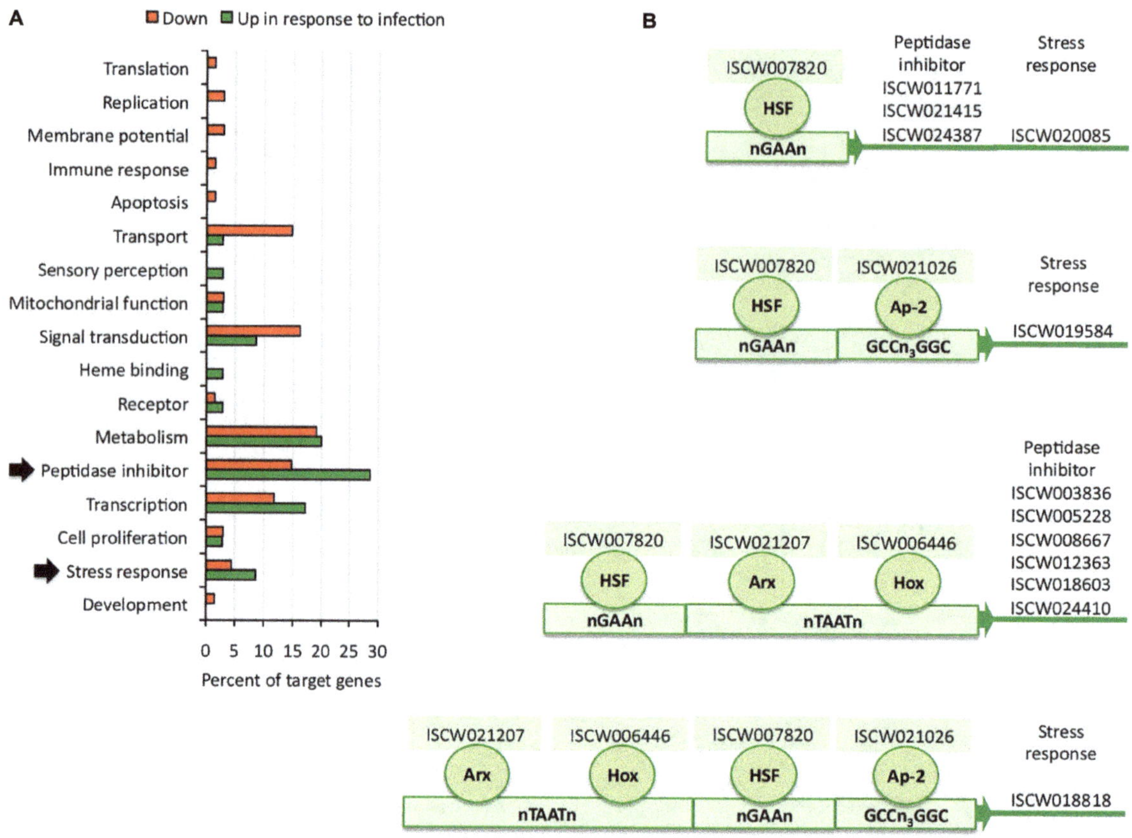

FIGURE 3 | Biological processes affected by the tick ISE6 cells regulome in response to *A. phagocytophilum* infection. **(A)** Upregulated and downregulated target genes in the *in silico* predicted tick ISE6 cells regulome in response to *A. phagocytophilum* infection were grouped according to their BP. The BP with higher representation in the upregulated than in downregulated regulome in response to infection (arrows) were selected for characterization of TF-TG interactions. **(B)** Predicted regulatory DNA motifs according to regulatory factors identified by RNAseq in infected cells only and involved in the control of upregulated target genes annotated in the peptidase inhibitor and stress response BP with higher representation in the upregulated than in downregulated regulome.

and stress response (**Figure 3A** and **Supplementary Dataset 2**). The stress response upregulated TG included genes coding for peroxinectin and uncharacterized protein with heme binding and peroxidase activity (n = 2), and glutathione peroxidase with glutathione peroxidase activity. The peptidase inhibitor TG encoded for a carboxypeptidase inhibitor precursor with carboxipeptidase and metalloendopeptidase inhibitor activity, uncharacterized protein, Kunitz-type proteinase inhibitor 5 II, serpin-2 precursors and secreted salivary gland peptides with serine-type endopeptidase inhibitor activity (n = 6), and cystatin and salivary cystatin-L with cysteine-type endopeptidase inhibitor activity (n = 2).

These proteins are involved in key physiological processes during tick life cycle such as heme/iron metabolism and detoxification and tick-host interactions (Chmelar et al., 2016; de la Fuente et al., 2016a). Glutathione peroxidase belongs to the glutathione antioxidant defense system and protects eukaryotic cells from oxidative damage (Espinosa-Diez et al., 2015). Glutathione peroxidase levels and activity are affected in different ways by *Anaplasma marginale* infection in both vertebrate and tick cells (Reddy et al., 1988; More et al., 1989; Kalil et al., 2017; Esmaeilnejad et al., 2018). While the activity and expression of glutathione peroxidase and other components of the antioxidant system was lower in *A. marginale*-infected cattle and water buffaloes (Reddy et al., 1988; More et al., 1989; Esmaeilnejad et al., 2018), glutathione peroxidase coding gene was upregulated in embryonic *Rhipicephalus microplus* BME26 cells in response to *A. marginale* infection (Kalil et al., 2017). These results showed that *A. marginale* infection induces a differential response of the glutathione antioxidant defense system in the vertebrate and tick hosts. RNAi-mediated gene silencing of glutathione peroxidase and other antioxidant defense system genes increased *A. marginale* infection in BME26 cells, suggesting that the antioxidant response mediated by this molecule might play a role in the control of infection in ticks (Kalil et al., 2017). Another of the identified tick TG, peroxinectin, is a cell adhesion protein involved in melanization of pathogens in invertebrates (Sritunyalucksana et al., 2001; Cerenius and Söderhäll, 2004), was upregulated in crayfish resistant to white spot syndrome virus, and susceptible crayfish failed to upregulate this gene in response to viral infection (Yi et al., 2017). Strong cellular adhesion in response to the invading agent during crustacean encapsulation defense reaction was proposed as a

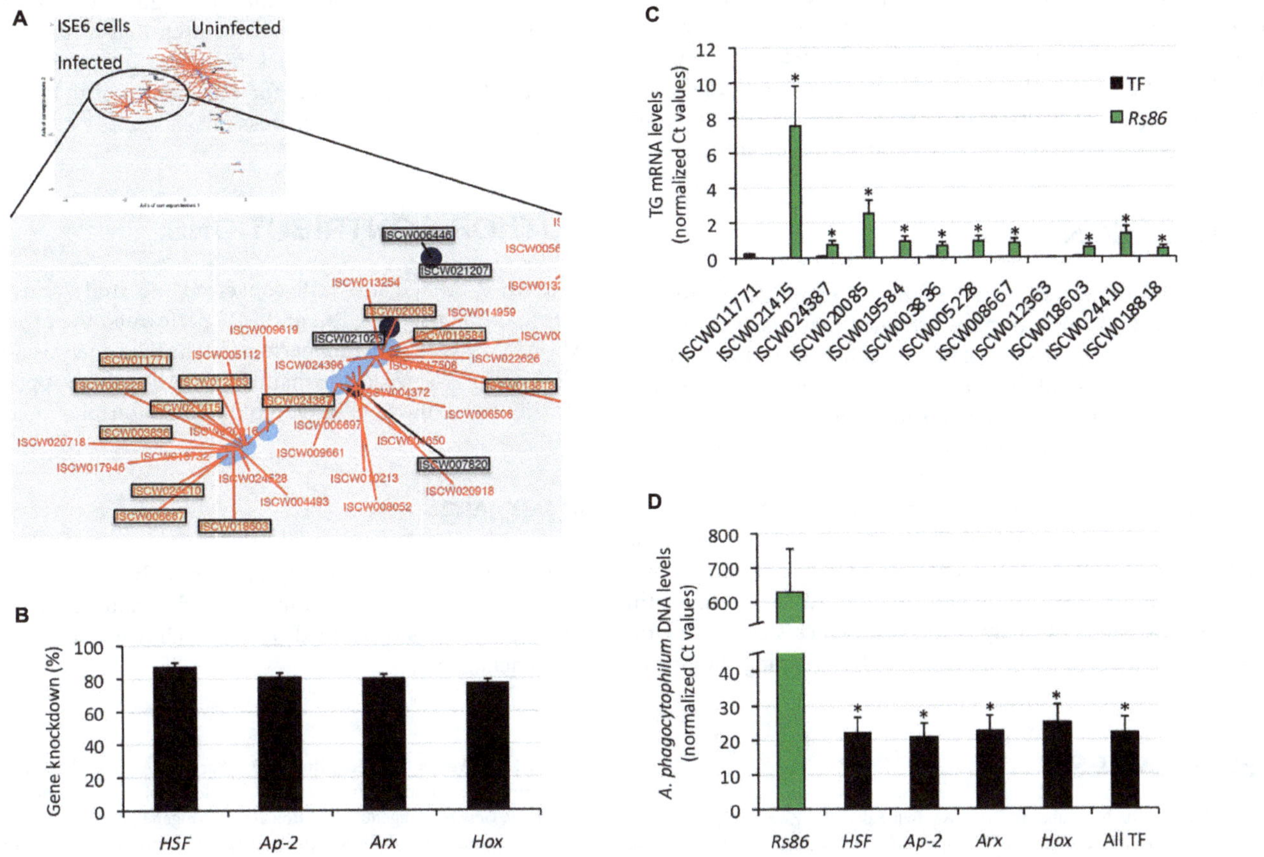

FIGURE 4 | Functional characterization of selected TF-TG components of the tick ISE6 cells regulome. **(A)** The predictive results of network analysis and *in silico* prediction of TF-TG interactions were compared in infected ISE6 cells. The TF-TG interactions predicted by both methods (squared in black letter for TF and red letter for TG) were then functionally characterized by RNAi in tick ISE6 cells. **(B)** Percentage of TF gene knockdown with respect to Rs86 siRNA control in ISE6 cells. Normalized against tick *rps4* Ct values were compared between test siRNAs-treated tick cells and controls treated with *Rs86* siRNA by Chi^2-test ($p < 0.05$; $n = 4$ biological replicates). **(C)** The TG mRNA levels were determined by qRT-PCR in ISE6 cells after TF gene knockdown or treatment with control *Rs86* siRNA. Normalized against tick *rps4* Ct values (average + S.E.) were compared between test siRNAs-treated tick cells and controls treated with *Rs86* siRNA by Chi^2-test (*$p < 0.001$; $n = 4$ biological replicates). **(D)** The *A. phagocytophilum* DNA levels were determined by qPCR in ISE6 cells after TF gene knockdown or treatment with control *Rs86* siRNA. Normalized against tick *rps4* Ct values (average + S.D.) were compared between test siRNAs-treated tick cells and controls treated with *Rs86* siRNA by Chi^2-test (*$p < 0.001$; $n = 2$–4 biological replicates).

protective mechanism mediated by peroxinectin in infected crayfish. The heme-binding lipoprotein (HELP), a transporter of heme in ticks, was previously found to be upregulated and downregulated in midguts and salivary glands, respectively, of *A. phagocytophilum*-infected ticks (Villar et al., 2016). HELP, together with Vitellogenin 1 and 2, was proposed to transport heme to other tick tissues such as salivary glands (Hajdusek et al., 2009). The uncharacterized protein with heme binding activity identified in this study may have a function similar to HELP, suggesting that *A. phagocytophilum* affects hemoglobin primary cleavage and heme transport in tick midguts and salivary glands, possibly to regulate the levels of heme in a tissue-specific manner with potential effects for pathogen and vector survival. The expression of Kunitz-type proteinase inhibitors have been found to be modified in several tick species in response to infection by tick-borne pathogens such as *Bartonella henselae* (Liu et al., 2014), flavivirus (McNally et al., 2012), *Babesia bigemina* (Antunes et al., 2012), and *A. marginale* (Zivkovic et al., 2010). Kunitz peptides are moonlighting proteins that perform multiple functions within the feeding lesion (Schwarz et al., 2014). Upregulation of Kunitz proteins in salivary glands of ticks infected with *B. henselae* (Liu et al., 2014) and flavivirus (McNally et al., 2012) may be associated with host immunity modulation at the feeding site. In contrast to upregulation, it is less clear why Kunitz peptides, including a Kunitz-type proteinase inhibitor 5, would be dowregulated in salivary glands following *A. marginale* infection (Zivkovic et al., 2010). Additional studies show that the expression of Kunitz peptides is complex and may be related to the tick and pathogen species (Rachinsky et al., 2007; Antunes et al., 2012).

These preliminary evidences based on selected TF-TG interactions support that the analysis of tick regulome in response to different stimuli such as pathogen infection could provide potential targets for the control of tick infestations and pathogen infection/transmission. Furthermore, some of these protein families have been proposed as protective antigens using a rational approach for the identification of tick vaccine protective antigens (de la Fuente et al., 2016a). As recently proposed (de la Fuente et al., 2018), the combination of regulomics with intelligent Big Data analytic techniques may contribute to the high throughput identification of candidate vaccine antigens.

CONCLUSION

Our modeling of the modulation of the tick regulome in response to *A. phagocytophilum* infection provided new insights into the mechanisms that target specific functions in different tick tissues. These results supported the use of network analysis for the study of regulome response to infection. Although general mechanisms affected by *A. phagocytophilum* infection may be conserved even between tick and human cells (de la Fuente et al., 2016b), the effect of vector-pathogen co-evolution on pathogen isolates adaptation to grow in tick cells (Alberdi et al., 2015) may result in differences between isolates in the modulation of the tick cell regulome. Future research should be directed at validating the results of the network analysis for regulomics studies and the characterization of TF-TG interactions. Deciphering the precise nature of circuits that shape the tick regulome in response to pathogen infection is an area of research that in the future will advance our knowledge of tick-pathogen interactions, and the identification of new targets for the control of tick infestations and pathogen infection/transmission.

AUTHOR CONTRIBUTIONS

MV, AE-P, AC-C, and JdlF conceived the study and designed the experiments. SA-J, PA, and MV performed the experiments. AE-P, MV, AC-C, and JdlF performed the data analysis. JdlF, SA-J, AE-P, and AC-C wrote the manuscript. All authors approved and contributed to the final version of the manuscript.

FUNDING

This research was financially supported by the Ministerio de Economía, Industria y Competitividad, Spain grant BFU2016-79892-P. MV was funded by the Universidad de Castilla La Mancha, Spain.

REFERENCES

Alberdi, P., Ayllón, N., Cabezas-Cruz, A., Bell-Sakyi, L., Zweygarth, E., Stuen, S., et al. (2015). Infection of *Ixodes* spp. tick cells with different *Anaplasma phagocytophilum* isolates induces the inhibition of apoptotic cell death. *Ticks Tick Borne Dis.* 6, 758–767. doi: 10.1016/j.ttbdis.2015.07.001

Antunes, S., Galindo, R. C., Almazán, C., Rudenko, N., Golovchenko, M., Grubhoffer, L., et al. (2012). Functional genomics studies of *Rhipicephalus (Boophilus) annulatus* ticks in response to infection with the cattle protozoan parasite, *Babesia bigemina*. *Int. J. Parasitol.* 42, 187–195. doi: 10.1016/j.ijpara.2011.12.003

Artigas-Jerónimo, S., de la Fuente, J., and Villar, M. (2018a). Interactomics and tick vaccine development: new directions for the control of tick-borne diseases. *Expert Rev. Proteomics* 15, 627–635. doi: 10.1080/14789450.2018.1506701

Artigas-Jerónimo, S., Villar, M., Cabezas-Cruz, A., Valdés, J. J., Estrada-Peña, A., Alberdi, P., et al. (2018b). Functional evolution of Subolesin/Akirin. *Front. Physiol.* 9:1612. doi: 10.3389/fphys.2018.01612

Ayllón, N., Villar, M., Busby, A. T., Kocan, K. M., Blouin, E. F., Bonzón-Kulichenko, E., et al. (2013). *Anaplasma phagocytophilum* inhibits apoptosis and promotes cytoskeleton rearrangement for infection of tick cells. *Infect. Immun.* 81, 2415–2425. doi: 10.1128/IAI.00194-13

Ayllón, N., Villar, M., Galindo, R. C., Kocan, K. M., Šíma R., López, J. A., et al. (2015). Systems biology of tissue-specific response to *Anaplasma phagocytophilum* reveals differentiated apoptosis in the tick vector *Ixodes scapularis*. *PLoS Genet.* 11:e1005120. doi: 10.1371/journal.pgen.1005120

Barthelemy, M. (2004). Betweenness centrality in large complex networks. *Eur. Phys. J. B* 38, 163–168. doi: 10.1140/epjb/e2004-00111-4

Bell-Sakyi, L., Darby, A., Baylis, M., and Makepeace, B. L. (2018). The Tick Cell Biobank: a global resource for in vitro research on ticks, other arthropods and the pathogens they transmit. *Ticks Tick Borne Dis.* 9, 1364–1371. doi: 10.1016/j.ttbdis.2018.05.015

Boyle, W. K., Groshong, A. M., Drecktrah, D., Boylan, J. A., Gherardini, F. C., Blevins, J. S., et al. (2019). DksA controls the response of the Lyme disease spirochete *Borrelia burgdorferi* to starvation. *J. Bacteriol.* 201:e00582-18. doi: 10.1128/JB.00582-18

Bugrysheva, J. V., Pappas, C. J., Terekhova, D. A., Iyer, R., Godfrey, H. P., Schwartz, I., et al. (2015). Characterization of the RelBbu regulon in *Borrelia burgdorferi* reveals modulation of glycerol metabolism by (p)ppGpp. *PLoS One* 10:e0118063. doi: 10.1371/journal.pone.0118063

Casella, L. G., Weiss, A., Pérez-Rueda, E., Ibarra, J. A., and Shaw, L. N. (2017). Towards the complete proteinaceous regulome of *Acinetobacter baumannii*. *Microb. Genom.* 3:mgen000107. doi: 10.1099/mgen.0.000107

Cerenius, L., and Söderhäll, K. (2004). The prophenoloxidase-activating system in invertebrates. *Immunol. Rev.* 198, 116–126. doi: 10.1111/j.0105-2896.2004.00116.x

Chmelar, J., Kotal, J., Karim, S., Kopacek, P., Francischetti, I. M. B., Pedra, J. H. F., et al. (2016). Sialomes and mialomes: a systems-biology view of tick tissues and tick-host interactions. *Trends Parasitol.* 32, 242–254. doi: 10.1016/j.pt.2015.10.002

Cho, S. J., Valles, Y., Kim, K. M., Ji, S. C., Han, S. J., and Park, S. C. (2012). Additional duplicated Hox genes in the earthworm: *Perionyx excavatus* Hox genes consist of eleven paralog groups. *Gene* 493, 260–266. doi: 10.1016/j.gene.2011.11.006

Contreras, M., Alberdi, P., Fernández de Mera, I. G., Krull, C., Nijhof, A., Villar, M., et al. (2017). Vaccinomics approach to the identification of candidate protective antigens for the control of tick vector infestations and *Anaplasma phagocytophilum* infection. *Front. Cell. Infect. Microbiol.* 7:360. doi: 10.3389/fcimb.2017.00360

de la Fuente, J. (2018). Controlling ticks and tick-borne diseases...looking forward. *Ticks Tick Borne Dis.* 9, 1354–1357. doi: 10.1016/j.ttbdis.2018.04.001

de la Fuente, J., Antunes, S., Bonnet, S., Cabezas-Cruz, A., Domingos, A., Estrada-Peña, A., et al. (2017). Tick-pathogen interactions and vector competence: identification of molecular drivers for tick-borne diseases. *Front. Cell. Infect. Microbiol.* 7:114. doi: 10.3389/fcimb.2017.00114

de la Fuente, J., Ayoubi, P., Blouin, E. F., Almazán, C., Naranjo, V., and Kocan, K. M. (2005). Gene expression profiling of human promyelocytic cells in response to infection with *Anaplasma phagocytophilum*. *Cell. Microbiol.* 7, 549–559. doi: 10.1111/j.1462-5822.2004.00485.x

de la Fuente, J., and Merino, O. (2013). Vaccinomics, the new road to tick vaccines. *Vaccine* 31, 5923–5929. doi: 10.1016/j.ttbdis.2018.04.001

de la Fuente, J., Villar, M., Estrada-Peña, A., and Olivas, J. A. (2018). High throughput discovery and characterization of tick and pathogen vaccine protective antigens using vaccinomics with intelligent Big Data analytic techniques. *Expert Rev. Vaccines* 17, 569–576. doi: 10.1080/14760584.2018

de la Fuente, J., Kopáček, P., Lew-Tabor, A., and Maritz-Olivier, C. (2016a). Strategies for new and improved vaccines against ticks and tick-borne diseases. *Parasite Immunol.* 38, 754–769. doi: 10.1111/pim.12339 de la Fuente, J., Villar, M., Cabezas-Cruz, A., Estrada-Peña, A., Ayllón, N., and Alberdi, P. (2016b). Tick-host-pathogen interactions: conflict and cooperation. *PLoS Pathog.* 12:e1005488. doi: 10.1371/journal.ppat.1005488

de la Fuente, J., Waterhouse, R. M., Sonenshine, D. E., Roe, M. R., Ribeiro, J. M., Sattelle, D. B., et al. (2016c). Tick genome assembled: new opportunities for research on tick-host-pathogen interactions. *Front. Cell. Infect. Microbiol.* 6:103. doi: 10.3389/fcimb.2016.00103

Deplancke, B., and Gheldof, N. (2012). *Gene Regulatory Networks Methods and Protocols.* New York, NY: Human Press.

Esmaeilnejad, B., Tavassoli, M., Samiei, A., Hajipour, N., Imani-Baran, A., and Farhang-Pajuh, F. (2018). Evaluation of oxidative stress and antioxidant status, serum trace mineral levels and cholinesterases activity in cattle infected with *Anaplasma marginale. Microb. Pathog.* 123, 402–409. doi: 10.1016/j.micpath.2018.07.039

Espinosa-Diez, C., Miguel, V., Mennerich, D., Kietzmann, T., Sánchez-Pérez, P., Cadenas, S., et al. (2015). Antioxidant responses and cellular adjustments to oxidative stress. *Redox Biol.* 6, 183–197. doi: 10.1016/j.redox.2015.07.008

Estrada-Peña, A., Villar, M., Artigas-Jerónimo, S., López, V., Alberdi, P., Cabezas-Cruz, A., et al. (2018). Use of graph theory to characterize human and arthropod vector cell protein response to infection. *Front. Cell. Infect. Microbiol.* 8:265. doi: 10.3389/fcimb.2018.00265

Forde, C. E., and McCutchen-Maloney, S. L. (2002). Characterization of transcription factors by mass spectrometry and the role of SELDI-MS. *Mass Spectrom. Rev.* 21, 419–439. doi: 10.1002/mas.10040

Gomez-Pastor, R., Burchfiel, E. T., and Thiele, D. J. (2018). Regulation of heat shock transcription factors and their roles in physiology and disease. *Nat. Rev. Mol. Cell Biol.* 19, 4–19. doi: 10.1038/nrm.2017.73

Gronostajski, R. M., Guaneri, J., Lee, D. H., and Gallo, S. M. (2011). The NFI-Regulome Database: a tool for annotation and analysis of control regions of genes regulated by Nuclear Factor I transcription factors. *J. Clin. Bioinforma.* 1:4. doi: 10.1186/2043-9113-1-4

Gulia-Nuss, M., Nuss, A. B., Meyer, J. M., Sonenshine, D. E., Roe, R. M., Waterhouse, R. M., et al. (2016). Genomic insights into the Ixodes scapularis tick vector of Lyme disease. *Nat. Commun.* 7:10507. doi: 10.1038/ncomms10507

Hajdusek, O., Sojka, D., Kopacek, P., Buresova, V., Franta, Z., Sauman, I., et al. (2009). Knockdown of proteins involved in iron metabolism limits tick reproduction and development. *Proc. Natl. Acad. Sci. U.S.A.* 106, 1033–1038. doi: 10.1073/pnas.0807961106

Kalil, S. P., Rosa, R. D. D., Capelli-Peixoto, J., Pohl, P. C., Oliveira, P. L., Fogaça, A. C., et al. (2017). Immune-related redox metabolism of embryonic cells of the tick *Rhipicephalus microplus* (BME26) in response to infection with *Anaplasma marginale. Parasit. Vectors.* 10:613. doi: 10.1186/s13071-017-2575-9

Liu, X. Y., de la Fuente, J., Cote, M., Galindo, R. C., Moutailler, S., Vayssier-Taussat, M., et al. (2014). IrSPI, a tick serine protease inhibitor involved in tick feeding and *Bartonella henselae* infection. *PLoS Negl. Trop. Dis.* 8:e2993. doi: 10.1371/journal.pntd.0002993

McNally, K. L., Mitzel, D. N., Anderson, J. M., Ribeiro, J. M., Valenzuela, J. G., Myers, T. G., et al. (2012). Differential salivary gland transcript expression profile in Ixodes scapularis nymphs upon feeding or flavivirus infection. *Ticks Tick Borne Dis.* 3, 18–26. doi: 10.1016/j.ttbdis.2011.09.003

Mitra, S., Dunphy, P. S., Das, S., Zhu, B., Luo, T., and McBride, J. W. (2018). *Ehrlichia chaffeensis* TRP120 effector targets and recruits host polycomb group proteins for degradation to promote intracellular infection. *Infect. Immun.* 86:e00845-17. doi: 10.1128/IAI.00845-17

More, T., Reddy, G. R., Sharma, S. P., and Singh, L. N. (1989). Enzymes of oxidant defence system of leucocytes and erythrocytes in bovine anaplasmosis. *Vet. Parasitol.* 31, 333–337. doi: 10.1016/0304-4017(89)90082-4

Munderloh, U., Liu, Y., Wang, M., Chen, C., and Kurtti, T. (1994). Establishment, maintenance and description of cell lines from the tick *Ixodes scapularis. J. Parasitol.* 80, 533–543.

Ogawa, N., and Biggin, M. D. (2012). High-throughput SELEX determination of DNA sequences bound by transcription factors *in vitro. Methods Mol. Biol.* 786, 51–63. doi: 10.1007/978-1-61779-292-2_3

Opsahl, T., Agneessens, F., and Skvoretz, J. (2010). Node centrality in weighted networks: generalizing degree and shortest paths. *Soc. Networks* 32, 245–251. doi: 10.1016/j.socnet.2010.03.006

Pellerin, I., Schnabel, C., Catron, K. M., and Abate, C. (1994). Hox proteins have different affinities for a consensus DNA site that correlate with the positions of their genes on the Hox cluster. *Mol. Cell Biol.* 14, 4532–4545. doi: 10.1128/mcb.14.7.4532

Peppenelli, M. A., Miller, M. J., Altman, A. M., Cojohari, O., and Chan, G. C. (2018). Aberrant regulation of the Akt signaling network by human cytomegalovirus allows for targeting of infected monocytes. *Antiviral Res.* 158, 13–24. doi: 10.1016/j.antiviral.2018.07.015

Potier, D., Atak, Z. K., Sanchez, M. N., Herrmann, C., and Aerts, S. (2012). Using cisTargetX to predict transcriptional targets and networks in *Drosophila. Methods Mol. Biol.* 786, 291–314. doi: 10.1007/978-1-61779-292-2_18

Rachinsky, A., Guerrero, F. D., and Scoles, G. A. (2007). Differential protein expression in ovaries of uninfected and *Babesia*-infected southern cattle ticks, *Rhipicephalus (Boophilus) microplus. Insect Biochem. Mol. Biol.* 37, 1291–1308. doi: 10.1016/j.ibmb.2007.08.001

Reddy, G. R., More, T., Sharma, S. P., and Singh, L. N. (1988). The oxidant defence system in water-buffaloes (*Bubalus bubalis*) experimentally infected with *Anaplasma marginale. Vet. Parasitol.* 27, 245–249. doi: 10.1016/0304-4017(88)90039-8

Rioualen, C., Da Costa, Q., Chetrit, B., Charafe-Jauffret, E., Ginestier, C., and Bidaut, G. (2017). HTS-Net: an integrated regulome-interactome approach for establishing network regulation models in high-throughput screenings. *PLoS One* 12:e0185400. doi: 10.1371/journal.pone.0185400

Rougemont, J., and Naef, F. (2012). Computational analysis of protein-DNA interactions from ChIP-seq data. *Methods Mol. Biol.* 786, 263–273. doi: 10.1007/978-1-61779-292-2_16

Schwarz, A., Cabezas-Cruz, A., Kopecký, J., and Valdés, J. J. (2014). Understanding the evolutionary structural variability and target specificity of tick salivary Kunitz peptides using next generation transcriptome data. *BMC Evol. Biol.* 14:4. doi: 10.1186/1471-2148-14-4

Severo, M. S., Pedra, J. H. F., Ayllón, N., Kocan, K. M., and de la Fuente, J. (2015). "*Anaplasma*," in *Molecular Medical Microbiology*, 2nd Edn, Vol. 3, eds Y. W. Tang, M. Sussman, D. Liu, I. Poxton, and J. Schwartzman (London: Academic Press), 2033–2042.

Shaw, D. K., Wang, X., Brown, L. J., Oliva Chávez, A. S., Reif, K. E., Smith, A. A., et al. (2017). Infection-derived lipids elicit an immune deficiency circuit in arthropods. *Nat. Commun.* 8:14401. doi: 10.1038/ncomms14401

Shih, H. Y., Sciumè, G., Mikami, Y., Guo, L., Sun, H. W., Brooks, S. R., et al. (2016). Developmental acquisition of regulomes underlies innate lymphoid cell functionality. *Cell* 165, 1120–1133. doi: 10.1016/j.cell.2016.04.029

Simpson, G. L. (2016). *cocorresp: Co-Correspondence Analysis Ordination Methods. R package version 0.3-0.* Available at: http://cran.r-project.org/package=cocorresp (accessed June, 2018).

Sritunyalucksana, K., Wongsuebsantati, K., Johansson, M. W., and Söderhäll, K. (2001). Peroxinectin, a cell adhesive protein associated with the proPO system from the black tiger shrimp, *Penaeus monodon. Dev. Comp. Immunol.* 25, 353–363. doi: 10.1016/s0145-305x(01)00009-x

Vaquerizas, J. M., Teichmann, S. A., and Luscombe, N. M. (2012). How do you find transcription factors? computational approaches to compile and annotate repertoires of regulators for any genome. *Methods Mol. Biol.* 786, 3–19. doi: 10.1007/978-1-61779-292-2_1

Villar, M., Ayllón, N., Alberdi, P., Moreno, A., Moreno, M., Tobes, R., et al. (2015). Integrated metabolomics, transcriptomics and proteomics identifies metabolic pathways affected by *Anaplasma phagocytophilum* infection in tick cells. *Mol. Cell. Proteomics* 14, 3154–3172. doi: 10.1074/mcp.M115.051938

Villar, M., López, V., Ayllón, N., Cabezas-Cruz, A., López, J. A., Vázquez, J., et al. (2016). The intracellular bacterium *Anaplasma phagocytophilum* selectively manipulates the levels of vertebrate host proteins in the tick vector Ixodes scapularis. *Parasit. Vectors* 9:467. doi: 10.1186/s13071-016-1747-3

Villar, M., Popara, M., Ayllón, N., Fernández de Mera, I. G., Mateos-Hernández, L., Galindo, R. C., et al. (2014). A systems biology approach to the characterization of stress response in *Dermacentor reticulatus* tick unfed larvae. *PLoS One* 9:e89564. doi: 10.1371/journal.pone.0089564

Williams, T., and Tjian, R. (1991). Analysis of the DNA-binding and activation properties of the human transcription factor AP-2. *Genes Dev.* 5, 670–682. doi: 10.1101/gad.5.4.670

Yang, V. W. (1998). Eukaryotic transcription factors: identification, characterization and functions. *J. Nutr.* 128, 2045–2051. doi: 10.1093/jn/128.11.2045

Yi, S., Li, Y., Shi, L., and Zhang, L. (2017). Novel Insights into Antiviral gene regulation of red swamp crayfish, *Procambarus clarkii*, infected with white spot syndrome virus. *Genes* 8:E320. doi: 10.3390/genes8110320

Zivkovic, Z., Esteves, E., Almazán, C., Daffre, S., Nijhof, A. M., Kocan, K. M., et al. (2010). Differential expression of genes in salivary glands of male *Rhipicephalus (Boophilus) microplus* in response to infection with *Anaplasma marginale*. *BMC Genomics* 11:186. doi: 10.1186/1471-2164-11-186

14

Transcriptional Immunoprofiling at the Tick-Virus-Host Interface during Early Stages of Tick-Borne Encephalitis Virus Transmission

Saravanan Thangamani [1,2,3], Meghan E. Hermance [1], Rodrigo I. Santos [1], Mirko Slovak [4], Dar Heinze [5], Steven G. Widen [6] and Maria Kazimirova [4]*

[1] Department of Pathology, The University of Texas Medical Branch, Galveston, TX, United States, [2] Institute for Human Infections and Immunity, The University of Texas Medical Branch, Galveston, TX, United States, [3] Center for Tropical Diseases, The University of Texas Medical Branch, Galveston, TX, United States, [4] Institute of Zoology, Slovak Academy of Sciences, Bratislava, Slovakia, [5] Department of Surgery, Center for Regenerative Medicine, Boston University and Boston Medical Center, Boston, MA, United States, [6] Department of Biochemistry and Molecular Biology, The University of Texas Medical Branch, Galveston, TX, United States

***Correspondence:**
Saravanan Thangamani
sathanga@utmb.edu

Emerging and re-emerging diseases transmitted by blood feeding arthropods are significant global public health problems. Ticks transmit the greatest variety of pathogenic microorganisms of any blood feeding arthropod. Infectious agents transmitted by ticks are delivered to the vertebrate host together with saliva at the bite site. Tick salivary glands produce complex cocktails of bioactive molecules that facilitate blood feeding and pathogen transmission by modulating host hemostasis, pain/itch responses, wound healing, and both innate and adaptive immunity. In this study, we utilized Illumina Next Generation Sequencing to characterize the transcriptional immunoprofile of cutaneous immune responses to *Ixodes ricinus* transmitted tick-borne encephalitis virus (TBEV). A comparative immune gene expression analysis of TBEV-infected and uninfected tick feeding sites was performed. Our analysis reveals that ticks create an inflammatory environment at the bite site during the first 3 h of feeding, and significant differences in host responses were observed between TBEV-infected and uninfected tick feeding. Gene-expression analysis reveals modulation of inflammatory genes after 1 and 3 h of TBEV-infected tick feeding. Transcriptional levels of genes specific to chemokines and cytokines indicated a neutrophil-dominated immune response. Immunohistochemistry of the tick feeding site revealed that mononuclear phagocytes and fibroblasts are the primary target cells for TBEV infection and did not detect TBEV antigens in neutrophils. Together, the transcriptional and immunohistochemistry results suggest that early cutaneous host responses to TBEV-infected tick feeding are more inflammatory than expected and highlight the importance of inflammatory chemokine and cytokine pathways in tick-borne flavivirus transmission.

Keywords: TBEV, flavivirus, tick, *Ixodes ricinus*, cutaneous, immune response

INTRODUCTION

Tick-borne encephalitis virus (TBEV) is a zoonotic tick-borne virus in the *Flaviviridae* family (genus *Flavivirus*). It is the causative agent of tick-borne encephalitis (TBE), a serious neurological disease in humans. During the last few decades, TBE has become a widespread public health concern in Eurasia with endemic regions extending from Western and Central Europe to Siberia and parts of Asia (Süss, 2011). The various strains of TBEV are subdivided into three main subtypes that are closely related genetically and antigenically: European (Eu), Siberian (Sib), and Far-Eastern (FE) (Gritsun et al., 2003a; Mansfield et al., 2009). TBEV-Eu is widely distributed in Europe, including the European regions of Russia, while TBEV-Sib is mainly found in Russia, the Baltic countries and Finland (Mansfield et al., 2009; Kovalev and Mukhacheva, 2014). TBEV-FE is present in Far-Eastern Russia and parts of China, Japan, and the Republic of Korea (Mansfield et al., 2009). Human infections with TBEV can range from mild flu-like symptoms to severe or fatal neuroinvasive disease, often with long-term neurological symptoms. There is a correlation between the TBEV subtype and severity of disease. TBEV-FE is associated with severe neurological disease and a case fatality rate of approximately 30–40%, while the case fatality rates for TBEV-Sib and TBEV-Eu are approximately 6–8% and 1–2%, respectively (Gritsun et al., 2003a; Tonteri et al., 2013). Although the incidence rates vary from year to year and between subtypes, several thousand human TBE cases are reported annually (CDC Tick-borne Encephalitis, 2017).

In nature, the *Ixodes ricinus* tick is the primary vector for TBEV-Eu while the *Ixodes persulcatus* tick is the main vector for the TBEV-Sib and TBEV-FE (Gritsun et al., 2003b). *I. ricinus* is widely distributed throughout Europe, extending to Turkey, and northern Iran, while *I. persulcatus* is distributed across the Urals, Siberia, Far-Eastern Russia, and parts of China and Japan (Gritsun et al., 2003a; Lindquist and Vapalahti, 2008). A sympatric zone exists in northern Baltics, western Finland and northwestern Russia where the habitats for *I. ricinus* and *I. persulcatus* overlap and multiple TBEV subtypes have been recorded (Lindquist and Vapalahti, 2008; Süss, 2011; Kovalev and Mukhacheva, 2014). TBEV is maintained in natural transmission cycles involving ixodid ticks and wild-living mammalian hosts. When infected with TBEV, a tick is supposed to remain infected throughout its life cycle (Gritsun et al., 2003a). Transovarial transmission of TBEV from an infected female tick to the egg mass can occur, but this route of tick infection is not entirely efficient at maintaining TBEV within the natural tick population (Danielová et al., 2002). During the tick feeding process, TBEV-infected ticks can transmit the virus to susceptible vertebrate hosts, but they can also transmit TBEV to uninfected ticks that are co-feeding on the same host (Mansfield et al., 2009; Randolph, 2011). During co-feeding, TBEV can be transmitted even non-viremically i.e., when the ticks feed on a non-viremic or virus-immune host (Labuda et al., 1993, 1997). The local skin site of tick feeding is understood to be an important focus for early TBEV replication, and immune cell infiltrates to this feeding site are believed to serve as vehicles for TBEV transmission between co-feeding ticks (Labuda et al., 1996).

Infectious agents transmitted by ticks are delivered to the vertebrate host together with saliva at the tick feeding site. Tick-borne viruses are transmitted to the host very early during the tick feeding process. TBEV can be transmitted from the saliva of an *I. ricinus* tick to the cement cone in the skin of a host as early as 1 h after the tick attaches and initiates feeding (Alekseev et al., 1996). As *I. ricinus* and *I. persulcatus* ticks feed, TBEV replicates to higher viral titers than in unfed ticks (Alekseev and Chunikhin, 1990; Belova et al., 2012; Slovák et al., 2014). The dynamic nature of TBEV replication in ticks has also been demonstrated in field-collected ticks. In partially engorged *I. ricinus* nymphs removed from humans, TBEV prevalence was higher than in questing, unfed nymphs collected in the same region (Süss et al., 2004). Experimental data suggest that in nature, ticks secrete repeated "pulses" of a few infectious virus particles over the course of feeding (Kaufman and Nuttall, 1996). Thus, virus transmission from an infected tick to a host is a very dynamic process that begins soon after the tick initiates feeding.

Ixodid ticks must remain attached to their hosts for several days to successfully acquire a bloodmeal and complete development, and have evolved salivary countermeasures directed against the host's immune and hemostatic defenses. Tick salivary glands produce complex cocktails of biologically active molecules that facilitate blood feeding and pathogen transmission by modulating host hemostasis, pain/itch responses, wound healing, and both innate and adaptive immunity. Bioactive tick salivary molecules include those with anti-pain/itch, antiplatelet, anticoagulation, vasodilatory, immunomodulatory, and anti-inflammatory activities (Ribeiro et al., 2006, Francischetti et al., 2009; Kazimírová and Štibrániová, 2013; Wikel, 2013; Šimo et al., 2017). As the course of tick feeding progresses, salivary gland genes are differentially expressed, reflecting the dynamic and complex composition of tick saliva (Ribeiro et al., 2006; Šimo et al., 2017).

The skin is the first host organ that tick saliva and a tick-borne pathogen contact during the tick feeding process. The cutaneous interface between the tick, pathogen, and host is crucial for influencing the initial host response to tick infestation and pathogen transmission (Kazimírová et al., 2017; Šimo et al., 2017). A prior study examined the tick-induced changes in cutaneous gene expression and histopathology during the early stages of uninfected *Ixodes scapularis* feeding. Early transcriptional and histopathological changes at the feeding site of uninfected *I. scapularis* nymphs are initially characterized by modulation of host responses in resident cells, followed by progression to a neutrophil-dominated immune response after 12 h of tick feeding (Heinze et al., 2012). Similarly, a complex proinflammatory environment was observed at the Powassan virus (POWV), a North American tick-borne flavivirus, infected tick feeding site. Together these findings from the cutaneous interface provide evidence of an immunologically privileged micro-environment at the tick feeding site that is established during the early stages of POWV-infected tick feeding (Hermance and Thangamani, 2014; Hermance et al., 2016).

In the present study, Illumina Next Generation Sequencing (NGS) and immunohistochemistry are utilized to understand host immunomodulation induced by TBEV-infected *I. ricinus* feeding at the earliest stages of TBEV transmission. By studying the interactions between the host immune response and tick-mediated immunomodulation during the early hours of infected tick feeding, we can begin to understand the immunologic processes that facilitate transmission of a tick-borne flavivirus to a host.

MATERIALS AND METHODS

Ethics Statement

All experiments involving mice were performed in accordance with the animal use protocol approved by the State Veterinary and Food Administration of the Slovak Republic (permit number 1335/12-221).

Animals

Five-week-old female BALB/c mice were purchased from Dobra Voda Breeding Station, Institute of Experimental Pharmacology and Toxicology, Slovak Academy of Sciences (SAS). The animals were housed at the Institute of Virology, Biomedical Research Center, SAS (Bratislava, Slovakia) under standard conditions. Food and water were provided *ad libitum*. Upon arrival, mice were allowed to adapt to the local environment before being incorporated into the study. Mice were 6 weeks old at the start of the study. At the end of the experiment animals were euthanized by cervical dislocation under anesthesia induced by carbon dioxide.

Virus and Tick Infection

I. ricinus ticks were obtained from a laboratory colony maintained at the Institute of Zoology SAS (Bratislava, Slovakia). The F1 generation of laboratory-bred *I. ricinus* females was used for virus inoculation. TBEV (Hypr strain prepared as a 10% mouse brain suspension of 1.1×10^9 PFU/ml in Leibovitz's L-15 medium) was provided by the Institute of Virology, Biomedical Research Center, SAS. Fasting *I. ricinus* females were inoculated into the haemocoel with TBEV (5.5×10^4 PFU per tick) through the coxal plate of the second pair of legs using a digital microinjector TM system (MINJ-D-CE; Tritech Research, Inc., USA) (Kazimírová et al., 2012). By this procedure, ~100% of the ticks were found to acquire TBEV infection (Slovák et al., 2014). Inoculated ticks were incubated at room temperature and 85% relative humidity in a desiccator for 21 days prior to the infestation experiments.

Infestation of Mice by Ticks

Two groups of mice ($n = 6$ per group) were infested with either TBEV-infected or uninfected (control) *I. ricinus* females. Ticks were placed in small neoprene capsules glued on the shaved backs of the mice (two capsules per mouse, four tick females per capsule) (Kazimírová et al., 2012; Hermance and Thangamani, 2014). Ticks in each capsule were allowed to feed for either 1 or 3 h. After the allotted feeding time, skin biopsies were taken from euthanized mice, at each tick feeding site using a Premier Uni-Punch (Premier Products Co., Plymouth Meeting, PA). For immunohistochemical analysis, skin biopsies ($n = 3$) were harvested with attached ticks and placed in 4% formaldehyde. For RNA extraction, the attached ticks were removed from the skin biopsies and the biopsies ($n = 3$) were placed in RNALater (Ambion, Life Technologies, Carlsbad, CA). Control biopsies were taken from the shaved skin of naïve tick-free mice and stored in either 4% formaldehyde or RNALater.

Cutaneous Immune Response

Total RNA was extracted as previously described (Heinze et al., 2012; Hermance and Thangamani, 2014) and RNAseq analysis (Illumina deep sequencing / NGS) was performed on these samples. Briefly, 1 μg of total RNA from mouse skin biopsies ($n = 3$) was poly A+ selected and fragmented using divalent cations and heat (94°C, 8 min). Illumina TruSeq v2 sample preparation kits (Illumina Inc., San Diego, CA) were used for the RNA-Seq library construction. Each sample library was uniquely indexed to allow combining libraries during sequencing and subsequent separation post-sequencing. NGS was performed at the NGS core facility, Sealy Center for Molecular Medicine, The University of Texas Medical Branch (UTMB). Sample libraries were analyzed by the Illumina HiSeq 1500 using a 2×50 base paired end run protocol, with TruSeq v3 sequencing-by-synthesis chemistry. Reads were aligned to the mouse mm10 reference genome using TopHat version v2.0.4. Cuffdiff version 2.0.2 was used to estimate differential gene expression between TBEV-infected and uninfected feeding sites after 1 or 3 h of tick feeding. The total dataset of 23,000 genes was filtered for p-values ≤ 0.05 and a fold change ≤ -1.5 or $\geq +1.5$. The Log_2(fold change) and p-value data for each gene expression comparison (Supplement Table 1) were then uploaded to Ingenuity Pathway Analysis (IPA) software (Ingenuity Systems, Redwood City, CA) for further transcriptional analysis of the early cutaneous immune response, as previously described (Heinze et al., 2012; Hermance and Thangamani, 2014).

Real-Time PCR Validation

Real-time PCR was used to validate the NGS data (Supplement Table 1). Skin biopsies were harvested from the feeding sites of TBEV-infected and uninfected ticks as described above. At each time point, biopsies from three mice were used for the real-time PCR validation. Fifteen gene targets were selected for real-time PCR analysis. We selected these genes based our previous studies with POWV where these genes were shown to be modulated genes of interest during the host anti-tick response to POWV infection (Hermance and Thangamani, 2014, 2015). This list also includes genes that were not differentially modulated as per RNASeq analysis. Primers were purchased from Integrated DNA Technologies and the primer sequences are provided in Supplement Table 2. Primers were mixed with IQ SYBR green supermix (Bio-Rad) and loaded into iCycler IQ PCR 96-well plates (Bio-Rad) to create customized PCR arrays where each gene was measured in triplicate. For each PCR plate, 1 μg of total RNA extracted from skin biopsies was converted into cDNA using the RT^2 First Strand kit (Qiagen). cDNA was loaded onto the 96-well PCR plates, which were run on an iCycler iQ5 real-time PCR instrument (Bio-Rad) with the following cycling protocol: 10 min at 95°C; 15 s at 95°C, 1 min 60°C for 40 cycles, and an 80-cycle (+0.5°C /cycle) 55–95°C melt curve. Every array included GAPDH as an endogenous control gene and a no-template control. The iCycler's software was used to calculate the threshold cycle (C_T) values for all analyzed genes. The delta-delta C_T method was used to calculate fold-changes in gene expression between TBEV-infected and uninfected tick feeding sites. Data normalization was achieved by correcting all C_T values to the average C_T values of the GAPDH housekeeping gene. Statistically significant differences in gene expression between the 1 vs. 3 h tick feeding time points were determined by the Student's *t*-test. *P*-values less than 0.05 were considered significant. SPSS statistical software was used.

Immunohistochemistry

The skin biopsies with attached ticks were formalin-fixed for a minimum of 48 h in 4% formaldehyde. These biopsy samples were treated with Decal (Decal Chemical Corp, Tallman, NY) for 2 h, and then paraffin-embedded (Heinze et al., 2012). Five micron paraffin sections were taken from each sample and adhered to glass slides. The slides were deparaffinized in xylene and then rehydrated in decreasing concentrations of ethanol (Hermance et al., 2016). For antigen retrieval, the slides were treated with 10 mM Tris Base + 0.05% Tween 20 (pH 10) for 20 min with microwave heating. Upon returning to room temperature, endogenous peroxidase quenching was performed by incubating the slides in 4% H_2O_2 for 30 min. The primary antibody for TBEV detection used in this study was a Hyper Mouse Immune Ascitic Fluid (HMIAF) antibody against TBEV; therefore, the Mouse-On-Mouse kit (MOM, Vector labs, Burlingame, CA) was used in order to reduce the endogenous mouse Ig background staining generated when mouse primary antibodies are used on mouse tissue (Santos et al., 2016). Slides were incubated for 1 h at room temperature with the MOM mouse Ig blocking reagent. The HMIAF primary antibody against TBEV was diluted 1:250 in the MOM diluent and incubated for 30 min at room temperature. Secondary antibody consisted of MOM biotinylated horse anti-mouse IgG reagent, which was incubated for 30 min at room temperature. The biotinylated secondary antibody was detected with a streptavidin-peroxidase ultrasensitive polymer (Sigma-Aldrich, St. Louis, MO) followed by staining with the NovaRED HRP substrate kit (Vector Laboratories Inc., Burlingame, CA). Slides were counterstained with Harris hematoxylin and coverslips were mounted using Permount (ThermoFisher Scientific, Waltham, MA). Uninfected skin and tick biopsy sections generated from uninfected tick feeding sites were used as negative controls to verify the specificity of the MIAF anti-TBEV primary antibody. Secondary antibody only (no primary antibody) controls were used to confirm that the MOM biotinylated anti-mouse IgG reagent did not bind non-specifically to cellular components.

RESULTS AND DISCUSSION

In the present study, the host cutaneous immune response to TBEV-infected *I. ricinus* feeding after 1 and 3 h of tick attachment was investigated by Illumina NGS and immunohistochemistry. No prior studies have examined the early host immune response at the feeding site of a TBEV-infected tick. We also used the RNASeq data to check for the presence of TBEV at the infected tick feeding site by aligning the sequences against a TBEV reference genome (NM_001672). TBEV sequences were detected in the 3 hpi (hours post infection), but not in the 1 hpi samples (**Figure 1A**).

The differences in the total number of significantly up- and downregulated host genes ($p \leq 0.05$) between TBEV-infected and uninfected tick feeding sites as well as between TBEV-infected feeding sites 1 and 3 h post tick attachment are shown in **Figure 1B**. When the TBEV-infected and uninfected tick feeding sites were compared, the total number of significantly upregulated genes decreased from 1 to 3 h, while there was an overall increase in significantly downregulated genes from 1 to 3 h tick attachment. An online tool (Oliveros, 2007) was used to generate a Venn diagram showing the overlap of significantly modulated genes between the 1 and 3 h comparison of the TBEV-infected vs. uninfected tick feeding sites (**Figure 1C**). 10.2% of significantly modulated genes were shared between the three comparisons; however, the majority of significantly modulated genes were unique to either the 1 h TBEV-infected vs. 1 h uninfected tick feeding site (18.7%), the 3 h TBEV-infected vs. 3 h uninfected tick feeding site (25.7%), or the 3 h TBEV-infected vs. 1 h TBEV-infected tick feeding site (14%). Additionally, a list of all modulated genes at either time point in the study was used to generate a heat map (**Figure 1D**). This heat map suggests that after 1 h of TBEV-infected tick feeding, there was a pattern of mostly upregulated cutaneous genes; however, after 3 h, the pattern changed to downregulation. This pattern of gene expression was further validated by the real-time PCR data. Though we could not recapitulate the exact fold changes of the selected immune genes observed by RNASeq data, our data clearly concur with the expression pattern of the selected genes: upregulation at 1 hpi and downregulation at 3 hpi (**Figure 1E**). Together these data suggest that a distinctive cutaneous immune response profile exists after 1 h of TBEV-infected tick feeding, but it changes to reflect a new and unique profile after 3 h. This change in gene expression profile could be attributed to the dynamic salivary secretion and physical injury during tick attachment/feeding mechanisms.

Ingenuity Pathway Analysis

In total, 1,548 genes were analyzed by Ingenuity Pathway Analysis (IPA) software (Supplement Table 1). The focus of the present study is on the cutaneous immune response observed at the TBEV-infected vs. the uninfected tick feeding sites after 1 and 3 h of tick feeding. The networks generated from IPA analysis illustrate the interrelationships between genes and the temporal changes in gene modulation. The top IPA-generated networks are shown for the TBEV-infected vs. uninfected tick feeding sites after 1 h of tick feeding (**Figure 2A**), the TBEV-infected vs. uninfected tick feeding sites after 3 h of tick feeding (**Figure 2B**), and the TBEV-infected tick feeding site after 3 h of tick feeding vs. the TBEV-infected tick feeding site after 1 h of feeding (**Figure 2C**). The three bio-functions most associated

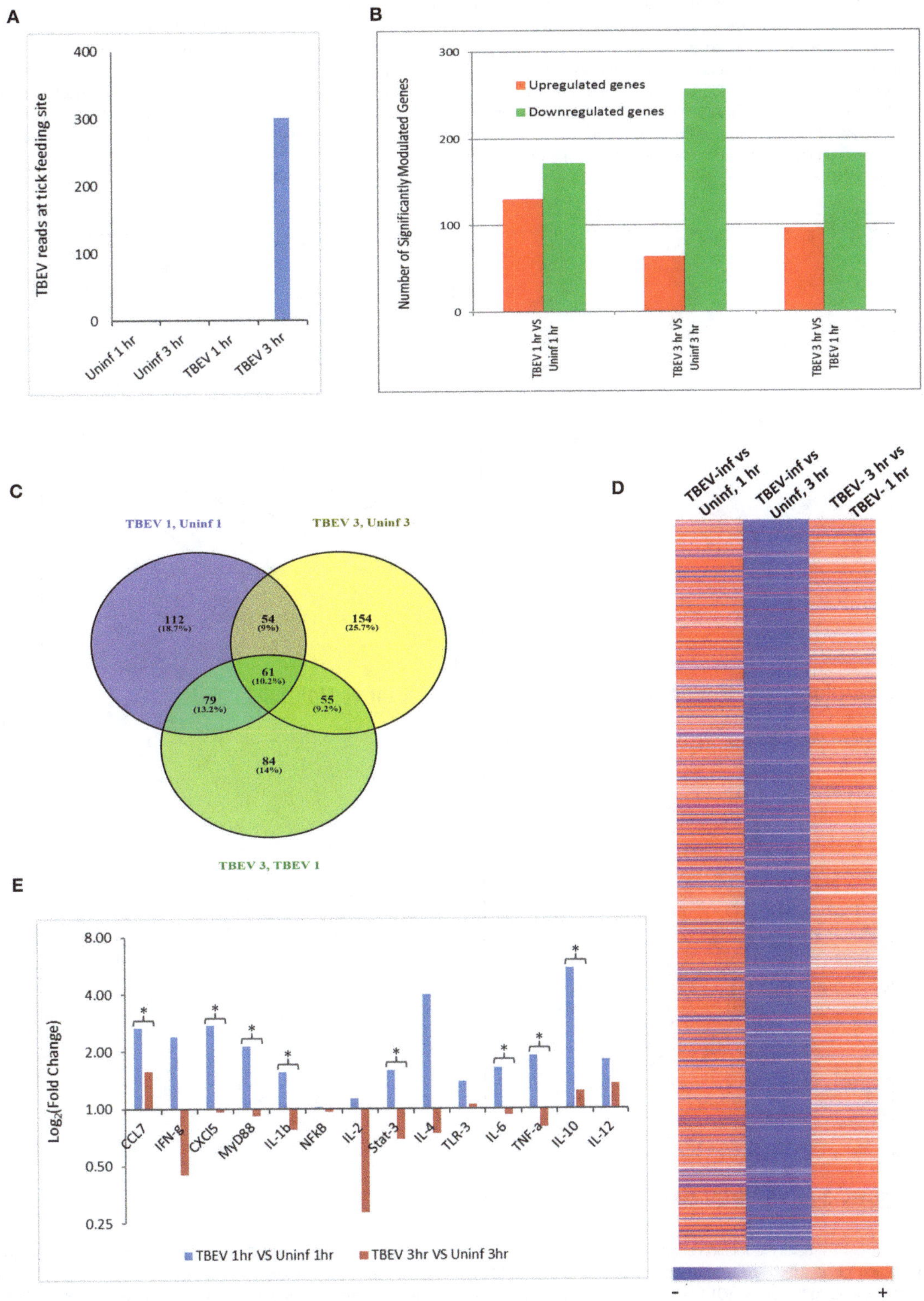

FIGURE 1 | Comparative transcriptional analysis of the TBEV-infected and uninfected *Ixodes ricinus* tick feeding loci. **(A)** The RNASeq data was screened for the presence of TBEV reads at the tick feeding site by aligning the sequences against a TBEV reference genome (MN_001672). The number of TBEV reads that match the TBEV reference genome is plotted for the uninfected tick feeding sites and the TBEV-infected tick feeding sites. **(B,C)** The following comparisons are depicted: TBEV-infected tick feeding loci at 1 h vs. uninfected tick feeding loci at 1 h, TBEV-infected tick feeding loci at 3 h vs. uninfected tick feeding loci at 3 h, TBEV-infected

(Continued)

FIGURE 1 | tick feeding loci at 3 h vs. TBEV-infected tick feeding loci at 1 h. **(B)** The total number of significantly up- or downregulated ($p \leq 0.05$) genes for each comparison. **(C)** Venn diagram showing overlap of significantly modulated genes for each of the three comparisons. **(D)** Heat map showing temporal changes in gene expression profiles. A list of all genes modulated at any time point in the study was used to generate a heatmap with Morpheus web server application (www.broadinstitute.org). **(E)** The immune genes selected for validation were shown to be modulated genes of interest during the host anti-tick response in previous studies. Pre-optimized primers were purchased from IDT and used for the real-time PCR validation. The delta-delta CT method was used to calculate fold-changes in gene expression between TBEV-infected and uninfected tick feeding sites as described in the methods section. GAPDH was used as an endogenous control gene. Statistically significant differences in gene expression between the 1 vs. 3 h tick feeding time points were determined by the Student's *t*-test. *P*-values less than 0.05 were considered significant. Significant differences are indicated by asterisks.

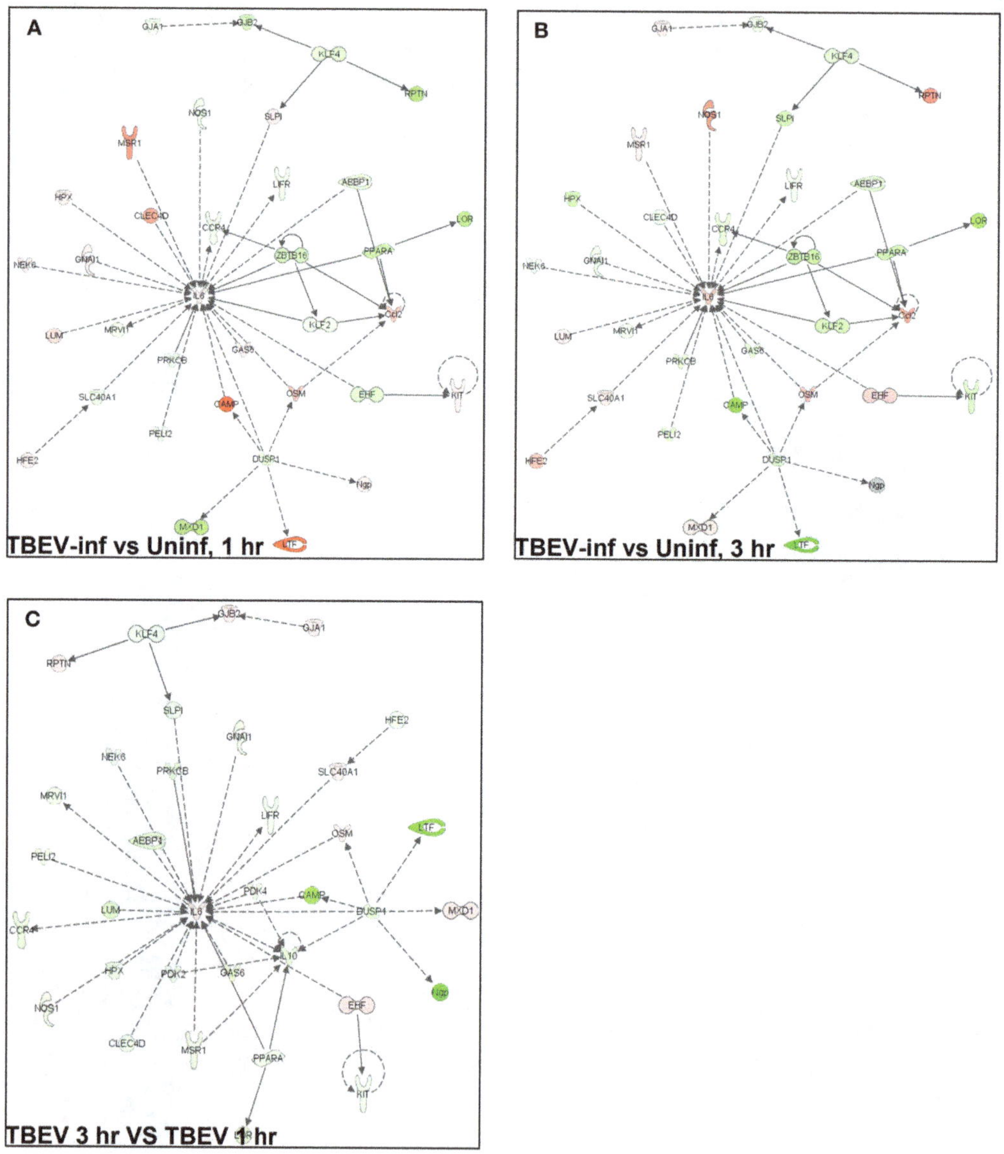

FIGURE 2 | An overview of host gene modulation after 1 and 3 h of TBEV-infected *Ixodes ricinus* tick feeding. **(A)** The top IPA-generated network is shown for the TBEV-infected tick feeding loci at 1 h vs. the uninfected tick feeding loci at 1 h **(B)** The top IPA-generated network is shown for the TBEV-infected tick feeding loci at 3 h vs. the uninfected tick feeding loci at 3 h. **(C)** The top-IPA-generated network is shown for the TBEV-infected tick feeding loci at 3 h vs. TBEV-infected tick feeding loci at 1 h. Note: Red/pink represents upregulated genes, green represents down-regulated genes, and gray represents unchanged or insignificant genes.

with the networks representing the TBEV-infected vs. uninfected comparisons (**Figures 2A,B**) are cellular movement, organismal injury and abnormalities, and hematological system development and function. After 1 h of TBEV-infected tick feeding, 19 host genes shown in the **Figure 2A** network were downregulated and 16 host genes were upregulated. After 3 h of TBEV-infected tick feeding, 22 host genes in the **Figure 2B** network were downregulated, 12 were upregulated, and one gene (Ngp) had a fold change of zero. Thus, as 1 h progressed to 3 h of TBEV-infected tick feeding, the network displayed a slight shift toward cutaneous gene downregulation (**Figure 2**). The IPA-generated network for the TBEV-infected 3 h vs. the TBEV-infected 1 h tick feeding site (**Figure 2C**) is unique from the **Figures 2A,B** networks, as it lacks Ccl2, KLF2, and ZBTB16, but instead includes 20 unique genes which contribute to this network's association with bio-functions such as molecular transport, organismal injury and abnormalities, and cellular movement.

In both the 1 and 3 h comparisons between TBEV-infected vs. uninfected tick feeding sites, inflammatory response was the primary predicted host response. Based on the IPA transcriptional immunoprofiling, the inflammatory response was projected to be activated in the 1 h comparison of the TBEV-infected vs. uninfected tick feeding site (activation z-score = 1.549), and inhibited in the 3 h comparison (activation z-score = −1.26). Temporal changes in gene expression for all genes predicted to have direct correlative relationships with the inflammatory response were plotted after 1 or 3 h of TBEV-infected vs. uninfected tick feeding (**Figure 3**). Transcriptional levels of cytokines Ccl2, Ccl12, Cxcl1, Cxcl2, Cxcl5, IL6, and IL10 were all upregulated after 1 h of TBEV-infected tick feeding, thus contributing to the overall activation of the inflammatory response (**Figure 3**). At the 3 h time point, the majority of these cytokine transcriptional level were still upregulated, with the exception of Cxcl5 and IL10, which were both slightly downregulated. Real-time PCR validation of a few selected immune genes followed the general pattern observed in the

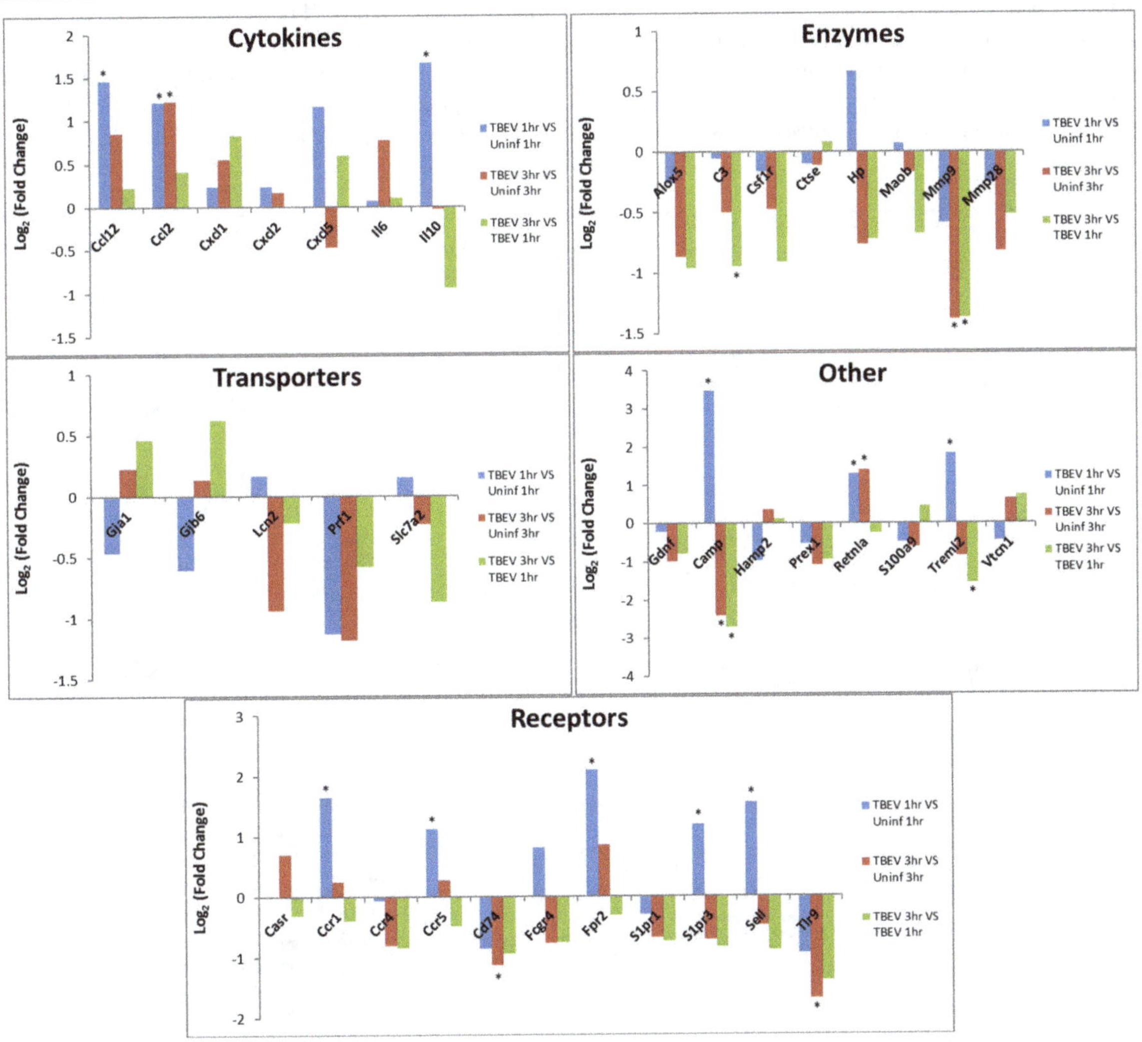

FIGURE 3 | Changes in gene expression related to the inflammatory response after 1 and 3 h of TBEV-infected *Ixodes ricinus* tick feeding. Temporal changes in gene expression data were analyzed by IPA software. Genes predicted to be directly involved in the "Inflammatory Response" were plotted to show temporal changes in gene expression for the following comparisons: TBEV-infected tick feeding loci at 1 h vs. uninfected tick feeding loci at 1 h, TBEV-infected tick feeding loci at 3 h vs. uninfected tick feeding loci at 3 h, TBEV-infected tick feeding loci at 3 h vs. TBEV-infected tick feeding loci at 1 h. Genes with significant modulation in expression ($p \leq 0.05$) are marked with an asterisk.

Illumina NGS analysis (**Figure 1E**). All of the enzymes projected to have a direct, correlative relationship with the inflammatory response were downregulated at 3 h, further contributing to the predicted inhibition of the inflammatory response at the feeding site of a TBEV-infected tick (**Figure 3**). Additionally, transcript expression of several receptors (CCR1, CCR5, and Sell) were all significantly upregulated after 1 h of TBEV-infected tick feeding (**Figure 3**), likely contributing to the overall accumulation of immune cells to the tick attachment site. In summary, the cutaneous gene expression analysis indicates that the inflammatory response is activated after only 1 h of TBEV-infected tick feeding, and that increased recruitment and accumulation of immune cells is expected at the 1 h time point. However, after 3 h of TBEV-infected tick feeding, the cutaneous inflammatory response is predicted to undergo slight inhibition, as demonstrated by the downregulated expression of over half of the genes shown to have a correlative relationship with the inflammatory response (**Figure 3**).

An IPA core comparison analysis was used to analyze changes in host cutaneous gene expression in response to TBEV-infected tick feeding vs. uninfected tick feeding observed across the two experimental time points (1 and 3 h). **Figure 4** shows activation status prediction networks for the top five immune responses or bio-functions generated from the IPA core comparison analysis. "Maintenance of leukocytes" was the top predicted bio-function in the core comparison analysis (**Figure 4**). This IPA category moniker refers to bio-functions associated with the normal cellular activities that maintain cellular homeostasis, including engulfment, phagocytosis, regulation, and stasis of cells. The maintenance of leukocytes was predicted to be inhibited at both the 1 and 3 h comparisons of TBEV-infected vs. uninfected tick feeding (activation z-score = −2 for both time points). At both the 1 and 3 h time points, GATA3 transcription was downregulated (**Figure 4**). GATA3 is a transcription factor required for both the maintenance and development of Th2 cells (Pai et al., 2004). Furthermore, IL34, which is highly expressed by keratinocytes in the epidermis and plays an important role in the maintenance and development of Langerhans cells (Greter et al., 2012), was also downregulated after 1 and 3 h of TBEV-infected tick feeding (**Figure 4**). CCR4 knockout ($CCR4^{-/-}$) bone marrow-derived dendritic cells are less efficient in the maintenance of Th17 responses compared to wild type dendritic cells (Poppensieker et al., 2012); therefore, the downregulation of CCR4 transcription in the present study contributes to the

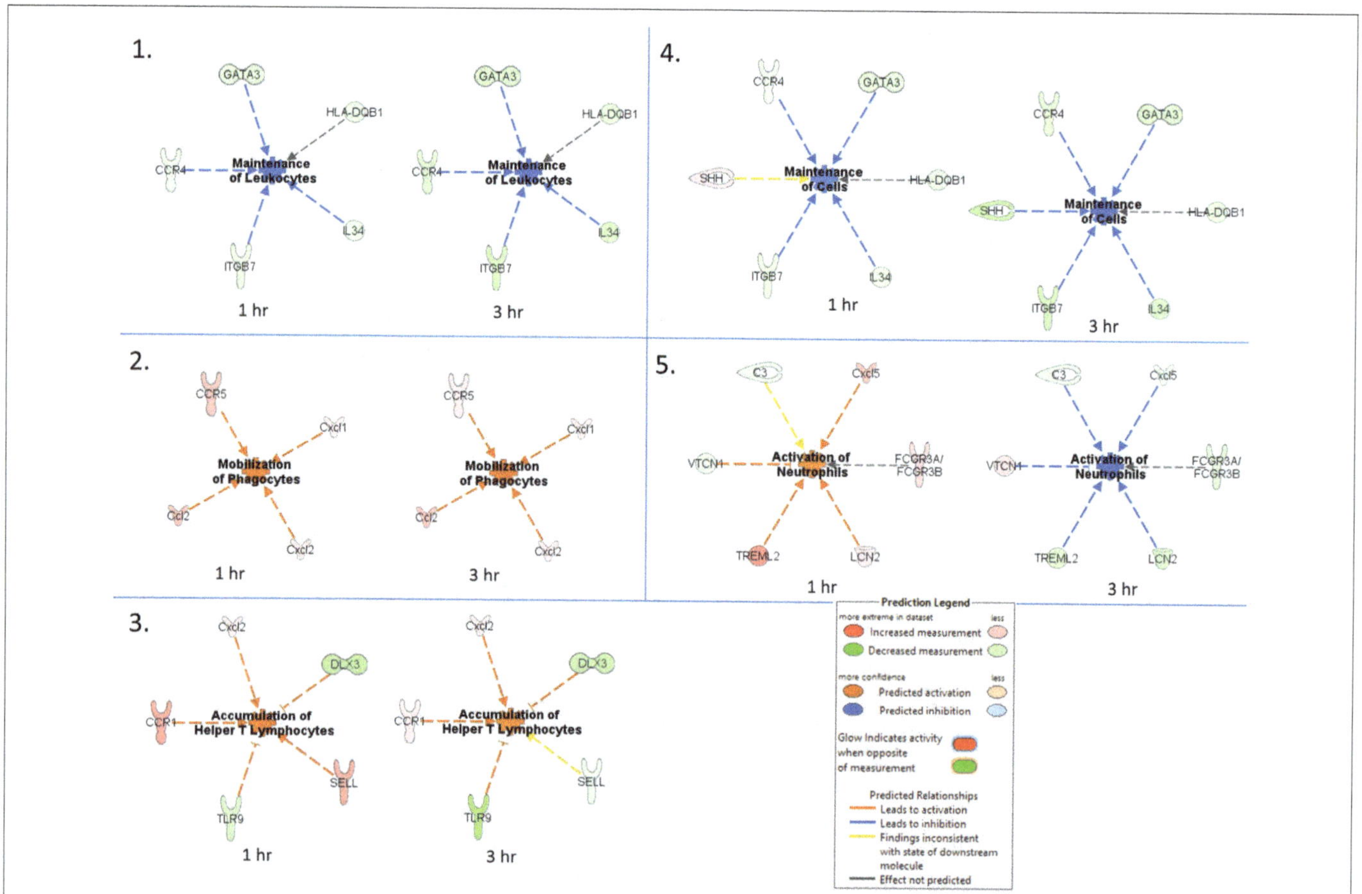

FIGURE 4 | Activation status prediction networks for the top five immune responses / bio-functions generated from the IPA core comparison analysis. An IPA core comparison analysis was used to analyze which biological processes are relevant at 1 and 3 h of TBEV-infected vs. uninfected tick feeding. The predicted activation status of each network is shown.

inhibition of leukocyte maintenance at the 1 and 3 h time points. Mouse integrin subunit beta 7 (ITGB7) is necessary for the maintenance of memory T lymphocytes expressing the CD4 protein (Yang et al., 2011). Since ITGB7 is downregulated in the present transcriptional immunoprofiling study, it likely contributes to the inhibited maintenance of memory CD4+ T cells after 1 and 3 h of TBEV-infected tick feeding.

"Mobilization of phagocytes" was the second predicted bio-function in the core comparison analysis. After 1 and 3 h of TBEV-infected vs. uninfected tick feeding, the mobilization of phagocytes was predicted to be activated (activation z-score = 1.982 for both time points) (**Figure 4**). Monocytes, macrophages, neutrophils, dendritic cells, and mast cells are several of the professional phagocytic cells. In mice, there are two Ccl2 homologs, Ccl2 and Ccl12, both of which are potent phagocyte chemoattractants. The transcript levels of these two chemokines are upregulated at both the 1 and 3 h time points, thereby increasing the mobilization and chemotaxis of phagocytes at the TBEV-infected tick feeding site (**Figures 3, 4**). CCR5 is known to regulate accumulation of activated macrophages in the West Nile virus-infected mouse brain (Glass et al., 2005), and upregulated transcription of this chemokine receptor in the present study likely contributes to the activated mobilization of phagocytes. Mast cells and tissue resident macrophages release the potent neutrophil chemoattractants, Cxcl1 and Cxcl2 (De Filippo et al., 2008, 2013). In response to tissue inflammation, mast cells positioned near the vasculature initiate neutrophil infiltration from the circulation by releasing Cxcl1 and Cxcl2, while tissue resident macrophages also release Cxcl1 and Cxcl2, recruiting neutrophils deeper into the inflamed tissue (De Filippo et al., 2013). In the present study transcript levels of both these chemokines are both upregulated during TBEV-infected tick feeding, thus contributing to the activated mobilization of neutrophils that infiltrate the tick feeding site very early (**Figures 3, 4**).

The third predicted bio-function generated in the IPA core comparison analysis was "accumulation of helper T lymphocytes." The activation z-score for this bio-function decreased from 2.19 at 1 h post-TBEV-infected tick feeding to 1.452 at the 3 h time point. Transcript levels of CCR1 and Cxcl2 are upregulated at both time points in the present study and these genes are associated with the recruitment and accumulation of helper T lymphocytes at the cutaneous site of TBEV-infected tick feeding (**Figure 4**). Selectin L (SELL) is a cellular adhesion molecule found on the surface of most lymphocytes that mediates lymphocyte capture and rolling at sites of inflammation (Tedder et al., 1995). In the present study, SELL transcription was upregulated at the 1 h time point, contributing to the IPA prediction that helper T lymphocytes are accumulating, but the downregulated transcription of SELL at 3 h is inconsistent with the predicted activation pattern, as depicted by the yellow arrow in **Figure 4**. TLR9, a receptor that preferentially binds unmethylated CpG sequences in bacterial and viral DNA, was downregulated in the present study (**Figure 4**). Here, the downregulation of TLR9 transcription is predicted to activate the accumulation of T lymphocytes at the skin feeding site of a TBEV-infected tick. This prediction is supported by a recently developed mouse model of cutaneous lupus that is dependent on the expression of TLR7 and the loss of TLR9, which ultimately results in extensive accumulation of IFNγ-producing T lymphocytes (Mande et al., 2017). Distal-less 3 (DLX3) is a transcription factor involved in the terminal differentiation of keratinocytes. In a

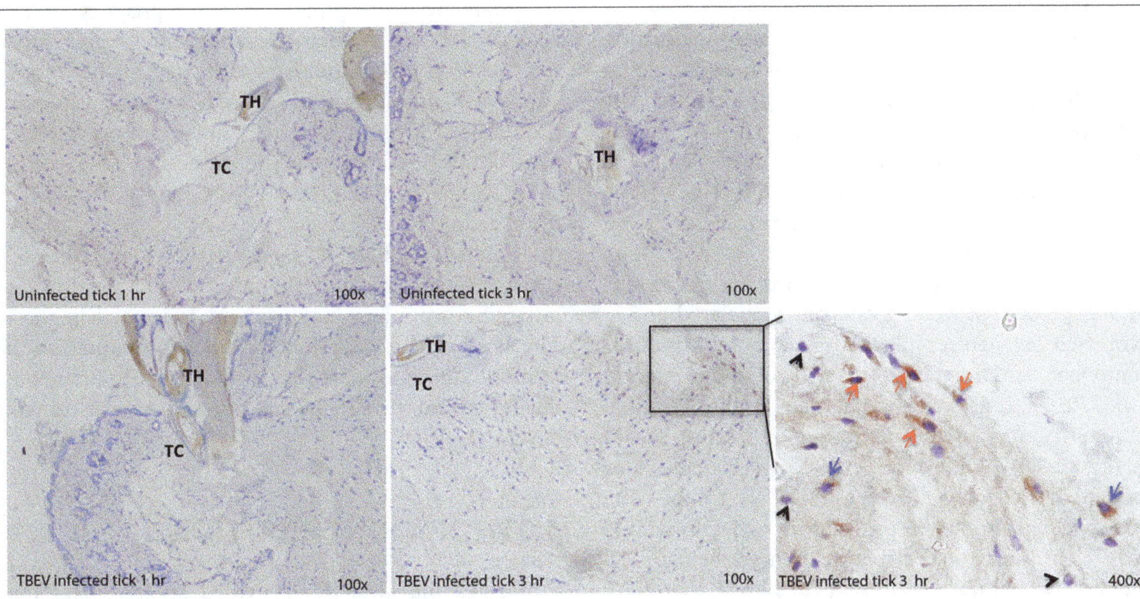

FIGURE 5 | Immunohistochemistry of the *Ixodes ricinus* feeding loci. Five micron sections from skin biopsies harvested at *I. ricinus* feeding sites were subjected to immunohistochemistry procedures to detect TBEV antigens. Red arrows point to TBEV infected fibroblasts; blue arrows point to TBEV infected mononuclear phagocytes, and black arrowheads point to uninfected neutrophils. TH, tick hypostome; TC, tick cement.

mouse model with epidermal ablation of DLX3, there was an increase of IL17-producing $CD4^+$ T cells, $CD8^+$ T cells, and γδ T cells in the skin and draining lymph nodes (Hwang et al., 2011); thus, the downregulated transcription of DLX3 in the skin biopsies from the present study likely contributes to the accumulation of helper T lymphocytes at the cutaneous feeding site of infected ticks (**Figure 4**).

"Maintenance of cells" was the fourth predicted bio-function in the IPA core comparison analysis. This bio-function was predicted to be inhibited at both experimental time points (1 h activation z-score = −1.342, 3 h activation z-score = −2.236). The "maintenance of cells" activation network is very similar to the top predicted network, "maintenance of leukocytes"; however, the only difference is that Sonic hedgehog (SHH) is present in the "maintenance of cells" network (**Figure 4**). The touch dome, a highly specialized mechanosensory epidermal structure composed of distinct keratinocytes in close association with innervated Merkel cells, is maintained by signaling with SHH to tissue-specific stem cells (Xiao et al., 2015). In the present study SHH transcription is upregulated after 1 h of TBEV-infected tick feeding, a finding that is inconsistent with the predicted pattern of inhibited cell maintenance (depicted by the yellow arrow in **Figure 4**); however, at the 3 h time point, SHH transcription was downregulated, contributing to the predicted inhibition of touch dome cell maintenance (**Figure 4**). Some damage to the perineural skin microenvironment is likely to occur because of the mechanical injury induced by tick feeding, and this could ultimately impact SHH signaling and the touch dome homeostasis.

The "activation of neutrophils" was the fifth predicted bio-function in the core comparison analysis. After 1 h of TBEV-infected vs. uninfected tick feeding, neutrophil activation was predicted to be activated (activation z-score = 1.342); however, after 3 h, neutrophils were predicted to be inhibited (activation z-score = −2.236) (**Figure 4**). The upregulated transcription of Cxcl5 and TREML2 at the 1 h time point, followed by the downregulation of these genes at the 3 h time point contribute to this phenomenon because Cxcl5 is a chemokine involved in the activation of neutrophils (Proost et al., 1993) and TREML2 potentiates neutrophil activation in response to G protein-coupled receptor signaling (Halpert et al., 2011). Likewise, Lipocalin-2 (LCN2) transcription was upregulated at 1 h post-TBEV-infected tick feeding and downregulated at 3 h. LCN2 is expressed in neutrophils and is a potent inducer of their chemotaxis and migration to sites of inflammation (Schroll et al., 2012); thus, its upregulation at the 1 h time point further contributes to the activation of neutrophils at the feeding site of TBEV-infected ticks. VTCN1 belongs to the B7 family of costimulatory proteins. VTCN1 inhibits the expansion of neutrophils from their progenitors, as demonstrated by VTCN1-deficient mice that display enhanced neutrophil-mediated innate immunity (Zhu et al., 2009); therefore, the downregulation of VTCN1 transcription after 1 h, and its upregulation after 3 h, contributes to the activation of neutrophils at the cutaneous feeding site of a TBEV-infected tick (**Figure 4**).

Immunohistochemistry

Immunohistochemical analysis was performed at the feeding sites of TBEV-infected and uninfected *I. ricinus* to determine if the gene expression data could be correlated to the tissue morphology and inflammation. The tick feeding site is characterized by extravasated erythrocytes and leucocytes, and with a steady influx of inflammatory cells. As early as 1 h post-TBEV-infected tick feeding, neutrophils were observed at both infected and uninfected tick feeding sites, with a marked increase at the infected tick feeding site. After 3 h of TBEV-infected tick feeding, increased recruitment of inflammatory cells was observed at the infected tick feeding site compared to the uninfected tick feeding site. Among these, TBEV antigens were localized in fibroblasts and mononuclear cells, but not in neutrophils (**Figure 5**). These immunohistochemistry observations support the cutaneous immune gene expression data, showing an inflammatory micro-environment at the feeding site of TBEV-infected ticks. The recruitment of inflammatory cells appears to be much more pronounced in the TBEV-infected tick feeding site than the uninfected tick feeding site.

CONCLUSIONS

The present study demonstrates that TBEV-infected *I. ricinus* adult ticks create an inflammatory environment at the murine cutaneous interface within 1 h of feeding. Significant differences in immune responses were observed between hosts infested with TBEV-infected vs. uninfected ticks. Furthermore, genes associated with neutrophil activation and mobilization were modulated in the presence of TBEV, suggesting that there is an influx of neutrophils and other phagocytic inflammatory cells to the tick feeding site after only 1 and 3 h of infected tick feeding. Immunohistochemistry further supported the cutaneous immune gene expression analysis, demonstrating pronounced recruitment of inflammatory cells, especially neutrophils, to the feeding site of TBEV-infected ticks. Taken together with our earlier study on POWV-infected tick feeding sites (Hermance and Thangamani, 2014), and the current study, it is clearly evident that during the earliest stages of flavivirus-infected tick feeding, a complex, inflammatory micro-environment is created in the host's skin. The present study serves to expand our understanding of the immunological events that occur at the cutaneous interface during the early stages of tick-borne flavivirus transmission to a host.

AUTHOR CONTRIBUTIONS

Conceived the idea: ST; Provided reagents and materials: ST and MK; Performed experiments: ST, MK, MH, RS, SW, MS, and DH; Data analysis: ST, MH, and SW; Wrote manuscript: ST and MH. All authors critically read and revised the manuscript.

FUNDING

ST is supported by NIH/NIAID grants R01AI127771 and R21AI113128. MK was supported by the Slovak Research and Development Agency (contract no. APVV-0737-12).

ACKNOWLEDGMENTS

The authors wish to thank Dr. Boris Klempa and Marta Siebenstichova from the Institute of Virology, Biomedical Research Center, Slovak Academy of Sciences (Bratislava, Slovakia) for providing TBEV MBS for tick inoculations.

REFERENCES

Alekseev, A. N., Burenkova, L. A., Vasilieva, I. S., Dubinina, H. V., and Chunikhin, S. P. (1996). Preliminary studies on virus and spirochete accumulation in the cement plug of ixodid ticks. *Exp. Appl. Acarol.* 20, 713–723. doi: 10.1007/BF00051556

Alekseev, A. N., and Chunikhin, S. P. (1990). The experimental transmission of the tick-borne encephalitis virus by ixodid ticks (the mechanisms, time periods, species and sex differences). *Parazitologiia* 24, 177–185.

Belova, O. A., Burenkova, L. A., and Karganova, G. G. (2012). Different tick-borne encephalitis virus (TBEV) prevalences in unfed versus partially engorged ixodid ticks -evidence of virus replication and changes in tick behavior. *Ticks Tick Borne Dis.* 3, 240–246. doi: 10.1016/j.ttbdis.2012.05.005

CDC Tick-borne Encephalitis (2017). *Tick-borne encephalitis (TBE). Risk of Exposure. 2017.* Available online at: https://www.cdc.gov/vhf/tbe/exposure/index.html

Danielová, V., Holubová, J., Pejcoch, M., and Daniel, M. (2002). Potential significance oftransovarial transmission in the circulation of tick-borne encephalitis virus. *Folia Parasitol.* 49, 323–325. doi: 10.14411/fp.2002.060

De Filippo, K., Dudeck, A., Hasenberg, M., Nye, E., van Rooijen, N., Hartmann, K., et al. (2013). Mast cell and macrophage chemokines CXCL1/CXCL2 control the early stage of neutrophil recruitment during tissue inflammation. *Blood* 121, 4930–4937. doi: 10.1182/blood-2013-02-486217

De Filippo, K., Henderson, R. B., Laschinger, M., and Hogg, N. (2008). Neutrophil chemokines KC and macrophage-inflammatory protein-2 are newly synthesized by tissue macrophages using distinct TLR signaling pathways. *J. Immunol.* 180, 4308–4315. doi: 10.4049/jimmunol.180.6.4308

Francischetti, I. M., Sa-Nunes, A., Mans, B. J., Santos, I. M., and Ribeiro, J. M. (2009). The role of saliva in tick feeding. *Front. Biosci.* 14:363. doi: 10.2741/3363

Glass, W. G., Lim, J. K., Cholera, R., Pletnev, A. G., Gao, J. L., and Murphy, P. M. (2005). Chemokine receptor CCR5 promotes leukocyte trafficking to the brain and survival in West Nile virus infection. *J. Exp. Med.* 202, 1087–1098. doi: 10.1084/jem.20042530

Greter, M., Lelios, I., Pelczar, P., Hoeffel, G., Price, J., Leboeuf, M., et al. (2012). Stroma-derived interleukin-34 controls the development and maintenance of Langerhans cells and the maintenance of microglia. *Immunity* 37, 1050–1060. doi: 10.1016/j.immuni.2012.11.001

Gritsun, T. S., Lashkevich, V. A., and Gould, E. A. (2003a). Tick-borne encephalitis. *Antiviral Res.* 57, 129–146. doi: 10.1016/S0166-3542(02)00206-1

Gritsun, T. S., Nuttall, P. A., and Gould, E. A. (2003b). Tick-borne flaviviruses. *Adv. Virus. Res.* 61, 317–371. doi: 10.1016/S0065-3527(03)61008-0

Halpert, M. M., Thomas, K. A., King, R. G., and Justement, L. B. (2011). TLT2 potentiates neutrophil antibacterial activity and chemotaxis in response to G protein-coupled receptor-mediated signaling. *J. Immunol.* 187, 2346–2355. doi: 10.4049/jimmunol.1100534

Heinze, D. M., Carmical, J. R., Aronson, J. F., and Thangamani, S. (2012). Early immunologic events at the tick-host interface. *PLoS ONE* 7:e47301. doi: 10.1371/journal.pone.0047301

Hermance, M. E., Santos, R. I., Kelly, B. C., Valbuena, G., and Thangamani, S. (2016). Immune cell targets of infection at the tick-skin interface during Powassan virus transmission. *PLoS ONE* 11:e0155889. doi: 10.1371/journal.pone.0155889

Hermance, M. E., and Thangamani, S. (2014). Proinflammatory cytokines and chemokines at theskin interface during Powassan virus transmission. *J. Invest. Dermatol.* 134, 2280–2283. doi: 10.1038/jid.2014.150

Hermance, M. E., and Thangamani, S. (2015). Tick saliva enhances Powassan virus transmission to the host, influencing its dissemination and the course of disease. *J. Virol.* 89, 7852–7860. doi: 10.1128/JVI.01056-15

Hwang, J., Kita, R., Kwon, H. S., Choi, E. H., Lee, S. H., Udey, M. C., et al. (2011). Epidermal ablation of Dlx3 is linked to IL-17-associated skin inflammation. *Proc. Natl. Acad. Sci. U.S.A.* 108, 11566–15671. doi: 10.1073/pnas.1019658108

Kaufman, W. R., and Nuttall, P. A. (1996). *Amblyomma variegatum* (Acari: Ixodidae): mechanism and control of arbovirus secretion in tick saliva. *Exp. Parasitol.* 82, 316–323. doi: 10.1006/expr.1996.0039

Kazimírová, M., and Štibrániová, I. (2013). Tick salivary compounds: their role in modulation of host defences and pathogen transmission. *Front. Cell. Infect. Microbiol.* 3:43. doi: 10.3389/fcimb.2013.00043

Kazimírová, M., Mantel, N., Raynaud, S., Slovák, M., Ustaniková, K., Lang, J., et al. (2012). Evaluation of chimeric yellow fever 17D/dengue viral replication in ticks. *Vector Borne Zoonot. Dis.* 12, 979–985. doi: 10.1089/vbz.2011.0947

Kazimírová, M., Thangamani, S., Bartíková, P., Hermance, M., Holíková, V., Štibrániová, I., et al. (2017). Tick-borne viruses and biological processes at the tick-host-virus interface. *Front. Cell. Infect. Microbiol.* 7:339. doi: 10.3389/fcimb.2017.00339

Kovalev, S. Y., and Mukhacheva, T. A. (2014). Tick-borne encephalitis virus subtypes emerged through rapid vector switches rather than gradual evolution. *Ecol. Evol.* 4, 4307–4316. doi: 10.1002/ece3.1301

Labuda, M., Austyn, J. M., Zuffova, E., Kozuch, O., Fuchsberger, N., Lysy, J., et al. (1996). Importance of localized skin infection in tick-borne encephalitis virus transmission. *Virology* 219, 357–366. doi: 10.1006/viro.1996.0261

Labuda, M., Jones, L. D., Williams, T., Danielova, V., and Nuttall, P. A. (1993). Efficient transmission of tick-borne encephalitis virus between cofeeding ticks. *J. Med. Entomol.* 30, 295–299. doi: 10.1093/jmedent/30.1.295

Labuda, M., Kozuch, O., Zuffová, E., Elecková, E., Hails, R. S., and Nuttall, P. A. (1997). Tick-borne encephalitis virus transmission between ticks cofeeding on specific immune natural rodent hosts. *Virology* 235, 138–143. doi: 10.1006/viro.1997.8622

Lindquist, L., and Vapalahti, O. (2008). Tick-borne encephalitis. *Lancet* 371, 1861–1871. doi: 10.1016/S0140-6736(08)60800-4

Mande, P., Taravati, K., Rosenblum, M., and Rothstein, A. M. (2017). Taking a 'Toll' on skin: a novel TLR9-deficient model of cutaneous lupus [Abstract]. *J. Immunol.* 198, 207.2.

Mansfield, K. L., Johnson, N., Phipps, L. P., Stephenson, J. R., Fooks, A. R., and Solomon, T. (2009). Tick-borne encephalitis virus - a review of an emerging zoonosis. *J. Gen. Virol.* 90, 1781–1794. doi: 10.1099/vir.0.011437-0

Oliveros, J. C. (2007). *Venny. An Interactive Tool for Comparing Lists with Venn Diagrams.* Available online at: http://bioinfogp.cnb.csic.es/tools/venny/index.html (Accessed February, 2017).

Pai, S. Y., Truitt, M. L., and Ho, I. C. (2004). GATA-3 deficiency abrogates the development and maintenance of T helper type 2 cells. *Proc. Natl. Acad. Sci. U.S.A.* 101, 1993–1998. doi: 10.1073/pnas.0308697100

Poppensieker, K., Otte, D. M., Schürmann, B., Limmer, A., Dresing, P., Drews, E., et al. (2012). CC chemokine receptor 4 is required for experimental autoimmune encephalomyelitis by regulating GM-CSF and IL-23 production in dendritic cells. *Proc. Natl. Acad. Sci. U.S.A.* 109, 3897–3902. doi: 10.1073/pnas.1114153109

Proost, P., Wuyts, A., Conings, R., Lenaerts, J. P., Billiau, A., Opdenakker, G., et al. (1993). Human and bovine granulocyte chemotactic protein-2: complete amino acid sequence and functional characterization as chemokines. *Biochemistry* 32, 10170–10177. doi: 10.1021/bi00089a037

Randolph, S. E. (2011). Transmission of tick-borne pathogens between co-feeding ticks: milan labuda's enduring paradigm. *Ticks Tick Borne Dis.* 2, 179–182. doi: 10.1016/j.ttbdis.2011.07.004

Ribeiro, J. M., Alarcon-Chaidez, F., Francischetti, I. M., Mans, B. J., Mather, T. N., Valenzuela, J. G., et al. (2006). An annotated catalog of salivary gland transcripts from *Ixodes scapularis* ticks. *Insect Biochem. Mol. Biol.* 36, 111–129. doi: 10.1016/j.ibmb.2005.11.005

Santos, R. I., Hermance, M. E., Gelman, B. B., and Thangamani, S. (2016). Spinal cord ventral horns and lymphoid organ involvement in *Powassan virus* infection in a mouse model. *Viruses* 8:220. doi: 10.3390/v8080220

Schroll, A., Eller, K., Feistritzer, C., Nairz, M., Sonnweber, T., Moser, P. A., et al. (2012). Lipocalin-2 ameliorates granulocyte functionality. *Eur. J. Immunol.* 42, 3346–3357. doi: 10.1002/eji.201142351

Slovák, M., Kazimírová, M., Siebenstichová, M., Ustaníková, K., Klempa, B., Gritsun, T., et al. (2014). Survival dynamics of tick-borne encephalitis virus in *Ixodes ricinus* ticks. *Ticks Tick Borne Dis.* 5, 962–969. doi: 10.1016/j.ttbdis.2014.07.019

Süss, J. (2011). Tick-borne encephalitis 2010: epidemiology, risk areas, and virus strains in Europe and Asia-an overview. *Ticks Tick Borne Dis.* 2, 2–15. doi: 10.1016/j.ttbdis.2010.10.007

Süss, J., Schrader, C., Falk, U., and Wohanka, N. (2004). Tick-borne encephalitis (TBE) in Germany - epidemiological data, development of risk areas and virus prevalence in field-collected ticks and in ticks removed from humans. *Int. J. Med. Microbiol.* 293, 69–79. doi: 10.1016/S1433-1128(04)80011-1

Šimo, L., Kazimirova, M., Richardson, J., and Bonnet, S. I. (2017). The essential role of tick salivary glands and saliva in tick feeding and pathogen transmission. *Front. Cell. Infect. Microbiol.* 7:281. doi: 10.3389/fcimb.2017.00281

Tedder, T. F., Steeber, D. A., and Pizcueta, P. (1995). L-selectin-deficient mice have impaired leukocyte recruitment into inflammatory sites. *J. Exp. Med.* 181, 2259–2264. doi: 10.1084/jem.181.6.2259

Tonteri, E., Kipar, A., Voutilainen, L., Vene, S., Vaheri, A., Vapalahti, O., et al. (2013). The three subtypes of tick-borne encephalitis virus induce encephalitis in a natural host, the bank vole (*Myodes glareolus*). *PLoS ONE* 8:e81214. doi: 10.1371/journal.pone.0081214

Wikel, S. (2013). Ticks and tick-borne pathogens at the cutaneous interface: host defenses, tick countermeasures, and a suitable environment for pathogen establishment. *Front. Microbiol.* 4:337. doi: 10.3389/fmicb.2013.00337

Xiao, Y., Thoresen, D. T., Williams, J. S., Wang, C., Perna, J., Petrova, R., et al. (2015). Neural Hedgehog signaling maintains stem cell renewal in the sensory touch dome epithelium. *Proc. Natl. Acad. Sci. U.S.A.* 112, 7195–7200. doi: 10.1073/pnas.1504177112

Yang, L., Yu, Y., Kalwani, M., Tseng, T. W., and Baltimore, D. (2011). Homeostatic cytokines orchestrate the segregation of CD4 and CD8 memory T-cell reservoirs in mice. *Blood* 118, 3039–3050. doi: 10.1182/blood-2011-04-349746

Zhu, G., Augustine, M. M., Azuma, T., Luo, L., Yao, S., Anand, S., et al. (2009). B7-H4-deficient mice display augmented neutrophil-mediated innate immunity. *Blood* 113, 1759–1767. doi: 10.1182/blood-2008-01-133223

15

Genomic Study of *Babesia bovis* Infection Level and its Association with Tick Count in Hereford and Braford Cattle

Ligia Cavani [1], Camila Urbano Braz [1*], Rodrigo Giglioti [2], Cintia Hiromi Okino [2], Claudia Cristina Gulias-Gomes [3], Alexandre Rodrigues Caetano [4], Márcia Cristina de Sena Oliveira [2], Fernando Flores Cardoso [3] and Henrique Nunes de Oliveira [1]*

[1] School of Agricultural and Veterinary Sciences, São Paulo State University (Unesp), Jaboticabal, Brazil, [2] Empresa Brasileira de Pesquisa Agropecuária, Embrapa Pecuária Sudeste, São Carlos, Brazil, [3] Empresa Brasileira de Pesquisa Agropecuária, Embrapa Pecuária Sul, Bagé, Brazil, [4] Empresa Brasileira de Pesquisa Agropecuária, Embrapa Recursos Genéticos e Biotecnologia, Brasília, Brazil

***Correspondence:**
Ligia Cavani
ligiacavani@hotmail.com
Camila Urbano Braz
camila_urbano@yahoo.com.br

Bovine babesiosis is a tick-borne disease caused by intraerythrocytic protozoa and leads to substantial economic losses for the livestock industry throughout the world. *Babesia bovis* is considered the most pathogenic species, which causes bovine babesiosis in Brazil. Genomic data could be used to evaluate the viability of improving resistance against *B. bovis* infection level (IB) through genomic selection, and, for that, knowledge of genetic parameters is needed. Furthermore, genome-wide association studies (GWAS) could be conducted to provide a better understanding of the genetic basis of the host response to *B. bovis* infection. No previous work in quantitative genetics of *B. bovis* infection was found. Thus, the objective of this study was to estimate the genetic correlation between IB and tick count (TC), evaluate predictive ability and applicability of genomic selection, and perform GWAS in Hereford and Braford cattle. The single-step genomic best linear unbiased prediction method was used, which allows the estimation of both breeding values and marker effects. Standard phenotyping was conducted for both traits. IB quantifications from the blood of 1,858 animals were carried using quantitative PCR assays. For TC, one to three subsequent tick counts were performed by manually counting adult female ticks on one side of each animal's body that was naturally exposed to ticks. Animals were genotyped using the Illumina BovineSNP50 panel. The posterior mean of IB heritability, estimated by the Bayesian animal model in a bivariate analysis, was low (0.10), and the estimations of genetic correlation between IB and TC were also low (0.15). The cross-validation genomic prediction accuracy for IB ranged from 0.18 to 0.35 and from 0.29 to 0.32 using k-means and random clustering, respectively, suggesting that genomic predictions could be used as a tool to improve genetics for IB, especially if a larger training population is developed. The top 10 single nucleotide polymorphisms from the GWAS explained 5.04% of total genetic variance for IB, which were located on chromosomes 1, 2, 5, 6, 12, 17, 18, 16, 24, and 26.

Some candidate genes participate in immunity system pathways indicating that those genes are involved in resistance to *B. bovis* in cattle. Although the genetic correlation between IB and TC was weak, some candidate genes for IB were also reported in tick infestation studies, and they were also involved in biological resistance processes. This study contributes to improving genetic knowledge regarding infection by *B. bovis* in cattle.

Keywords: babesiosis, cross-validation, genetic parameters, genomic selection, genome-wide association studies

INTRODUCTION

Bovine babesiosis is a tick-borne disease caused by intraerythrocytic protozoa of the *Babesia* genus leading to substantial economic losses for the livestock industry throughout the world (1–3). In Brazil, bovine babesiosis is caused by *Babesia bovis* and *Babesia bigemina*, which are exclusively transmitted by the one-host tick *Rhipicephalus microplus* (4, 5). *B. bovis* is the most pathogenic species (6). The infective forms, which are in tick saliva, invade the host's erythrocytes, multiply until hemolysis, and invade new erythrocytes until the host dies or develops immunity (7). Calves have an innate age-related resistance to babesiosis. Thus, in regions where there is endemic stability, calves are exposed to babesiosis and develop immunity to the disease (6). On the other hand, in regions of endemic instability, where climatic conditions prevent the survival of ticks during a certain period of the year, calves may not be infected when they are young, and outbreaks of babesiosis may occur when ticks reinfest the pastures (8).

Bock et al. (9) and Jonsson et al. (10) observed that zebu (*Bos taurus indicus*) were more resistant to *B. bovis* than taurine (*Bos taurus taurus*) breeds. More recently, the levels of *B. bovis* infection in bovine blood samples have been successfully quantified through quantitative PCR (qPCR) assays (11–14). Differences in these levels were observed between zebu (*B. taurus indicus*) and taurine (*B. taurus taurus*) breeds (12), corroborating previous findings. Phenotypic variation of the level of *B. bovis* infection has been reported (12, 15). However, no quantitative genetic studies have been found in the literature, and little is known regarding its association with tick resistance.

Advances in molecular genetic techniques have allowed the incorporation of genetic markers such as single nucleotide polymorphisms (SNPs) into the breeding analysis, enabling earlier accurate predictions (16). Genomic selection is a powerful strategy to increase the rate of genetic gain, especially in traits where selection based on phenotypic records is difficult, such as disease resistance traits and low heritability traits (17, 18). Cardoso et al. (19) showed that it is possible to control tick infestation through the genomic selection of tick-resistant animals. Therefore, the genetic improvement could be an important tool for *B. bovis* infection control. Moreover, using SNP information allows the detection of genomic regions associated with *B. bovis* infection level through genome-wide association studies (GWAS) (20) and, thus, contributes to a better understanding of the genetic basis of this economically important and complex trait. Regarding a tick resistance trait in cattle, many studies have identified genomic regions through association studies (21–26).

The objective of this study was to estimate the genetic correlation between *B. bovis* infection level (IB) and tick count (TC), evaluate predictive ability and application of genomic selection, and perform GWAS for IB in Hereford and Braford cattle to better understand the biological mechanisms underlying IB and its association with tick resistance.

MATERIALS AND METHODS

Phenotype Data

The data set was provided by the Delta G Connection breeding program (Gensys Associated Consultants, Porto Alegre, RS, Brazil), which included Hereford and Braford cattle raised on pastures in southern Brazil. The Braford breed is a combination of 3/8 indicine breeds and 5/8 Hereford; however, in Brazil, the breeders are allowed to vary the relative proportion of the component breeds. In addition to phenotypic records on IB and TC, pedigree information for the last three generations and genotype data were included. A total of 5,867 (1,915 Hereford and 3,952 Braford) animals provided TC records, and 1,858 animals (225 Hereford and 1,633 Braford) provided IB records, between the years 2010–2013. The average age of the animals during the evaluation period was 17.5 months (10.9–23.1 months).

Babesia bovis Infection Level

The IB was assessed by determining the number of copies of *B. bovis* target DNA sequence (cytochrome b gene). For that, DNA was extracted from blood samples of each animal collected on FTA cards using the Gensolve DNA recovery kit (Gentegra, Pleasanton, CA, USA). The concentration and quality of this DNA were determined in a NanoDrop spectrophotometer (NanoDrop Technologies Inc., Wilmington, Delaware, USA). The DNA samples were kept at −80°C until further analysis. After that, the qPCR was performed using the CFX™ Real-Time PCR Detection System (BioRad, Hercules, CA, USA), according to Giglioti et al. (14). The primers cbosg 1 (F): 5′ -TGTTCCTGGAAGCGTTGATTC-3′ and cbosg 2 (R): 5′-AGCGTGAAAATAACGCATTGC-3′ amplify an 88-bp fragment from the cytochrome b gene of *B. bovis* (11, 27). The standard curves were plotted using 10-fold dilutions of synthetic DNA gBlocks® Gene Fragments (IDT, Coralville, IA, USA), which contain known concentrations of the *B. bovis* target sequence. To estimate the number of copies of the target DNA sequence (NC), the samples and controls were submitted to qPCR tests together with dilutions of synthetic DNA gBlocks®. Then, using software native to the CFX96 system, NC values for dilutions were utilized as a reference for the estimation of NC in the samples. Default settings were used for all parameters, except for the threshold line that was set to the same value, at 200 relative fluorescence unit, for all qPCR tests. All samples and controls were tested in duplicate, and samples with a standard deviation >0.5 were retested. Samples presenting NC > 0 and specific temperature melting (Tm) (77.5 ± 0.5°C) were considered positive.

Tick Count

The animals were naturally exposed to ticks, and after weaning, when the visual estimate of the average infestation across all animals in a management group (animals raised together, receiving the same feeding and sanitary management) exceeded about 20 engorged female ticks, counts were performed by manual counting adult female ticks (4.5–8 mm in length) on the right side of each animal (28). This process was carried out one to three times in each management group. Tick counts were performed in late spring, summer, and early fall, and the minimum period between counts was 30 days.

For the analyses, the IB and TC records were transformed in log10(x + 1) due to normality assumptions of the models used in this study. The descriptive statistics are shown in **Table 1**.

Genotype Data

A total of 4,496 animals were genotyped with the Illumina BovineSNP50 BeadChip (50K; Illumina, San Diego, CA). Genotype quality control was performed using the R *snpStats* package (29) to remove samples with a call rate < 0.90, heterozygosity 3.0 SD above or below the observed mean, mismatching sex, and duplicated records. Only SNPs mapped to the autosomes, with call rates > 0.98, minor allele frequencies > 0.03, and not in a highly significant deviation from the Hardy–Weinberg equilibrium ($P > 10^{-7}$), were considered for the analyses. Additionally, only the SNP with the highest minor allele frequency was retained when two SNPs were highly correlated ($r > 0.98$). After quality control, 39,919 SNP markers and 4,388 samples remained for the statistical analysis.

Statistical Models

The genetic parameter estimations for IB and TC were performed by Bayesian inference in a bivariate analysis using an animal model. The Bayesian approach was chosen because the sample size was not large, and, to our knowledge, this is the first quantitative genetic study for IB, which is a new phenotype. The advantage of Bayesian methods, in this case, is that interpretation of the results and uncertainties about the estimates are facilitated, as all results are presented in terms of probabilities (30).

The model can be represented as follows:

$$\mathbf{y}=\mathbf{X}\boldsymbol{\beta}+\mathbf{Z_1 a}+\mathbf{Z_2 p}+\mathbf{e}$$

with the joint distribution of vectors **a**, **p**, and **e** as:

$$\begin{bmatrix}\mathbf{a}\\\mathbf{p}\\\mathbf{e}\end{bmatrix}\sim N\left\{\begin{bmatrix}0\\0\\0\end{bmatrix},\begin{bmatrix}\mathbf{G_0}\otimes\mathbf{H} & 0 & 0\\ 0 & \mathbf{P_0}\otimes\mathbf{I} & 0\\ 0 & 0 & \mathbf{R_0}\otimes\mathbf{I}\end{bmatrix}\right\},$$

where $\mathbf{y}$ is a vector of observations; $\boldsymbol{\beta}$ is a vector of systematic (fixed) effects; $\mathbf{a}$ is a vector of random additive genetic direct effects; $\mathbf{p}$ is the vector of random permanent environmental effects; $\mathbf{e}$ is a vector of random residuals; $\mathbf{X}$, $\mathbf{Z_1}$, and $\mathbf{Z_2}$ are known incidence matrices; $\mathbf{G_0}$ and $\mathbf{P_0}$ are the additive genetic direct and environmental permanent effects (co)variance matrices, respectively; $\mathbf{H}$ is the additive genetic relationship matrix; $\mathbf{R_0}$ is the residual (co)variance matrix; and $\mathbf{I}$ is an identity matrix with suitable dimensions. Only the permanent environmental effects were included in the model for TC; therefore, $\mathbf{p}$, $\mathbf{Z_2}$, and $\mathbf{P_0}$ were not considered for IB.

The $\mathbf{H}$ matrix combines genotype and pedigree information (31, 32), and its inverse ($\mathbf{H^{-1}}$) can be described in matrix notation as:

$$\mathbf{H}^{-1}=\mathbf{A}^{-1}+\begin{bmatrix}0 & 0\\ 0 & \mathbf{G}^{-1}-\mathbf{A}_{22}^{-1}\end{bmatrix},$$

where $\mathbf{G}$ is a genomic relationship matrix constructed as in VanRaden (33) using current allele frequencies, and $\mathbf{A_{22}}$ is a numerator relationship matrix only for genotyped animals.

Concerning the systematic effects, contemporary groups (CGs) were included for IB and TC, as well as the effect of racial composition (zebu proportion, heterozygosity, and recombination loss computed from pedigree information). Linear and quadratic effects of animal age were considered only for TC. For IB, the linear effect of total DNA concentration available for qPCR assays was considered. The CG was composed of the animal from the same farm, sex, year and season of birth, and management group. For TC, the date of the phenotypic evaluations was also included in the CG. CGs with less than three observations were excluded from the data set. The total numbers of CGs for IB and TC were 15 and 227, respectively.

TABLE 1 | Descriptive statistics for *Babesia bovis* infection level (IB) and tick counts (TC) in Braford and Hereford cattle.

Traits	N[a]	Mean[b]	SD[b]	Minimum	Median[b]	Maximum[b]
IB	1,858	719.9 (1.6)	5,920.68 (1.14)	0	79.2 (1.9)	154,199.5 (5.2)
TC	13,874	38.9 (1.4)	48.46 (0.47)	0	25 (1.4)	600 (2.8)

[a] *Number of records.*
[b] *Log-transformed scale data is shown in parentheses.*

The GIBBS2F90 program (34) was used to obtain samples from the posterior distributions of genetic, permanent environmental, and residual (co)variances. A Gibbs sampling chain with 500,000 samples was generated, with the initial 50,000 samples discarded as burn-in based on visual inspection of trace plots and the convergence tests of Gelman and Rubin (35) and Geweke (36) as well as of Heidelberg and Welch (37) using the *coda* package (38) of the R software (39). The posterior distributions of the variance and covariance components were approximated based on the remaining 450,000 samples.

Genomic selection and GWAS were performed just for IB using the single-step genomic best linear unbiased prediction (ssGBLUP) approach, and the effects considered in the model were the same as previously described for the IB trait. The ssGBLUP method allows estimation of both breeding values and marker effects and combines genomic and pedigree relationships using the **H** matrix, as described earlier.

To estimate the genomic selection accuracy, cross-validation was applied. Furthermore, two animal grouping methods were used: k-means and random. More details are described later.

The predictive ability of genomic selection for IB was assessed by cross-validation, where 1,855 animals (1,631 Braford and 224 Hereford) with genotypes and IB phenotypes were divided into three groups by two strategies using R software (39). The strategies to divide the groups were k-means clustering of marker relationship distances and replicated 10 times at random. Average genomic relationships of each animal with all others within and between groups were calculated to characterize relatedness between training and validation sets (40). For each grouping strategy, 3-fold cross-validations were performed by alternately using records of two groups as training sets to derive genomic predictions for the third (validation) group, whose data were omitted in the analyses for marker effect estimation. Prediction accuracies, within a cluster *c*, were estimated as the correlation between predicted ($\hat{\mathbf{a}}$) and estimated true (**a**) breeding values ($\hat{r}_{\mathbf{a}\hat{\mathbf{a}}c}$), as proposed by Legarra et al. (41):

$$\hat{r}_{\mathbf{a}\hat{\mathbf{a}}c} = PA / \sqrt{h^2}$$

in which PA is the predictive ability defined as the correlation between IB of animals from group *c* adjusted for the fixed effects and predicted values from cross-validation, represented by direct genomic value. Moreover, h^2 is the heritability for IB.

The GWAS for IB were performed using the method proposed by Wang et al. (42), which is based on the ssGBLUP. The effects of the SNPs ($\hat{\mathbf{u}}$) were obtained using the equation described as:

$$\hat{u} = \lambda \mathbf{D}\mathbf{Z}'\mathbf{G}^{*-1}\hat{\mathbf{a}}_{\mathbf{g}}$$

where $\hat{\mathbf{u}}$ is the vector of estimated SNP effects; λ is the variance ratio calculated according to VanRaden et al. (43); $\hat{\mathbf{a}}_g$ is the animal effect of genotyped animals; $\mathbf{Z}'$ is a transpose matrix that relates the genotypes of each locus; $\mathbf{G}^*$ is the weighted genomic relationship matrix; **D** is a diagonal matrix of the weights of SNP variances obtained by the algorithm with the following steps, where *t* is an iteration number, *p* is the allele frequency of the second allele, and *i* is the *i-th* SNP:

1. $t = 0$; $\mathbf{D}_{(t)} = \mathbf{I}$; $\mathbf{G}_{(t)} = \mathbf{Z}\mathbf{D}_{(t)}\mathbf{Z}'\lambda$
2. Compute $\hat{\mathbf{a}}_g$ by ssGBLUP;
3. Calculate $\hat{\mathbf{u}}_{(t)} = \lambda \mathbf{D}_{(t)}\mathbf{Z}'\mathbf{G}_{(t)}^{-1}\hat{\mathbf{a}}_g$;
4. Calculate the weight for each SNP: $d^*_{i_{(t+1)}} = \hat{u}^2_{i_{(t)}} 2p_i(1 - p_i)$ (44);
5. Normalize $\mathbf{D}_{(t+1)} = (\mathrm{tr}(\mathbf{D}_{(0)})/\mathrm{tr}(\mathbf{D}^*_{(t+1)}))\mathbf{D}^*_{(t+1)}$;
6. Calculate $\mathbf{G}_{(t+1)} = \mathbf{Z}\mathbf{D}_{(t+1)}\mathbf{Z}'\lambda$;
7. Loop to step 3 for 3 times.

The analyses were carried out using the BLUPF90 family of programs (34). The results of GWAS are reported as the proportion of variance explained by a single SNP. A Manhattan plot was created using the R package "ggplot2" (45). Once the SNPs that explain the largest amount of IB genetic variance were identified, they were assigned to the candidate genes. The candidate genes were identified through the Ensembl genome database project, available at https://useast.ensembl.org/index.html, based on the *Bos taurus* ARS.120 reference assembly. For that, the genomic coordinates were expanded by 500 kb upstream and downstream; in this sense, an SNP was assigned to a candidate gene if it was located within or near to the gene. Gene ontology and biological pathway annotations of the genes were retrieved using the biomaRt package (46) and Reactome Pathway Knowledgebase (47), respectively.

RESULTS AND DISCUSSION

Genetic Parameters

Estimates of heritability and repeatability for TC were low (0.127) and moderate (0.267), respectively (**Table 2**). The proportion of phenotypic variance explained by genetic variance of TC evaluated in the population of Hereford and Braford cattle was lower than other studies in Brazil with the same breeds that reported a heritability of 0.19 (19, 48). These differences between estimated heritability can be explained by population sample differences and by the model. The main model difference is the matrix relationships; in this study, we used genomic information (SNPs) to build the matrix relationships (H matrix). Lower

TABLE 2 | Posterior mean and 95% highest posterior density intervals (within parentheses) of (co)variance components for *Babesia bovis* infection level (IB) tick counts (TC), and genetic correlation between IB and TC in Braford and Hereford cattle performed by Bayesian animal model in bivariate analysis.

Parameter	IB	TC
Additive genetic variance, σ^2_a	0.088 (0.040, 0.141)	0.012 (0.009, 0.016)
Permanent environmental variance, σ^2_p	–	0.014 (0.010, 0.071)
Residual variance, σ^2_e	1.048 (0.168, 0.890)	0.072 (0.070, 0.074)
Heritability, h^2	0.077 (0.037, 0.124)	0.127 (0.093, 0.160)
Repeatability, r^2	–	0.267 (0.245, 0.289)
Genetic correlation, $r_{IB,TC}$	0.152 (−0.147, 0.445)	

estimates of genetic variance based on genomic relationships compared with those using pedigree relationships may occur; however, the estimates based on genomic relationships are frequently more accurate (49). Further, higher heritabilities would be expected in experimental stations' environmental conditions, as shown by Burrow (50), who reported a heritability of 0.42 for TC in a composite breed, as the conditions of the collection are more controlled. In the present study, the tick counts were carried out through collection by several technicians, and although all were trained for collection, this can be a factor in increasing experimental error. From this perspective, Ayres et al. (51) estimated heritabilities of 0.12 and 0.11 for TC in Brazilian Nellore × Hereford crossbred cattle, and Budeli et al. (52), in South African Bonsmara breed cattle, found heritabilities ranging from 0.03 to 0.17 in groups of animals divided according to mean tick count.

Despite the low posterior mean for IB heritability (0.077), there is additive genetic variability for this trait, and therefore, selection responses may be obtained. No previous information on quantitative genetics for IB was found in the literature; however, low to moderate values for repeatability of IB in Angus (13) and Canchim (14) have been reported. Usually, the heritability estimates for disease traits are low mainly because of the complexity behind these phenotypes (53, 54). Moreover, the genetic correlation between IB and TC was weak (0.152). This suggests that selection for TC would not change IB considerably in the population of this study. Although no quantitative genetic studies were found for levels of babesiosis infection in cattle, Giglioti et al. (14) found the phenotypic correlation between tick count and *B. bovis* levels ranging from 0.02 to 0.17, in different ages. It is important to note that the number of records for IB is much lower than for TC; besides, IB is a new phenotype related to a disease.

Genomic Selection for *Babesia bovis* Infection Level

The k-means clustering yielded three unbalanced groups with 830, 770, and 255 animals in groups 1, 2, and 3, respectively (**Table 3**). A multidimensional scaling bidimensional scatter plot according to the k-means groups is presented in **Figure 1**. Groups 1 and 2 were composed mainly by Braford breed with an average of 35% zebu contribution, whereas group 3 contained primarily Hereford breed (11% zebu contribution). As expected, the average genomic relationship was larger within than between groups. The average number of animals for the groups divided at random replicated 10 times was 618.33 animals (74.67 ± 6.18 Hereford, 12.33 ± 3.36 1/2 Braford, 496.67 ± 6.51 3/8 Braford, and 34.67 ± 3.51 1/4 Braford). Random groups had a similar average genomic relationship within groups (0.011 ± 0.045), and between groups, with the average close to zero.

The accuracy of prediction for groups divided at random was higher than k-means clustering for groups 1 and 2 (**Table 4**). The groups generated by the k-means method had a larger number of crossbred animals, mainly in group 1 (800 animals of Braford breed, **Table 3**). For group 3, the accuracy of the predictions for k-means clustering and random methods was almost the same (0.3). Although, to our knowledge, there is no published genomic predictive study for *B. bovis* in cattle, the superiority of prediction accuracy using random clustering compared with k-means was also observed by Bock et al. (19) for tick resistance in

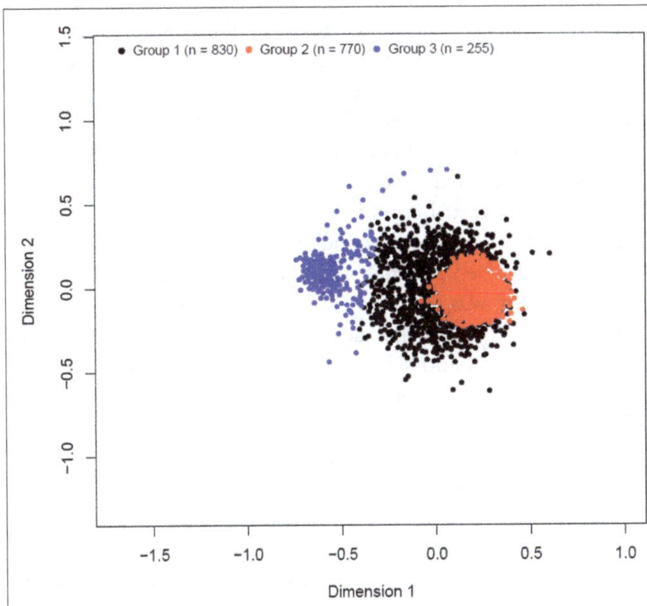

FIGURE 1 | Multidimensional scaling bidimensional scatter plot of k-means clustering cross-validation groups.

TABLE 3 | Number of individuals (N) and averages (±SD) of genomic relationship (*Gij*) within and between-group of Hereford breed and Braford composition breed for k-means clustering groups.

Groups; *N*	Hereford	Braford			*Gij* within group	*Gij* between group
		1/2[a]	3/8[a]	1/4[a]		
1; 830	30	18	734	48	0.009 ± 0.035	0.000 ± 0.030
2; 770	30	18	696	26	0.054 ± 0.042	−0.008 ± 0.049
3; 255	164	1	60	30	0.070 ± 0.054	−0.003 ± 0.056

[a] *Zebu proportion.*

TABLE 4 | Prediction accuracy of direct genomic value predictions for each k-means clustering and random cross-validation group using the ssGBLUP method for *Babesia bovis* infection level.

	Prediction accuracy		
	Group 1	**Group 2**	**Group 3**
k-means	0.180	0.225	0.346
Random	0.293	0.317	0.316

Braford and Hereford cattle. Based on these results, the number of animals used for training the model is more important to achieve better prediction accuracy than the difference between the breed composition of group 3 and the other two groups. This is in agreement with a previous study that reported that a large number of animals in the training population is an important factor that improves the accuracy of genomic selection (18). The lower number of animals could explain the low accuracy for group 1 under k-means clustering in the training population and also the larger genetic relationship distance of groups 2 and 3. Accuracies of genomic predictions are related to the training data size and genetic relatedness between training and validation individuals (55, 56). Furthermore, the low IB heritability (**Table 2**) could be a determinant to the low prediction accuracies found in this study, as genomic selection reliability also depends on trait heritability (57). In this same population, Sollero et al. (58) found much higher accuracy for tick resistance (0.27 to 0.44), even when a specific SNP panel for TC with very low density was used. In dairy cattle, some traits related to resistance to infectious diseases have already been included in genetic evaluations and selection programs using genomic data (59), for example, the overall immune response (60, 61) that has higher heritability and prediction accuracy than results in the present study and the incidence of clinical mastitis (62) showing accuracies and heritability values for the predicted breeding values comparable with those found here. Other traits such as *Mycobacterium avium* subspecies paratuberculosis infection (63) or bovine respiratory disease in Holstein (64) also present low heritability and predictive accuracy. Despite low accuracy, genomic predictions could still be used as a viable tool to obtain a selection response for IB for replacement candidates. However, the expected genetic progress for this trait would be slow.

Genome-Wide Association Studies for *Babesia bovis* Infection Level

Figure 2 shows the Manhattan plot with the percentages of additive genetic variance explained by each SNP for the IB trait. The top 10 SNPs (**Table 5**) explained 5.05% of IB additive genetic variance and identified 42 candidate genes involved in biological mechanisms that may underlie *B. bovis* resistance in cattle. Defense against parasites is mediated by sequential and coordinated immune responses called innate and adaptative (65), and several of the candidate genes participate in immune system pathways (*ATP8A1, LCP1, LRCH1, QSOX1, FGF2, DSC1, DSC3, FGFR2,* and *CEBPG*), which include adaptive and innate immune systems, and cytokine signaling pathways, indicating that genetic variations in these genes can alter the immune response and consequently, influence susceptibility and outcome of babesiosis in cattle. An essential aspect of *B. bovis* infection is that young calves have strong innate immunity, which lasts until about 6 months of age (66). Animals that survive infection with *B. bovis* become persistently infected and resistant to the clinical form of the disease, a phenomenon known as concomitant immunity (67). Adaptative immunity mechanisms are responsible for the absence of clinical signs in persistently infected animals.

LCP1 is a protein of the plastin family. This family is composed of actin-binding proteins that are conserved evolutionarily and expressed in different types of plants and animals (68). In mammals, three isoforms have been identified: T, I, and L-plastin. This latter group includes LCP1 that is expressed in hematopoietic cell lines, with essential functions in the activation of macrophages (69), lymphocytes, and granulocytes (70). According to Brown (71), the immune response against babesiosis depends on the activation of CD4+ T lymphocytes in the development of acquired protein antigen-specific responses. CD4+ T cells are essential for coordinating high-affinity IgG production and activating macrophages through the production of IFN-ɣ.

LRCH1 also encodes proteins that influence the migration of CD4+ T cells (72). These cells play a regulatory role in the immune response and result in higher resistance to *R. microplus* in cattle, although other genes have been reported as mediators for T cell regulation (73, 74). Piper et al. (75) reported that Brahman animals (*B. indicus*) had higher percentages of T cells than did the Holstein–Friesians (*B. taurus*). Constantinoiu et al. (76) observed an increase of T cells in the skin around the site of *R. microplus* larvae attachment in both *B. indicus* and *B. taurus* cattle. Moré et al. (23) observed the participation of CD4+ T cell subtypes in Braford animals classified as tick-resistant. Another type of cell that influences the immune system is the B cell, which plays a role in the humoral immunity component of the adaptive immune system by secreting antibodies (77). The B cells are activated by the proteins encoded by *FGF2* and *FGFR2* genes through the signaling process, and *CEBPG* genes are involved in B cell differentiation. An increase of B lymphocytes in the dermis of tick-resistant cattle breeds was also observed, and differential B-lymphocyte regulation in lymph node tissue was associated with tick susceptibility (78).

The *FGF2* and *FGFR2* genes are involved in interleukins, fibroblast growth factor receptor, cytokine, and MAPK signaling pathways. The *SPRY1* gene also participates in fibroblast growth factor receptor and MAPK signaling pathways. Inflammatory interleukins, growth factors, and cytokines activate the MAPK signaling pathway, which regulates the immune response against intracellular parasites (79, 80). Moreover, cytokines stimulate natural killer cells to produce interferon-gamma (IFN-γ) during the chronic phase of *B. bovis* infection. The IFN-γ activates macrophages that synthesize and release nitric oxide, which inhibits *B. bovis* replication (81–84). The *CEBPG* gene also influences the natural killer cell process.

DSC1, DSC2, and *DSC3* are involved in the keratinization pathway and have been reported in tick resistance studies.

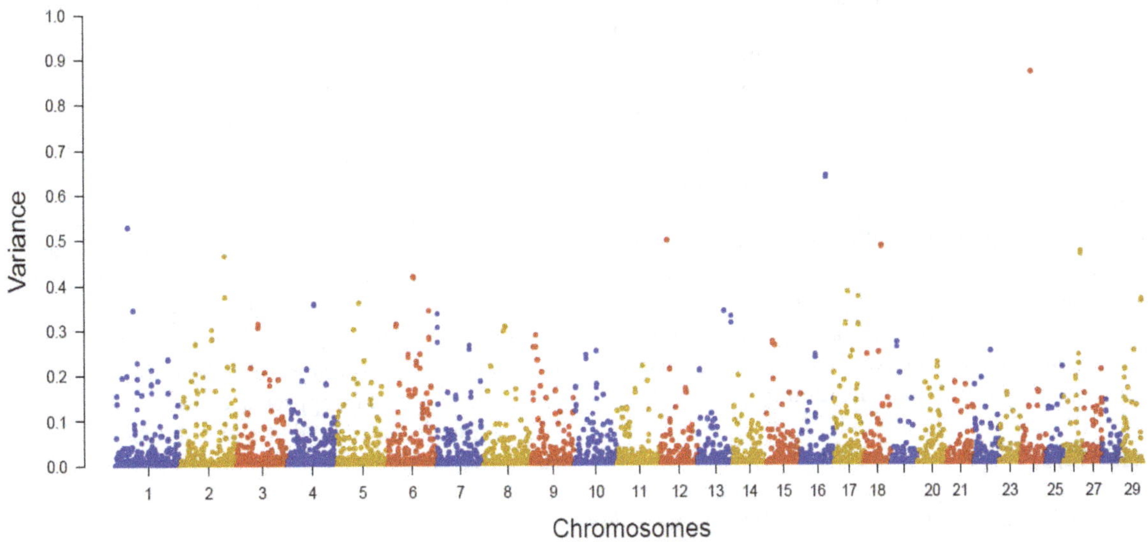

FIGURE 2 | Manhattan plot of additive genetic variance explained by single SNP for *Babesia bovis* infection level.

TABLE 5 | Description of the SNPs with the largest effects on *Babesia bovis* infection level in Hereford breed and Braford composition breed.

BTA	SNP position	Genes[a]	Var (%)
24	26,698,515	*DSC1, DSC2, DSC3*	0.853
16	62,734,784	*CEP350, QSOX1, LHX4, ACBD6, TOR1AIP1, TOR1AIP2, FAM163A*	0.640
1	32,883,377	*CADM2*	0.548
12	16,641,931	*LRCH1, ESD, HTR2A, RUBCNL, LRRC63, LCP1*	0.508
18	44,019,061	*PEPD, CEBPG, CHST8, KCTD15, SLC7A10, LRP3, WDR88, GPATCH1, FAAP24*	0.487
26	42,178,883	*ATE1, NSMCE4A, TACC2, BTBD16, FGFR2*	0.479
6	62,979,121	*ATP8A1, SHISA3, BEND4, SLC30A9, TMEM33, GRXCR1*	0.408
2	109,327,881	*Intergenic region*	0.377
17	34,752,485	*SPRY1, SPATA5, NUDT6, FGF2*	0.377
5	53,704,130	*SLC16A7*	0.367

[a]*Genomic coordinates for each gene based on the Bos taurus ARS.120 reference assembly were expanded by 500 kb upstream and downstream.*
BTA, Bos taurus autosome; Var, proportion of additive genetic variance explained by the single SNP.

Terminal differentiation of keratinocytes is important for the renewal of the stratum corneum, which plays an essential role in defense against the pathogen (85). According to the authors, tick bite lesions led to an increase of keratinocyte differentiation and the promotion of stratum corneum formation. Wang et al. (86) suggested that a dramatic reduction in keratin transcripts may occur in response to tick infestation. Also, *DSC1*, *DSC2*, *DSC3*, and *CADM2* genes participate in the cell adhesion process, which plays a critical role in initiating and sustaining the immune response against foreign pathogens (87). Piper et al. (88) reported that *DSC2* was detected as differentially expressed between tick-infested Holstein–Friesian and Brahman animals at the tick-attachment site. Moreover, a gene with an important biological function in controlling cellular adhesion and migration was associated with tick burden in cattle (89).

Genes involved in the hemostasis pathway, such as *SLC7A10* and *QSOX1*, were also found to harbor the regions identified as influencing IB. Sustained heavy *R. microplus* infestation has been shown to alter host hemostatic mechanisms by inhibiting platelet aggregation and coagulation functions (90). Several putative genes (*SPRY1*, *NUDT6*, *FGF2*, *FGFR2*, and *TACC2*) influencing IB participate in the cell proliferation process. In response to a heavy tick burden, many different types of cells proliferate to present exogenously derived antigens to the immune system (75). The authors identified genes differentially expressed between tick-infested Holstein–Friesian and Brahman animals that were involved in the cell proliferation process.

HTR2A is involved in inflammatory mediator regulation of transient receptor potential (TRP) channels and calcium signaling pathways. Modifications in intracellular calcium concentrations represent a fundamental mechanism in the control of inflammatory and immune cell functions (91). Intracellular calcium influx is a key process for lymphocyte activation and proliferation and cytokine synthesis (92, 93). Cytokine is involved in the immune process against *B. bovis* infection and replication, as discussed previously. As TRP channels favor intracellular calcium permeability, it is conceivable that, in association with other prominent molecular pathways, TRP channels could contribute to immune and inflammatory responses (91). Bagnall et al. (85) demonstrated that genes involved in the intracellular calcium regulation pathway are upregulated in response to cattle tick infestation in bovine skin. Also, the *HTR2A* gene participates in the ERK1 and ERK2 cascade process, which has control over inflammatory mediator synthesis and survival of innate immune cells (94).

CONCLUSIONS

Predictive accuracies are related to the size of training populations, and despite its low heritability, genomic predictions could be used as a tool to improve genetics for *B. bovis* infection level in Hereford and Braford cattle. The effectiveness of this process would rely on generating a larger reference population than that used in the present study. Moreover, some candidate genes that participate in immunity system pathways were identified and could contribute to improving the genetic knowledge regarding *B. bovis* infection in cattle. Although the genetic correlation between *B. bovis* infection level and tick count was weak, some candidate genes for IB were also reported in tick infestation studies, and they were also involved in biological resistance processes.

AUTHOR CONTRIBUTIONS

LC: conception, analysis and interpretation of data, writing the draft, and approval of the version to be published. CB: analysis and interpretation of data and approval of the version to be published. RG and CO: sample preparation, laboratory analysis, interpretation of results, and approval of the version to be published. CG-G: experimental planning and design, data collection, sample preparation, and approval of the version to be published. AC: experimental planning and design, laboratory analysis, and critical revising of the manuscript. MO: technical and conceptual guidance, supervision of laboratory analysis, critical revising of the manuscript, and approval of the version to be published. FC: experimental planning and design, data collection, and approval of the version to be published. HO: experimental planning, critical revising of the manuscript, and approval of the version to be published. All authors contributed to the article and approved the submitted version.

FUNDING

São Paulo Research Foundation supported this work (grant number 2015/13024-0 and grant number 2016/07216-7). Also, this study was financed in part by the Coordenação de Aperfeiçoamento de Pessoal de Nível Superior - Brazil (CAPES) - Finance Code 001.

ACKNOWLEDGMENTS

This work is part of LC's doctoral dissertation (95) (Genetic study of *Babesia bovis* infection level and the association with tick resistance in Hereford and Braford cattle) at São Paulo State University (Unesp), School of Agricultural and Veterinarian Sciences.

REFERENCES

McCosker PJ. The global importance of babesiosis. In: Ristic M, Kreier JP, editors. *Babesiosis*. New York, NY: Academic Press (1981). p. 1–24.

Nari A. Strategies for the control of one-host ticks and relationship withtick-borne diseases in South America. *Vet Parasitol.* (1995) 57:153–65. doi: 10.1016/0304-4017(94)03117-F

Grisi L, Leite RC, Martins JRS, Barros ATM, Andreotti R, Cançado PHD, et al. Reassessment of the potential economic impact of cattle parasites in Brazil. *Rev Brasil Parasitol Vet.* (2014) 23:150–6. doi: 10.1590/S1984-29612014042

Guglielmone AA. Epidemiology of babesiosis and anaplasmosis in Southand Central America. *Vet Parasitol.* (1995) 57:109–19. doi: 10.1016/0304-4017(94)03115-D

Oliveira-Sequeira TCG, Oliveira MCS, Araujo JP, Amarante AFT. PCR- based detection of *Babesia bovis* and *Babesia bigemina* in their natural host *Boophilus microplus* and cattle. *Int J Parasitol.* (2005) 35:105–11. doi: 10.1016/j.ijpara.2004.09.002

Bock R, Jackson L, De Vos AJ, Jorgensen W. Babesiosis of cattle. *Parasitology.* (2004) 129:247–69. doi: 10.1017/S0031182004005190

Hunfeld KP, Hildebrandt A, Gray JS. Babesiosis: recent insights into an ancient disease. *Int J Parasitol.* (2008) 38:1219–37. doi: 10.1016/j.ijpara.2008.03.001

Barros SL, Madruga CR, Araujo FR, Menk CF, Almeida MA, Melo EPS, et al. Serological survey of *Babesia bovis, Babesia bigemina* and *Anaplasma marginale* antibodies in cattle from the semi-arid region of Bahia, Brazil, by enzyme linked immunosorbent assays. *Mem Inst Oswaldo Cruz.* (2005) 100:613–7. doi: 10.1590/S0074-02762005000600003

Bock RE, De Vos AJ, Kingston TG, Mclellan DJ. Effect of breed of cattle on innate resistance to infection with *Babesia bovis*, *B. bigemina* and *Anaplasma marginale*. *Aust Vet J.* (1997) 75:337–40. doi: 10.1111/j.1751-0813.1997.tb15706.x

Jonsson NN, Bock RE, Jorgensen WK. Productivity and health effects of anaplasmosis and babesiosis on *Bos indicus* cattle and their crosses, and the effects of differing intensity of tick control in Australia. *Vet Parasitol.* (2008) 155:1–9. doi: 10.1016/j.vetpar.2008.03.022

Buling A, Criado-Fornelio A, Acenzo G, Benitez D, Barbacarretero JC, Florin-Cristensen M. A quantitative PCR assay for the detection and quantification of *B. bovis* and *B. bigemina. Vet Parasitol.* (2007) 147:16–25. doi: 10.1016/j.vetpar.2007.03.031

Bilhassi TB, Oliveira HN, Ibelli AMG, Giglioti R, Regitano LCA, Oliveira-Siqueira TCG, et al. Quantitative study of *Babesia bovis* infection in beef cattle from São Paulo state, Brazil. *Ticks Tick Borne Dis.* (2014) 5:234–8. doi: 10.1016/j.ttbdis.2013.11.002

Giglioti R, Oliveira HN, Santana CH, Ibelli AM, Néo TA, Bilhassi TB, et al. *Babesia bovis* and *Babesia bigemina* infection levels estimated by qPCR in Angus cattle from an endemic area of São Paulo state, Brazil. *Ticks Tick Borne Dis.* (2016) 7:657–62. doi: 10.1016/j.ttbdis.2016.02.011

Giglioti R, Oliveira HN, Bilhassi TB, Portilho AI, Okino CH, Marcondes CR, et al. Estimates of repeatability and correlations of hemoparasites infection levels for cattle reared in endemic areas for Rhipicephalus microplus. *Vet Parasitol.* (2018) 250:78–84. doi: 10.1016/j.vetpar.2017.12.010

Benavides MV, Sacco AM. Differential *Bos taurus* cattle response to *Babesia bovis* infection. *Vet Parasitol.* (2007) 150:54–64. doi: 10.1016/j.vetpar.2007.08.022

De Los Campos G, Hickey JM, Pong-Wong R, Daetwyler HD, Calus MPL. Whole-genome regression and prediction methods applied to plant and animal breeding. *Genetics.* (2013) 193:327–45. doi: 10.1534/genetics.112.143313

Meuwissen THE, Hayes BJ, Goddard ME. Prediction of total genetic value using genome-wide dense marker maps. *Genetics.* (2001) 157:1819–29. Available online at: https://www.genetics.org/content/157/4/1819.full

Van Eenennaam AL, Weigel KA, Young AE, Cleveland MA, Dekkers JCM. Applied animal genomics: results from the field. *Ann Rev Anim Biosci.* (2014) 2:105–39. doi: 10.1146/annurev-animal-022513-114119

Cardoso FF, Gomes CCG, Sollero BP, Oliveira MM, Roso VM, Picolli ML, et al. Genomic prediction for tick resistance in Braford and Hereford cattle. *J Anim Sci.* (2015) 93:2693–705. doi: 10.2527/jas.2014-8832

Visscher PM, Brown MA, Mccarthy MI, Yang J. Five years of GWAS discovery. *Am J Hum Genet.* (2012) 90:7–24. doi: 10.1016/j.ajhg.2011.11.029

Barendse W. *Assessing Tick Resistance in a Bovine Animal for Selecting Cattle for Tick Resistance by Providing a Nucleic Acid From the Bovine Animal and Assaying for the Occurrence of a Single Nucleotide Polymorphism (SNP).* Patent application WO2007051248-A1 1–146. Geneva: World Intellectual Property Organization (WIPO) (2010).

Mapholi NO, Maiwashe A, Matika O, Riggio V, Bishop SC, MacNeil MD, et al. Genome-wide association study of tick resistance in South African Nguni cattle. *Ticks Tick Borne Dis.* (2016) 7:487–97. doi: 10.1016/j.ttbdis.2016.02.005

Moré DD, Cardoso FF, Mudadu M, Malagó W Jr., Gulias-Gomes CC, Sollero BP, et al. Network analysis uncovers putative genes affecting resistance to tick infestation in Braford cattle skin. *BMC Genomics.* (2019) 20:998. doi: 10.1186/s12864-019-6360-3

Porto-Neto LR, Jonsson NN, D'Occhio MJ, Barendse W. Molecular genetic approaches for identifying the basis of variation in resistance to tick infestation in cattle. *Vet Parasitol.* (2011) 180:165–72. doi: 10.1016/j.vetpar.2011.05.048

Porto-Neto LR, Reverter A, Prayaga KC, Chan EKF, Johnston DJ, Bolormaa S, et al. The genetic architecture of climatic adaptation in tropical cattle. *PLoS ONE.* (2014) 9:e113284. doi: 10.1371/journal.pone.0113284

Turner LB, Harrison BE, Bunch RJ, Porto Neto LR, Li Y, Barendse W. A genome-wide association study of tick burden and milk composition in cattle. *Anim Prod Sci.* (2010) 50:235–45. doi: 10.1071/AN09135

Salem GH, Liu X, Johnsrude JD, Dame JB, Roman Reddy G. Development and evaluation of an extra chromosomal DNA-based PCR test for diagnosing bovine babesiosis. *Mol Cell Probes.* (1999) 13:107–13. doi: 10.1006/mcpr.1998.0223

Wharton RH, Utech KBW. The relation between engorgement and dropping of *Boophilus microplus* (canestrini) (ixodidae) to the assessment of tick numbers on cattle. *J Aust Entomol Soc.* (1970) 9:171–82. doi: 10.1111/j.1440-6055.1970.tb00788.x

Clayton D. *snpStats: SnpMatrix and XSnpMatrix Classes and Methods.* R package version 1.18.0 (2014). Available online at: http://www.bioconductor. org/packages/release/bioc/html/snpStats.html (accessed October 6, 2016).

Gianola D, Rosa GJM. One Hundred years of statistical developments in animal breeding. *Ann Rev Anim Biosci.* (2015) 3:19–56. doi: 10.1146/annurev-animal-022114-110733

Aguilar I, Misztal I, Johnson DL, Legarra A, Tsuruta S, Lawlor TJ. Hot topic: a unified approach to utilize phenotypic, full pedigree, and genomic information for genetic evaluation of Holstein final score. *J Dairy Sci.* (2010) 93:743–52. doi: 10.3168/jds.2009-2730

Legarra A, Aguilar I, Misztal I. A relationship matrix including full pedigree and genomic information. *J Dairy Sci.* (2009) 92:4656–63. doi: 10.3168/jds.2009-2061

VanRaden PM. Efficient methods to compute genomic predictions. *J Dairy Sci.* (2008) 91:4414–23. doi: 10.3168/jds.2007-0980

Misztal I, Tsuruta S, Strabel T, Auvray B, Druet T, Lee DW. BLUPF90 and related programs (BGF90). In: *Proceedings of the 7th World Congress on Genetics Applied to Livestock Production.* Montpellier: French Commune. (2002). p. 28–07.

Gelman A, Rubin DB. Inference from iterative simulation using multiple sequences. *Stat Sci.* (1992) 7:457–72. Available online at: https://projecteuclid. org/download/pdf_1/euclid.ss/1177011136

Geweke J. Evaluating the accuracy of sampling-based approaches to the calculation of posterior moments. In: Bernardo JM, Berger JO, Dawid AP, Smith AFM, editors. *Bayesian Statistic.* New York, NY: Oxford University (1992). p. 625–31.

Heidelberger P, Welch PD. Simulation run length control in the presence of an initial transient. *Oper Res.* (1983) 31:1109–44. doi: 10.1287/opre.31. 6.1109

Plummer M, Best N, Cowles K, Vines K. Coda: convergence diagnosis and output analysis for MCMC. *R News.* (2006) 6:7–11. Available online at: https:// cran.r-project.org/doc/Rnews/Rnews_2006-1.pdf#page=7

R Core Team. *The R Project for Statistical Computing.* (2013). Available online at: http://www.R-project.org/ (accessed September 10, 2016).

Saatchi M, Schnabel RD, Rolf MM, Taylor JF, Garrick DJ. Accuracy of direct genomic breeding values for nationally evaluated traits in US Limousin and Simmental beef cattle. *Genet Select Evol.* (2012) 44:38. doi: 10.1186/1297-9686-44-38

Legarra A, Robert-Granie C, Manfredi E, Elsen JM. Performance of genomic selection in mice. *Genetics.* (2008) 180:611–8. doi: 10.1534/genetics.108.088575

Wang H, Misztal I, Aguilar I, Legarra A, Muir WM. Genome-wide association mapping including phenotypes from relatives without genotypes. *Genet Res.* (2012) 94:73–83. doi: 10.1017/S0016672312 000274

VanRaden PM, Van Tassell CP, Wiggans GR, Sonstegard TS, Schnabel RD, Taylor JF, et al. Invited review: reliability of genomic predictions for North American Holstein bulls. *J Dairy Sci.* (2009) 92:16–24. doi: 10.3168/jds.2008-1514

Zhang Z, Liu J, Ding X, Bijma P, de Koning DJ, Zhang Q. Best linear unbiased prediction of genomic breeding values using a trait- specific marker-derived relationship matrix. *PLoS ONE.* (2010) 5:e12648. doi: 10.1371/journal.pone.0012648

Wickham H. *ggplot2: Elegant Graphics for Data Analysis.* New York, NY: Springer (2009).

Durinck S, Spellman P, Birney E, Huber W. Mapping identifiers for the integration of genomic datasets with the R/Bioconductor package biomaRt. *Nat Protoc.* (2009) 4:1184–91. doi: 10.1038/nprot.2009.97

Fabregat A, Jupe S, Matthews L, Sidiropoulos K, Gillespie M, Garapati P, et al. The reactome pathway knowledgebase. *Nucleic Acids Res.* (2018) 44:D649–55. doi: 10.1093/nar/gkx1132

Biegelmeyer P, Gulias-Gomes CC, Roso VM, Dionello NJL, Cardoso FF. Tick resistance genetic parameters and its correlations with production traits in Hereford and Braford cattle. *Livest Sci.* (2017) 202:96–100. doi: 10.1016/j.livsci.2017.05.019

Veerkamp RF, Mulder HA, Thompson R, Calus MPL. Genomic and pedigree-based genetic parameters for scarcely recorded traits when some animals are genotyped. *J Dairy Sci.* (2011) 94:4189–97. doi: 10.3168/jds.2011-4223

Burrow HM. Variances and covariances between productive and adaptive traits and temperament in a composite breed of tropical beef cattle. *Livestock Prod Sci.* (2001) 70:213–33. doi: 10.1016/S0301-6226(01) 00178-6

Ayres DR, Pereira RJ, Boligon AA, Baldi F, Roso VM, Albuquerque LG. Genetic parameters and investigation of genotype × environment interactions in Nellore × Hereford crossbred for resistance to cattle ticks in different regions of Brazil. *J Appl Genet.* (2015) 56:107–13. doi: 10.1007/s13353-014-0238-5

Budeli MA, Nephawe KA, Norris D, Selapa NW, Bergh L, Maiwashe A. Genetic parameter estimates for tick resistance in Bonsmara cattle. *S Afr J Anim Sci.* (2009) 39:321–7. doi: 10.4314/sajas.v39i4.51125

Berry DP, Bermingham ML, Good M, More SJ. Genetics of animal health and disease in cattle. *Ir Vet J.* (2011) 64:5. doi: 10.1186/2046-0481-64-5

Raszek MM, Guan LL, Plastow GS. Use of genomic tools to improve cattle health in the context of infectious diseases. *Front Genet.* (2016) 7:30. doi: 10.3389/fgene.2016.00030

Habier D, Fernando RL, Garrick DJ. Genomic BLUP decoded: a look into the black box of genomic prediction. *Genetics.* (2013) 194:597–607. doi: 10.1534/genetics.113.152207

Taylor JF. Implementation and accuracy of genomic selection. *Aquaculture.* (2014) 420–21, S8–14. doi: 10.1016/j.aquaculture.2013.02.017

Hayes BJ, Bowman PJ, Chamberlain AJ, Goddard ME. Invited review: genomic selection in dairy cattle – progress and challenges. *J Dairy Sci.* (2009) 92:433– 43. doi: 10.3168/jds.2008-1646

Sollero BP, Junqueira VS, Gomes CCG, Caetano AR, Cardoso FF. Tag SNP selection for prediction of tick resistance in Brazilian Braford and Hereford cattle breeds using Bayesian methods. *Genet Sel Evol.* (2017) 49:49. doi: 10.1186/s12711-017-0325-2

Chesnais JP, Cooper TA, Wiggans GR, Sargolzaei M, Pryce JE, Miglior F. Using genomics to enhance selection of novel traits in North American dairy cattle. *J Dairy Sci.* (2016) 99:2413–27. doi: 10.3168/jds. 2015-9970

Thompson-Crispi KA, Sewalem A, Miglior F, Mallard B. Genetic parameters of adaptive immune response traits in Canadian holsteins. *J Dairy Sci.* (2012) 95:401–9. doi: 10.3168/jds.2011-4452

Thompson-Crispi KA, Sargolzaei M, Ventura R, Abo-Ismail M, Miglior F, Schenkel F, et al. A genome-wide association study of immune response traits in Canadian Holstein cattle. *BMC Genomics.* (2014) 15:559. doi: 10.1186/1471-2164-15-559

Martin P, Barkema HW, Brito LF, Narayana SG, Miglior F. Symposium review: novel strategies to genetically improve mastitis resistance in dairy cattle. *J Dairy Sci.* (2018) 101:2724–36. doi: 10.3168/jds.2017-13554

Zare Y, Shook GE, Collins MT, Kirkpatrick BW. Genome-wide association analysis and genomic prediction of *Mycobacterium avium* subspecies paratuberculosis infection in US Jersey Cattle. *PLoS ONE.* (2014) 9:e88380. doi: 10.1371/journal.pone.0088380

Hoff JL, Decker JE, Schnabel RD, Seabury CM, Neibergs HL, Taylor JF. QTL-mapping and genomic prediction for bovine respiratory disease in U.S. Holsteins using sequence imputation and feature selection. *BMC Genomics.* (2019) 20:555. doi: 10.1186/s12864-019-5941-5

Abbas AK, Lichtman AH, Pober JS. *Cellular and Molecular Immunology.* Philadelphia: WB Saunders Company (2018).

Goff WL, Johnson WC, Parish SM, Barrington GM, Tuo W, Valdez RA. The age-related immunity in cattle to *Babesia bovis* infection involves the rapid induction of interleukin-12, interferon-gamma and inducible nitric oxide synthase mRNA expression in the spleen. *Parasite Immunol.* (2001) 23:463–71. doi: 10.1046/j.1365-3024.2001.00402.x

Brown WC, Norimine J, Knowles DP, Goff WL. Immune control of *Babesia bovis* infection. *Vet Parasitol.* (2006) 138:75–87. doi: 10.1016/j.vetpar.2006.01.041

Adams AE, Shen W, Lin C-S, Leavitt J, Matsudaira P. Isoform-specific complementation of the yeast sac6 null mutation by human fimbrin. *Mol Cell Biol.* (1995) 15:69–75. doi: 10.1128/MCB.15.1.69

Shinomiya H. Plastin family of actin-bundling proteins: its functions in leukocytes, neurons, intestines, and cancer. *Int J Cell Biol.* (2012) 2012:213492. doi: 10.1155/2012/213492

Lin CS, Aebersold RH, Kent SB, Varma M, Leavitt J. Molecular cloning and characterization of plastin, a human leukocyte protein expressed in transformed human fibroblasts. *Mol Cell Biol.* (1988) 8:4659–68. doi: 10.1128/MCB.8.11.4659

Brown WC. Molecular approaches to elucidating innate and acquired immune responses to *Babesia bovis*, a protozoan parasite that causes persistent infection. *Vet Parasitol.* (2001) 101:233–48. doi: 10.1016/S0304-4017(01)00569-6

Xu X, Han L, Zhao G, Xue S, Gao Y, Xiao J, et al. LRCH1 interferes with DOCK8-Cdc42–induced T cell migration and ameliorates experimental autoimmune encephalomyelitis. *J Exp Med.* (2017) 214:209–26. doi: 10.1084/jem.20160068

Domingues R, Wohlres-Viana S, Reis DR, Teixeira HC, Ferreira AP, Guimarães SE, et al. Expression of immune response genes in peripheral blood of cattle infested with *Rhipicephalus microplus*. *Genet Mol Res.* (2014) 13:4013–21. doi: 10.4238/2014.May.23.12

Jonsson NN, Piper EK, Constantinoiu CC. Host resistance in cattle to infestation with the cattle tick *Rhipicephalus microplus*. *Parasite Immunol.* (2014) 36:551–7. doi: 10.1111/pim.12140

Piper EK, Jonsson NN, Gondro C, Lew-Tabor AE, Moolhuijzen P, Vance ME, et al. Immunological profiles of *Bos taurus* and *Bos indicus* cattle infested with the cattle tick, *Rhipicephalus (Boophilus) microplus*. *Clin Vaccine Immunol.* (2009) 16:1074–86. doi: 10.1128/CVI.00157-09

Constantinoiu CC, Jackson LA, Jorgensen WK, Lew-Tabor AE, Piper EK, Mayer DG, et al. Local immune response against larvae of *Rhipicephalus (Boophilus) microplus* in *Bos taurus indicus* and *Bos taurus Taurus* cattle. *Int J Parasitol.* (2010) 40:865–75. doi: 10.1016/j.ijpara.2010.01.004

Sasaki S, Ito E, Toki T, Maekawa T, Kanezaki R, Umenai T, et al. Cloning and expression of human B cell-specific transcription factor BACH2 mapped to chromosome 6q15. *Oncogene.* (2000) 19:3739–49. doi: 10.1038/sj.onc.1203716

Robbertse L, Richards SA, Clift SJ, Barnard AC, Leisewitz A, Crafford JE, et al. Comparison of the differential regulation of T and B lymphocyte subsets in the skin and lymph nodes amongst three cattle breeds as potential mediators of immune-resistance to *Rhipicephalus microplus*. *Ticks Tick Borne Dis.* (2018) 9:976–87. doi: 10.1016/j.ttbdis.2018.03.034

Soares-Silva M, Diniz FF, Gomes GN, Bahia D. The mitogen-activated protein kinase (MAPK) pathway: role in immune evasion by trypanosomatids. *Front Microbiol.* (2016) 7:183. doi: 10.3389/fmicb.2016.00183

Chen L, Deng H, Cui H, Fang J, Zuo Z, Deng J, et al. Inflammatory responses and inflammation-associated diseases in organs *Oncotarget.* (2017) 9:7204–18. doi: 10.18632/oncotarget.23208

Shoda LK, Palmer GH, Florin-Christensen J, Florin-Christensen M, Godson DL, Brown WC. *Babesia bovis*-stimulated macrophages express interleukin-1beta, interleukin-12, tumor necrosis factor alpha, and nitric oxide and inhibit parasite replication *in vitro*. *Infect Immun.* (2000) 68:5139–45. doi: 10.1128/IAI.68.9.5139-5145.2000

Goff WL, Johnson WC, Parish SM, Barrington GM, Elsasser TH, Davis WC, et al. IL-4 and IL-10 inhibition of IFN-gamma- and TNF-alpha-dependent nitric oxide production from bovine mononuclear phagocytes exposed to *Babesia bovis* merozoites. *Vet Immunol Immunopathol.* (2002) 84:237–51. doi: 10.1016/S0165-2427(01)00413-5

Goff WL, Johnson WC, Horn RH, Barrington GM, Knowles DP. The innate immune response in calves to *Boophilus microplus* tick transmitted *Babesia bovis* involves type-1 cytokine induction and NK-like cells in the spleen. *Parasite Immunol.* (2003) 25:185–8. doi: 10.1046/j.1365-3024.2003.00625.x

Goff WL, Storset AK, Johnson WC, Brown WC. Bovine splenic NK cells synthesize IFNgamma in response to IL-12-containing supernatants from *Babesia bovis*-exposed monocyte cultures. *Parasite Immunol.* (2006) 28:221–8. doi: 10.1111/j.1365-3024.2006.00830.x

Bagnall N, Gough J, Cadogan L, Burns B, Kongsuwan K. Expression of intracellular calcium signalling genes in cattle skin during tick infestation. *Parasite Immunol.* (2009) 31:177–87. doi: 10.1111/j.1365-3024.2008.01092.x

Wang YH, Reverter A, Kemp D, McWilliam SM, Ingham A, Davis CA, et al. Gene expression profiling of Hereford Shorthorn cattle following challenge with *Boophilus microplus* tick larvae. *Aust J Exp Agric.* (2007) 47:1397–407. doi: 10.1071/EA07012

Vestweber D. Adhesion and signaling molecules controlling the transmigration of leukocytes through endothelium. *Immunol Rev.* (2007) 218:178–96. doi: 10.1111/j.1600-065X.2007.00533.x

Piper EK, Jackson LA, Bielefeldt-Ohmann H, Gondro C, Lew-Tabor AE, Jonsson NN. Tick-susceptible *Bos taurus* cattle display an increased cellular response at the site of larval *Rhipicephalus (Boophilus) microplus* attachment, compared with tick-resistant *Bos indicus* cattle. *Int J Parasitol.* (2010) 40:431–41. doi: 10.1016/j.ijpara.2009.09.009

Porto-Neto L, Bunch R, Harrison BE, Prayaga K, Barendse W. Haplotypes that include the integrin alpha 11 gene associated with tick burden in cattle. *BMC Genet.* (2010) 11:55. doi: 10.1186/1471-2156-11-55

Reck J, Berger M Jr., Terra RMS, Marks FS, da Silva Vaz I, Guimaraes JA Jr., et al. Systemic alterations of bovine hemostasis due to *Rhipicephalus (Boophilus) microplus* infestation. *Res Vet Sci.* (2009) 86:56–62. doi: 10.1016/j.rvsc.2008.05.007

Parenti A, De Logu F, Geppetti P, Benemei S. What is the evidence for the role of TRP channels in inflammatory and immune cells?. *Br J Pharmacol.* (2016) 173:953–69. doi: 10.1111/bph.13392

Oh-hora M, Rao A. Calcium signaling in lymphocytes. *Curr Opin Immunol.* (2008) 20:250–8. doi: 10.1016/j.coi.2008.04.004

Feske S, Skolnik EY, Prakriya M. Ion channels and transporters in lymphocyte function and immunity. *Nat Rev Immunol.* (2012) 12:532–47. doi: 10.1038/nri3233

Liu Y1, Shepherd EG, Nelin LD. MAPK phosphatases–regulating the immune response. *Nat Rev Immunol.* (2007) 7:202–12. doi: 10.1038/nri2035

Cavani L. *Genetic study of Babesia bovis infection level and the association with tick resistance in Hereford and Braford cattle* [dissertation]. São Paulo State University (Unesp), School of Agricultural and Veterinarian Sciences, Jaboticabal, Brazil (2019).

16

Cattle Tick *Rhipicephalus microplus*-Host Interface: A Review of Resistant and Susceptible Host Responses

Ala E. Tabor[1,2*], *Abid Ali*[3,4†], *Gauhar Rehman*[3†], *Gustavo Rocha Garcia*[5], *Amanda Fonseca Zangirolamo*[5], *Thiago Malardo*[5] and *Nicholas N. Jonsson*[6*]

[1] Centre for Animal Science, Queensland Alliance for Agriculture and Food Innovation, The University of Queensland, St. Lucia, QLD, Australia, [2] Centre for Comparative Genomics, Murdoch University, Perth, WA, Australia, [3] Department of Zoology, Abdul Wali Khan University Mardan, Mardan, Pakistan, [4] Escola de Enfermagem de Ribeirão Preto, University of São Paulo, Ribeirão Preto, Brazil, [5] Ribeirão Preto School of Medicine, University of São Paulo, Ribeirão Preto, Brazil, [6] Institute of Biodiversity, Animal Health and Comparative Medicine, The University of Glasgow, Glasgow, United Kingdom

***Correspondence:**
Ala E. Tabor
a.lewtabor@uq.edu.au
Nicholas N. Jonsson
nicholas.jonsson@glasgow.ac.uk

†Equal first authors.

Ticks are able to transmit tick-borne infectious agents to vertebrate hosts which cause major constraints to public and livestock health. The costs associated with mortality, relapse, treatments, and decreased production yields are economically significant. Ticks adapted to a hematophagous existence after the vertebrate hemostatic system evolved into a multi-layered defense system against foreign invasion (pathogens and ectoparasites), blood loss, and immune responses. Subsequently, ticks evolved by developing an ability to suppress the vertebrate host immune system with a devastating impact particularly for exotic and crossbred cattle. Host genetics defines the immune responsiveness against ticks and tick-borne pathogens. To gain an insight into the naturally acquired resistant and susceptible cattle breed against ticks, studies have been conducted comparing the incidence of tick infestation on bovine hosts from divergent genetic backgrounds. It is well-documented that purebred and crossbred *Bos taurus indicus* cattle are more resistant to ticks and tick-borne pathogens compared to purebred European *Bos taurus taurus* cattle. Genetic studies identifying Quantitative Trait Loci markers using microsatellites and SNPs have been inconsistent with very low percentages relating phenotypic variation with tick infestation. Several skin gene expression and immunological studies have been undertaken using different breeds, different samples (peripheral blood, skin with tick feeding), infestation protocols and geographic environments. Susceptible breeds were commonly found to be associated with the increased expression of toll like receptors, MHC Class II, calcium binding proteins, and complement factors with an increased presence of neutrophils in the skin following tick feeding. Resistant breeds had higher levels of T cells present in the skin prior to tick infestation and thus seem to respond to ticks more efficiently. The skin of resistant breeds also contained higher numbers of eosinophils, mast cells and basophils with up-regulated proteases, cathepsins, keratins, collagens and extracellular matrix proteins in response to feeding ticks. Here we review immunological and molecular determinants that explore the cattle tick *Rhipicephalus microplus*-host resistance phenomenon as well as contemplating new insights and future directions to study tick resistance and susceptibility, in order to facilitate interventions for tick control.

Keywords: ticks, immunity, tick resistance, tick susceptibility, cattle breeds, genetic variation, gene expression profiling, immune responses

INTRODUCTION

Vector-borne pathogens cause diseases with a great impact on public and veterinary health and have accounted for 22% of emerging infections between 1940 and 2004 (Jones et al., 2008). As obligate hematophagous arthropod pests of vertebrates, ticks pose serious threats to beef and dairy cattle producers. It has been estimated that 80% of the world's cattle population is at risk from tick and tick-borne diseases (TBDs) causing estimated annual losses of US$ 22–30 billion (Lew-Tabor and Rodriguez Valle, 2016). The negative impact of ticks on cattle production is due to the direct effects of feeding, such as weight loss and damage of leather, and indirect effects, such as the transmission of tick-borne pathogens. The resulting diseases can potentially cause major production losses in livestock, thereby reducing farm incomes, increasing costs to consumers, and threatening trade between regions and/or world markets.

Since the establishment of extensive vector control programs, a steady decline in vector-borne diseases was observed last century, however recently the emergence and re-emergence of vector-borne diseases has been observed. This re-emergence may be linked to new global trends associated with changes in animal husbandry, urbanization, animal transboundary transportation, and globalization (Ogden and Lindsay, 2016). In this scenario, various approaches for tick control are in practice around the world in accordance with local legislation, environmental conditions, price based selection, and geography. Acaricide (synthetic pesticides) application is the most common component of tick control strategies, however the use of acaricides impose numerous limitations including the selective pressure for the development of more resistant ticks, environmental contamination, drug residues in food products, the expense of developing new acaricides, and the difficulty of producing tick-resistant cattle while maintaining desirable production characteristics (Willadsen, 2004; Abbas et al., 2014). Anti-tick vaccines are a very promising alternative to acaricide usage, however are still insufficient to confer protection against multiple tick species in various geographical regions (de la Fuente and Contreras, 2015; de la Fuente et al., 2016; Schetters et al., 2016).

Anti-tick immunity has been described in guinea pigs, cattle and rabbits, and refers to the capacity of previously exposed hosts to interfere with tick feeding and reproductive fecundity (Nuttall, 1911; Trager, 1939; Hewetson, 1972). A reduction in tick weight, duration of attachment, number of ticks feeding, egg mass, and molting success are some of the parameters measured to determine host anti-tick immunity (Trager, 1939). For the first time, Nuttall (1911) demonstrated host immunity to ticks as a phenomenon of natural immunity in humans. Experimentally, acquired resistance to tick infestation was observed by Trager (1939), who noticed that after repeated infestation of *Dermacentor variabilis* on guinea pigs, the host developed resistance to subsequent tick infestation, shown by the decreasing number of successfully feeding larvae. Furthermore, it was found that as compared with larvae infesting a host with no previous exposure to ticks, larvae infesting resistant hosts weighed less. Several researchers continued to observe host resistance to tick feeding affecting each tick life stage (Gregson, 1941; Feldman-Muhsam, 1964; Wikel, 1996). Various immunological determinants have been examined that influence host resistance to tick infestation including a high level of eosinophils, basophils, T cells, mast cells, specific immunoglobulins, histamine, and changes to gene transcription profiles (Kemp and Bourne, 1980; de Castro and Newson, 1993; Kashino et al., 2005; Veríssimo et al., 2008; Kongsuwan et al., 2010; Piper et al., 2010; Engracia Filho et al., 2017).

Bovines present contrasting, heritable phenotypes for infestation with *Rhipicephalus microplus* and related tick species as a consequence of co-evolution of resistant cattle with ticks and also decades of selective breeding. The *R. microplus* tick has a strong preference for *Bos taurus taurus* cattle over highly resistant *Bos taurus indicus* cattle (Wambura et al., 1998; Porto Neto et al., 2011b; Jonsson et al., 2014; Biegelmeyer et al., 2015). In this article we review the tick:host physical interface, genetic and molecular studies, and immunological determinants of bovine host resistance to ticks.

TICK-HOST PHYSICAL INTERFACE

The cattle tick *R. microplus* co-evolved with Asian bovines (zebu breeds) and due to the global migration of *B. t. taurus* European breeds for dairy production during the eighteenth–nineteenth centuries, this tick spread across tropical and sub-tropical regions of the world (Frisch, 1999; Estrada-Peña et al., 2006; Barré and Uilenberg, 2010). Currently *R. microplus* is considered to be a species complex, in which there are recognized geographic differences between the 5 clades including 3 clades of *R. microplus* (A, B, and C), as well as *R. australis* and *R. annulatus* (Burger et al., 2014; Low et al., 2015). Each taxa transmits both anaplasmosis and babesiosis and each have a parasitic life cycle on cattle for ~21 days. They will be described collectively as *R. microplus* or simply as cattle ticks in this review. Cattle ticks are attracted to their hosts through stimuli such as carbon dioxide, temperature, vibrations, visual stimuli, and odor (Osterkamp et al., 1999). The susceptible European (*B. t. taurus*) breeds which were introduced into regions in which *R. microplus* is endemic failed to resist tick infestation to the same extent as tropical *B. t. indicus* breeds, which have developed an effective anti-tick immune response (Frisch, 1999).

The immune response varies among newly introduced European cattle (Taurine breeds, susceptible hosts) whereas Asian bovines (zebuine breeds or resistant hosts) co-evolved with ticks (Utech et al., 1978). Physical barriers that affect tick resistance include density of the fur coat, skin thickness, skin pigmentation (light or dark), skin vibration and/or self-cleaning ability, tongue papillae, and odor (de Castro et al., 1985; Spickett et al., 1989; Veríssimo et al., 2002, 2015; Martinez et al., 2006; Gasparin et al., 2007). In addition to physical differences between resistant and susceptible hosts, their behavior also affects the *R. microplus* parasitic load. Self-grooming is widely used by cattle as an important defense mechanism against ticks (Riek, 1956; Snowball, 1956; Bennett, 1969) and the level of resistance may possibly be associated with tongue morphology. For example the papillae from tick-resistant breeds have smaller spacing, which is more effective in removing *R. microplus* larvae from the skin (Veríssimo et al., 2015). However, there is also conjecture that resistant breeds simply groom more often (Kemp et al., 1976). It has been suggested that innate characteristics such as thinner coats and lower fur density have direct impacts in decreasing tick preferential attachment and infestation (Spickett et al., 1989; Veríssimo et al., 2002; Gasparin et al., 2007; Marufu et al., 2011). However, other studies have shown that skin features have no influence on tick infestation (Wagland, 1978; Doube and Wharton, 1980). Evidence for resistance of cattle to ticks due to physical parameters is scarce and further studies to examine the mechanisms that govern these physical phenomena are still needed.

IMMUNOLOGICAL DETERMINANTS ASSOCIATED WITH HOST RESISTANCE: HOST COUNTER ATTACK?

It is well-established that cattle have three subclasses of IgG (IgG1, IgG2, and IgG3), and during blood meals ticks ingest a substantial amount of IgG (Knight et al., 1988; Symons et al., 1989; Kacskovics and Butler, 1996; Rabbani et al., 1997; Gudderra et al., 2002; Saini et al., 2007). Host IgGs can be found in the tick hemolymph and are potentially biologically active against specific tick proteins (Ben-Yakir et al., 1987). Furthermore, specific host antibodies neutralize the tick salivary pharmacopeia and can damage the tick by binding to tick internal organs such as salivary glands, midgut, or ovaries (Ackerman et al., 1981; Willadsen and Kemp, 1988; Tellam et al., 1992). In other tick-host systems (*Dermacentor andersoni* and guinea pigs), antibodies have been shown to mediate inflammatory reactions by triggering effector-cell recruitment and cellular immune response as a consequence of both Fc receptor activation of leukocytes and complement activation that are harmful to the tick, also an immune mechanism in human auto-immune disease syndromes (Wikel and Whelen, 1986; Hogarth, 2002).

It was documented previously that the passive transfer of plasma from genetically immune resistant animals to naïve hosts, increases resistance to tick challenge and this response was believed to be mediated by antibodies (Roberts and Kerr, 1976; Shapiro et al., 1986). The pattern of antibody responses to immunogens from tick salivary glands and guts have been reviewed by different research groups (Willadsen, 1980; Wikel, 1982; Kaufman, 1989; Kashino et al., 2005; Cruz et al., 2008; Piper et al., 2009, 2010; Garcia et al., 2017).

Some studies have shown that during laboratory animal infestations, such as guinea pigs, rabbits and mice, reactive antibody titers to tick salivary antigens increased (Allen and Humphreys, 1979; Allen, 1989). The densities of *Amblyomma hebraeum, Rhipicephalus appendiculatus,* and *Rhipicephalus evertsi evertsi* ticks was higher on the susceptible breed (*B. t. taurus* Hereford) as compared to resistant cattle (*B. t. indicus* Brahman) with a positive correlation between the level of tick infestation and the level of IgG in susceptible hosts (Rechav, 1987). Piper and colleagues confirmed this correlation noting that susceptible cattle (Holstein-Friesian) have higher levels of tick specific IgGs compared to Brahmans suggesting that these antibodies do not confer immunity to ticks (Piper et al., 2008, 2009, 2010). As with other immune parameters in high and low resistance animals, the interpretation of data can be problematic as a susceptible animal will have more ticks feeding at any time, which would in turn be expected to result in a higher antigenic challenge. However, the negative relationship between IgG levels and host resistance was later confirmed and shown to be independent of the number of feeding ticks, using Santa Gertrudis cattle [a stable composite breed of *B. t. taurus* (5/8) and *B. t. indicus* (3/8)], in which there is wide variation in host resistance to ticks (Piper et al., 2017). Susceptible animals had significantly higher tick-specific IgG1 antibody titres (to several tick antigens including adult female salivary glands and guts, and whole larvae) compared to tick resistant cattle (Piper et al., 2017). In contrast, Kashino et al reported that tick saliva-specific IgG1 and IgG2 antibodies decreased in susceptible (Holstein) compared to resistant (Nelore) cattle where the IgG levels remained the same, however, only IgG levels to tick salivary antigens were examined (Kashino et al., 2005). Previous studies have surmised that there are genetic differences in the bovine host's ability to elicit antibody responses to antigens in *R. microplus* and *D. andersoni* tick saliva (Whelen et al., 1986; Opdebeeck and Daly, 1990). Despite the fact that differences in the IgG levels against tick antigens between heavy or light infestations have been reported, there is individual variation in the same bovine breed with respect to humoral immune responses to tick antigenic molecules (Cruz et al., 2008). In addition, despite most studies reporting increased total IgG production against wide ranging tick antigens in susceptible breeds compared to resistant, IgG responses to salivary proteins were significantly higher in tick naïve resistant hosts (Nelore) at the first larval challenge (Garcia et al., 2017).

Variation in IgG2 allotypes has been associated with variation in immune responses to pathogens. When two allotypes IgG2a and IgG2b were found to differ in sequence at the CH1–CH3 regions it was reported that IgG2b was more able to initiate the bovine complement cascade while animals with the IgG2a allotype were more susceptible to extracellular pyogenic pathogens (Heyermann and Butler, 1987; Bastida-Corcuera et al., 1999). Other studies have shown that the distribution and presence of IgG2 allotypes differed significantly between taurine and indicine breeds (Butler et al., 1994; Carvalho et al., 2011). Blakeslee et al. (1971) described that ~80% of susceptible bovines (Holstein) have the IgG2a allotype and that the IgGγ2b was rare in these animals (Blakeslee et al., 1971). Recently, it was shown that the IgGγ2a allotype was significantly more frequent in taurine hosts (tick susceptible) and IgGγ2b was significantly frequent in indicine cattle (tick resistant) (Carvalho et al., 2011). Male tick saliva contains IgG-binding proteins (IGBPs) secreted into the host which assists the female tick to evade the host immune response (Wang and Nuttall, 1999; Santos et al., 2004; Gong et al., 2014). Carvalho et al. (2011) suggested that certain IgG2 allotypes may hinder the function of these tick IGBPs.

Aside from IGBPs, other tick specific proteins have been examined in terms of their immune recognition by tick resistant and susceptible cattle. A *R. microplus* recombinant serine protease inhibitor (Serpin- rRMS-3) was recognized by resistant bovines and not susceptible, suggesting that RMS-3 could be a protective antigen (Rodriguez-Valle et al., 2012). Another study by the same group demonstrated that host responses to six *R. microplus* lipocalins (LRMs which include tick histamine binding proteins) were higher in resistant cattle (Rodriguez-Valle et al., 2013). Both RMS-3 and the LRM proteins were identified based on the *in silico* identification of B cell binding epitopes. In addition, predicted T cell epitopes from 3 LRMs stimulated the generation of a significantly higher number of interferon gamma (IFN-γ) secreting cells (consistent with a Th1 response) in tick-susceptible Holstein–Friesians compared with tick-resistant Brahman cattle. In contrast, expression of the Th2-associated cytokine interleukin-4 (IL4) was lower in Holstein–Friesian (susceptible) cattle when compared with Brahman (resistant) cattle (Rodriguez-Valle et al., 2013). IL4 is known to decrease the production of Th1 cells and IFN-γ, and is thus a key regulator of both the humoral and adaptive immune responses.

The immunological parameters of tick resistance have been shown to differ between tick susceptible and tick resistant breeds as well as within the same breeds. The studies reported differ in the parameters of trials and tick infestations, for example, the use of tick naïve cattle artificially infested or the use of cattle naturally exposed to ticks (Kashino et al., 2005; Piper et al., 2008, 2009). The study undertaken by Kashino et al. (2005) used susceptible cattle that had been treated with acaricides when high tick numbers were observed and the cattle had been vaccinated with GAVAC (Bm86 based tick vaccine), introducing additional variables to the study. Further studies examining specific tick proteins to compare divergent host immune responses are still warranted.

MOLECULAR GENETIC VARIANTS ASSOCIATED WITH HOST RESISTANCE

Numerous studies have attempted to identify genetic markers for host resistance to tick infestation and they are summarized and discussed by Porto Neto et al. (2011b) and Mapholi et al. (2014). Approaches have included immunological methods (Stear et al., 1984, 1989, 1990); protein-based analyses (Ashton et al., 1968; Carvalho et al., 2008); candidate gene sequence or genotype (Acosta-Rodriguez et al., 2005; Martinez et al., 2006; Untalan et al., 2007); genomic detection of quantitative trait loci (QTL) using SNPs or microsatellites, with or without fine mapping (Barendse, 2007; Gasparin et al., 2007; Regitano et al., 2008; Prayaga et al., 2009; Machado et al., 2010; Porto Neto et al., 2010a, 2011a; Turner et al., 2010; Cardoso et al., 2015; Mapholi et al., 2016; Sollero et al., 2017). There is one example of a meta-analysis of genomic association with transcriptome in tick infestation (Porto Neto et al., 2010b). Although this appears to represent a large body of science, it has generated relatively little data which can be used for improved genetic selection. It can be concluded from the studies on the major histocompatibility complex (MHC, also referred to as the bovine lymphocyte antigen (BoLA) system) that the MHC makes a contribution to variation in resistance however there is no single, consistent genotype of any gene in the MHC that is associated with high or low resistance to ticks across breeds and production systems. A number of QTL markers have been identified using microsatellites and SNPs, however these have mostly been inconsistent and the loci have had relatively weak effects. The research of Barendse (2007) and Turner et al. (2010) found several significant loci but most of them had effects in the order of 1% of the phenotypic variation in tick infestation. The lack of consistent and strong findings is not surprising. Counting ticks is difficult and time consuming thus studies resort to scoring systems, which are less precise than counts, and this can have an effect on heritability. Alternatively, the numbers used tend to be relatively small and studies are underpowered. The most robust report is that by Turner et al. (2010), who reported on a study in which ticks were counted and heritability was a respectable 37%, and which used 1,960 cattle. In contrast, Prayaga et al. (2009) used a scoring system, 900 animals and estimated heritability of tick score to be 9%. Furthermore, a study examining the genomic prediction for tick resistance in Braford (Brahman x Hereford/tick resistant x tick susceptible breed, respectively) and Hereford cattle in Brazil showed that genomic selection for tick resistant Braford cattle may be achievable (Cardoso et al., 2015). A recent trait tag-SNP approach by the same group reported 914 SNPs explaining more than 20% of the estimated genetic variance for tick resistance (Sollero et al., 2017).

Despite the challenges of the genomic approach to identifying either mechanisms or markers for host resistance to ticks in cattle, they have enabled the identification of allelic variation in genes that are very likely to influence the trait. The *ELTD1* gene (EGF, latrophilin, and seven transmembrane domain containing 1) was identified from GWAS in dairy and beef cattle (Prayaga et al., 2009; Turner et al., 2010). Its association with the host resistance phenotype was confirmed but its effect was limited to <1% of the total phenotypic variation in the trait (Porto Neto et al., 2011a). Similarly, haplotypes that included the *ITGA11* gene (integrin alpha 11) were significantly associated with tick burden and explained about 1.5% of the variation in the trait. Finally, the potential functional role of allelic variation in a gene identified by the same GWAS studies (Prayaga et al., 2009;

Turner et al., 2010) *RIPK2* (serine-threonine kinase 2) was further examined using knock out mice (Porto Neto et al., 2012). This gene is known to play an essential role in the modulation of innate and adaptive immune responses and it was found that it influenced the recognition of tick salivary antigens by mice.

Limited association of tick burden or phenotype to the genotype is currently available and large bovine genomic meta-analyses may contribute to the identification of within breed markers for tick resistance in the future.

VARIATION IN GENE EXPRESSION AMONG RESISTANT AND SUSCEPTIBLE HOSTS AND RELATIONSHIP WITH IMMUNE RESPONSES

Bioactive molecules secreted by *R. microplus* ticks into the skin of the host during attachment and blood feeding stimulate host effective responses. The variation in the mechanisms by which each host breed responds to each of these bioactive molecules likely results in different levels of resistance. It is well-established that the resistance to tick infestation is due to a complex set of responses, however the specific mechanisms and their relative importance continues to be the subject of debate.

Table 1 summarizes selected up-regulated genes including those that are potentially associated with immune responsiveness, blood coagulation, calcium regulation, and/or wound healing from several studies undertaken to date. The parameters of all of the studies differ from each other including: the number of biological replicates, the number of larvae used in infestations, the breeds and subspecies used, their prior exposure, the methodology and platform used to measure host responses (immunohistochemistry, microarray platforms, qPCR), the timing of sample collection, and the samples analyzed (skin or blood). Without undertaking a formal meta-analysis of the original data, we have attempted to summarize differences and similarities in relation to susceptible vs. resistant animals among reports. The similarities identified are presented diagrammatically in **Figure 1** with text listing commonly up-regulated cells or genes in susceptible (**Figure 1A**) and resistant (**Figure 1B**) cattle.

Gene expression studies have been undertaken using peripheral blood leukocytes (PBL) and skin tick bite sites. These studies have included host qPCR, EST libraries, microarray analyses and cDNA library/next generation sequencing. The findings are summarized in **Table 1**.

Studies on PBL suggest that resistant hosts are more likely to develop a stable T-cell-mediated response against *R. microplus*, while susceptible cattle demonstrated cellular and gene expression profiles consistent with innate and inflammatory responses to tick infestation (Kashino et al., 2005; Piper et al., 2009). The up-regulation of genes in tick susceptible cattle involved in inflammatory and other important immunological responses mediate a greater natural potential to develop higher pro-inflammatory responses in comparison to tick resistant animals.

Gene expression studies on skin taken from larval attachment sites have demonstrated that cytokines, chemokines, and complement factors were differentially expressed between naïve-skin and infested skin in susceptible Holstein–Friesian cattle. It was also found that immunoglobulin transcripts were differentially expressed in infested skin from Holstein-Friesian compared to resistant Brahman cattle. Therefore, the chronic pathology established in *B. t. taurus* cattle might facilitate the tick feeding process (Piper et al., 2010). In addition, extracellular matrix genes such as: keratocan, osteoglycin, collagen, and lumican were up-regulated in infested-skin from *B. t. indicus* resistant Brahman cattle. In a study involving coagulation in skin from resistant and susceptible cattle infested with *R. microplus* (Carvalho et al., 2010b), susceptible hosts had an increased blood clotting time at tick hemorrhagic feeding pools in comparison to normal skin and the skin of resistant hosts. Furthermore, the host resistant phenotype affects the transcript of genes associated with anti-hemostatic proteins in the salivary glands of *R. microplus*, with transcripts coding for anti-coagulant proteins expressed at a higher level in ticks fed on susceptible hosts compared to ticks fed on resistant hosts (Carvalho et al., 2010b).

In the same experiment where PBL gene expression was studied in infested indicine and taurine cattle, the authors examined the response to infestation and larval attachment in bovine skin (Piper et al., 2010). The susceptible cattle displayed an intense cellular inflammatory response at the tick attachment site, i.e., genes involved in inflammatory processes and immune responses including those which encode for matrix proteins were up-regulated in tick-infested susceptible cattle, but not in resistant hosts. Nascimento et al. (2010) constructed cDNA libraries from skin biopsies from resistant and susceptible cattle to evaluate the pattern of gene expression of three calcium-binding-proteins. The results showed that genes coding for translationally controlled tumor protein (*1-TPT1*), calcium channel protein transient receptor potential vanilloid 6 (*TRPV6*) and cysteine proteinase inhibitor (*CST6*) were highly expressed in susceptible cattle compared to resistant cattle (Nascimento et al., 2010). Also, a microarray study using samples from tick infested cattle to evaluate the profile of gene expression during *R. microplus* larvae attachment showed differentially expressed genes involved in lipid metabolism, inflammation control and impairment of tick infestation in resistant cattle (*B. t. indicus* Nelore) (Carvalho et al., 2014). Conversely, in susceptible cattle (*B. t. taurus* Holstein) the acute phase response appeared impaired but this study confirmed the up-regulation of calcium ion control genes which correlates with the calcium binding proteins reported by Nascimento et al. (2010). Franzin et al. (2017) also report the up-regulation of protein S100G, another calcium binding protein, in susceptible cattle. An earlier qPCR study showed higher up-regulation of calcium signaling genes in a tick resistant composite breed in response to ticks most predominantly at 24 h post-infestation with larvae (Belmont Red) (Bagnall et al., 2009). Calcium signaling, calcium binding and/or calcium ion control genes and their functions in tick resistant and tick susceptible cattle warrant further specific examination.

Another host gene expression study was reported recently demonstrating that resistant cattle (*B. t. indicus* Nelore breed)

TABLE 1 | Summary of differentiating characteristics of tick susceptible vs. tick resistant cattle (bold font indicates correlation between studies of certain transcripts and or other markers—genetic, cellular, immunohistochemistry) in response to *Rhipicephalus microplus* ticks.

Methodology (cattle breeds compared)	Susceptible	Resistant	Main conclusion and reference
Cellular IgG isotyping; Cattle naturally infested on pasture; susceptible cattle treated with acaricide when tick counts were >500. Cattle vaccinated with GAVAC. (Holstein and Aberdeen *B. t. taurus* vs. Nelore *B. t. indicus*)	IgG1 and IgG2 decrease (anti-salivary gland antibodies only)	IgG1 and IgG2 no change	IgG suppression by tick infestation on susceptible cattle. Kashino et al., 2005
Genetics study, cattle naturally infested in pasture and at 10–14 months infested with 10,000 tick larvae, PCR to determine allele frequency (F2 population of composites *B. t. indicus* Gyr 1/2 x *B. t. taurus* Holstein 1/2)		**BoLA Class II** DRB3.2	The MHC Class II DRB3.2 allele is associated with tick resistance. Martinez et al., 2006
Microarray gene expression, natural tick infestation for ~6 months ("naïve" sample taken post field infest), followed by 5 artificial tick challenges over 17 months with 20,000–25,000 larvae (Hereford Shorthorn cattle- tropically adapted *B. t. taurus*)	**B-cell CLL/lymphoma 10** **Collagen**, pro α **Apolipoprotein** **Keratin** **Immunoglobulins** IL13 receptor α 1 precursor	**Cathepsin** B **Collagens** (type I α2; type III pro; type VI, α 3) **Complement** component 1, q subcomponent, α	Susceptible cattle upregulated immune responsive genes and those involved in protein synthesis. **BDA20, Odorant Binding Protein (OBP)** and the dendritic cell protein-B5 over expressed by both groups. Wang Y. H. et al., 2007
Genetic microsatellite and cytokine qPCR of 4 breeds, 17 months natural tick infestation (*B. t. indicus* Nelore, Composite Canchim 5/8 *B.taurus* 3/8 *B. t. indicus* × Nelore, *B. t. taurus* Aberdeen Angus × Nelore, and *B. t. taurus* Simmental x Nelore)	IL4	**IL8** and **IL2** down-regulated	Tick counts were associated with IL4, IL2 is down-regulated in 3 genetically different groups of infested bovines compared to pre-infestation, and IL8 was down-regulated in resistant bovines compared to susceptible animals Regitano et al., 2008
RT-PCR gene expression of peripheral white blood cells, previous natural exposure to ticks, 7 weekly artificial infestations of 10,000 larvae while held in tick infested pasture. (Holstein Friesian *B.taurus* vs. Brahman cattle *B. t. indicus*)	Toll-like receptor pathway (TLR5, TLR7, TLR9, **NFKBp50**, MyD88, Traf-6, CD14, IL-1β) Chemokine ligands and receptors (**CCL2**, CCL26; CCR-1) **IL-10** **bovine dander allergen 20 (BDA20)**		15 transcripts increased significantly in the susceptible breed to suggest innate inflammatory processes Piper et al., 2008
Cellular, RT-PCR and microarray gene expression (microarray) of leukocytes–infestation as described above (Piper et al., 2008) (Holstein Friesian *B. t. taurus* vs. Brahman cattle *B. t. indicus*)	Higher WBC counts Low hemoglobin CD14+ and **MHC Class II** (macrophage cells) High tick specific immunoglobulins (larvae, adult female salivary gland and gut)—high IgG1 **CXCL10**	**CD4+, CD25+** and **γδ T cells** **IL2**, IL2Rα, IL4Rα, TNFα, CCR-1, CCR-7, CXCL4, CD28, CD3E CD40 ligand	Susceptible cattle produce an innate inflammatory type response with high IgG1 titers suggesting also a T cell response. Resistant cattle produce a stable T cell mediated response. Piper et al., 2009
RT-PCR gene expression of calcium signaling genes in skin biopsies. Natural field exposure to ticks, followed by treatment and at 8 months artificial infestation of 10,000 larvae. Skin biopsies at 0, 3, and 24h post infestation (Belmont Red—composite breed ~ 1/2 *B. t. taurus* and 1/2 *B. t. indicus*, tropically adapted)		**Calcium signaling genes** (significant at 24 h post-exposure): *AHNAK* nucleoprotein (desmoyokin) *CASQ* (Calsequestrin) **IL2** (Interleukin-2) NFAT2CIP (nuclear factor of activated T-cells, calcineurin-dependent) PLCG1 (phospholipase C, γ1)	The significant elevation of some calcium dependent genes following tick exposure suggests that the calcium pathway might be responsive to parasite exposure and could contribute to host immune response. Bagnall et al., 2009

(Continued)

TABLE 1 | Continued

Methodology (cattle breeds compared)	Susceptible	Resistant	Main conclusion and reference
Protein and mRNA expression- infestation as described above (Bagnall et al., 2009) of skin biopsies at 0, 3 and 24 h post-infestation. (Belmont Red – composite breed ~ 1/2 *B. t. taurus* and 1/2 *B. t. indicus*, tropically adapted)		**Keratins** lipocalin 9 epidermal barrier catalyzing enzyme transglutaminase 1 transcriptional regulator B lymphocyte-induced maturation protein 1 lipid processing proteins	Resistant cattle have physically stronger epidermal layers of the skin Kongsuwan et al., 2010
Host gene expression microarrays (skin); infestation as described above Piper et al., 2008 (Holstein Friesian *B. t. taurus* vs. Brahman *B. t. indicus* cattle)	**Chemokine ligands** (C-X-C motif) 2 and 5; (C-C motif) 2 and 8 – CXCL2, CXCL5, **CCL2**, CCL8 **Complement** component 1 and 3; Complement factor D (adipsin) **IL8** **Major histocompatibility complex Class II DRB3** Chemokine Regakine 1 (chemotactic activity for neutrophils) Spleen trypsin inhibitor; Plasminogen activator, tissue; Serpin peptidase inhibitor, clade F; Proapoptotic caspase adapter protein (inflammatory role, recruitment of immune cells to infected tissue); Peptidoglycan recognition protein 1 (inducer of TNFα and IFN γ); **Apolipoprotein D** **Lysozyme** Prostaglandin D2 synthase (inhibitor of platelet aggregation)	Keratocan, osteoglycin, lumican, **Collagen**, (types I and III); Lysyl oxidase-like 4 (formation of collagen) Down-regulated **Cytochrome P450** (**CYP4F3**, CYP11A1) Serpin peptidase inhibitor, clade A (alpha-1 antiproteinase, antitrypsin); Phospholipase A2, group VII (platelet-activating factor acetylhydrolase, plasma); Secreted phosphoprotein 2 (cystatin); Procollagen C-endopeptidase enhancer Lipid metabolism Amino acid metabolism Oxidoreductases	Genes involved with inflammatory processes and immune responsiveness upregulated in susceptible cattle. Genes encoding consistuents of the extracellular matrix were up-regulated in resistant cattle. Piper et al., 2010
qPCR analysis after artificial tick infestation, skin biopsies from tick lesions. (Gyr -*B. t. indicus* × Holstein - *B. t. taurus*)	**Calcium-dependent signal transduction** (**S100A7**), histamine releasing protein (TPT1), epithelial calcium channel 2 (TRPV6) cysteine proteinase inhibitor (CST6)		Susceptible cattle develop hypersensitive reaction which is not protective Nascimento et al., 2010
EST analysis, natural tick infestation followed by acaricide treatment and artificial infestation of 10,000 larvae, biopsies collected at Days 5 and 12 from base of tail (F2 population from Gyr -*B. t. indicus* × Holstein - *B. t. taurus*)	CD44 antigen (lymphocyte activation) CD63 antigen (marker for activated basophils and IgE-mediated allergy) ADAM metallopeptidase **odorant binding protein** poly A binding protein ribosomal proteins	MHC Class antigen 1 **Cathepsin** L2 precursor **Collagen** (type I alpha; type III alpha) **Keratins** Ribosomal proteins	Structural proteins and MHC Class I in resistant cattle; Immune response transcripts in susceptible cattle Nascimento et al., 2011
Immunohistochemistry, infestation of Holstein Friesian and Brahmans as described by (Piper et al., 2008) above. Infestation of tick naïve Santa Gertrudis cattle–10,000 larvae artificially weekly for 13 weeks followed by natural infestation on pasture (Holstein Friesian *B. t. taurus* vs. Brahman *B. t. indicus*) (Composite Santa Gertrudis breed *B. t. taurus* 5/8 × *B. t. indicus* 3/8)	CD45, CD45RO (Holstein-Friesian) Mixed CD45 and CD45RO reactions (Santa Gertrudis)	**CD4+,** CD8+, **CD25+** and **γδ T cells** **MHC Class II cells** Mixed CD45 and CD45RO reactions (Santa Gertrudis)	Higher number of γδ T cells present in the skin of tick naïve resistant cattle. Epitopes recognized by some antibodies might not be present on the cell populations from all breeds of cattle or might be expressed in different levels. Santa Gertrudis resistance associated with lower cellular reaction at the larval attachment sites. Constantinoiu et al., 2010, 2013; Jonsson et al., 2014

(Continued)

TABLE 1 | Continued

Methodology (cattle breeds compared)	Susceptible	Resistant	Main conclusion and reference
Microarray gene expression (skin), natural infestation on pasture (10 months), acaricide treatment, followed by artificial infestation 10,000 larvae, skin biopsies 0, 24 and 48 h post-artificial infestation. (F2 of composite Gyr -*B. t. indicus* × Holstein - *B. t. taurus*)	**Calcium ion control genes** **Cytochrome P450** (CYP4F3)—**leukotriene** (allergy inducing chemical mediator) degradation	**Complement factors** 1, 2 and 3 complexes (C1, C2, C3); complement factor 4 binding protein; complement factor B properdin, galectin-1 Coagulation Factor XIIIa Lipid metabolism	Lipid metabolism in inflammation control in resistant cattle. Acute phase response impaired in susceptible cattle. Carvalho et al., 2014
RT-PCR gene expression of peripheral white blood cells, natural tick infestation followed by acaricide treatment, subsequent artificial infestation with 20,000 larvae, blood samples taken at 0, 24, and 48 h post-infestation. (F2 of composite Gyr -*B. t. indicus* × Holstein - *B. t. taurus*)	**CXCL10** and CXCL8 were down-regulated	**CD4+, CD25+** and **γδ T cells** **IL10**, FoxP3, **CXCL10**, CD25	A correlation between T γδ cell activity and immunological mechanisms in resistant cattle Domingues et al., 2014
Cellular and humoral responses (blood), 10,000 larvae artificially weekly for 13 weeks followed by natural infestation on pasture, blood collected 21 days post 1st infestation and weekly to measure changes in measure parameters (Composite Santa Gertrudis breed *B. t. taurus* 5/8 x *B. t. indicus* 3/8)	High tick-specific (anti-salivary and gut, anti-larval) **IgG1 titers**; variable IgG2 responses Decreased hemoglobin, decreased RBC count Increased **CD25+**, **CD4+**, WC1+	No IgG2 Increased **CD4+ cells** (prior to infestation) Decreased CD3+, **CD4+**, CD8+ Increased **MHCII+**, WC3+ and CD14+ cells	A non-protective high level of IgG1 in tick susceptible cattle. Piper et al., 2017
Microarray gene expression (skin) and histology Acaricide treatment of calves prior to artificial tick infestation with 10,000, skin biopsies with and without feeding ticks were taken prior to infestation (day 0) followed by 2 days (larvae) and 9 days (nymphs). Biopsies without feeding ticks to emulate "stressed" phenotype. Selected immune response genes differentially expressed (>2-fold) by larvae in comparison to baseline and stress responses (no ticks) in susceptible and resistant cattle (Table S5). (Holstein *B. t. taurus* vs. Nelore *B. t. indicus*)	CD209 antigen (leads to **IL10** production) Fibroleukin (fibrinogen type 2) Secretogranin-2 Secretoneurin (chemotaxis of monocytes and eosinophils) CXC6 (downregulated); CCL3, CCL4 high affinity **immunoglobulin** epsilon receptor subunit alpha precursor (**NF-kB**, MAPK activation) **Complement factor** D **Complement** C1q tumor necrosis factor-related protein 7 precursor T-cell surface glycoprotein CD3 delta chain platelet-derived growth factor receptor-like protein precursor (wound healing) Serine/threonine-protein kinase 1 Secreted phosphoprotein 24 (endopeptidase, platelet degranulation) **Keratin** **Protein S100**-G (calcium binding) **Lysozyme**	CD3+ and **γδ T cells** WC1+ Activation of basophils interferon-induced GTP-binding protein Mx2 Interferon alpha-inducible proteins 6 and 27 IL3 **cathepsin** D precursor	Susceptible cattle produce more tick attracting volatiles. Resistant hosts expose ticks to an earlier inflammatory response. Franzin et al., 2017

up-regulated the expression of fewer genes encoding enzymes producing volatile compounds that render them less "attractive" to ticks compared with susceptible cattle (*B. t. taurus* Holstein breed) (Franzin et al., 2017). This finding is consistent with the theory associated with odor (Osterkamp et al., 1999) described above. The study also reported that resistant hosts when exposed to ticks mount an earlier inflammatory response than susceptible cattle (gene expression studies undertaken at 2 days post larval infestation using tick naïve cattle) (Franzin et al., 2017) which appears to disappear later (feeding nymphs at 9 days) but lingers in susceptible cattle.

Franzin et al. (2017) identified numerous novel immune response genes that were up-regulated in susceptible Holstein cattle including *FCER1A* the high affinity immunoglobulin epsilon receptor subunit alpha precursor which is known to be responsible for initiating an allergic response. The up-regulation

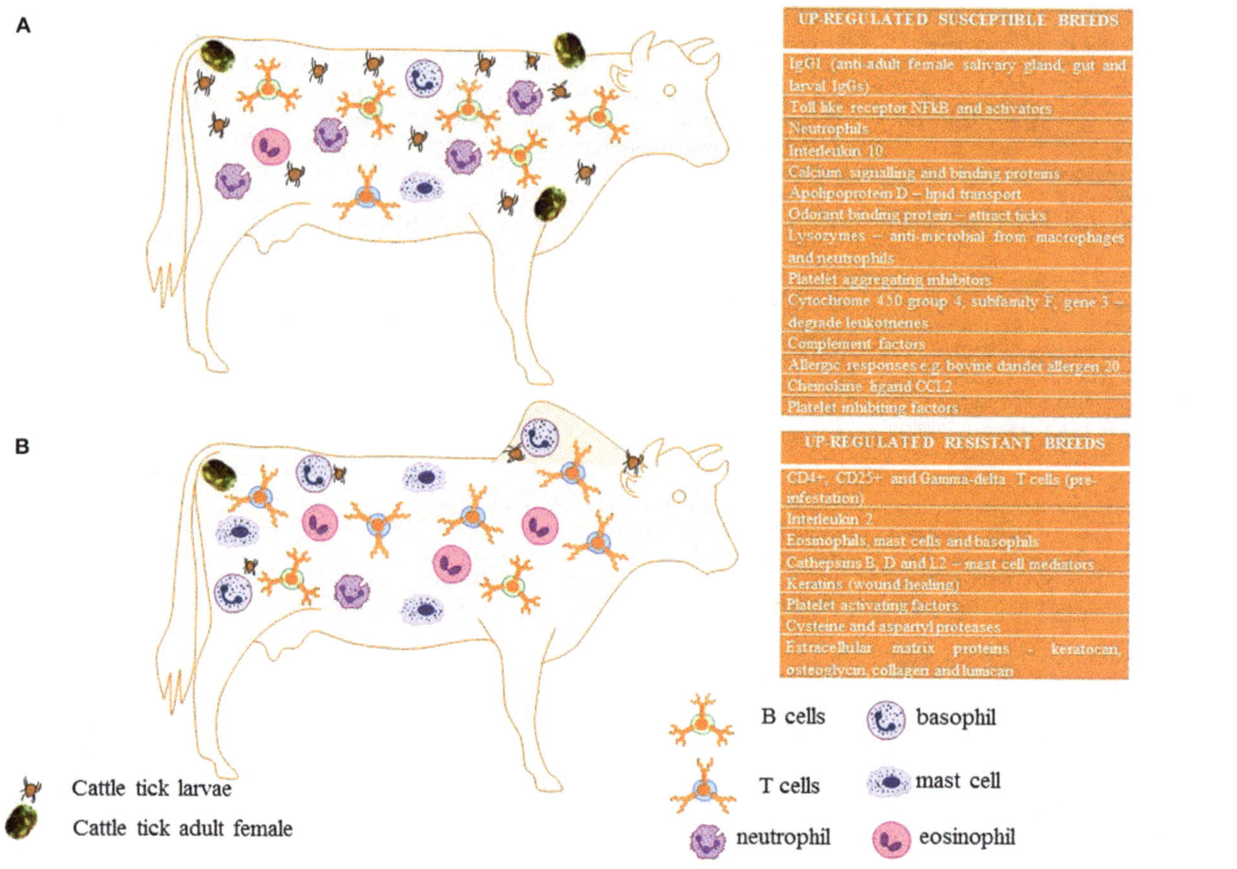

FIGURE 1 | Summary of expression and immunological profiles *commonly* associated in tick susceptible **(A)** compared to tick resistant breeds **(B)** of cattle as identified in **Table 1**. This diagram was created using images from Motifolio Inc.

of complement *C1QTNF7* (C1q tumor necrosis factor-related protein 7 precursor), an inducer of pro-inflammatory activators (Kishore et al., 2004) also concurs with the conclusions of tick susceptible cattle responding in a pro-inflammatory manner (Piper et al., 2010). Piper et al. (2008) had identified the up-regulation of Toll-like receptors (i.e., *NFkB*, nuclear factor kappa-light-chain-enhancer of activated B cells) that correlates with the activity of the complement C1Q identified by Franzin et al. (2017). In addition, *BCL10* (B-cell CLL/lymphoma 10) was up-regulated in susceptible cattle (Franzin et al., 2017) and is also known to activate *NFkB* (Wang M. et al., 2007). In addition fibroleukin is known to have a dual prothrombinase and immunoregulatory activity and was up-regulated in tick naïve (tick susceptible) cattle by larvae (Franzin et al., 2017). Immunoregulatory activity includes the suppression of T cell proliferation and cytokine production, mainly of Th1 and Th17 cells but not Th2 cells (Bézie et al., 2015), which is in contrast to other observations above suggesting that susceptible cattle mount a Th1 response. Functionally, Bézie et al. (2015) found that fibroleukin induced long-term allograft survival in a rat model through regulatory B cells which in turn suppress the proliferation of CD4+T cells. These cells are up-regulated in tick resistant cattle in the majority of studies undertaken. To summarize the results presented by Franzin et al. (2017), early responses to larvae (48 h post-infestation by naïve tick susceptible cattle) appear to show a mixed Th1 and Th2 response with tick susceptibility being associated with a Th1 response.

Several differences are noted among the comparisons of gene expression studies and as noted by Regitano et al. (2008) we generally concur that "*differences in gene expression of resistant cows compared to susceptible cows were breed-specific.*" However, there are some consistencies identified in the above studies. The presence of high densities of CD4+, CD25+, and $\gamma\delta$ T cells are seen relatively consistently in resistant indicine cattle (see **Table 1**). The up-regulation of keratins and collagens is also common in resistant indicine cattle, with some divergent upregulation in susceptible breeds in fewer studies. The up-regulation of IgGs in susceptible cattle was reported by most researchers. MHC Class II and calcium binding proteins seem to be mostly up-regulated in susceptible breeds, with the latter commonly associated with susceptible breeds studied in Brazil. The expression of chemokine ligands varied greatly between studies and breeds with no identifiable consistency. Other genes that were up-regulated consistently in susceptible cattle include: apolipoproteins (lipid transport), lysozymes (anti-microbial, also found in macrophages and polymorphonuclear neutrophils), Toll like receptors, *NFkB* and NFkB activators *C1QTNF7* (complement C1q tumor necrosis factor –related protein 7) and *BCL10* (B-cell CLL/lymphoma 10) and several complement factors. IL10 is considered an anti-inflammatory cytokine perhaps induced early in susceptible cattle but IL10 appears to be associated with long term resistance in *B. t. indicus* Gyr cattle in Brazil (Domingues et al., 2014; Franzin et al., 2017). Cytochrome P450 enzymes are a superfamily of hemoproteins known to be involved in the synthesis or metabolism of various molecules and chemicals within cells. A P450 gene called CYP4F3 (cytochrome 450 group 4, subfamily F, gene 3) is known to degrade leukotrienes which are the chemical mediators of allergic responses (Karasuyama et al., 2011). CYP4F3 was downregulated in the skin of tick exposed resistant cattle (Brahmans, Piper et al., 2010) yet up-regulated in the skin of susceptible cattle (Holsteins, Carvalho et al., 2014) thus showing a correlation for the activity of this enzyme in tick susceptible cattle. A summary of all of these factors is presented in **Figure 1**.

Differential expression of genes coding for other host modifying enzymes were associated with resistant and susceptible phenotypes (**Table 1**). Although not identified in more than one study, the up-regulation of these factors appears to correlate to the relevant phenotype and are thus worthy of further description. For example the following were identified in different studies as up-regulated in tick resistant breeds: Cathepsin B (Wang Y. H. et al., 2007), Cathepsin L2 precursor (cysteine proteases, mast cell mediators) (Nascimento et al., 2011), Cathepsin D (aspartyl protease, mast cell mediator) (Franzin et al., 2017), serine peptidase inhibitor clade A (inhibits neutrophil elastase), phospholipase A2, group VII (platelet activating factor) (Piper et al., 2010), coagulation factors, and procollagen C-endopeptidase enhancer (metalloprotease inhibitor) (Piper et al., 2010); and conversely in tick susceptible breeds: serine peptidase inhibitor clade F (negative regulation of inflammatory response), spleen trypsin inhibitor, plasminogen activator (serine protease which produces plasmin which catalyzes the degradation of fibrin polymers in blood clots), prostaglandin D2 synthase (platelet aggregation inhibitor) (Piper et al., 2010), and phosphoprotein 24 (endopeptidase associated with platelet degranulation) (Franzin et al., 2017) were up-regulated.

Comparative transcriptomic studies of different life stages (larvae and adult females) have shown that ticks respond differentially according to whether they are sensing or feeding on a tick-susceptible or tick-resistant breed of cattle. A microarray study based on a *R. microplus* EST database (Wang M. et al., 2007), using sensing larvae (not attached to the host but contained within a fabric bag and able to sense the host) and feeding, adult females, which were collected from naïve, tick-susceptible Holstein Friesian *B. t. taurus*, and tick-resistant Brahman *B. t. indicus* cattle has been reported (Rodriguez-Valle et al., 2010). Ticks that were feeding on resistant cattle demonstrated the up-regulation of serpin 2, lipocalins and histamine binding proteins. A recent study utilized next generation sequencing to compare tick expression differences from larvae, nymph salivary glands and larval offspring of females - all fed on tick-resistant Nelore *B. t. indicus* and tick-susceptible Holstein *B. t. taurus* (Franzin et al., 2017). That study showed an increased number of transcripts that included evasins, immunosuppressant proteins, lipocalins (including histamine, serotonin, and odorant binding proteins), and reprolysin metalloproteases from ticks associated with susceptible cattle, and an increased number of chitinases and cysteine proteases from ticks associated with resistant cattle. The analysis also included larvae exposed to volatile compounds prepared from the same breeds of cattle and showed that resistant breeds produce less attractive volatiles (Franzin et al., 2017). The latter was thought to be correlated to the fact that ticks on susceptible cattle up-regulated odorant binding proteins. Not enough studies have been undertaken to draw any similarities between the molecular profiles of ticks from susceptible vs. resistant hosts particularly when different stages and breeds are compared. It is clear however that the tick gene expression profiles associated with tick-resistant vs. tick-susceptible cattle appear to be divergent.

Acquired immunity to tick infestation is established after a period of susceptibility to a primary infestation (Wagland, 1978). As confirmed above, gene expression profiles from tick resistant breeds appear to be congruent with a T-cell mediated response, while susceptible cattle exhibit innate and inflammatory responses with higher levels of tick specific IgG1. One quite consistent fact is that resistant cattle appear to be primed to respond to ticks with a higher presence of $\gamma\delta$ T cells in the skin of tick naïve resistant cattle in comparison to susceptible. A formal meta-analysis of all gene expression studies where the data are in the public domain is theoretically possible but would likely be compromised by variation in the conditions of each of the studies. Each gene expression comparison study was undertaken using quite different conditions. The variable factors include: environment, season, naïve vs. tick exposed cattle, the use of acaricides post exposure prior to artificial infestations, infestation protocols including frequency and numbers of larvae, and comparative breeds including within breed studies.

CELLULAR PHYSIOLOGY ASSOCIATED WITH HOST RESISTANCE

Granulocytes (or polymorphonuclear leukocytes) are white blood cells characterized by the presence of granules in their cytoplasm and which perform different immune functions. They include neutrophils (most abundant), eosinophils, mast cells, and basophils. The inflammatory profile of the host skin contributes to resistance or susceptibility to tick infestation. Marufu et al. (2013) showed that tick susceptibility (*B. t. taurus* Bonsmara cattle) is associated with an immediate type hypersensitivity reaction. On the other hand, the resistance phenotype was linked to a delayed hypersensitivity reaction in *B. t. indicus* Nguni breed (Marufu et al., 2013) confirming the observations of Constantinoiu et al. (2010) with *B.t.taurus* Holstein Friesian (susceptible) and *B.t.indicus* Brahman (resistant) cattle. **Table 2** summarizes the cellular profiles obtained in response to ticks with differences associated with: the tick stage (larvae, nymph and adults), use of previously tick-exposed or naïve cattle, timing of sample collection post-infestation, blood or skin samples, and methodologies used.

Neutrophils are usually found in the blood stream and are the most abundant phagocyte. During host infection, neutrophils are quickly recruited to the site of infection i.e., skin in response to tick infestation. Neutrophils may favor infestation by destroying the extracellular matrix around the attached tick and thereby allowing access to blood for feeding (Tatchell and Bennett, 1969; Tatchell and Moorhouse, 1970). Similar numbers of neutrophils were found to be recruited in Holstein (susceptible, *B. t. taurus*) and Nelore cattle (resistant, *B. t. indicus*) (Carvalho et al., 2010a), with slightly higher neutrophils in the skin of susceptible cattle at early stages of infestation using naïve cattle of the same breeds (Franzin et al., 2017). Marufu et al. (2014) showed higher counts of neutrophils at the attachment sites of *R. microplus* in both resistant and susceptible breeds compared to non-infested skin, with higher counts also found in tick susceptible Bonsmara cattle compared to tick resistant Nguni cattle (Marufu et al., 2014). Higher levels of neutrophils do not seem to show a protective role against *R. microplus* infestation and feeding larvae demonstrated a high ingestion of neutrophils in susceptible *B. t. taurus* Holstein Friesian cattle (Constantinoiu et al., 2010). Moreover, activated neutrophils lead to a calcium ion influx which could correlate with the common up-regulation of calcium binding proteins in susceptible cattle gene expression studies (**Table 1**). Overall, higher neutrophil densities in the skin at the site of a tick attachment appear to be associated with the tick susceptible phenotype.

Eosinophils have long been known to be associated with parasite infections and allergy, with several immune functions having been only recently elucidated. For example, recent evidence suggests that eosinophils suppress Th17 and Th1 responses via dendritic cell regulation and also activate basophil degranulation (Wen and Rothenberg, 2016). Eosinophils may influence the tick resistant phenotype due to their role in the translocation of mast cell histamine and lysosomal enzymes to the feeding site lesion, and by impairing tick attachment (Schleger et al., 1981). *B. t. taurus* show higher eosinophil counts during secondary infestations compared with *B. t. indicus* breeds in early studies (Tatchell and Moorhouse, 1968). Marufu et al. (2013) confirmed this observation with higher eosinophil counts in tick susceptible Bonsmara cattle, in contrast to other studies which showed higher eosinophil counts in tick resistant cattle (Nelore *B. t. indicus*) in Brazil and Australian Shorthorn breed (*B. t. taurus* tropically adapted cattle) (Schleger et al., 1976; Carvalho et al., 2010b). Using the same breeds as Carvalho et al. (2010b), Franzin et al. (2017) showed higher eosinophil counts in susceptible cattle during the first infestation of tick naïve cattle, yet higher eosinophil counts at nymph feeding sites in the tick resistant breed. Suppression of Th1 responses by eosinophils may be logically associated with the response of resistant cattle and may also correlate with mast cell activity.

Mast cells (including tissue basophils) are a multifunctional cell population involved in maintaining local homeostasis of connective tissue, control of blood coagulation and defensive functions of innate and adaptive immunity. In addition mast cell dysfunction is associated with several chronic allergic/inflammatory disorders (da Silva et al., 2014). Mast cells contain granules rich in histamine and heparin, and are the main effectors of allergic reactions. Host resistance to ticks appears to concur with mast cell functions such as allergic responses, wound healing and immune tolerance, and a potential mast cell dysfunction in tick-susceptible cattle. Most studies on cattle have shown higher mast cell counts in resistant breeds in response to ticks (**Table 2**). However, one study comparing several breeds found that the Nelore *B. t. indicus* resistant breed had the highest number of mast cells in response to ticks while the Gyr *B. t. indicus* tick resistant breed had similar levels as two tick susceptible *B. t. taurus* breeds, Holstein and Brown Swiss (Veríssimo et al., 2008). In contrast, previously Gyr *B. t. indicus* cattle showed a higher number of mast cells in the dermis compared to susceptible European breeds (Moraes et al., 1992; Veríssimo et al., 2008). A few mast cell activators (da Silva et al., 2014) have been noted in resistant host gene expression studies above including Cathepsins B, D, and L2, platelet activating factors, complement factor C3, IL10, IL2, and TNFα (**Table 1**).

Basophils are known for their allergic effector function and were first described in response to ticks by Trager in 1939. Basophils notably accumulated at tick bite sites causing cutaneous hypersensitivity (Trager, 1939). In the 1950s, it was confirmed that histamines are stored in basophil granules (Graham et al., 1955). Basophils have been associated with immunity against parasites including ticks and helminths, reviewed by Karasuyama et al. (2011). It is thus logical as described above for mast cells, that high levels of circulating basophils would be associated with the tick resistant phenotype, which has been confirmed by two groups (Carvalho et al., 2010a; Marufu et al., 2014; Franzin et al., 2017). The release of histamine has been postulated as a mechanism which dislodges feeding ticks. This was confirmed when mice were injected with cultured mast cells which resulted in tick rejection following infestation of *Haemophysalis longicornis* ticks, with no tick rejection in mast cell deficient mice (Matsuda et al., 1987). A recent review of basophil functions confirms their effector role in allergic reactions, however basophils also share features of innate and adaptive immunity (Steiner et al., 2016) which again associates well with the tick resistant bovine phenotype. Steiner et al. (2016) examined the ever expanding function of basophils including the modulation of several cytokines, Toll-like receptors and chemokines (including CXCL10, CCR1, CCR7 described as up-regulated in certain tick resistant cattle studies, **Table 1**).

The correlation of granulocyte activity (and their immune effector mechanisms) in the skin of tick resistant cattle could further be examined to attempt to correlate immunity with gene expression studies described above. The existence of tick histamine-binding salivary lipocalins have been associated with inhibiting histamines from their receptors (Paesen et al., 1999; Mans et al., 2008) with specific lipocalins up-regulated in resistant vs. susceptible breeds in response to ticks (Rodriguez-Valle et al., 2013). In addition, the central role of histamine in tick resistance was supported by antihistamine administration to cattle which led to increased tick loads on

TABLE 2 | Summary of inflammatory profile between susceptible and resistant breeds of cattle.

Methodology (cattle breeds compared)	Susceptible	Resistant	Main conclusion and reference
Histology of skin using larvae—several different breeds (*B. t. taurus* vs. *B. t. indicus*)	Higher **eosinophils** during secondary infestation		Wide variations in the magnitude of the lesions between different hosts Tatchell and Moorhouse, 1968
Skin histology at larval tick lesions, 3 h feeding on previously tick exposed cattle (tropically adapted Illawarra Shorthorn *B. t. taurus* susceptible vs. resistant)		Higher **mast cells** Higher **eosinophils** Higher **neutrophils**	Degree of mast cell disruption, eosinophil concentration and degranulation and the extent of epidermal vesiculation were all significantly higher in highly resistant hosts. Schleger et al., 1976
Skin biopsies from tick lesions (Gyr -*B. t. indicus* vs Holstein - *B. t. taurus*)	Lower mast cell counts	Higher **mast cell** counts	Mast cells important in host resistance Moraes et al., 1992
Dermal (upper and deep) mast cell counts (Nelore and Gyr -*B. t. indicus* vs. Holstein, Brown-Swiss and Jersey - *B. t. taurus*)	Holsten and Brown Swiss similar to Gyr Lowest mast cell counts – Brown-Swiss	High **mast cells** cell counts– Nelore Gyr - Similar to Holstein and Brown Swiss	Negative correlation between the number of mast cells in the upper dermis and tick counts. Mast cells important in tick resistance. Veríssimo et al., 2008
Immuno staining of skin sections (Brahman *B. t. indicus* vs. Holstein-Friesian *B. t. taurus*)	Higher **neutrophils**	Delayed hypersensitivity	γδ T cells might have a role in limiting the inflammatory process and preservation of the skin homeostasis in *B. t. indicus* cattle. Constantinoiu et al., 2010
In vitro binding of leukocytes and skin histology (Nelore -*B. t. indicus* vs. Holstein - *B. t. taurus*)	Adhesion molecules: leukocyte adhesion glycoprotein 1	Higher **basophils** Higher **eosinophils** Adhesion molecules: E-selectin (promotes adhesion of memory T cells)	Resistant cattle had significantly higher counts of basophils and eosinophils compared to susceptible breeds. Adhesion molecules indicate differences in resistant and susceptible hosts. Carvalho et al., 2010a
Cutaneous hypersensitivity responses to tick larval antigens in previously exposed cattle (Bonsmara *B. t. taurus* vs. Nguni *B. t. indicus*)	Intense cutaneous hypersensitivity response	Delayed hypersensitivity response	Marufu et al., 2013
Cellular responses to adult *R. microplus* in skin biopsies (Bonsmara *B. t. taurus* vs. Nguni *B. t. indicus*)	Higher basophils (lower than resistant cattle) Higher mast cells (lower than resistant cattle) Higher mononuclear cells (lower than resistant cattle) Higher **neutrophils** Higher **eosinophils**	Higher **basophils** Higher **mast cells** Higher mononuclear cells Higher neutrophils (lower than susceptible cattle) Higher eosinophils (lower than susceptible cattle)	Cellular responses showed higher counts of basophils, mast and mononuclear cells and lower neutrophil and eosinophil counts in resistant breeds. Marufu et al., 2014
Histopathology larvae and nymph with naïve cattle. (Holstein *B. t. taurus* vs. Nelore *B. t. indicus*)	Higher **eosinophils** (larvae) Higher **mast** cells (nymph, slightly higher compared to larvae bite site)	Higher **mast** cells (larvae), mast cells degranulated and decreased (nymph) Higher **eosinophils** (nymph) Higher **basophils** (nymphs)	Resistant hosts expose ticks to an earlier inflammatory response which is delayed in susceptible breeds. Franzin et al., 2017

Bold fonts highlight common trends across different publications.

both *B. t. taurus* (Hereford) and *B. t. indicus* (Brahman) breeds (Tatchell and Bennett, 1969).

In summary, these studies confirm that cattle breeds behave differently during *R. microplus* infestation, presenting various intrinsic mechanisms to provide protection against ticks. Overall, resistant cattle appear to be associated with increased mast cells, eosinophils, and basophils in the skin, while the recruitment of neutrophils is potentially associated with tick susceptibility. The release of histamines from these cells appears to be associated with the resistant phenotype. Histamine is thought to inhibit tick attachment and leads to itching, which subsequently leads to more grooming and tick removal.

MICROBIOTA ROLE IN TICK RESISTANCE

The microbiome contributes to the architecture and function of tissues, host energy metabolism, and also plays an important role in the balance between health and disease as demonstrated recently for intracellular protozoa (Yilmaz et al., 2014; Bär et al., 2015). In vertebrates, semiochemicals can be generated by the activity of the microbiota upon amino acids, short chain fatty acids or hormones secreted in body emissions, such as sweat, tears, sebum, saliva, breath, urine, and feces (Amann et al., 2014; Fischer et al., 2015). This volatile repertoire is of paramount importance with evidence that they can direct host-vector specificity (Smallegange et al., 2011; Davis et al., 2013). The variation in the host chemical production thus causes differential attractiveness to vectors between species and in turn, the bacterial profiles differ according to human genetic background (Benson et al., 2010; Prokop-Prigge et al., 2015). Microbial composition can be affected by diet and other management strategies, such as those used for beef and dairy cattle (Durso et al., 2012; Thoetkiattikul et al., 2013). The differences in the composition of their microbiota (Dowd et al., 2008; Durso et al., 2010, 2012; de Oliveira et al., 2013; Mao et al., 2015), as well as the distinct volatile organic compounds (VOC) produced by *B. t. taurus* and *B. t. indicus* cattle may corroborate the contrasting tick infestation phenotypes observed among these animals (Steullet and Gnerin, 1994; Osterkamp et al., 1999; Borges et al., 2015; Ferreira et al., 2015). Although a few studies have demonstrated that host VOCs play a role in attracting *Rhipicephalus* spp. ticks (Louly et al., 2010; Borges et al., 2015; de Oliveira Filho et al., 2016; Franzin et al., 2017), research is still needed to investigate the interrelationship of host microbiota with VOC production related with tick attraction or repulsion. This may potentially reveal yet other factors contributing to tick susceptibility thereby presenting new opportunities to develop control methods for the livestock ectoparasite, *R. microplus*.

FUTURE RESEARCH AGENDA

Understanding the mechanisms behind genetic resistance to ticks and tick-borne diseases in livestock could improve breeding programs to develop cattle that are more resistant and productive (reviewed by Mapholi et al., 2014). Research to identify host genetic markers associated with tick susceptibility or resistance have been limited and compounded by the comparison of local breeds in different geographic regions as summarized here in this review. In addition, several studies reviewed here applied gene expression analysis of tick resistant breeds such as Nelore or Brahman. Brahman cattle have diverged through "up-breeding" in Australia and are thought to contain ~7–10% *B. t. taurus* in their genomes (Bolormaa et al., 2011), whereas the Nelore breed is viewed as highly pure *B. t. indicus* in comparison (<1% *B. t. taurus* content). High throughput genomics is increasingly affordable and thus prior to the identification of tick resistance markers, it would be practical to first determine the genomic differences between and within breeds under study.

Further research assessing tick:host preference mechanisms are still needed. Whether these can be manipulated to protect susceptible cattle from ticks is yet to be determined. The volatile organic compounds of susceptible cattle could be influenced by the microbiome which in turn may be controlled by diet. Recently it was demonstrated that butyric acid (also a VOC, commonly found in feces) stimulates bovine neutrophils and potentiates platelet activating factors thus modulating the innate immune response (Carretta et al., 2016). Indeed, to identify links between tick host attraction and bovine immune responses would be interesting. The potential to manipulate volatiles through probiotic treatments and/or diet could be a future option for tick control.

Within the host immune studies compared in this review, it was apparent that the conditions of the experiments preclude direct comparisons of in particular, gene expression data. Nonetheless some similarities were identified. Future research could focus on proteomic analyses of tick lesions between resistant and susceptible breeds with the recommendation to use tick naïve cattle with multiple skin sampling from early infestations (i.e., initial attachment of larvae) until tick resistance is achieved after several infestations. The studies reported most likely are hampered by the costs associated with long cattle experiments. This could be why many studies held cattle in tick infested pastures during artificial tick infestations as this is the most economical option for long term studies.

Tick vaccines can potentially protect the host from tick infestations and tick borne diseases. This review concentrated less on the development of tick vaccines as it was considered that to develop a successful tick vaccine it would be wise to understand the most common immune effectors to emulate this outcome when using a new anti-tick vaccine candidate(s). Perhaps CRISPR/Cas9 gene editing technologies (parasite CRISPR/Cas9 models recently reviewed by (Cui and Yu, 2016) could be manipulated to examine host-tick relationships in order to demonstrate the most effective tick resistance pathway(s) to be exploited for vaccine development. Indeed CRISPR/Cas9 host editing to favor tick resistance could also be exploited in the future. Further insights into the immunomodulatory processes between ticks and tick susceptible/resistant hosts could identify major genes which would facilitate tick control strategies and the development a broad-spectrum anti-tick vaccine.

CONCLUSIONS

Taking advantage of recent advances from new approaches and technologies as applied to the field of vector biology, such as transcriptomics, proteomics, immune-molecular characterization, elucidation of naturally acquired resistance, and the development of innovative arthropod and animal models, may lead to improved investigations of naturally acquired resistant breeds against tick and tick-borne pathogens. Immune-proteomic, sialotranscriptome and reverse genetics/gene editing (RNAi, CRISPR/Cas9) may help to identify new vaccine candidates that resist ticks and tick-borne pathogens. By understanding the tick:host interface and the most common denominators of immunity to ticks, this acquired immune response could be manipulated to improve the efficacy of novel anti-tick vaccines. Conversely, the knowledge obtained may assist in the selection of tick resistant cattle or the manipulation of susceptible cattle to develop a protective tick immune response. Furthermore, the in depth analysis of host microbiota and volatile organic compounds could lead to probiotic or diet changes or inhibitory chemicals which could render susceptible cattle less attractive to ticks. Future research may lead to a combination of several of these technologies as novel tick and tick-borne disease control options by first identifying viable biological targets and dissecting pathways leading to vaccination or pharmaceutical therapies or cattle management opportunities for tick control.

AUTHOR CONTRIBUTIONS

AA, GR, and AT conceived the research review. AT prepared the comparative Tables/Figures and with NJ revised all sections written by other co-authors. GRG, AZ, TM and NJ wrote or contributed to specific sections within the review.

FUNDING

The contribution by AT was supported by Meat & Livestock Australia MDC project: P.PSH.0798.

ACKNOWLEDGMENTS

The authors gratefully acknowledge the financial support of the FAPESP and CAPES (Brazil) and Pakistan Science Foundation (PSF) for the financial support in ongoing research and fellowships.

REFERENCES

Abbas, R. Z., Zaman, M. A., Colwell, D. D., Gilleard, J., and Iqbal, Z. (2014). Acaricide resistance in cattle ticks and approaches to its management: the state of play. *Vet. Parasitol.* 203, 6–20. doi: 10.1016/j.vetpar.2014.03.006

Ackerman, S., Clare, F. B., McGill, T. W., and Sonenshine, D. E. (1981). Passage of host serum components, including antibody, across the digestive tract of *Dermacentor variabilis* (Say). *J. Parasitol.* 67, 737–740. doi: 10.2307/3280459

Acosta-Rodriguez, R., Alonso-Morales, R., Balladares, S., Flores-Aguilar, H., Garcia-Vazquez, Z., and Gorodezky, C. (2005). Analysis of BoLA class II microsatellites in cattle infested with *Boophilus microplus* ticks: class II is probably associated with susceptibility. *Vet. Parasitol.* 127, 313–321. doi: 10.1016/j.vetpar.2004.10.007

Allen, J. R. (1989). Immunology of interactions between ticks and laboratory animals. *Exp. Appl. Acarol.* 7, 5–13. doi: 10.1007/BF01200448

Allen, J. R., and Humphreys, S. J. (1979). Immunisation of guinea pigs and cattle against ticks. *Nature* 280, 491–493. doi: 10.1038/280491a0

Amann, A., de Lacy Costello, B., Miekisch, W., Schubert, J., Buszewski, B., Pleil, J., et al. (2014). The human volatilome: volatile organic compounds (VOCs) in exhaled breath, skin emanations, urine, feces and saliva. *J. Breath. Res.* 8:034001. doi: 10.1088/1752-7155/8/3/034001

Ashton, G. C., Seifert, G. W., and Francis, J. (1968). An association between serum amylase phenotype and tick infestation in cattle. *Aust. J. Biol. Sci.* 21, 303–308.

Bagnall, N., Gough, J., Cadogan, L., Burns, B., and Kongsuwan, K. (2009). Expression of intracellular calcium signalling genes in cattle skin during tick infestation. *Parasite Immunol.* 31, 177–187. doi: 10.1111/j.1365-3024.2008.01092.x

Bär, A.-K., Phukan, N., Pinheiro, J., and Simoes-Barbosa, A. (2015). The interplay of host microbiota and parasitic protozoans at mucosal interfaces: implications for the outcomes of infections and diseases. *PLoS Negl. Trop. Dis.* 9:e0004176. doi: 10.1371/journal.pntd.0004176

Barendse, W. (2007). *Assessing Tick Resistance in a Bovine Animal for Selecting Cattle for Tick Resistance by Providing a Nucleic Acid from the Bovine Animal and Assaying for the Occurrence of a Single Nucleotide Polymorphism (SNP).* Patent No. WO2007051248 A1.

Barré, N., and Uilenberg, G. (2010). Spread of parasites transported with their hosts: case study of two species of cattle tick. *Rev. Sci. Tech.* 29, 149–160. Available online at: https://www.oie.int/doc/ged/D7236.PDF

Bastida-Corcuera, F. D., Butler, J. E., Yahiro, S., and Corbeil, L. B. (1999). Differential complement activation by bovine IgG2 allotypes. *Vet. Immunol. Immunopathol.* 71, 115–123. doi: 10.1016/S0165-2427(99)00095-1

Bennett, G. F. (1969). Boophilus microplus (Acarina: Ixodidae): experimental infestations on cattle restrained from grooming. *Exp. Parasitol.* 26, 323–328. doi: 10.1016/0014-4894(69)90125-8

Benson, A. K., Kelly, S. A., Legge, R., Ma, F., Low, S. J., Kim, J., et al. (2010). Individuality in gut microbiota composition is a complex polygenic trait shaped by multiple environmental and host genetic factors. *Proc. Natl. Acad. Sci. U.S.A.* 107, 18933–18938. doi: 10.1073/pnas.1007028107

Ben-Yakir, D., Fox, C. J., Homer, J. T., and Barker, R. W. (1987). Quantification of host immunoglobulin in the hemolymph of ticks. *J. Parasitol.* 73, 669–671. doi: 10.2307/3282157

Bézie, S., Picarda, E., Tesson, L., Renaudin, K., Durand, J., Ménoret, S., et al. (2015). Fibrinogen-like protein 2/fibroleukin induces long-term allograft survival in a rat model through regulatory B Cells. *PLoS ONE* 10:e0119686. doi: 10.1371/journal.pone.0119686

Biegelmeyer, P., Nizoli, L. Q., da Silva, S. S., dos Santos, T. R. B., Dionello, N. J. L., Gulias-Gomes, C. C., et al. (2015). Bovine genetic resistance effects on biological traits of *Rhipicephalus (Boophilus) microplus*. *Vet. Parasitol.* 208, 231–237. doi: 10.1016/j.vetpar.2015.01.010

Blakeslee, D., Butler, J. E., and Stone, W. H. (1971). Serum antigens of cattle. II. Immunogenetics of two immunoglobulin allotypes. *J. Immunol.* 107, 227–235.

Bolormaa, S., Hayes, B. J., Hawken, R. J., Zhang, Y., Reverter, A., and Goddard, M. E. (2011). Detection of chromosome segments of zebu and taurine origin and their effect on beef production and growth. *J. Anim. Sci.* 89, 2050–2060. doi: 10.2527/jas.2010-3363

Borges, L. M. F., de Oliveira Filho, J. G., Ferreira, L. L., Louly, C. C. B., Pickett, J. A., and Birkett, M. A. (2015). Identification of non-host semiochemicals for the brown dog tick, *Rhipicephalus sanguineus* sensu lato (Acari: Ixodidae), from tick-resistant beagles, Canis lupus familiaris. *Ticks Tick Borne Dis.* 6, 676–682. doi: 10.1016/j.ttbdis.2015.05.014

Burger, T. D., Shao, R., and Barker, S. C. (2014). Phylogenetic analysis of mitochondrial genome sequences indicates that the cattle tick, *Rhipicephalus (Boophilus) microplus*, contains a cryptic species. *Mol. Phylogenet. Evol.* 76, 241–253. doi: 10.1016/j.ympev.2014.03.017

Butler, J. E., Navarro, P., and Heyermann, H. (1994). Heterogeneity of bovine IgG2. VI. Comparative specificity of monoclonal and polyclonal capture antibodies for IgG2a (A1) and IgG2a (A2). *Vet. Immunol. Immunopathol.* 40, 119–133. doi: 10.1016/0165-2427(94)90028-0

Cardoso, F. F., Gomes, C. C. G., Sollero, B. P., Oliveira, M. M., Roso, V. M., Piccoli, M. L., et al. (2015). Genomic prediction for tick resistance in Braford and Hereford cattle. *J. Anim. Sci.* 93, 2693–2705. doi: 10.2527/jas.2014-8832

Carretta, M. D., Hidalgo, A. I., Burgos, J., Opazo, L., Castro, L., Hidalgo, M. A., et al. (2016). Butyric acid stimulates bovine neutrophil functions and potentiates the effect of platelet activating factor. *Vet. Immunol. Immunopathol.* 176, 18–27. doi: 10.1016/j.vetimm.2016.05.002

Carvalho, W. A., Bechara, G. H., More, D. D., Ferreira, B. R., da Silva, J. S., and de Miranda Santos, I. K. (2008). *Rhipicephalus (Boophilus) microplus*: distinct acute phase proteins vary during infestations according to the genetic composition of the bovine hosts, *Bos taurus* and *Bos indicus*. *Exp. Parasitol.* 118, 587–591. doi: 10.1016/j.exppara.2007.10.006

Carvalho, W. A., Domingues, R., de Azevedo Prata, M. C., da Silva, M. V. G. B., de Oliveira, G. C., Guimarães, S. E. F., et al. (2014). Microarray analysis of tick-infested skin in resistant and susceptible cattle confirms the role of inflammatory pathways in immune activation and larval rejection. *Vet. Parasitol.* 205, 307–317. doi: 10.1016/j.vetpar.2014.07.018

Carvalho, W. A., Franzin, A. M., Abatepaulo, A. R. R., de Oliveira, C. J. F., Moré, D. D., da Silva, J. S., et al. (2010a). Modulation of cutaneous inflammation induced by ticks in contrasting phenotypes of infestation in bovines. *Vet. Parasitol.* 167, 260–273. doi: 10.1016/j.vetpar.2009.09.028

Carvalho, W. A., Ianella, P., Arnoldi, F. G. C., Caetano, A. R., Maruyama, S. R., Ferreira, B. R., et al. (2011). Haplotypes of the bovine IgG2 heavy gamma chain in tick-resistant and tick-susceptible breeds of cattle. *Immunogenetics* 63, 319–324. doi: 10.1007/s00251-011-0515-y

Carvalho, W. A., Maruyama, S. R., Franzin, A. M., Abatepaulo, A. R. R., Anderson, J. M., Ferreira, B. R., et al. (2010b). *Rhipicephalus (Boophilus) microplus*: clotting time in tick-infested skin varies according to local inflammation and gene expression patterns in tick salivary glands. *Exp. Parasitol.* 124, 428–435.

Constantinoiu, C. C., Jackson, L. A., Jorgensen, W. K., Lew-Tabor, A. E., Piper, E. K., Mayer, D. G., et al. (2010). Local immune response against larvae of *Rhipicephalus (Boophilus) microplus* in *Bos taurus indicus* and *Bos taurus taurus* cattle. *Int. J. Parasitol.* 40, 865–875. doi: 10.1016/j.ijpara.2010.01.004

Constantinoiu, C. C., Jonsson, N. N., Jorgensen, W. K., Jackson, L. A., Piper, E. K., and Lew-Tabor, A. E. (2013). Immuno-fluorescence staining patterns of leukocyte subsets in the skin of taurine and indicine cattle. *Res. Vet. Sci.* 95, 854–860. doi: 10.1016/j.rvsc.2013.08.014

Cruz, A. P. R., Silva, S. S., Mattos, R. T., Da Silva Vaz Jr, I., Masuda, A., and Ferreira, C. A. S. (2008). Comparative IgG recognition of tick extracts by sera of experimentally infested bovines. *Vet. Parasitol.* 158, 152–158. doi: 10.1016/j.vetpar.2008.08.016

Cui, Y., and Yu, L. (2016). Application of the CRISPR/Cas9 gene editing technique to research on functional genomes of parasites. *Parasitol. Int.* 65, 641–644. doi: 10.1016/j.parint.2016.08.011

da Silva, E. Z. M., Jamur, M. C., and Oliver, C. (2014). Mast cell function. *J. Histochem. Cytochem.* 62, 698–738. doi: 10.1369/0022155414545334

Davis, T. S., Crippen, T. L., Hofstetter, R. W., and Tomberlin, J. K. (2013). Microbial volatile emissions as insect semiochemicals. *J. Chem. Ecol.* 39, 840–859. doi: 10.1007/s10886-013-0306-z

de Castro, J. J., Cunningham, M. P., Dolan, T. T., Dransfield, R. D., Newson, R. M., and Young, A. S. (1985). Effects on cattle of artificial infestations with the tick *Rhipicephalus appendiculatus*. *Parasitology* 90, 21–33. doi: 10.1017/S0031182000048988

de Castro, J. J., and Newson, R. M. (1993). Host resistance in cattle tick control. *Parasitol. Today* 9, 13–17. doi: 10.1016/0169-4758(93)90154-8

de la Fuente, J., and Contreras, M. (2015). Tick vaccines: current status and future directions. *Expert Rev. Vaccines* 14, 1367–1376. doi: 10.1586/14760584.2015.1076339

de la Fuente, J., Kopacek, P., Lew-Tabor, A., and Maritz-Olivier, C. (2016). Strategies for new and improved vaccines against ticks and tick-borne diseases. *Parasite Immunol.* 38, 754–769. doi: 10.1111/pim.12339

de Oliveira Filho, J. G., Sarria, A. L. F., Ferreira, L. L., Caulfield, J. C., Powers, S. J., Pickett, J. A., et al. (2016). Quantification of brown dog tick repellents, 2-hexanone and benzaldehyde, and release from tick-resistant beagles, *Canis lupus* familiaris. *J. Chromatogr. B* 1022, 64–69. doi: 10.1016/j.jchromb.2016.03.014

de Oliveira, M. N. V., Jewell, K. A., Freitas, F. S., Benjamin, L. A., Tótola, M. R., Borges, A. C., et al. (2013). Characterizing the microbiota across the gastrointestinal tract of a Brazilian Nelore steer. *Vet. Microbiol.* 164, 307–314. doi: 10.1016/j.vetmic.2013.02.013

Domingues, R., Wohlres-Viana, S., Reis, D. R., Teixeira, H. C., Ferreira, A. P., Guimarães, S. E., et al. (2014). Expression of immune response genes in peripheral blood of cattle infested with Rhipicephalus microplus. *Genet. Mol. Res.* 13, 4013–4021. doi: 10.4238/2014.May.23.12

Doube, B. M., and Wharton, R. H. (1980). The effect of locality, breed and previous tick experience on seasonal changes in the resistance of cattle to *Boophilus microplus* (Ixodoidea: Ixodidae). *Experientia* 36, 1178–1179. doi: 10.1007/BF01976112

Dowd, S. E., Callaway, T. R., Wolcott, R. D., Sun, Y., McKeehan, T., Hagevoort, R. G., et al. (2008). Evaluation of the bacterial diversity in the feces of cattle using 16S rDNA bacterial tag-encoded FLX amplicon pyrosequencing (bTEFAP). *BMC Microbiol.* 8:125. doi: 10.1186/1471-2180-8-125

Durso, L. M., Harhay, G. P., Smith, T. P. L., Bono, J. L., DeSantis, T. Z., Harhay, D. M., et al. (2010). Animal-to-animal variation in fecal microbial fiversity among beef cattle. *Appl. Environ. Microbiol.* 76, 4858–4862. doi: 10.1128/AEM.00207-10

Durso, L. M., Wells, J. E., Harhay, G. P., Rice, W. C., Kuehn, L., Bono, J. L., et al. (2012). Comparison of bacterial communities in faeces of beef cattle fed diets containing corn and wet distillers' grain with solubles. *Letts Appl. Microbiol.* 55, 109–114. doi: 10.1111/j.1472-765X.2012.03265.x

Engracia Filho, J. R., Araújo, C. D., Pinto, G. N., Mendes, Y. H., and Bechara, G. H. (2017). Cellular response in the tick feeding site in crossbred cattle artificially infested by *Rhipicephalus microplus*. *Exp. Appl. Acarol.* 72, 171–178. doi: 10.1007/s10493-017-0143-9

Estrada-Peña, A., Bouattour, A., Camicas, J. L., Guglielmone, A., Horak, I., Jongejan, F., et al. (2006). The known distribution and ecological preferences of the tick subgenus Boophilus (Acari: Ixodidae) in Africa and Latin America. *Exp. Appl. Acarol.* 38, 219–235. doi: 10.1007/s10493-006-0003-5

Feldman-Muhsam, B. (1964). Laboratory colonies of Rhipicephalus. *Bull. World Health Organ.* 31, 587–589.

Ferreira, L. L., Soares, S. F., de Oliveira Filho, J. G., Oliveira, T. T., Pérez de León, A. A., and Borges, L. M. F. (2015). Role of *Rhipicephalus microplus* cheliceral receptors in gustation and host differentiation. *Ticks Tick Borne Dis.* 6, 228–233. doi: 10.1016/j.ttbdis.2014.12.008

Fischer, S., Trefz, P., Bergmann, A., Steffens, M., Ziller, M., Miekisch, W., et al. (2015). Physiological variability in volatile organic compounds (VOCs) in exhaled breath and released from faeces due to nutrition and somatic growth in a standardized caprine animal model. *J. Breath Res.* 9:027108. doi: 10.1088/1752-7155/9/2/027108

Franzin, A. M., Maruyama, S. R., Garcia, G. R., Oliveira, R. P., Ribeiro, J. M. C., Bishop, R., et al. (2017). Immune and biochemical responses in skin differ between bovine hosts genetically susceptible and resistant to the cattle tick *Rhipicephalus microplus*. *Parasit. Vectors* 10:51. doi: 10.1186/s13071-016-1945-z

Frisch, J. E. (1999). Towards a permanent solution for controlling cattle ticks. *Int. J. Parasitol.* 29, 57–71. doi: 10.1016/S0020-7519(98)00177-5

Garcia, G. R., Maruyama, S. R., Nelson, K. T., Ribeiro, J. M. C., Gardinassi, L. G., Maia, A. A. M., et al. (2017). Immune recognition of salivary proteins from the cattle tick *Rhipicephalus microplus* differs according to the genotype of the bovine host. *Parasit. Vectors* 10:144. doi: 10.1186/s13071-017-2077-9

Gasparin, G., Miyata, M., Coutinho, L. L., Martinez, M. L., Teodoro, R. L., Furlong, J., et al. (2007). Mapping of quantitative trait loci controlling tick *Riphicephalus (Boophilus) microplus* resistance on bovine chromosomes 5, 7and 14G. *Anim. Genet.* 38, 453–459. doi: 10.1111/j.1365-2052.2007.01634.x

Gong, H., Qin, S., Wan, X., Zhang, H., Zhou, Y., Cao, J., et al. (2014). Immunoglobulin G binding protein (IGBP) from *Rhipicephalus haemaphysaloides*: identification, expression, and binding specificity. *Parasitol. Res.* 113, 4387–4395. doi: 10.1007/s00436-014-4115-2

Graham, H. T., Lowry, O. H., Wheelwright, F., Lenz, M. A., and Parish, H. H. (1955). Distribution of histamine among leukocytes and platelets. *Blood* 10:467.

Gregson, J. D. (1941). Host immunity to ticks (Acarina). *J. Entomol. Soc.* 38, 12–13.

Gudderra, N. P., Sonenshine, D. E., Apperson, C. S., and Roe, R. M. (2002). Hemolymph proteins in ticks. *J. Insect Physiol.* 48, 269–278. doi: 10.1016/S0022-1910(02)00050-1

Hewetson, R. W. (1972). "The inheritance of resistance by cattle to cattle tick," in *Australian Veterinary Association Conference Paper* (Brisbane, QLD).

Heyermann, H., and Butler, J. E. (1987). the heterogeneity of bovine IgG2—IV. Structural differences between IgG2a molecules of the A1 and A2 allotypes. *Mol. Immunol.* 24, 1327–1334. doi: 10.1016/0161-5890(87)90128-3

Hogarth, P. M. (2002). Fc receptors are major mediators of antibody based inflammation in autoimmunity. *Curr. Opin. Immunol.* 14, 798–802. doi: 10.1016/S0952-7915(02)00409-0

Jones, K. E., Patel, N. G., Levy, M. A., Storeygard, A., Balk, D., Gittleman, J. L., et al. (2008). Global trends in emerging infectious diseases. *Nature* 451, 990–993. doi: 10.1038/nature06536

Jonsson, N. N., Piper, E. K., and Constantinoiu, C. C. (2014). Host resistance in cattle to infestation with the cattle tick *Rhipicephalus microplus*. *Parasite Immunol.* 36, 553–559. doi: 10.1111/pim.12140

Kacskovics, I., and Butler, J. E. (1996). The heterogeneity of bovine IgG2—VIII. The complete cDNA sequence of bovine IgG2a (A2) and an IgG1. *Mol. Immunol.* 33, 189–195. doi: 10.1016/0161-5890(95)00107-7

Karasuyama, H., Wada, T., Yoshikawa, S., and Obata, K. (2011). Emerging roles of basophils in protective immunity against parasites. *Trends Immunol.* 32, 125–130. doi: 10.1016/j.it.2010.11.006

Kashino, S. S., Resende, J., Sacco, A. M. S., Rocha, C., Proenca, L., Carvalho, W. A., et al. (2005). *Boophilus microplus*: the pattern of bovine immunoglobulin isotype responses to high and low tick infestations. *Exp. Parasitol.* 110, 12–21. doi: 10.1016/j.exppara.2005.01.006

Kaufman, W. R. (1989). Tick-host interaction: a synthesis of current concepts. *Parasitol. Today* 5, 47–56. doi: 10.1016/0169-4758(89)90191-9

Kemp, D. H., and Bourne, A. (1980). *Boophilus microplus*: the effect of histamine on the attachment of cattle-tick larvae–studies *in vivo* and *in vitro*. *Parasitology* 80, 487–496. doi: 10.1017/S0031182000000950

Kemp, D. H., Koudstaal, D., Roberts, J. A., and Kerr, J. D. (1976). Boophilus microplus: the effect of host resistance on larval attachments and growth. *Parasitology* 73, 123–136. doi: 10.1017/S0031182000051386

Kishore, U., Gaboriaud, C., Waters, P., Shrive, A. K., Greenhough, T. J., Reid, K. B. M., et al. (2004). C1q and tumor necrosis factor superfamily: modularity and versatility. *Trends Immunol.* 25, 551–561. doi: 10.1016/j.it.2004.08.006

Knight, K. L., Suter, M., and Becker, R. S. (1988). Genetic engineering of bovine Ig. Construction and characterization of hapten-binding bovine/murine chimeric IgE, IgA, IgG1, IgG2, and IgG3 molecules. *J. Immunol.* 140, 3654–3659.

Kongsuwan, K., Josh, P., Colgrave, M. L., Bagnall, N. H., Gough, J., Burns, B., et al. (2010). Activation of several key components of the epidermal differentiation pathway in cattle following infestation with the cattle tick, *Rhipicephalus (Boophilus) microplus*. *Int. J. Parasitol.* 40, 499–507. doi: 10.1016/j.ijpara.2009.10.013

Lew-Tabor, A. E., and Rodriguez Valle, M. (2016). A review of reverse vaccinology approaches for the development of vaccines against ticks and tick borne diseases. *Ticks Tick Borne Dis.* 7, 573–585. doi: 10.1016/j.ttbdis.2015.12.012

Louly, C. C. B., Soares, S. F., da Nóbrega Silveira, D., Guimarães, M. S., and Borges, L. M. F. (2010). Differences in the behavior of Rhipicephalus sanguineus tested against resistant and susceptible dogs. *Exp. Appl. Acarol.* 51, 353–362. doi: 10.1007/s10493-009-9334-3

Low, V. L., Tay, S. T., Kho, K. L., Koh, F. X., Tan, T. K., Lim, Y. A. L., et al. (2015). Molecular characterisation of the tick *Rhipicephalus microplus* in Malaysia: new insights into the cryptic diversity and distinct genetic assemblages throughout the world. *Parasit. Vectors* 8:341. doi: 10.1186/s13071-015-0956-5

Machado, M. A., Azevedo, A. L., Teodoro, R. L., Pires, M. A., Peixoto, M. G., de Freitas, C., et al. (2010). Genome wide scan for quantitative trait loci affecting tick resistance in cattle (*Bos taurus* x *Bos indicus*). *BMC Genomics* 11:280. doi: 10.1186/1471-2164-11-280

Mans, B. J., Anderson, J. F., Francischetti, I. M. B., Valenzuela, J. G., Schwan, T. G., Pham, V. M., et al. (2008). Comparative sialomics between hard and soft ticks: implications for the evolution of blood-feeding behavior. *Insect Biochem. Mol. Biol.* 38, 42–58. doi: 10.1016/j.ibmb.2007.09.003

Mao, S., Zhang, M., Liu, J., and Zhu, W. (2015). Characterising the bacterial microbiota across the gastrointestinal tracts of dairy cattle: membership and potential function. *Sci. Rep.* 5:16116. doi: 10.1038/srep16116

Mapholi, N. O., Maiwashe, A., Matika, O., Riggio, V., Bishop, S. C., MacNeil, M. D., et al. (2016). Genome-wide association study of tick resistance in South African *Nguni cattle*. *Ticks Tick Borne Dis.* 7, 487–497. doi: 10.1016/j.ttbdis.2016.02.005

Mapholi, N. O., Marufu, M. C., Maiwashe, A., Banga, C. B., Muchenje, V., MacNeil, M. D., et al. (2014). Towards a genomics approach to tick (Acari:Ixodidae) control in cattle: a review. *Ticks Tick Borne Dis.* 5, 475–483. doi: 10.1016/j.ttbdis.2014.04.006

Martinez, M. L., Machado, M. A., Nascimento, C. S., Silva, M. V. G. B., Teodoro, R. L., Furlong, J., et al. (2006). Association of BoLA-DRB3.2 alleles with tick (*Boophilus microplus*) resistance in cattle. *Genet. Mol. Res.* 5, 513–524. Available online at: http://www.funpecrp.com.br/gmr/year2006/vol3-5/pdf/gmr0211.pdf

Marufu, M. C., Chimonyo, M., Mans, B. J., and Dzama, K. (2013). Cutaneous hypersensitivity responses to *Rhipicephalus tick* larval antigens in pre-sensitized cattle. *Ticks Tick Borne Dis.* 4, 311–316. doi: 10.1016/j.ttbdis.2012.12.001

Marufu, M. C., Dzama, K., and Chimonyo, M. (2014). Cellular responses to *Rhipicephalus microplus* infestations in pre-sensitised cattle with differing phenotypes of infestation. *Exp. Appl. Acarol.* 62, 241–252. doi: 10.1007/s10493-013-9723-5

Marufu, M. C., Qokweni, L., Chimonyo, M., and Dzama, K. (2011). Relationships between tick counts and coat characteristics in Nguni and *Bonsmara cattle* reared on semiarid rangelands in South Africa. *Ticks Tick Borne Dis.* 2, 172–177. doi: 10.1016/j.ttbdis.2011.07.001

Matsuda, H., Nakano, T., Kiso, Y., and Kitamura, Y. (1987). Normalization of anti-tick response of mast cell-deficient W/Wv mice by intracutaneous injection of cultured mast cells. *J. Parasitol.* 73, 155–160. doi: 10.2307/3282361

Moraes, F. R., Moraes, J. R. E., Costa, A. J., Rocha, U. F., and Ardisson, F. A. (1992). A Comparative study of lesions eauscd by different parasitic stages of *Boophilus microplus* (Canestrini) in the skins of naturally inffcstcd taurine and zebuine hosts. The correlation of tick resistance with mast cell counts in the host's skin. *Braz. J. Vet Res. Anim.* 29, 378–383 Suplemento.

Nascimento, C. S., Machado, M. A., Guimarães, S. E., Guimarães, M. F., Peixoto, J. O., Furlong, J., et al. (2010). Differential expression of genes in resistant versus susceptible Gyr x Holstein cattle challenged with the tick *Rhipicephalus (Boophilus) microplus*. *Genet. Mol. Res.* 9, 1974–1979. doi: 10.4238/vol9-4gmr905

Nascimento, C. S., Machado, M. A., Guimarães, S. E., Martins, M. F., Peixoto, J. O., Furlong, J., et al. (2011). Expressed sequenced tags profiling of resistant and susceptible Gyr x Holstein cattle infested with the tick *Rhipicephalus (Boophilus) microplus*. *Genet. Mol. Res.* 10, 3803–3816. doi: 10.4238/2011.November.8.3

Nuttall, G. H. F. (1911). On the adaptation of ticks to the habits of their hosts. *Parasitology* 4, 46–67. doi: 10.1017/S0031182000002456

Ogden, N. H., and Lindsay, L. R. (2016). Effects of climate and climate change on vectors and vector-borne diseases: ticks are different. *Trends Parasitol.* 32, 646–656. doi: 10.1016/j.pt.2016.04.015

Opdebeeck, J. P., and Daly, K. E. (1990). Immune responses of infested and vaccinated Hereford cattle to antigens of the cattle tick, *Boophilus microplus*. *Vet. Immunol. Immunopathol.* 25, 99–108. doi: 10.1016/0165-2427(90)90113-7

Osterkamp, J., Wahl, U., Schmalfuss, G., and Haas, W. (1999). Host-odour recognition in two tick species is coded in a blend of vertebrate volatiles. *J. Comp. Physiol. A* 185, 59–67. doi: 10.1007/s003590050366

Paesen, G. C., Adams, P. L., Harlos, K., Nuttall, P. A., and Stuart, D. I. (1999). Tick histamine-binding proteins: isolation, cloning, and three-dimensional structure. *Mol. Cell* 3, 661–671. doi: 10.1016/S1097-2765(00)80359-7

Piper, E. K., Jackson, L. A., Bagnall, N., Kongsuwan, K., Lew, A. E., and Jonsson, N. N. (2008). Gene expression in skin of *Bos taurus* and *Bos indicus* cattle infested with the cattle tick. *Vet. Immunol. Immunopathol.* 126, 110–119. doi: 10.1016/j.vetimm.2008.06.011

Piper, E. K., Jackson, L. A., Bielefeldt-Ohmann, H., Gondro, C., Lew-Tabor, A. E., and Jonsson, N. N. (2010). Tick-susceptible *Bos taurus* cattle display an increased cellular response at the site of larval *Rhipicephalus (Boophilus) microplus* attachment, compared with tick-resistant *Bos indicus* cattle. *Int. J. Parasitol.* 40, 865–875. doi: 10.1016/j.ijpara.2009.09.009

Piper, E. K., Jonsson, N. N., Gondro, C., Lew-Tabor, A. E., Moolhuijzen, P., Vance, M. E., et al. (2009). Immunological profiles of *Bos taurus* and *Bos indicus* cattle infested with the cattle tick, *Rhipicephalus (Boophilus) microplus*. *Clin. Vaccine Immunol.* 16, 1074–1086. doi: 10.1128/CVI.00157-09

Piper, E. K., Jonsson, N. N., Gondro, C., Vance, M. E., Lew-Tabor, A., and Jackson, L. A. (2017). Peripheral cellular and humoral responses to infestation with the cattle tick *Rhipicephalus microplus* in Santa Gertrudis cattle. *Parasite Immunol.* 39:e12402. doi: 10.1111/pim.12402

Porto Neto, L. R., Bunch, R. J., Harrison, B. E., and Barendse, W. (2011a). DNA variation in the gene ELTD1 is associated with tick burden in cattle. *Anim. Genet.* 42, 50–55. doi: 10.1111/j.1365-2052.2010.02120.x

Porto Neto, L. R., Bunch, R. J., Harrison, B. E., Prayaga, K. C., and Barendse, W. (2010a). Haplotypes that include the integrin alpha 11 gene are associated with tick burden in cattle. *BMC Genet.* 11:55. doi: 10.1186/1471-2156-11-55

Porto Neto, L. R., Jonsson, N. N., D'Occhio, M. J., and Barendse, W. (2011b). Molecular genetic approaches for identifying the basis of variation in resistance to tick infestation in cattle. *Vet. Parasitol.* 180, 165–172. doi: 10.1016/j.vetpar.2011.05.048

Porto Neto, L. R., Jonsson, N. N., Ingham, A., Bunch, R. J., Harrison, B. E., and Barendse, W. (2012). The RIPK2 gene: a positional candidate for tick burden supported by genetic associations in cattle and immunological response of knockout mouse. *Immunogenetics* 64, 379–388. doi: 10.1007/s00251-012-0601-9

Porto Neto, L. R., Piper, E. K., Jonsson, N. N., Barendse, W., and Gondro, C. (2010b). "Meta-analysis of genome wide association and gene expression studies to identify candidate genes for tick burden in cattle," in *9th World Congress of Genetics Applied to Livestock Production* (Leipzig), 0664.

Prayaga, K. C., Corbet, N. J., Johnston, D. J., Wolcott, M. L., Fordyce, G., and Burrow, H. M. (2009). Genetics of adaptive traits in heifers and their relationship to growth, pubertal and carcass traits in two tropical beef cattle genotypes. *Anim. Prod. Sci.* 49, 413–425. doi: 10.1071/EA08247

Prokop-Prigge, K. A., Mansfield, C. J., Parker, M. R., Thaler, E., Grice, E. A., Wysocki, C. J., et al. (2015). Ethnic/racial and genetic influences on cerumen odorant profiles. *J. Chem. Ecol.* 41, 67–74. doi: 10.1007/s10886-014-0533-y

Rabbani, H., Brown, W. R., Butler, J. E., and Hammarström, L. (1997). Genetic polymorphism of the IGHG3 gene in cattle. *Immunogenetics* 46, 326–331. doi: 10.1007/s002510050279

Rechav, Y. (1987). Resistance of Brahman and Hereford Cattle to African ticks with reference to serum gamma globulin levels and blood composition. *Exp. Appl. Acarol.* 3, 219–232. doi: 10.1007/BF01270458

Regitano, L. C. A., Ibelli, A. M. G., Gasparin, G., Miyata, M., Azevedo, A. L. S., Coutinho, L. L., et al. (2008). On the search for markers of tick resistance in bovines. *Dev. Biol.* 132, 225–230. Available online at: https://ainfo.cnptia.embrapa.br/digital/bitstream/item/40968/1/PROCILCAR2008.00167.pdf

Riek, R. F. (1956). Factors influencing the susceptibility of cattle to tick infestation. *Aust. Vet. J.* 32, 204–209. doi: 10.1111/j.1751-0813.1956.tb05660.x

Roberts, J. A., and Kerr, J. D. (1976). *Boophilus microplus*: passive transfer of resistance in cattle. *J. Parasitol.* 62, 485–488. doi: 10.2307/3279162

Rodriguez-Valle, M., Lew-Tabor, A., Gondro, C., Moolhuijzen, P., Vance, M., Guerrero, F. D., et al. (2010). Comparative microarray analysis of *Rhipicephalus (Boophilus) microplus* expression profiles of larvae pre-attachment and feeding adult female stages on Bos indicus and Bos taurus cattle. *BMC Genomics* 11:437. doi: 10.1186/1471-2164-11-437

Rodriguez-Valle, M., Moolhuijzen, P., Piper, E. K., Weiss, O., Vance, M., Bellgard, M., et al. (2013). *Rhipicephalus microplus* lipocalins (LRMs): genomic identification and analysis of the bovine immune response using *in silico* predicted B and T cell epitopes. *Int. J. Parasitol.* 43, 739–752. doi: 10.1016/j.ijpara.2013.04.005

Rodriguez-Valle, M., Vance, M., Moolhuijzen, P. M., Tao, X., and Lew-Tabor, A. E. (2012). Differential recognition by tick-resistant cattle of the recombinantly expressed *Rhipicephalus microplus* serine protease inhibitor-3 (RMS-3). *Ticks Tick Borne Dis.* 3, 159–169. doi: 10.1016/j.ttbdis.2012.03.002

Saini, S. S., Farrugia, W., Muthusamy, N., Ramsland, P. A., and Kaushik, A. K. (2007). Structural evidence for a new IgG1 antibody sequence allele of cattle. *Scand. J. Immunol.* 65, 32–38. doi: 10.1111/j.1365-3083.2006.01865.x

Santos, I. K. F. M., Valenzuela, J. G., Ribeiro, J. M. C., Castro, M., Costa, J. N., Costa, A. M., et al. (2004). Gene discovery in Boophilus microplus, the cattle tick: the transcriptomes of ovaries, salivary glands, and hemocytes. *Ann. N. Y. Acad. Sci.* 1026, 242–246. doi: 10.1196/annals.1307.037

Schetters, T., Bishop, R., Crampton, M., Kopacek, P., Lew-Tabor, A., Maritz-Olivier, C., et al. (2016). Cattle tick vaccine researchers join forces in CATVAC. *Parasit. Vectors* 9:105. doi: 10.1186/s13071-016-1386-8

Schleger, A. V., Lincoln, D. T., and Kemp, D. H. (1981). A putative role for eosinophils in tick rejection. *Experientia* 37, 49–50. doi: 10.1007/BF01965562

Schleger, A. V., Lincoln, D. T., McKenna, R. V., Kemp, D. H., and Roberts, J. A. (1976). *Boophilus microplus*: cellular responses to larval attachment and their relationship to host resistance. *Aust. J. Biol. Sci.* 29, 499–512. doi: 10.1071/BI9760499

Shapiro, S. Z., Voigt, W. P., and Fujisaki, K. (1986). Tick antigens recognized by serum from a guinea pig resistant to infestation with the tick *Rhipicephalus appendiculatus*. *J. Parasitol.* 72, 454–463. doi: 10.2307/3281686

Smallegange, R. C., Verhulst, N. O., and Takken, W. (2011). Sweaty skin: an invitation to bite? *Trends Parasitol.* 27, 143–148. doi: 10.1016/j.pt.2010.12.009

Snowball, G. (1956). The effect of self-licking by cattle on infestations of cattle tick, *Boophilus microplus* (Canestrini). *Aust. J. Agric. Res.* 7, 227–232. doi: 10.1071/AR9560227

Sollero, B. P., Junqueira, V. S., Gomes, C. C. G., Caetano, A. R., and Cardoso, F. F. (2017). Tag SNP selection for prediction of tick resistance in Braford and Hereford cattle breeds using Bayesian methods. *Genet. Sel. Evol.* 49:49. doi: 10.1186/s12711-017-0325-2

Spickett, A. M., De Klerk, D., Enslin, C. B., and Scholtz, M. M. (1989). Resistance of Nguni, Bonsmara and Hereford cattle to ticks in a Bushveld region of South Africa. *Onderstepoort J. Vet. Res.* 56, 245–250.

Stear, M. J., Hetzel, D. J., Brown, S. C., Gershwin, L. J., Mackinnon, M. J., and Nicholas, F. W. (1990). The relationships among ecto- and endoparasite levels, class I antigens of the bovine major histocompatibility system, immunoglobulin E levels and weight gain. *Vet. Parasitol.* 34, 303–321. doi: 10.1016/0304-4017(90)90077-O

Stear, M. J., Newman, M. J., Nicholas, F. W., Brown, S. C., and Holroyd, R. G. (1984). Tick resistance and the major histocompatibility system. *Aust. J. Exp. Biol. Med. Sci.* 62, 47–52. doi: 10.1038/icb.1984.4

Stear, M. J., Nicholas, F. W., Brown, S. C., and Holroyd, R. G. (1989). Class I antigens of the bovine major histocompatibility system and resistance to the cattle tick (*Boophilus microplus*) assessed in three different seasons. *Vet. Parasitol.* 31, 303–315. doi: 10.1016/0304-4017(89)90080-0

Steiner, M., Huber, S., Harrer, A., and Himly, M. (2016). The evolution of human basophil biology from neglect towards understanding of their immune functions. *BioMed Res. Int.* 2016:16. doi: 10.1155/2016/8232830

Steullet, P., and Gnerin, P. M. (1994). Identification of vertebrate volatiles stimulating olfactory receptors on tarsus I of the tick *Amblyomma variegatum* Fabricius (Ixodidae). *J. Comp. Physiol. A* 174, 39–47. doi: 10.1007/BF00192004

Symons, D. B. A., Clarkson, C. A., and Beale, D. (1989). Structure of bovine immunoglobulin constant region heavy chain gamma 1 and gamma 2 genes. *Mol. Immunol.* 26, 841–850. doi: 10.1016/0161-5890(89)90140-5

Tatchell, R. J., and Bennett, G. F. (1969). *Boophilus microplus*: antihistaminic and tranquilizing drugs and cattle resistance. *Exp. Parasitol.* 26, 369–377. doi: 10.1016/0014-4894(69)90130-1

Tatchell, R. J., and Moorhouse, D. E. (1968). The feeding processes of the cattle tick *Boophilus microplus* (Canestrini). *Parasitology* 58, 441–459. doi: 10.1017/S0031182000069468

Tatchell, R. J., and Moorhouse, D. E. (1970). Neutrophils: their role in the formation of a tick feeding lesion. *Science* 167, 1002–1003. doi: 10.1126/science.167.3920.1002

Tellam, R. L., Smith, D., Kemp, D. H., and Willadsen, P. (1992). "Vaccination against ticks," in *Animal Parasite Control Utilizing Biotechnology*, ed W.K. Yong (Boca Raton, FL: CRC Press Inc.), 303–331.

Thoetkiattikul, H., Mhuantong, W., Laothanachareon, T., Tangphatsornruang, S., Pattarajinda, V., Eurwilaichitr, L., et al. (2013). Comparative analysis of microbial profiles in cow rumen fed with different dietary fiber by tagged 16S rRNA gene pyrosequencing. *Curr. Microbiol.* 67, 130–137. doi: 10.1007/s00284-013-0336-3

Trager, W. (1939). Acquired immunity to ticks. *J. Parasitol.* 25, 57–81. doi: 10.2307/3272160

Turner, L. B., Harrison, B. E., Bunch, R. J., Neto, L. R. P., Li, Y., and Barendse, W. (2010). A genome-wide association study of tick burden and milk composition in cattle. *Anim. Prod. Sci.* 50, 235–245. doi: 10.1071/AN09135

Untalan, P. M., Pruett, J. H., and Steelman, C. D. (2007). Association of the bovine leukocyte antigen major histocompatibility complex class II DRB3*4401 allele with host resistance to the Lone Star tick, *Amblyomma americanum*. *Vet. Parasitol.* 145, 190–195. doi: 10.1016/j.vetpar.2006.12.003

Utech, K., Wharton, R., and Kerr, J. (1978). Resistance to *Boophilus microplus* (Canestrini) in different breeds of cattle. *Aust. J. Agric. Res.* 29, 885–895. doi: 10.1071/AR9780885

Veríssimo, C. J., Bechara, G. H., Mukai, L. S., Otsuk, I. P., and Pozzi Arcaro, J. R. (2008). Mast cell counts correlate with *Rhipicephalus (Boophilus) microplus* tick load in different cattle breeds. *Braz. J. Vet. Pathol.* 1, 81–87. Available online at: http://revistas.bvs-vet.org.br/bjvp/article/view/35972

Veríssimo, C. J., D'Agostino, S. M., Pessoa, F. F., de Toledo, L. M., and de Miranda Santos, I. K. F. (2015). Length and density of filiform tongue papillae: differences between tick-susceptible and resistant cattle may affect tick loads. *Parasit. Vectors* 8:594. doi: 10.1186/s13071-015-1196-4

Veríssimo, C. J., Nicolau, C. V. J., Cardoso, V. L., and Pinheiro, M. G. (2002). Haircoat characteristics and tick infestation on Gyr (Zebu) and crossbred (Holstein × Gyr) cattle. *Arch. Zootech.* 51, 389–392. Available online at: http://citeseerx.ist.psu.edu/viewdoc/download?doi=10.1.1.514.7304&rep=rep1&type=pdf

Wagland, B. (1978). Host resistance to cattle tick (*Boophilus microplus*) in Brahman (*Bos indicus*) cattle. III.* Growth on previously unexposed animals. *Aust. J. Agric. Res.* 29, 401–409. doi: 10.1071/AR9780401

Wambura, P. N., Gwakisa, P. S., Silayo, R. S., and Rugaimukamu, E. A. (1998). Breed-associated resistance to tick infestation in *Bos indicus* and their crosses with *Bos taurus*. *Vet. Parasitol.* 77, 63–70. doi: 10.1016/S0304-4017(97)00229-X

Wang, H., and Nuttall, P. A. (1999). Immunoglobulin-binding proteins in ticks: new target for vaccine development against a blood-feeding parasite. *Cell. Mol. Life Sci.* 56, 286–295. doi: 10.1007/s000180050430

Wang, M., Guerrero, F. D., Pertea, G., and Nene, V. M. (2007). Global comparative analysis of ESTs from the southern cattle tick, *Rhipicephalus (Boophilus) microplus*. *BMC Genomics* 8, 368–382. doi: 10.1186/1471-2164-8-368

Wang, Y. H., Reverter, A., Kemp, D., McWilliam, S. M., Ingham, A., Davis, C. A., et al. (2007). Gene expression profiling of Hereford Shorthorn cattle following challenge with *Boophilus microplus* tick larvae. *Aust. J. Exp. Agric.* 47, 1397–1407. doi: 10.1071/EA07012

Wen, T., and Rothenberg, M. E. (2016). The regulatory function of eosinophils. *Microbiol. Spectrum* 4, 1–12. doi: 10.1128/microbiolspec.MCHD-0020-2015

Whelen, A. C., Richardson, L. K., and Wikel, S. K. (1986). Dot-ELISA assessment of guinea pig antibody responses to repeated *Dermacentor andersoni* infestations. *J. Parasitol.* 72, 155–162. doi: 10.2307/3281809

Wikel, S. K. (1982). Immune resonses to arthropods and their products. *Ann Rev. Entomol.* 27, 21–48. doi: 10.1146/annurev.en.27.010182.000321

Wikel, S. K. (1996). Host immunity to ticks. *Ann. Rev. Entomol.* 41, 1–22. doi: 10.1146/annurev.en.41.010196.000245

Wikel, S. K., and Whelen, A. C. (1986). Ixodid-host immune interaction. Identification and characterization of relevant antigens and tick-induced host immunosuppression. *Vet. Parasitol.* 20, 149–174. doi: 10.1016/0304-4017(86)90098-1

Willadsen, P. (1980). Immunity to ticks. *Adv. Parasitol.* 18, 293–311. doi: 10.1016/S0065-308X(08)60402-9

Willadsen, P. (2004). Anti-tick vaccines. *Parasitology* 129, S367–387. doi: 10.1017/S0031182003004657

Willadsen, P., and Kemp, D. H. (1988). Vaccination with 'concealed' antigens for tick control. *Parasitol. Today* 4, 196–198. doi: 10.1016/0169-4758(88)90084-1

Yilmaz, B., Portugal, S., Tran, T. M., Gozzelino, R., Ramos, S., Gomes, J., et al. (2014). Gut microbiota elicits a protective immune response against malaria transmission. *Cell* 159, 1277–1289 doi: 10.1016/j.cell.2014.10.053

Permissions

All chapters in this book were first published by Frontiers; hereby published with permission under the Creative Commons Attribution License or equivalent. Every chapter published in this book has been scrutinized by our experts. Their significance has been extensively debated. The topics covered herein carry significant findings which will fuel the growth of the discipline. They may even be implemented as practical applications or may be referred to as a beginning point for another development.

The contributors of this book come from diverse backgrounds, making this book a truly international effort. This book will bring forth new frontiers with its revolutionizing research information and detailed analysis of the nascent developments around the world.

We would like to thank all the contributing authors for lending their expertise to make the book truly unique. They have played a crucial role in the development of this book. Without their invaluable contributions this book wouldn't have been possible. They have made vital efforts to compile up to date information on the varied aspects of this subject to make this book a valuable addition to the collection of many professionals and students.

This book was conceptualized with the vision of imparting up-to-date information and advanced data in this field. To ensure the same, a matchless editorial board was set up. Every individual on the board went through rigorous rounds of assessment to prove their worth. After which they invested a large part of their time researching and compiling the most relevant data for our readers.

The editorial board has been involved in producing this book since its inception. They have spent rigorous hours researching and exploring the diverse topics which have resulted in the successful publishing of this book. They have passed on their knowledge of decades through this book. To expedite this challenging task, the publisher supported the team at every step. A small team of assistant editors was also appointed to further simplify the editing procedure and attain best results for the readers.

Apart from the editorial board, the designing team has also invested a significant amount of their time in understanding the subject and creating the most relevant covers. They scrutinized every image to scout for the most suitable representation of the subject and create an appropriate cover for the book.

The publishing team has been an ardent support to the editorial, designing and production team. Their endless efforts to recruit the best for this project, has resulted in the accomplishment of this book. They are a veteran in the field of academics and their pool of knowledge is as vast as their experience in printing. Their expertise and guidance has proved useful at every step. Their uncompromising quality standards have made this book an exceptional effort. Their encouragement from time to time has been an inspiration for everyone.

The publisher and the editorial board hope that this book will prove to be a valuable piece of knowledge for researchers, students, practitioners and scholars across the globe.

List of Contributors

Hajer Aounallah
Institut Pasteur de Tunis, LR19IPTX, Service d'Entomologie Médicale, Université de Tunis El Manar, Tunis, Tunisia
Innovation and Development Laboratory, Innovation and Development Center, Instituto Butantan, São Paulo, Brazil

Chaima Bensaoud
Institute of Parasitology, Biology Centre, Czech Academy of Sciences, České Budějovice, Czechia

Youmna M'ghirbi
Institut Pasteur de Tunis, LR19IPTX, Service d'Entomologie Médicale, Université de Tunis El Manar, Tunis, Tunisia

Fernanda Faria
Innovation and Development Laboratory, Innovation and Development Center, Instituto Butantan, São Paulo, Brazil

Jindrich Chmelar
Department of Medical Biology, Faculty of Science, University of South Bohemia in České Budějovice, České Budějovice, Czechia

Michail Kotsyfakis
Institute of Parasitology, Biology Centre, Czech Academy of Sciences, České Budějovice, Czechia
Department of Medical Biology, Faculty of Science, University of South Bohemia in České Budějovice, České Budějovice, Czechia

Iveta Štibrániová, Pavlína Bartíková and Viera Holíková
Biomedical Research Center, Institute of Virology, Slovak Academy of Sciences, Bratislava, Slovakia

Mária Kazimírová
Institute of Zoology, Slovak Academy of Sciences, Bratislava, Slovakia

José de la Fuente
Department of Veterinary Pathobiology, Center for Veterinary Health Sciences, Oklahoma State University, Stillwater, OK, USA
SaBio, Instituto de Investigación en Recursos Cinegéticos (IREC), CSIC, Universidad de Castilla-La Mancha (UCLM), Junta de Comunidades de Castilla – La Mancha (JCCM), Ciudad Real, Spain

Daniel E. Sonenshine
Department of Biological Sciences, Old Dominion University, Norfolk, VA, USA

Robert M. Waterhouse
Department of Genetic Medicine and Development, University of Geneva Medical School, Geneva, Switzerland
Swiss Institute of Bioinformatics, Geneva, Switzerland
Computer Science and Artificial Intelligence Laboratory, Massachusetts Institute of Technology, Cambridge, MA, USA
Broad Institute of MIT and Harvard, Cambridge, MA, USA

R. Michael Roe
Department of Entomology, North Carolina State University, Raleigh, NC, USA

Jose M. Ribeiro
Laboratory of Malaria and Vector Research, National Institute of Allergy and Infectious Diseases, Rockville, MD, USA

David B. Sattelle
Division of Medicine, University College London, London, UK

Alejandro Cabezas-Cruz
Institute of Parasitology, Biology Center, Czech Academy of Sciences, Ceské Budejovice, Czechia
Faculty of Science, University of South Bohemia, Ceské Budejovice, Czechia
UMR BIPAR, INRA, ANSES, Ecole Nationale Vétérinaire d'Alfort, Université Paris-Est, Maisons-Alfort, France

Pilar Alberdi and Margarita Villar
SaBio, Instituto de Investigación en Recursos Cinegéticos IREC-CSIC-UCLM-JCCM, Ciudad Real, Spain

James J. Valdés
Institute of Parasitology, Biology Center, Czech Academy of Sciences, Ceské Budejovice, Czechia
Department of Virology, Veterinary Research Institute, Brno, Czechia
Faculty of Science, University of South Bohemia, České Budějovice, Czechia

Andréa C. Fogaça, Géssica Sousa, Daniel B. Pavanelo, Eliane Esteves and Sirlei Daffre
Department of Parasitology, Institute of Biomedical Sciences, University of São Paulo, São Paulo, Brazil

Larissa A. Martins
Institute of Parasitology, Biology Centre, Czech Academy of Sciences, Ceske Budejovice, Czechia
Laboratory of Bacteriology, Tick-Pathogen Transmission Unit, National Institute of Allergy and Infectious Diseases, Hamilton, MT, United States

Veronika Urbanová and Petr Kopáček
Institute of Parasitology, Biology Centre, Czech Academy of Sciences, Ceske Budejovice, Czechia

Ahmed Al-Rofaai and Lesley Bell-Sakyi
Department of Infection Biology, Institute of Infection and Global Health, University of Liverpool, Liverpool, United Kingdom

Sara Artigas-Jerónimo
SaBio, Instituto de Investigación en Recursos Cinegéticos (IREC), CSIC, Universidad de Castilla-La Mancha (UCLM), Junta de Comunidades de Castilla - La Mancha (JCCM), Ciudad Real, Spain

Agustín Estrada-Peña
Facultad de Veterinaria, Universidad de Zaragoza, Zaragoza, Spain

Jéssica Fiorotti, Caio Junior Balduino Coutinho-Rodrigues and Ricardo Oliveira Barbosa Bitencourt
Programa de Pós-Graduação em Ciências Veterinárias, Instituto de Veterinária, Universidade Federal Rural do Rio de Janeiro, Seropédica, Brazil

Rubem Figueiredo Sadok Menna-Barreto
Laboratório de Biologia Celular, IOC, Fundação Oswaldo Cruz, Rio de Janeiro, Brazil

Patrícia Silva Gôlo and Vânia Rita Elias Pinheiro Bittencourt
Departamento de Parasitologia Animal, Instituto de Veterinária, Universidade Federal Rural do Rio de Janeiro, Seropédica, Brazil

Diva Denelle Spadacci-Morena
Laboratório de Fisiopatologia, Instituto Butantan, São Paulo, Brazil

Isabele da Costa Angelo
Departamento de Epidemiologia e Saúde Pública, Instituto de Veterinária, Universidade Federal Rural do Rio de Janeiro, Seropédica, Brazil

Sarah I. Bonnet
UMR BIPAR INRA-ENVA-ANSES, Maisons-Alfort, France

Jindřich Chmelař
Faculty of Science, University of South Bohemia in České Budějovice, České Budějovice, Czechia

Florian Binetruy and Olivier Duron
Laboratoire MIVEGEC (Maladies Infectieuses et Vecteurs: Écologie, Génétique, Évolution et Contrôle), Centre National de la Recherche Scientifique (UMR5290), IRD (UMR224), Université de Montpellier, Montpellier, France

Angelica M. Hernández-Jarguín
SaBio Instituto de Investigación en Recursos Cinegéticos CSIC-UCLM-JCCM, Ciudad Real, Spain

Kristin L. Rosche, Lindsay C. Sidak-Loftis, Joanna Hurtado, Elizabeth A. Fisk and Dana K. Shaw
Program in Vector-borne Disease, Department of Veterinary Microbiology and Pathology, Washington State University, Pullman, WA, United States

Jan Kotál and Helena Langhansová
Faculty of Science, University of South Bohemia in České Budějovice, České Budějovice, Czechia
Institute of Parasitology, Biology Center, Czech Academy of Sciences, České Budějovice, Czechia

Karen L. Mansfield
Animal and Plant Health Agency, Addlestone, United Kingdom
Institute of Infection and Global Health, University of Liverpool, Liverpool, United Kingdom

Lv Jizhou
Animal and Plant Health Agency, Addlestone, United Kingdom
Chinese Academy of Inspection and Quarantine, Beijing, China

L. Paul Phipps
Animal and Plant Health Agency, Addlestone, United Kingdom

Nicholas Johnson
Animal and Plant Health Agency, Addlestone, United Kingdom
Faculty of Health and Medicine, University of Surrey, Guildford, United Kingdom

Saravanan Thangamani
Department of Pathology, The University of Texas Medical Branch, Galveston, TX, United States
Institute for Human Infections and Immunity, The University of Texas Medical Branch, Galveston, TX, United States
Center for Tropical Diseases, The University of Texas Medical Branch, Galveston, TX, United States

Meghan E. Hermance and Rodrigo I. Santos
Department of Pathology, The University of Texas Medical Branch, Galveston, TX, United States

Mirko Slovak and Maria Kazimirova
Institute of Zoology, Slovak Academy of Sciences, Bratislava, Slovakia

Dar Heinze
Department of Surgery, Center for Regenerative Medicine, Boston University and Boston Medical Center, Boston, MA, United States

Steven G. Widen
Department of Biochemistry and Molecular Biology, The University of Texas Medical Branch, Galveston, TX, United States

Ligia Cavani, Camila Urbano Braz and Henrique Nunes de Oliveira
School of Agricultural and Veterinary Sciences, São Paulo State University (Unesp), Jaboticabal, Brazil

Rodrigo Giglioti, Cintia Hiromi Okino and Márcia Cristina de Sena Oliveira
Empresa Brasileira de Pesquisa Agropecuária, Embrapa Pecuária Sudeste, São Carlos, Brazil

Claudia Cristina Gulias-Gomes and Fernando Flores Cardoso
Empresa Brasileira de Pesquisa Agropecuária, Embrapa Pecuária Sul, Bagé, Brazil

Alexandre Rodrigues Caetano
Empresa Brasileira de Pesquisa Agropecuária, Embrapa Recursos Genéticos e Biotecnologia, Brasília, Brazil

Ala E. Tabor
Centre for Animal Science, Queensland Alliance for Agriculture and Food Innovation, The University of Queensland, St. Lucia, QLD, Australia
Centre for Comparative Genomics, Murdoch University, Perth, WA, Australia

Abid Ali
Department of Zoology, Abdul Wali Khan University Mardan, Mardan, Pakistan
Escola de Enfermagem de Ribeirão Preto, University of São Paulo, Ribeirão Preto, Brazil

Gauhar Rehman
Department of Zoology, Abdul Wali Khan University Mardan, Mardan, Pakistan

Gustavo Rocha Garcia, Amanda Fonseca Zangirolamo and Thiago Malardo
Ribeirão Preto School of Medicine, University of São Paulo, Ribeirão Preto, Brazil

Nicholas N. Jonsson
Institute of Biodiversity, Animal Health and Comparative Medicine, The University of Glasgow, Glasgow, United Kingdom

Index

www.ingramcontent.com/pod-product-compliance
Lightning Source LLC
LaVergne TN
LVHW082213200926
848484LV00008B/2245